The Nursing Associate's Handbook of Clinical Skills

Edited by

Ian Peate OBE FRCN

Principal, School of Health Studies, Gibraltar

WILEY Blackwell

This edition first published 2021

Registered Office(s)
John Wiley & Sons, Inc., 111 River Street, Hoboken, NJ 07030, USA
John Wiley & Sons Ltd, The Atrium, Southern Gate, Chichester, West Sussex, PO19 8SQ, UK

Editorial Office
9600 Garsington Road, Oxford, OX4 2DQ, UK

For details of our global editorial offices, customer services and more information about Wiley products, visit us at www.wiley.com.

Wiley also publishes its books in a variety of electronic formats and by print-on-demand. Some content that appears in standard print versions of this book may not be available in other formats.

Library of Congress Cataloging-in-Publication Data
Names: Peate, Ian, editor.
Title: The nursing associate's handbook of clinical skills / edited by Ian Peate.
Description: Hoboken, NJ : Wiley-Blackwell, 2021. | Includes bibliographical references and index.
Identifiers: LCCN 2020028481 (print) | LCCN 2020028482 (ebook) | ISBN 9781119642305 (paperback) | ISBN 9781119642329 (adobe pdf) | ISBN 9781119642350 (epub)
Subjects: MESH: Nursing Assistants | Nursing Care–methods | Nursing Process | Nurse's Role | Nurse-Patient Relations | United Kingdom
Classification: LCC RT84 (print) | LCC RT84 (ebook) | NLM WY 193 | DDC 610.7306/98–dc23
LC record available at https://lccn.loc.gov/2020028481
LC ebook record available at https://lccn.loc.gov/2020028482

Cover Design: Wiley
Cover Image: © sturti/Getty Images

Set in 9.5/11pts MinionPro by SPi Global, Pondicherry, India
Printed and bound by CPI Group (UK) Ltd, Croydon, CR0 4YY

C9781119642305_020421

The Nursing Associate's Handbook of Clinical Skills

Dedication

This text is dedicated to the early trainee nursing associates who dared to take the plunge and became the trailblazers, becoming practitioners in their own right.

Contents

Unit 2
Procedures for Provision of Person-Centred Nursing Care 161

Unit 3
Provide Care and Support with Hygiene and The Maintenance of Skin Integrity 197

Unit 4
Provide Support with Nutrition and Hydration 263

Unit 5
Provide Support with Maintaining Bladder and Bowel Health 291

Unit 6
Provide Support with Mobility and Safety 323

Unit 7
Provide Support with Respiratory Care 359

Unit 8
Preventing and Managing Infection 403

Unit 9
Meeting Needs for Care and Support at the End of Life 463

Unit 10
Procedural Competencies for Administering Medicine Safely 483

Contributors

Janine Archer

PhD, MRes, PgCAP, BSc (Hons), DPSN (MH), RNT, FHEA

Head of Apprenticeships for the School of Health & Society, University of Salford, Greater Manchester

Janine Archer is Head of Apprenticeships for the School of Health & Society at the University of Salford, Greater Manchester. Janine, a Registered Mental Health Nurse, joined the University of Salford in November 2016 as Programme Lead for the Nursing Associate programme. Janine has worked in Higher Education since 2004, having previously been Programme Lead for the Improving Access to Psychological therapies (IAPT) low-intensity programme at the University of Manchester.

Having previously worked for the National Institute for Mental Health England (NIMHE-NW) as Project Lead of a Collaborative to embed Graduate Mental Health Workers (Psychological Wellbeing Practitioners) within Primary Healthcare services, Janine has a passion for supporting new ways of working within mental health.

Janine was awarded a prestigious Department of Health Researcher Development Award, enabling doctorate-level studies, and her PhD examined 'Collaborative Care for Depression in Primary Care'.

Janine has been engaged in a wide range of research and has led a Cochrane systematic review into Collaborative Care for common mental health problems (CMHPs). Awarded a prestigious Florence Nightingale Travel Award, Janine developed links with experts in Australia; this work cumulated into educational outputs and research exploring the management of long-term conditions and CMHPs.

Stuart Baker

RGN, BSc (Hons), MSc, TCH, PGCE, FHEA

Senior Lecture in Nursing (Adult), University of South Wales

Stuart is a Senior Lecture in Nursing (Adult) at the University of South Wales. He is part of the team responsible for the CertHE Health Care Nursing Support Worker course, and also works closely with the independent sector. Stuart began his nursing career in 1987 at Peterborough and Stamford School of Nurse Education. After several years as a staff nurse in acute surgery, he moved to Surrey as a deputy charge nurse. From here, he moved to Wales to complete a computer studies degree at the University of Glamorgan before returning to nursing in an educational role. Stuart also delivered training in nursing homes for almost 10 years before taking up a position as a senior lecturer at the University of South Wales in 2015.

Nicole Blythe

RGN BSc (Hons) Cert Nurse (Germany)

Clinical Educator. University of Salford

Nicole began her nursing career in 1989 in Erlenbach am Main, Germany. She undertook 3 years' student nurse training at the 'Krankenpflegeschule St. Hildegard' before becoming a staff nurse and then Deputy Ward Manager on a neurology/neurosurgical unit in a large district general hospital in Aschaffenburg, Germany. Nicole moved to England in 1997, working mainly in the Greater Manchester area as a staff nurse and Sister in Haematology, Acute Stroke Services, Cardiology and Cardiac Catheterisation. She completed her BSc (Hons) from the University of Manchester in 2010. Her areas of interest are staff and student education, pressure ulcer prevention and tissue viability. In 2017, Nicole started her full-time educational career as a Clinical Educator for the nursing associate pilot programme. She joined the University of Salford in 2018, where she continues to work as a Clinical Educator on the Nursing Associate Degree Apprenticeship.

Angelina L. Chadwick

RGN RMN DipN BSc (Hons) PGCE MSc SFEA

Lecturer in Mental Health Nursing, School of Health and Society, The University of Salford

Angelina began her career in 1986, starting with 3 years of general nurse training followed by a staff nurse position in the area of surgery at Bury General Hospital. She later retrained for a further 2 years to become a mental health nurse and continued to progress in a variety of clinical and management roles. These were held in acute inpatient, older people and community practitioner roles within the field of mental health nursing. Later, she moved into education as a training manager with National Health Service (NHS) Mental Health Trust, before moving into higher education as a nurse lecturer in 2010. She is currently a module leader with the pre-registration degree nursing programme and teaches on both pre-registration and post-qualifying programmes. Her keen interest areas are around physical health in mental health and the use of simulation in education. She gained Senior Fellow status with the Higher Education Academy in 2017.

Jacqueline Chang

SFHEA, MA Medical Ethics and Law, BSc Adult Nursing

Course Lead for Nursing Associates at Kingston University and St Georges University of London

Jacqueline has 20 years of nursing experience, specialising in palliative care in the community. She has been teaching nursing for 10 years and supports trainee and student nurse associates through their degree.

Angela Chick

RN DipHE

Ward Manager/Sister, Chelsea and Westminster NHS Foundation Trust

Angela is the ward manager on the stroke unit where she has worked since 2016 at Chelsea and Westminster NHS Foundation Trust. She joined the Trust in 2001 as a cadet nurse and completed her Diploma in Adult Nursing in 2006. Angela has a vast amount of nursing clinical expertise, having worked in medicine and surgery with a focus on stroke as well as elective and emergency admissions, with a strong interest in caring for colorectal patients. Working within the NHS, her passion is to enhance patient care through innovation and quality improvement. Angela has many scholarly outputs to her credit, including developing a poster to educate staff on managing high-output stomas to improve care standards. Alongside her colleague, she entered the trust's Dragons' Den–style competition with the idea to improve mouth care on her ward. They both won this and went on to develop a Trust-wide policy and protocol for mouth care across Chelsea and Westminster NHS Foundation Trust. This innovation was selected as a high-scoring abstract for the 2019 stroke conference, and most recently, the work has been highlighted by NHS providers with an output of an article.

Carl Clare

Programme Lead MSc Nursing, University of Hertfordshire

Carl began his nursing a career in 1990 as a nursing auxiliary. He later undertook student nurse training for 3 years at Selly Oak Hospital (Birmingham), moving to the Royal Devon and Exeter Hospitals, then Northwick Park Hospital, and finally the Royal Brompton and Harefield NHS Trust as a Resuscitation Officer and Honorary Teaching Fellow of Imperial College (London). Since 2006, he has worked at the University of Hertfordshire as a Senior Lecturer in Adult Nursing. His key areas of interest are long-term illness, physiology, sociology, and cardiac care. Carl has previously published work in cardiac care, resuscitation, and pathophysiology.

Nigel Davies

MSc, BSc (Hons), RN, FHEA

Principal Lecturer in Nursing, University of East London

Nigel began his nursing career in 1986, undertaking a degree in nursing at the then Polytechnic of the South Bank in London and at Wolfson School of Nursing at Westminster Hospital. His post-registration experience was predominately in cardiac care before moving into management positions and working as a chief nurse and director of infection prevention and control. He has maintained links or worked directly in higher education throughout his career, holding appointments as a lecturer–practitioner, senior lecturer, head of nursing, research fellow and professor. He joined the University of East London in 2017 to set up its new nursing courses, including apprentice and direct-entry nursing associate programmes. Nigel's qualifications include BSc (Hons) in nursing, MSc in health science, PGDip in practitioner research and a certificate in teaching in higher education.

Esme Elloway

RN Adult Nursing BSc (Hons), PGCAP, FHEA

Lecturer in Adult Nursing, Plymouth University

Esme has nursing experience in the United Kingdom and as a student nurse in Tanzania. She graduated from Keele University with an Honours Degree in Adult Nursing. Since then, she has gained a wealth of experience from working in a variety of specialties. Previous roles include working in stroke rehabilitation, renal, community, neurosurgical and trauma intensive care and research. She was part of the first cohort to complete the National Institute of Health Research Advanced Leadership Programme. Esme is enjoying her current role as a lecturer in Adult Nursing and is passionate about the development of student nurses as they progress throughout their degree programme.

Joanne Greenwood

Clinical Practice Educator, Oldham Care Organisation District Nurses, Northern Care Alliance

Joanne qualified as an adult nurse in 2010 from Keele University. Joanne started her career in accident and emergency at North Staffordshire NHS trust. Joanne went on to work in a community hospital and later moved to the community working both in district nursing and chronic disease management. Joanne worked on the nursing associate programme at Salford university as a clinical educator. Joanne moved back into a community teaching role for Oldham Care Organisation as a clinical practice educator. Joanne is passionate about professionalism within nursing practice.

Barry Hill

MSc. BSc (Hons) DipHE O.A. Dip, RN, NMC RNT/TCH, FHEA, V300.

Director of Education (Employability) and Programme Leader, Northumbria University; Clinical Editor, *British Journal of Nursing*

Barry began his career working as Health Care Assistant. He completed his Common Foundation Programme training as a student nurse at Northumbria University. He completed his adult branch nurse training at Buckinghamshire Chilterns University College (BCUC). Barry has worked as a staff nurse and senior staff nurse in cardiac and general intensive care not (ICU) at the Milne unit at St Mary's Hospital, London Paddington. He worked in neuro trauma and general intensive care as a charge nurse at Charing Cross Hospital, London. Following this role, he worked as a senior charge nurse at General ICU at Hammersmith Hospital, London. Lastly, he worked as a matron within the surgical division at Charing Cross Hospital, London, within Plastics, Orthopaedics, ENT, and Major Trauma (POEM) at Charing Cross Hospital, London. Educationally, Barry had worked as a clinical mentor in intensive care nursing, and has worked in Higher Education, teaching both undergraduate and postgraduate students. His key areas of interest include acute and critical care, advancing clinical skills, pharmacology and advanced-level practice. Barry has published widely in journals and books and is a Fellow with the Higher Education Academy.

Phill Hoddinott

RN DipHE, BSc, MSc, DIC, PGDip

Senior Lecturer and Academic Lead for Nursing Programmes, Buckinghamshire New University

Phill is a senior lecturer in adult nursing at Buckinghamshire New University within the School of Nursing & Allied Health. He works across the nursing programmes and is Programme Leader for the BSc (Hons) Nursing programme. Phill has over 20 years' experience as an adult registered nurse and has held a number of clinical, leadership and educational roles within the NHS and overseas. His clinical expertise lies in acute and emergency medicine, and he still works clinically in these settings within North West London. His research interest is centred on service user engagement within education, and he has conducted research on the impact of patient feedback given to nursing student learners in the clinical environment. Phill is a champion for the 'Men in Nursing Together' campaign and has an interest in the promotion of nursing as a career for men.

Abby Hughes

RN (Adult), BN, MSc, PGCAP, FHEA

Lecturer, University of Salford

Abby joined the University of Salford in 2016, where she is currently a lecturer on the Nursing Associate Programme. Abby's clinical background includes posts as Falls Lead Nurse, Ward Manager and Clinical Educator, as well as posts in Medical Wards, the Emergency Department and Medical Assessment Unit.

Graham Patrick Jones

MSc, BSc, PgCTLHE, RN (Adult)

Senior Lecturer, Teesside University School of Health & Life Science.

Graham is a Senior Lecturer at Teesside University School of Health & Life Science and is currently studying for a Doctorate in Health and Social Care. Graham is also a trustee of 'Transform Healthcare Cambodia', a UK non-profit-making charity that supports the healthcare system in Cambodia by facilitating medical and nursing teams to undertake 2-week clinical placements. In July 2019, two trainee nursing associates became the first to join a 20-strong team working in Battambang Referral Hospital in Cambodia.

Lesley Jones

RMN, PhD (Nursing), MSc Advanced Practice, MA Gerontology, PGCAP, FHEA

Programme Lead (Nursing Associate Higher Apprenticeship), University of Salford, Greater Manchester

Lesley started her career in 1987 and was initially an Enrolled Nurse before completing a conversion course in the 1990s to become a Registered Mental Health Nurse. Lesley initially worked in acute adult mental health services before moving to work in older people's mental health services, where she worked clinically for over 20 years. Lesley has held a number of clinical and leadership roles, including working as an advanced practitioner and non-medical prescriber in NHS inpatient mental health wards for people with dementia. Lesley was awarded a National Institute of Health Research Clinical Doctoral Research Fellowship in 2013. Her PhD was clinically focused and explored the meaning, presentation and assessment of complexity in dementia within the setting of NHS dementia inpatient wards. Lesley's interests include advanced dementia, understanding behaviour in dementia, end-of-life care and life story work. In 2018, Lesley moved to the University of Salford as a Nurse Lecturer on the TNA programme before becoming programme lead in 2020.

Hamish MacGregor

RN, BA (Hons), MSc

Director, Docklands Training Consultants Ltd.

Hamish started his nurse training in 1972, both in adult and psychiatric nursing. He later specialised in neurosurgical nursing, becoming a charge nurse in the area. He then went into nurse management with Lothian Health Board, and then Harrow Health Authority. In 1988, he joined the commissioning team of London Lighthouse, a palliative care facility for people with HIV and AIDS, first as Residential Services Manager then Assistant Director for Operational Services. In 1995, he moved into education, working part time, in order to develop his skills as a freelance trainer. At this time, Hamish developed an interest in moving and handling. In 1998, he worked part time, first in a community health trust and then in an acute health trust as a moving and handling advisor, as well as a freelance trainer for a range of organisations. In 2005, he set up Docklands Training Consultants, the company that provides moving and handling training and consultancy to healthcare and social care, universities and case managers for children and adults with complex needs. He is the author of *Moving and Handling Patients at a Glance*.

Louise McErlean

RGN, BSc (Hons), MA (Herts), FHEA

Louise began her nursing career in Glasgow in 1986, qualifying as a staff nurse in 1989. She has worked in hospitals in Glasgow, Belfast and London, specialising in intensive care nursing. She has worked in nurse education since 2005. Louise has a wide range of nursing interests including general surgery, medicine and intensive care. She has an interest in simulation, anatomy and physiology.

Claire Pryor

RN Adult MSc, BSc (Hons), FHEA, TCH

Senior Lecturer, Northumbria University

Claire Pryor is a senior lecturer in adult nursing at Northumbria University. Claire's educational interests lie predominantly in nursing care for the older person, and she is the module lead for non-medical prescribing. Her teaching activity spans both adult pre- and post-registration professional development. Claire's specialist areas of interest include delirium and delirium superimposed on dementia, which forms the basis of her PhD research, and integrating physical health and mental healthcare education and service provision. Prior to lecturing, Claire worked in a variety of primary and secondary care settings, including acute medical assessment, critical care, intermediate care and as an older persons' nurse practitioner in a mental health setting.

Joanna Regan

SEN, RN

Head of Nursing for Emergency and Specialty Medicine (ESM)

Jo began her nursing career in 1985 at Leeds Teaching Hospital, becoming an enrolled nurse, working in acute and elective orthopaedics. She later undertook a conversion course at Bradford University, continuing her career in orthopaedics as a staff nurse and ward sister. Jo continued in her career at Leeds, working as a matron in a number of adult specialities, then as Head of Nursing in Cardio Respiratory, Neurosciences and now in ESM, including emergency departments, acute assessment, elderly, general medicine, infectious diseases, HIV and sexual health services. Jo is particularly interested in advancing the Quality Improvement in nursing practice, using the Leeds Improvement methodology. She also takes a keen interest in patient experience and public involvement.

Hazel Ridgers

RN, Dip He Nursing, PGCAP, MA, FHEA

Freelance Writer, Researcher and Lecturer in Nursing and Public Health

Hazel trained as a nurse with King's College, London, and took up her first staff nurse post in older people's care at Guys and St Thomas' in 2006. She developed an interest in the health and well-being of older people living with HIV and undertook sexual health and HIV specialisation courses early in her nursing career. She has worked in HIV and sexual health as a nurse, research nurse and clinical teacher. Hazel began her career in education in 2010. She has worked as a clinical teacher both in acute hospital and university settings, and as a senior lecturer with a focus on clinical skills and simulated learning. Most recently, Hazel was the Programme Lead for the first Nursing Associate cohorts at the University of East London. Hazel is now a freelance writer, researcher and lecturer in Nursing and Public Health.

Ally Sanderson

MA, PGCE LTHE, ECP, RN

Senior Lecturer, Nursing and Midwifery Department, School of Health and Life Sciences, Teesside University

Ally is responsible for the preregistration skills (Year 2) module and works as part of a team within the optometry and midwifery department. Ally began her nursing career in Newcastle upon Tyne, Freeman Hospital School of Nursing in 1987, qualifying and beginning work on an ophthalmic ward at the Royal Victoria Infirmary. She has travelled during her nursing career and has worked in several specialist ophthalmic hospitals including Moorfield's in London. Ally branched out into the role of emergency care Practitioner (ECP) and non-medical prescriber in 2005, working in primary and acute care. In 2009, she moved to academia and has recently commenced her doctorate in professional practice.

Dominic Simpson

BSc (Hons), RN(Adult), PGCLTHE, AFHEA

Senior Lecturer in Adult Nursing and PhD Candidate, School of Health and Life Sciences, Northumbria University

Dominic is a registered adult nurse, having gained his degree at Northumbria University Newcastle. Dominic has held a number of clinical nursing roles across the North East of England, and his clinical expertise is within emergency medicine and critical care. His research interests focus on how to create cultures that promote safety and quality within the NHS. Dominic has previously been the simulation lead for Teesside

Universities Nursing Associate Programme. Dominic is a member of the Royal College of Nursing, and he is currently the co-chair of the Northern Research Network. Dominic is an active member of the British Association of Critical Care Nurses (BACCN). He uses his affiliation with the BACCN to provide a national voice to shape the strategy for critical care nursing and to promote safe, quality evidence-based nursing care to the critically ill patient. In 2019, Dominic was awarded membership of the Health Foundation's Q network, an initiative connecting people who have improvement expertise across the United Kingdom.

Daniel Soto-Prieto

RN, MEd, FHEA, PhD Candidate
Lecturer, University of East London

Qualified in Nursing, master's in education and currently PhD candidate, Daniel has developed his professional activity as a clinical nurse, project manager and academic in both Spain and the United Kingdom. Daniel has broad experience in surgical and anaesthetic areas, and he has led the implementation of innovative electronic systems within the NHS.

Over the years, he has gained vast experience in simulation, both in clinical and academic settings. Daniel is ambassador of the Nursing Now global campaign to raise the profile of nursing internationally.

Karen Sumpter

RN, DipMan, RNT, PGCHE, MA Management & Leadership, FHEA
Senior Lecturer in Adult Nursing, University of Hertfordshire

Karen began her nursing career in 1985 at Kings College Hospital and stayed for 2 years after qualifying as a registered nurse, working in a surgical ward environment. A love of ENT nursing and Head and Neck Cancer took Karen off to undertake a specialist course in this field at the Royal National Throat Nose & Ear Hospital. Karen remained in this specialty for many years working as a staff nurse, ward manager and Directorate Lead Nurse in the acute sector. Karen left the NHS in 2003 and moved to the voluntary sector, working for 10 years as the Deputy Director of Patient Services in a hospice, followed by 3 years as Clinical Lead for a national cancer charity. Through these senior roles, Karen has developed a passion for service development and redesign, team working, and staff development. Karen has a continued interest in cancer and end-of-life care and is a trustee for the charity Compassion in Dying.

Matthew van Loo

RN, FHEA, Dip Nur, BSc (Hons), PgDip, MSc
Clinical Matron, South Tees Hospitals NHS Foundation Trust

Matthew completed his undergraduate nursing education in 2003, graduating with a Diploma in Nursing. He took up employment with South Tees NHS Foundation Trust as a staff nurse and then charge nurse in Accident and Emergency. Following the completion of a BSc and non-medical prescribing, Matthew developed and led a nurse practitioner service within the Accident and Emergency Department. In 2010, he changed clinical areas and entered the speciality of Cardiac Surgery. As a trainee surgical care practitioner, he underwent 2 years of intensive training alongside completing an MSc. On completion of the MSc, he worked in an advanced clinical role in the Cardiac Surgery team. In 2015, Matthew left the NHS for a senior lecturer post at Teesside University; later, he became a principal lecturer, and recently Head of Department for Nursing and Midwifery. He completed a postgraduate certificate in Higher Education in 2016 and also became a Fellow of the Higher Education Academy. During his time at Teesside University, Matthew gained extensive experience in leading the design and delivery of curriculums in the fields of nursing associate, nursing, and several post-registration courses. Matthew also holds two external examiner roles at UK universities. He has strong interest in many aspects of education and specifically relating to cardiac care, clinical skills, the science of nursing, modern and digital pedagogy, and widening participation to education and the healthcare professions. Following a 5-year period in higher education, Matthew returned to clinical practice and is currently a clinical matron in a large NHS trust.

Tom Walvin

BSc (Hons), PGCert, RN, RNT, FHEA
Lecturer in Adult Nursing, University of Plymouth

Tom graduated from Bournemouth University as a registered nurse in 2010, training at Salisbury District Hospital. He practised in the Emergency Department, Cardiology and Research Nursing across Royal Hampshire County Hospital, Winchester; Royal Bournemouth Hospital and Royal Cornwall Hospital, Truro. Throughout this time, he also became experienced in various pre-hospital care roles. Tom enjoyed supporting the development of students across all these roles, and this led to him joining the University of Plymouth in 2015. Tom enjoys teaching clinical skills and clinical simulation, focusing on resuscitation and deteriorating patient care. He leads on the pathophysiology and contributes to anatomy, physiology and pharmacology teaching. Tom also continues to practise at University Hospitals NHS Trust, Plymouth and volunteers with the South Western Ambulance Service. Tom enjoys publishing and engaging in research across these teaching and clinical interests.

Kathy Whayman

RGN, DipN, MSc, PGDip Healthcare Education
Senior Lecturer University of Hertfordshire

Kathy began her nursing career in 1988. Her clinical background has developed in surgical, gastrointestinal and latterly colorectal nursing. An educator since 2005 Kathy has worked in partnership with a number of clinical teams within gastrointestinal (GI) nursing, helping to establish education and research programmes for nurses within this specialty. She is also a member of the Gastrointestinal Nursing Forum Steering Committee at the Royal College of Nursing. Her current job involves a variety of roles, including teaching on nursing practice, GI conditions, cancer and end-of-life care. She has a keen interest in nursing research, clinical skills teaching, service user involvement, student experience, and supporting learning in specialist clinical placements. Kathy enjoys teaching at all academic levels,. and is the current Field Tutor for the BSc (Hons) Pre-Registration Programme in Adult Nursing at the University of Hertfordshire.

Anthony Wheeldon

MSc (Lond), PGDE, BSc (Hons), DipHE, RN

Associate Subject Group Lead for Adult Nursing, University of Hertfordshire

Anthony began his nursing career at Barnet College of Nursing and Midwifery in 1992. After qualification, he worked as a staff nurse and senior staff nurse in the Respiratory Directorate at the Royal Brompton and Harefield NHS Trust in London. In 2000, he started teaching on post-registration cardio-respiratory courses before moving into full-time nurse education at Thames Valley University in 2002. Anthony has a wide range of interests including the promotion of inclusivity; success and attainment in nurse education; as well as cardio-respiratory care, anatomy and physiology, respiratory assessment and the application of bioscience in nursing practice. Since 2006, Anthony has worked at the University of Hertfordshire, where he teaches in pre- and post-registration nursing courses. He is currently an Associate Subject Group Lead for adult nursing.

Karen Wild

RN, HV, RNT, MA

Formerly a senior lecturer in adult nursing, Karen's career has inspired her interest in adult health and well-being, health promotion and education, and leadership skills at the master's level. Although recently retired from higher education, she maintains an interest in adult nursing and is a member of the editorial board of the *British Journal of Nursing.*

Julia Williams

RN, PhD, MA Ed, BSc (Hons), Dip D/N, SFHEA

Senior Lecturer in Adult Nursing, Academic Lead for Nursing Research

Julia's educational and research profile spans over 20 years, demonstrating a commitment to the development of academic nursing and in ensuring the delivery of knowledge in a meaningful way. Julia is currently Senior Lecturer and Academic Lead for Nursing Research, where through research and educational innovation, a caring and compassionate undergraduate nurse, can be prepared for qualified practice.

Julia's main area of clinical interest lies in colorectal nursing. Having worked as a specialist and lead nurse for many years, Julia now contributes to research with a focus on understanding the patient's experience in this specialist field.

Julia is currently Module Leader for three research modules in the nursing programmes offered at Bucks New University, at level 5, 6, and 7. These modules introduce students to approaches in research, enabling them to demonstrate critical thinking and an understanding of the research process. An awareness of different learning styles has equipped Julia to offer creative teaching to best enhance the students' learning of research. Julia's role also includes dissertation supervision for both undergraduate and postgraduate nursing students.

Julia's current activities outside of the university include roles such as the external examiner for University of Hull, consultant editor for *Gastrointestinal Nursing Journal*, and editorial board member for *British Journal of Nursing.*

Carol Wills

MSc Multidisciplinary Professional Development and Education, PGDip Advanced Practice, Bsc (Hons), Specialist Community Public Health Nursing (SCPHN) (Health Visiting), DipHE Adult Nursing, Registered Nurse (RN), Enrolled Nurse (EN), Registered Health Visitor (HV), Community Practitioner Prescriber (NP), Registered Lecturer/Practice Educator (RLP), Senior Fellow (SFHEA)

Subject and Programme Leader, Non-Medical Prescribing at Northumbria University

Carol began her career undertaking enrolled nurse training in 1983 at Hexham Hospital in Northumberland. She then worked within neuro trauma at Newcastle General Hospital and then several years in coronary care and intensive care at Hexham Hospital. This experience and additional training to complete registered nurse qualification then stimulated her to focus on primary care and prevention of ill health. Carol worked as a practice nurse and nurse practitioner in Newcastle city centre and as a staff nurse within Northumberland community nursing teams before going on to complete a health visiting degree and working in Newcastle as a health visitor for several years. During this time, she undertook several leadership and teaching roles, including as Immunisation Training Co-Ordinator, Community Practice Teacher and Trust Lead Mentor. Carol has been a senior lecturer at Northumbria University since 2002 and has led several postgraduate professional programmes including MSc Education in Professional Practice (NMC Teacher programme), PGDip SCPHN and the Non-Medical Prescribing programme. She has also undertaken national roles including as Policy Advice Committee member and Treasurer for the UK Standing Conference SCPHN Education and Subject Expert for several quality approval panels and External Examiner roles. Her key areas of interest and research are around developing learning and teaching and advanced-level practice.

Preface

The Nursing Associate's Handbook of Clinical Skills has been written for trainee nursing associates, whose numbers are continually growing. Those who have contributed to the 59 chapters are experienced clinicians and academics. The text aims to help trainee nursing associates develop and hone their skills in order to demonstrate proficiency as they offer care and support to people.

The *nursing associate*, in England, is a new member of the nursing team. The role has been devised in order to help bridge the gap between the health and care assistant and the registered nurse; it is a stand-alone role providing a progression route into graduate-level nursing, should the nursing associate desire this.

The nursing associate works with a variety of people of all ages and in a range of settings in both healthcare and social care. A review undertaken by Health Education England (2015), the Shape of Caring Review, revealed a discrepancy in skills and knowledge between healthcare assistants and registered nurses. In England, the creation of a new healthcare role was announced – the nursing associate. The role helps to meet the changing health and care needs of patients and the public. In July 2018, the Nursing and Midwifery Council (NMC) became the legal regulator for the nursing associate, and on 28 January 2019, the nursing associate part of the NMC's register was opened.

By law, the NMC was required to set standards of proficiency for nursing associates, and they did this (NMC, 2018a). The nursing associate is required to demonstrate proficiency in these standards in order to join and remain on the register. The standards set out what nursing associates are required to know and what they can do when they join the register. These standards are the minimum that are necessary to join the nursing associate part of the register.

This book is framed around annexes A and B of the proficiencies (NMC, 2018a). There are two parts reflecting the NMCs annexes, with subdivisions/units and the chapters. Providing the information in this way will make the parts, units and chapters easier to relate with and help the student make links with their programme of study; this is a core text.

In annexe A, the nursing associate is required to demonstrate communication and relationship management skills. At the point of registration, the nursing associate must be able to communicate effectively, with sensitivity and compassion, and to manage relationships with people which are key requirements to the provision of safe, high-quality person-centred care. The proficiencies must be adapted to ensure that they meet the needs of people across their lifespan, and in order to do this, the nursing associate requires a diverse range of communication skills and strategies that will ensure that individuals, their families and carers are supported to be actively involved in their own care wherever this is appropriate.

Annexe B of the proficiencies (NMC, 2018a) focuses on procedures that are to be undertaken by the nursing associate. The nursing associate is required to demonstrate proficiency in being able to carry out the procedures that have been described in this book in order to gain entry to the NMCs register along with an awareness of how requirements for procedures can differ across various health and care settings.

The nursing associate must apply evidence-based best practice with all procedures that they undertake regardless of the care setting. The ability to carry out these procedures safely, effectively, with sensitivity and compassion are key requirements outlined in the NMC's Code (NMC, 2018b).

The nursing associate contributes to most elements of care provision, including delivery and monitoring, the registered nurse takes the lead on assessment, planning and evaluation. Nursing associates contribute by reassessing, re-evaluating and reviewing.

In demonstrating the procedures, the nursing associate must do this with an awareness of variations that may be required in different practice settings and for people across the lifespan. In doing this effectively and with expertise, the procedures are carried out in such a way that they reflect cultural awareness and ensure that the needs, priorities, expertise and preferences of people are always valued and incorporated into care provision.

The chapters engage the reader by using a range of teaching and learning tools. Tools include pre and post-test questions, take note boxes and supporting evidence features that steer you towards the appropriate literature or provide links to electronic resources. Integrated throughout the chapters are the NMC proficiencies (NMC, 2018).

At the point of registration, the nursing associate must demonstrate cultural awareness when caring for people, ensuring that the needs, priorities, expertise and preferences of people are always valued and taken into account. Where appropriate, there are a series of flags that are used to highlight the fact that the nursing associate offers care and support to a number of people, in various settings. These flags are used to draw your attention to key issues. Red flags denote serious pathology; orange flags represent the equivalent of red flags for mental health and psychological problems; yellow flags are associated with beliefs values, emotions, fears and cultural consideration; blue flags highlight relationship issues; green flags are linked to the Code and legal issues; and violet flags have been used to represent issues that are concerned with housing or social issues, acknowledging, for example, that nursing associates care for people in places of detention and in secure environments, as well as for those who are homeless.

Using a range of full-colour illustrations, photographs, line drawings, tables, and graphs, the book engages readers, providing them with the skills to be able to demonstrate proficiency and to make the important link with theory and practice.

The terms that are used to describe people and communities are important. The importance of these terms is that they have the potential to create a particular perception of an individual or community that may be positive and enriching or harmful and stigmatising. Addressing people and communities how they wish to be addressed can enhance the therapeutic relationship.

There is and has been much debate about the best words to describe those people who use the services of healthcare professionals (including nursing associates). 'Patient' has been the traditional term; for some, the word 'patient' conjures up an image of passivity and the implied inequality in the relationship between the parties. It should also be pointed out that many people using the services of the nursing associate are not ill, but may be attending with lifestyle concerns, for example, fertility issues or for vaccination against illness.

There is a multiplicity of terms used in practice and in the literature, for example, 'person', 'survivor', 'service user', 'users', 'patient', 'expert', 'consumer', 'recipient' and 'client'. In this text, we have employed a number of terms to describe those who use the services of the nursing associate.

We have taken on writing this book for you with delight as we respond to the needs of the growing numbers of nursing associates. This book provides you with information that will empower you to develop and master your skills, and grow in confidence and competence, enabling you to offer care to people that is safe, effective and responsive to their needs.

Our aim was to produce a helpful, informative resource that provides you with the principles of care that can be adapted to meet the needs of people in dynamic healthcare and social care environments. Our aim was also to help you understand and perfect the care and support you offer as you realise that your contribution to the health and well-being of communities and nations is essential and is a combination of both art and science.

Ian Peate
Gibraltar

References

Health Education England (2015) "Raising the Bar. Shape of Caring: A Review of the Future Education and Training of Registered Nurses and Care Assistants" https://www.hee.nhs.uk/sites/default/files/documents/2348-Shape-of-caring-review-FINAL.pdf last accessed November 2019

Nursing and Midwifery Council (2018a) "Standards for Proficiency for Nursing Associates" https://www.nmc.org.uk/globalassets/sitedocuments/education-standards/nursing-assciates-proficiency-standards.pdf last accessed November 2019

Nursing and Midwifery Council (2018b) "The Code Professional standards of Practice and Behaviour for Nurses, Midwives and Nursing Associates" https://www.nmc.org.uk/globalassets/sitedocuments/nmc-publications/nmc-code.pdf last accessed November 2019

Acknowledgements

My thanks go to my partner Jussi Lahtinen and Mrs Frances Cohen, who have continually supported all of my endeavours, to the library staff at the Gibraltar Health Authority and also to the staff at the library at the Royal College of Nursing, London.

I am grateful to the contributors for giving their time to support me in the editing process. Thank you for imparting your knowledge and wisdom.

Two trainee nursing associates (now registered nursing associates) require very special acknowledgement: Nikki and Laura, your motivation and enthusiasm encouraged me to edit this text, and I am indebted to you both for that.

Thanks also to Magenta Styles at Wiley who has been unfaltering in her support and encouragement – an absolute pleasure to work with.

About the Editor

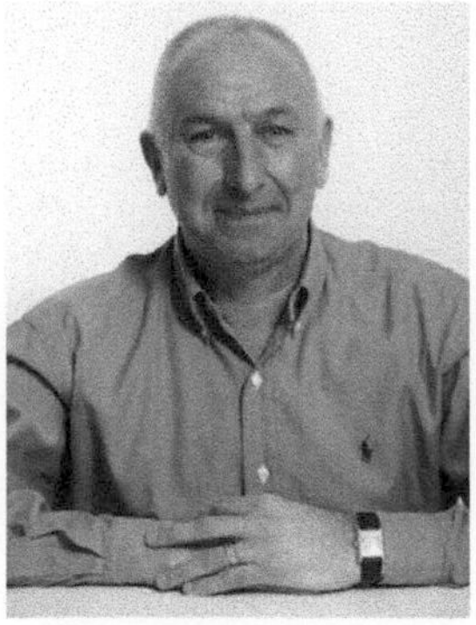

Ian Peate OBE FRCN

Principal, School of Health Studies, Gibraltar

Visiting Professor of Nursing at St George's University of London and Kingston University, London; Visiting Professor at Northumbria University; Visiting Senior Clinical Fellow at the University of Hertfordshire; Head of School, School of Health Studies, Gibraltar; and Editor in Chief of the *British Journal of Nursing*.

Ian began his nursing career at Central Middlesex Hospital, becoming an enrolled nurse practising in an intensive care unit. He later undertook 3 years' student nurse training at Central Middlesex and Northwick Park Hospitals, becoming a staff nurse and then a charge nurse. He has worked in nurse education since 1989. Ian's key areas of interest are nursing practice and theory, and he has published widely. He was awarded an OBE in the Queen's 90th Birthday Honours List for his services to Nursing and Nurse Education, and was bestowed a Fellowship from the Royal College of Nursing in 2017.

About the Companion Website

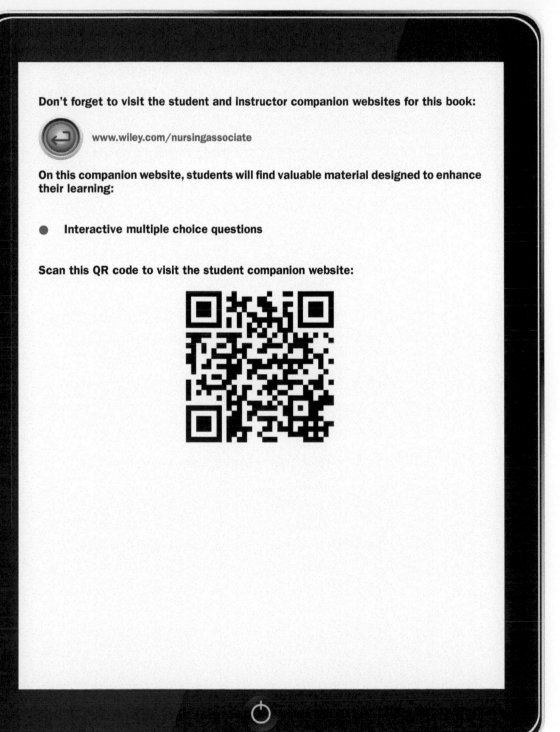

Don't forget to visit the student and instructor companion websites for this book:

www.wiley.com/nursingassociate

On this companion website, students will find valuable material designed to enhance their learning:

- **Interactive multiple choice questions**

Scan this QR code to visit the student companion website:

Annexe A

Communication and Relationship Management Skills

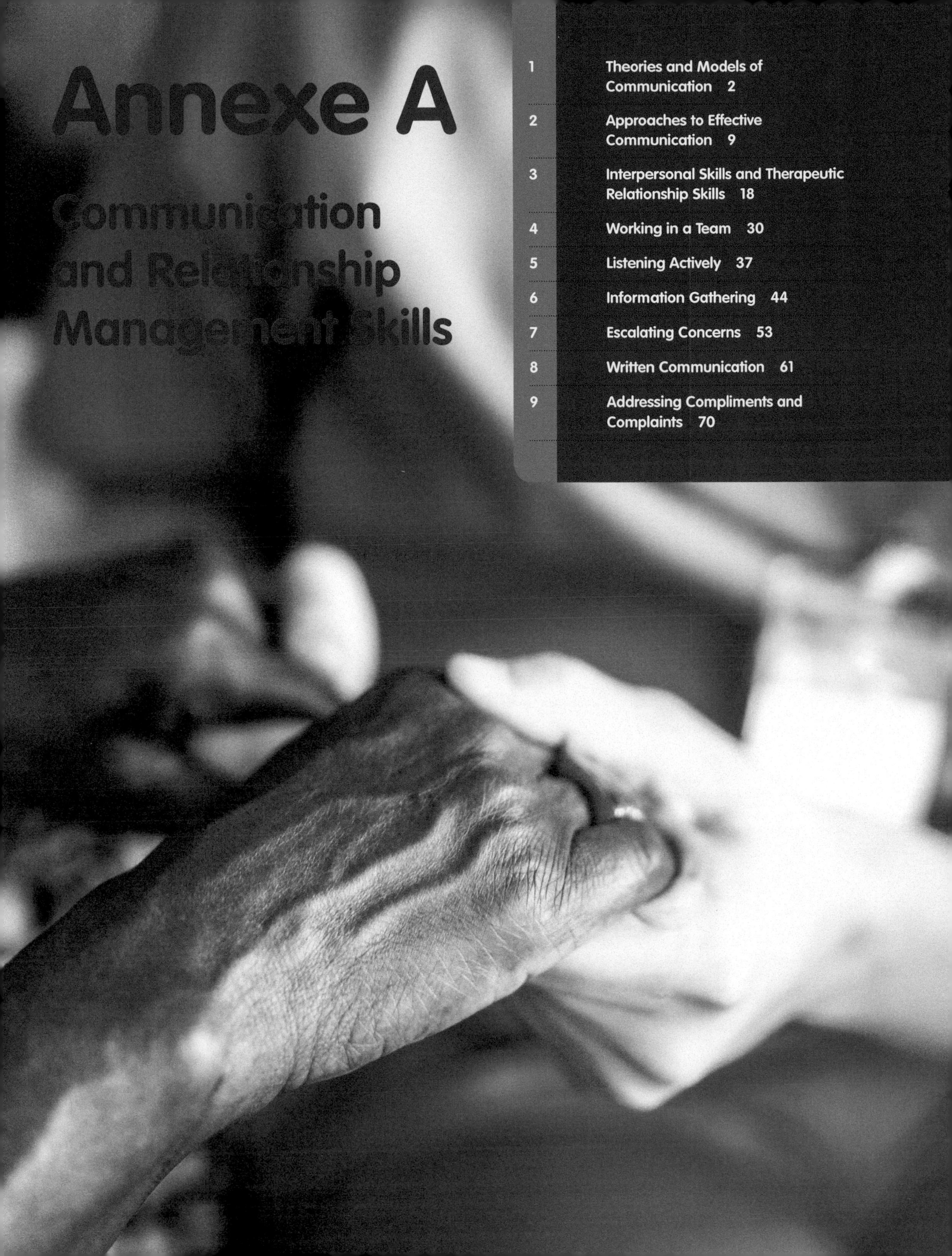

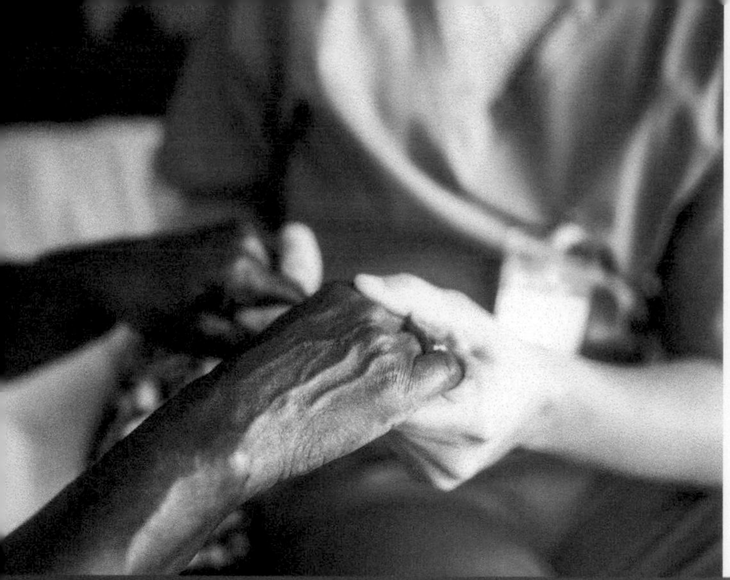

1

Theories and Models of Communication

Janine Archer and Lesley Jones

University of Salford, UK

Chapter Aim

- To explore the theories and models that underpin communication relevant to the role of a nursing associate

Learning Outcomes

By the end of this chapter, the reader will be able to:

- Identify and define the components of the three models of communication
- Describe contextual factors that affect communication
- Understand the importance of effective communication within the role of a nursing associate

Test Yourself Multiple Choice Questions

1. What are the three key communication models?
   A) Transgression, interaction and transaction
   B) Transmission, interaction and transaction
   C) Transport, interaction and transaction
   D) Transmission, intervention and transaction
2. Which of the following is/are the result(s) of poor communication?
   A) Medication error
   B) Poor patient outcomes
   C) Low staff morale
   D) All of the above

The Nursing Associate's Handbook of Clinical Skills, First Edition. Edited by Ian Peate.

Companion website: www.wiley.com/nursingassociate

3. **Which of the following terms is used to describe a communication barrier?**
   A) Channel
   B) Code
   C) Noise
   D) Receiver
4. **Which of the following represents the contexts considered important in the Transactional Model of Communication?**
   A) Psychological, social, cultural and relational
   B) Physical, psychological, social and cultural
   C) Physical, psychological, social, cultural and relational
   D) Physical, social, cultural and relational
5. **In Peplau's interpersonal relations theory, which of the following indicates when the nurse and patient begin to work collaboratively to enable the patient to become an active recipient of treatment?**
   A) Orientation phase
   B) Identification phase
   C) Exploitation phase
   D) Resolution phase

Introduction

Nursing associates provide safe and effective holistic patient-centred care that is underpinned by the 6Cs of caring (Department of Health 2012). Communication, one of the 6Cs, is a complex yet critical element in all areas of nursing activity. The nursing process, the assessment, diagnosing, planning, implementation and evaluation of care, is achieved only through careful attention to interpersonal relationships, the environment and the specific skills of verbal and non-verbal communication. Nursing associates are required to communicate with a wide variety of patients across their lifespan, including babies, children and young people, carers and families, and adults and older people. They are expected to provide prevention, treatment, rehabilitation and end-of-life care while working in a broad range of settings, such as at home, close to home and in hospital. They do not work in isolation and so require excellent communication skills to work effectively with not just patients and carers but also health and social care colleagues within a multidisciplinary team. Many of the people nursing associates communicate with will have communication challenges requiring them to make reasonable adjustments and adapt their style of communication.

There is a well-established link between team communication, worker morale and patient safety. Poor team communication has been directly linked to high nurse turnover rates and low morale (Brinkert 2010). Low morale contributes to high levels of stress, burnout, poor job satisfaction and an overall poor quality of life (Khamisa et al. 2015).

Supporting Evidence

The National Institute for Health and Care Excellence (2016) has provided guidance for health and social care professionals to enhance the transition between inpatient mental health settings and community or care home settings https://www.nice.org.uk/guidance/ng53/resources/tailored-resources-4429245855/chapter/2-Ensuring-effective-communication-between-teams-and-with-people-using-services-families-and-carers

Poor communication is often a feature in healthcare related events (Burgener 2017) with communication issues frequently featuring in National Health Service (NHS) complaints and medication related events. Within hospital and community health services, Ombudsman data identifies communication issues as one of the five most common complaint factors in cases which were fully or partially upheld in 2018–19 (Parliamentary and Health Service Ombudsman 2019).

In recent years, a number of serious failings in healthcare provision have made national news, for example, the Francis enquiry. This public enquiry reviewed reports on poor care in the Mid Staffordshire Foundation NHS Trust between 2005 and 2009, which was believed to have contributed to the avoidable death of many patients and highlighted communication failings in sharing information and concerns (Francis 2013).

Poor communication between healthcare professionals, poor communication with patients and limited communication between primary and secondary care have all been identified as factors which influence medication errors (World Health Organization 2016). Keers et al. (2013), in a systematic review of causes of medication administration errors in hospital, also identified inadequate written communication as a factor.

Take Note

Ineffective communication among healthcare professionals is one of the leading causes of error and patient harm, as well as reducing staff morale

Good communication is essential in meeting patients' needs and providing safe, quality patient care. Improvements in communication can lessen healthcare errors and make a positive impact on patient outcomes. For the nursing associate, it is important that they develop underpinning knowledge about communication as well as the skills to deliver effective communication to provide high quality care.

Red Flag

Poor communication between nursing associates and those they offer care and support to can occur for a variety of reasons. The provision of health and social care can be very unpredictable, complicated and stressful. The needs of patients can arise unexpectedly, and their condition can change very rapidly; when there is a communication breakdown, this can lead to negative care outcomes.

This chapter will focus on the underpinning knowledge of communication and will be followed by a series of chapters that will examine the specific communication skills required by the nursing associate. The Nursing and Midwifery Council (NMC) (2018) standards of proficiency for nursing associates require, at the point of registration, the nursing associate to communicate effectively using a range of skills and strategies with colleagues and people at all stages of life and with a range of mental, physical, cognitive and behavioural health challenges; this is closely related to platform 1, that is, being an accountable professional.

The World Health Organisation (WHO) defines communication as 'the transfer of information, ideas or feelings' (World Health Organization 2009, p.16). More recently, communication has been described as 'the exchange of information between people by sending and receiving it through speaking, writing or by using any other medium' (Sibiya 2018, p. 20). Effective communication means that information is conveyed clearly between people. To be an excellent nursing associate requires communication skills to engage effectively with patients using two-way communication. Failure to recognise this two-way communication could lead to negative conclusions, negative attitudes and dissatisfaction. The nursing associate must, therefore, continuously try to improve their communication skills to ensure high quality patient-centred care.

Models of communication help us to consider the processes involved when communicating in several arenas with a variety of people. They provide a visual representation of the different aspects of a communication encounter, simplifying the numerous steps the nursing associate needs to consider. Having this underpinning knowledge can help the nursing associate think about their current communication encounters, plan for future communication encounters and reflect and learn from the previous ones. The three main models that will be discussed in this chapter are the transmission/linear, interaction and transaction models of communication.

Transmission Model of Communication

In 1949, Shannon and Weaver first described the transmission, or linear, model of communication which consists of a sender creating a message which they send to the receiver without any feedback (see Figure 1.1.). This model describes communication as one way, from sender to receiver, which suggested that the sender and receiver had little to do with the interpretation of the message. The model does recognise physical noise as a communication barrier.

The main issue with one-way communication is that it does not include feedback which enables the sender and receiver to ensure that the meaning within the message has been understood. Relying on one-way communication can have an impact on patient outcomes. An example of this might be where a nursing associate advises the patient how to apply a cream but does not check whether the patient has understood the information. This could lead to the cream being applied incorrectly and delaying or even worsening the patient's condition. Communicating in this way has been described as something you do 'to' someone.

Communication models have evolved since the linear model was first described over 70 years ago, but the model was useful in that it established some terms which have subsequently been adopted and developed further (see Table 1.1).

The nursing associate will already have thought about the different aspects of communication. They may have realised that they communicate with colleagues differently when they are tired (sender) and that they adapt their tone of voice when talking to a young child (receiver). They may have considered the message being conveyed by avoiding medical terminology when telling patients about their treatment. They may have considered providing written and verbal instructions to convey the information (code). They will have considered the channel of communicating, for example, if a patient cannot hear, they may have written down the message or have taken the patient into a side room away from the noise of the ward environment.

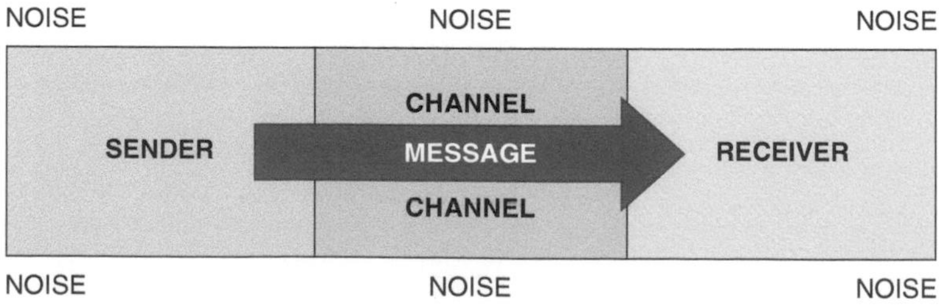

Figure 1.1 Transmission model of communication. *Source:* Adapted from Shannon & Weaver (1949).

Table 1.1 Common communication terms.

TERM	MEANING
Sender/receiver	The sender is the source of the communication. Anyone who is audience to the message is referred to as the receiver.
Message	The information being conveyed.
Code	Sometimes referred to as *encoding* and *decoding*. Encoding can be defined as transforming an abstract idea into a communicable message, using words, symbols, pictures, symbols and sounds. Decoding is when the receiver interprets the message and comes to an understanding about what the source is communicating.
Channel	The way the code is conveyed, for example, it may be easier to present complex information in a graph rather than written word alone.
Noise	Communication barrier.

Source: Adapted from Kiernan (2015).

The Interactive Model of Communication

The interactive or interaction model of communication relies on an exchange of communication from the sender to the receiver and back again creating two-way communication within physical and psychological contexts (Schramm 1997). The main difference between one- and two-way communication is that two-way communication provides feedback which enables the sender and receiver to ensure that the meaning within the information has been understood. It, therefore, closes the communication loop and is one way of minimising misunderstandings in the receiver's interpretation of the original meaning of the message.

This model is more interaction focused and concerned with the communication process itself. This model acknowledges that with so many messages being sent at one time, many of them may not even be received and some messages may be sent unintentionally.

The interactive model also takes into consideration the communicator's fields of experience and physical barriers. It also introduces semantic and psychological barriers. Physical barriers are vitally important as nursing associates must be able to care for people in a broad range of settings, including at home, close to home and in hospital, within a context of challenging environments. Nursing associates work with patients and their carers and families during times of heightened stress, anxiety and fear, and these emotions can affect our communication. Feedback and context help make this model of communication more useful than the transmission model for exploring individual communication encounters. The interactive model is depicted in Figure 1.2.

Orange Flag

Psychological barriers include the mental and emotional factors in a communication encounter

One of the main issues with the interactive model of communication is that it suggests communication is predictable and orderly, that is, A asks B a question and B responds. The reality of communication, especially in healthcare, is that it is much more disorganised with interruptions and people talking at the same time.

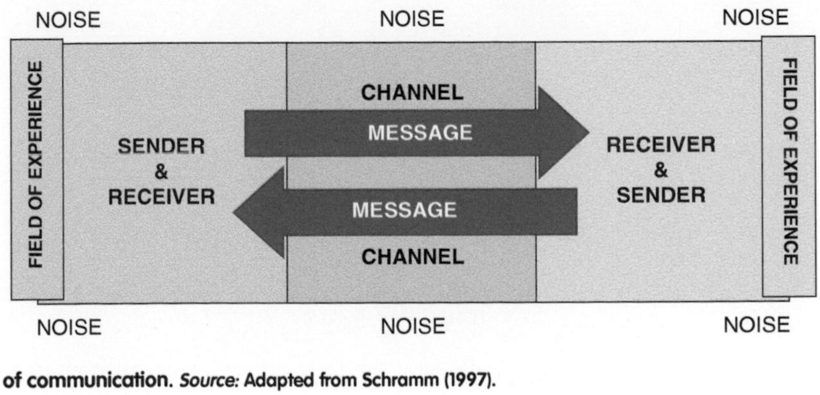

Figure 1.2 Interaction model of communication. *Source:* Adapted from Schramm (1997).

The Transactional Model of Communication

As the study of communication progressed, models expanded to account for more of the complex elements of the communication process. The transactional model of communication places emphasis on the concurrent and continuous nature of communication. In this model, all those involved in the communication experience are simultaneously the sender and receiver, continuously sending and receiving information and feedback from each other using verbal and non-verbal communication (Barnlund 1970).

The transactional model describes communication as a process in which communicators (can be more than two people) generate social realities within social, relational and cultural contexts. The purpose of communication is not simply to exchange messages but to also create relationships, develop intercultural relations, shape self-concepts and engage with others to create communities.

Blue Flag

The therapeutic relationship is an essential prerequisite to effective communication between health professionals and patients in order to not only transmit information but also effectively address mental processes that become activated by it. The communication between the nursing associate and the patient includes the ability to express genuine concern for the care of the patient, with the patient becoming a participant.

The transactional model also considers the context in which the communication occurs, which shapes the way you communicate; consideration is given not only to the content of the message (the what) but also to the relational dynamics (the how it is said). Like the interactional model of communication, the transactional model acknowledges the participants' field of experience but includes a more complex understanding of communication across physical, psychological, social, cultural and relational contexts. Figure 1.3 outlines the transactional model.

The transactional model agrees that physical and psychological contexts are important but in isolation are too simplistic. The transactional model argues that communication is more complex, as it shapes a person's reality before and after specific interactions occur, and, therefore, emphasis is placed on the importance of contextual influences outside of the single interaction, namely social, cultural and relational contexts.

Social context focuses on the stated rules and unstated norms that guide communication. There are many examples we can draw on from healthcare here. For example, a trainee nursing associate observes that the ward round is monopolised by the consultant and the nurse in charge and the trainee nursing associate may only realise they break this norm from the reaction of others, for example, being told not to talk again during ward round. These types of norms are traditional and have no place in the future of healthcare; the role of the nursing associate is to be resilient and advocate for best patient care.

Green Flag

The Nursing and Midwifery Council (NMC) (2018) Standards of proficiency for nursing associates

The NMC standards of proficiency require the nursing associate to understand the importance of courage and transparency and apply the duty of candour, recognising and reporting any situations, behaviours or errors that could result in poor care outcomes (Platform 1: Being an accountable professional; 1.3)

Relational context includes the historical and current relationship you have with an individual. The nursing associate will communicate differently with colleagues compared with family and friends and similarly with people they have just met versus someone they have known for

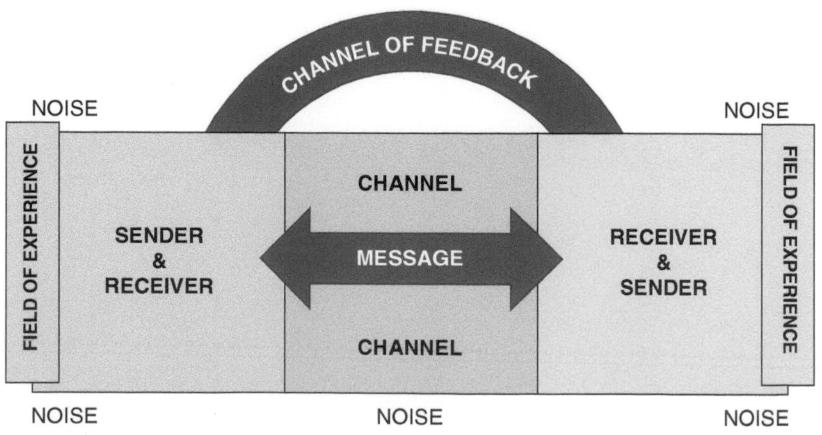

Figure 1.3 Transactional model of communication. *Source:* Adapted from Barnlund (1970).

some time. Early interactions are more likely to be governed by the social context of rules and norms but these maybe less apparent as relationships develop. Consider the nursing associates differing response when a patient says 'Get me a drink' compared to if a partner were to say it.

Cultural context includes, for example, ethnicity, gender, nationality, sexual orientation, class, ability and ethnicity, and we all have multiple aspects of cultural identity which influence our communication. The nursing associate needs to be aware of unconscious bias, as it harms patients and staff (Kapur 2015). Unconscious (or implicit) bias occurs when the way information is processed is influenced by stereotypes, and, therefore, those stereotypes impact actions and judgements. A stereotype is a belief that associates a group of people with certain traits or characteristics and is a prejudgement of a person based on the group they are associated with. Unconscious bias is a natural method of cognitive processing, so we all possess it. In healthcare, unconscious bias can lead to false assumptions and negative patient outcomes, especially in minority groups. An example might be that the nursing associate inadvertently spends less time with the patient with mental health issues because of the stereotype they hold that all people with mental health issues are violent. It is important for the nursing associate to be aware of unconscious bias and, while it will always exist, develop strategies to overcome it.

Yellow Flag

Health Education England have developed a Cultural Competence e-learning package to support health professionals in developing cultural competence https://www.e-lfh.org.uk/programmes/cultural-competence/

The three models of communication (transmission, interactive and transactional) while relevant to the role of the nursing associate, as they apply to all forms of human interaction, were developed to describe communication in general. The nurse-patient relationship is, by its very nature, embedded in interpersonal communication. There are a number of communication theories that have been developed in nursing to help explain and guide interactions between nurses and patients (Bylund et al. 2012). One such theory is Peplau's interpersonal relations theory (1997) which focuses on the nurse-patient relationship and the therapeutic process that takes place. Although the focus is on the nurse-patient relationship, it is similar to the transactional model in that communication that occurs in this context involves complex factors such as environment, attitudes and beliefs and culture. Peplau's interpersonal relations theory defines four stages of the relationship that achieve a common goal:

- Orientation phase: This is the initial stage of the relationship where the nursing associate demonstrates patient-centred care that enables the patient to ask questions and develop trust in the nursing associate. First impressions of the nursing associate and the healthcare provision begin to evolve. This phase sets the stage for a more trusting relationship and is where the nursing associate would introduce themselves (Granger 2014), collect information about the patient's needs, potential, interests and the patient's susceptibility to experience fear or anxiety (Fawcett 2010).
- Identification phase: This is when the nursing associate and patient begin to work collaboratively to enable the patient to become an active recipient of treatment. The nursing associate uses knowledge, skills, attitudes and values while consistently providing compassionate, non-judgemental care and empathy. This is an important stage during which the power shifts from the nursing associate to the patient as the patient becomes more independent. The nursing associate uses their communication skills as an educator and a leader to enable better patient outcomes.
- Exploitation phase: The patient maximises wider opportunities, exploiting the nurse-patient relationship to address treatment goals. The patient feels like an integral part of the relationship and may make requests to the nursing associate to gain a greater understanding of their own health and social care needs.
- Resolution phase: As a product of effective communication, patient issues are resolved, and they become independent. The patient no longer relies on the nursing associate's support, and the relationship ends. The skills here are for the nursing associate to enhance the patient's ability to become more self-reliant in leading a productive and healthier life (Fawcett 2010).

Conclusion

Excellent communication skills are critical in the development of effective relationships with patients, their carers and families and when working with other health and social care professionals. While it is important for nursing associates to develop the underpinning knowledge that governs communication experiences, it is equally necessary for them to develop the skills and behaviours that are prerequisite to effective communication. Chapter 2 highlights key approaches and identifies common barriers to effective communication.

References

Barnlund, D.C. (1970) A transactional model of communication, in Sereno, K.K. & Mortenson, C.D. (eds.) *Foundations of communication theory*, New York, NY: Harper and Row, 83–92.

Brinkert, R. (2010) A literature review of conflict communication causes, costs, benefits and interventions in nursing, *Journal of Nursing Management*, 18(2): 145–156. doi: 10.1111/j.1365-2834.2010.01061.x.

Burgener, M. (2017) Enhancing communication to improve patient safety and to increase patient satisfaction, *Health Care Management*, 36(3): 238–243. doi: 10.1097/HCM.0000000000000165.
Bylund, C.L., Peterson, E.B. & Cameron, K.A. (2012) A practitioner's guide to interpersonal communication theory: an overview and exploration of selected theories, *Patient Education and Counseling*, 87(3): 261–267. doi: 10.1016/j.pec.2011.10.006.
Department of Health. (2012) *Compassion in practice.* [online] Available: https://www.england.nhs.uk/wp-content/uploads/2012/12/compassion-in-practice.pdf. Accessed 6 September 2020.
Fawcett, J. (2010) *Contemporary nursing knowledge: Analysis and evaluation of nursing models and theories* (2nd ed), Philadelphia: F.A. Davies.
Francis, R. (2013) *Report of the Mid Staffordshire NHS foundation trust public inquiry*, London: The Stationery Office.
Granger, K. (2014) *Hello my name is.* [online] Available: http://hellomynameis.org.uk/home. Accessed 6 September 2020.
Kapur, N. (2015) Unconscious bias harms patients and staff, *British Medical Journal*, 351: h6347. doi: 10.1136/bmj.h6347.
Keers, R.N., Williams, S.D., Cooke, J. & Ashcroft, D.M. (2013) Causes of medication administration errors in hospitals: a systematic review of quantitative and qualitative evidence, *Drug Safety*, 36(110): 1045–1067. doi: 10.1007/s40264-013-0090-2.
Khamisa, N., Oldenburg, B., Peltzer, K. & Ilic, D. (2015) Work related stress, burnout, job satisfaction and general health of nurses, *International Journal of Environmental Research and Public Health*, 12(1): 652–666. doi: 10.3390/ijerph120100652.
Kiernan, E. (2015) Communication theory and its application in nursing and healthcare, in Lawrence, J., Perrin, C. & Keirnan, E. (eds.) *Building professional nursing communication*, Melbourne: Cambridge University Press.
NMC. (2018) *Standards of proficiency for nursing associates*, London: NMC.
Parliamentary and Health Service Ombudsman. (2019) *Complaints about the NHS in England 201819*, Parliamentary and Health Service Ombudsman. [online] Available: https://www.ombudsman.org.uk/publications/complaints-about-nhs-england-quarter-4-2018-19. Accessed 6 September 2020.
Peplau, H.E. (1997) Peplau's theory of interpersonal relations, *Nursing Science Quarterly*, 10(4): 162–167. doi.org/10.1177/089431849701000407.
Schramm, W. (1997) *The beginnings of communication study in America*, Thousand Oaks, CA: Sage.
Shannon, C. and Weaver, W. (1949) *The mathematical theory of communication*, Urbana, IL: University of Illinois Press.
Sibiya, M.N. (2018) *Effective communication in nursing*, London: Intechopen.
World Health Organization. (2009) *Human factors in patient safety: review of topics and tools*, Geneva: World health Organization.
World Health Organization. (2016) *Medication errors: technical series on safer primary care*, Geneva: World Health Organization.

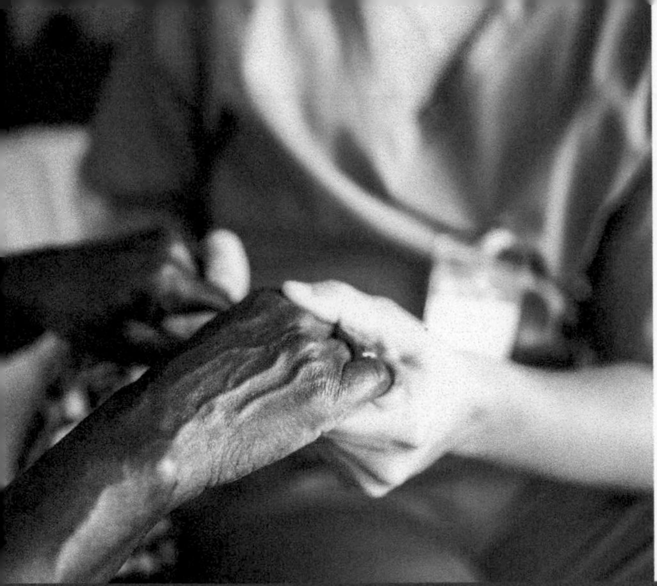

2

Approaches to Effective Communication

Janine Archer[1] *and Joanne Greenwood*[2]

[1] University of Salford, UK
[2] Oldham Care Organisation District Nurses, Northern Care Alliance, UK

Chapter Aim

- To equip the reader with the knowledge, skills and behaviours to communicate effectively and overcome obstacles to effective communication

Learning Outcomes

By the end of this chapter, the reader will be able to:

1. Describe a range of communication techniques
2. Describe common barriers to effective communication and consider the role of a nursing associate in overcoming these obstacles

Test Yourself Multiple Choice Questions

1. The Royal College of Nursing identified three reasons why communication is important. These are:
   A) It helps patients feel valued, special and engaged
   B) It helps patients feel alone, desperate and angry
   C) It helps patients feel valued, in control and at ease
2. Richardson (2017) developed a tool to aid healthcare professionals in effective communication, which is:
   A) Personal, enhanced and requested
   B) Propose, engage and reflect
   C) Proper, elaborate and realistic

The Nursing Associate's Handbook of Clinical Skills, First Edition. Edited by Ian Peate.

Companion website: www.wiley.com/nursingassociate

3. **It is good practice for healthcare professionals to prepare prior to any meaningful conversation**
   A) True
   B) False
4. **According to Laswell (1948), when healthcare professionals plan communication encounters, what should they consider?**
   A) 3P's, 2H's & 1W
   B) 4H's & 2P's
   C) 5W's & 1H
   D) 6Q's
5. **The four different types of communication are:**
   A) Verbal, non-verbal, written and drawn
   B) Verbal, non-verbal, written and observed
   C) Verbal, non-verbal, written and visual
   D) Verbal, non-verbal, written and picture

Introduction

To be a successful nursing associate, excellent communication skills are required. Effective communication requires the nursing associate to develop and maintain the required knowledge, skills and behaviours that enable them to work effectively with a wide range of people across the lifespan and during times where there are challenges to effective communication. The Nursing and Midwifery Council (NMC) (2018a) Nursing Associate Standards of Proficiency, at the point of registration, require the registered nursing associate to have the underpinning knowledge and communication skills to provide and monitor care. The NMC standards of proficiency also require the nursing associate to communicate effectively using a range of skills and strategies with colleagues and people at all stages of life and with a range of mental, physical, cognitive and behavioural health challenges.

In chapter 1, the underpinning theories and models of communication were discussed. This chapter will explore a range of communication approaches and the skills required to overcome some of the obstacles to effective communication. It will highlight the skills required when communicating with different age groups and the actions to be performed in challenging or complex situations.

As humans, we thrive on interaction with others. We learn to communicate at a very early age; as babies, we are able to communicate our wants and needs through cries and smiles (Grainger 2018). Those positive connections give us a sense of belonging and value. When done well, communication is a two-way process that involves listening, observation, body language, facial expressions and speech from all parties involved. Effective communication is extremely important at times of ill health or crisis (Raphael-Grimm 2014). Yet, communication is one of the five most common reasons for complaints in the National Health Service (NHS) in England (Parliamentary and Health Service Ombudsman 2019). It is vital for all healthcare professionals to understand the impact of their communication with the people they are caring for. Nursing associates have a legal and professional obligation to develop the skills to ensure that each interaction is effective and meaningful (Nursing and Midwifery Council 2018a).

Green Flag

Nursing and Midwifery Council (2018b) The Code: Professional standards of practice and behaviour for nurses, midwives and nursing associates

Practice effectively:

7.0 Communicate clearly. To achieve this, you must:
7.1 use terms that people in your care, colleagues and the public can understand
7.2 take reasonable steps to meet people's language and communication needs, providing, wherever possible, assistance to those who need help to communicate their own or other people's needs
7.3 use a range of verbal and non-verbal communication methods and consider cultural sensitivities to better understand and respond to people's personal and health needs
7.4 check people's understanding from time to time to keep misunderstanding or mistakes to a minimum
7.5 be able to communicate clearly and effectively in English

Every communication is important, however insignificant it may seem, especially when working in healthcare. The Royal College of Nursing (2016) identified three reasons why communication is important:

- Good communication helps patients/clients feel at ease
- Good communication helps patients/clients to feel in control
- Good communication makes patients/clients feel valued

Richardson (2017) developed a tool to aid healthcare professionals in effective communication, the PER tool (**Propose, Engage and Reflect**). This advocates that prior to any conversation, the healthcare professional **proposes** what they are planning to discuss to ensure that they have all the information needed and are aware of who will be involved in the conversation. This also includes ensuring there is a suitable place for the conversation to happen, as it is difficult for anyone to focus in a busy, noisy environment. The **engagement** aspect is the professional's opportunity to introduce themselves, gain the other person's attention, clarify who else is there and ensure the person(s) receiving the information is/are responding appropriately. The final element is for the healthcare professionals to **reflect** on whether they achieved what they set out to, if it went well and what they could have done differently (Richardson 2017).

In preparing for communication, the nursing associate can consider the 5Ws and 1H, derived from Lasswell's (1948) 5W model of communication.

- What
- Why
- When
- Where
- Who
- How

Careful planning of communication encounters can result in more meaningful and effective communication. See Table 2.1 for an overview of planning communication encounters.

It is important to have an awareness of the different formats of communication when proposing planned communication with patients and colleagues. There are generally four different types of communication to consider, namely verbal, non-verbal, written and visual (Table 2.2). Each of these will be described in detail in subsequent chapters of this book.

The **engagement** aspect of communication is when the nursing associate will work collaboratively with patients, families and carers to develop therapeutic relationships. As nursing associates work across all four fields of nursing practice (adult, mental health, children and young people and learning disabilities), as well as with people across the lifespan, they will need to consider the target audience when engaging in communication.

The NMC's (2018a) standards of proficiency require the nursing associate to demonstrate the skills and abilities required to develop, manage and maintain appropriate relationships with people, their families, carers and colleagues. The trainee nursing associate needs to be deemed proficient in this aspect of care provision.

When working with children and young people, family-centred care is a key concept, and the nursing associate needs to be aware that while the child is a pivotal member within the family unit, care must extend to involve the parents and wider family (Roberts et al. 2015). Children, more than any other age group, are keen observers and easily detect when a person is being disingenuous or impatient (Edwards & Coyne 2019). The nursing associate can strive to achieve a trusting and collaborative therapeutic relationship by demonstrating a genuine interest in the child and paying attention to all aspects of verbal and non-verbal communication.

Table 2.1 Planning communication encounters.

What – The 'What' question answers:
What am I required to communicate? What should the message be? What action is the audience required to take as a result of the communication?
Why – The 'Why' question deals with:
Why communicate now? Why this audience? Why is this important?
When – The 'When' explores:
When is the communication required? When is the action or result required?
Where – The 'Where' question answers:
Where is the venue or location of communication? Where can I get more information? Where is this communication going to lead?
Who – The 'Who' question defines the audience:
Who is the audience? Who does it impact? Who needs to take the required action? Who is in charge?
How – The 'How' question is about:
How am I going to communicate? (consider channel and reasonable adjustments) How am I going to handle any challenges? How should action be taken?

Table 2.2 The four different types of communication.

Verbal	• Spoken word • Vocal gestures e.g. sighs and gasps • Face-to-face and telephone
Non-verbal	• Body language • Gestures e.g. pointing
Written	• Patient notes • Email • Text
Visual	• Graphs and charts • Symbols e.g. sign on toilet door • Posters

Table 2.3 Tips for effective communication with children and young people.

DO	DO NOT
• Get to know a child's developmental level • Learn the child's interests based on your observations of their activities • Talk at the child's level and with vocabulary they will understand • Involve the child in decision-making appropriately • Maintain a calm, unhurried, caring and gentle approach • Use concrete examples and/or link information to activities of daily living • Allow opinions to be expressed • Be an active, attentive listener	• Make a child self-conscious by drawing attention to them • Use abstractions with a child who is a concrete thinker (e.g., for a child who does not understand time, tell them 'after lunch', not 'later' or 'at 2 o'clock') • Jump to conclusions • Get 'in the middle' between a child and a parent, especially in front of the child

When communicating with children and young people, the nursing associate must recognise the variable needs of children in relation to their age, development and ability. They must draw on their knowledge of the stages of child development and utilise communication skills, such as active listening, paraphrasing, summarising, reflecting and questioning, that are fundamental to the development of rapport and empathic therapeutic relationships (Nelson 2012). They should find out what children, young people and their parents want and need to know, what issues are important to them and what opinions or fears they have about their health or treatment.

Babies, when in infancy, communicate via sounds such as gurgles and cries. They also use facial expressions such as smiles, grimaces and eye contact to communicate their needs (Grainger 2018). As children develop, they begin to use single words to express their needs. When communicating at this stage, it is important to make use of pictures and objects to convey meaning as well as simple language (Edwards & Coye 2019). When communicating with adolescence, it can be difficult to develop rapport due to the challenges physiologically, psychologically and socially for this age group. Templeman (2019) explains how to foster a rapport with adolescents by introducing yourself, offering a hand to shake and making small talk. This can also be done by showing an interest in the individual, what do they enjoy doing, how is school and so forth. This will encourage the therapeutic relationship, as the individual is given time to talk about themselves to someone who is interested in them. The nursing associate needs to listen carefully and respond appropriately without being directive to show the adolescents that they are being taken seriously, which will develop their confidence (Templeman 2019).

It is imperative that children and young people are involved in discussions about their care and that the nursing associate explains things using language or other forms of communication they can understand. Some tips for communicating with children adapted from Boggs (2016) are listed in Table 2.3.

When communicating with adults, nursing associates need to be aware of the vocabulary they use, but also the words that are not spoken by the patient. The words left unspoken can be an indicator of feelings of low self-worth or fear of judgement. For example, a patient who is withdrawn and does not talk about their future may be contemplating suicide, or patients when talking about spirituality may not give any details about their beliefs due to fear of being judged (Richardson 2017).

The vocabulary used when talking to patients should change dependent on the person being spoken to, as those words needs to be understood. Parnell (2015) refers to this as 'plain language' – it should be to the point, clear and accurate. Nursing associates have a professional responsibility to communicate with colleagues, patients, patients' family and other professionals. When delivering information or explaining a procedure, it is difficult to gauge how much the person who is receiving the information has understood. Quite often, the information that is being communicated is complex and the population receiving this information is more diverse than ever. An effective technique is to keep it simple and ask the person to repeat back what they have understood. By doing this, the nursing associate can adapt the language used to clarify any points of misunderstanding (Parnell 2015).

Currently in the United Kingdom, approximately 1.5 million people have a learning disability (Mental Health Foundation 2019), and for this group of people, it is more likely that communication may be difficult. People with learning disabilities access mainstream healthcare, and as they are significantly more likely than the general population to be diagnosed with a wide range of conditions, the nursing associate will undoubtedly care for people with a learning disability throughout their nursing career. It is important that the nursing associate take the time to get to know their patients and see them, not the disability, and listen to them and their family/carers. Where people have communication needs or a disability, it is essential that nursing associates make reasonable adjustments, providing and sharing information in a way that promotes good health and health outcomes and does not prevent people from having equal access to the highest quality of care.

To be a good communicator with people with a learning disability, the nursing associate will need to:

- Always use accessible language and speak clearly
- Keep their head up and be on the same level as the person
- Avoid jargon or long words that might be hard to understand
- Be creative and prepared to use different communication tools such as visual cues to support understanding
- Take time and follow the lead of the person
- Go at their pace
- Check out understanding
- Ask for help if they need to

For people with profound and multiple learning disabilities (PMLD), it can be difficult to communicate intentionally, making this group of people particularly vulnerable. Nursing associates need to adapt the way they communicate with people with PMLD to find a way of listening and communicating in a way that is individualised and appropriate (Mansell 2010). This will involve being creative; it may be through the use of hand gestures and movements, or through picture and music. The purpose of communication, although via a more creative mode, is the same; it should remain a two-sided process where both parties are able to express themselves and communicate their needs. Mansell (2010) talks about other specialities in assisting people with PMLD such as speech and language therapists, family and carers, as each of these can provide insight into effective ways of communicating, be this a particular gesture, sign, object, sound or behaviour. A communication passport can be a useful tool, not only for people with PMLD but for a variety of people who have difficulty communicating. Communication passports should contain everything about the way that individual communicates. These should be updated regularly and readily available for anyone in contact with or involved in that person's care (Mansell 2010).

Supporting Evidence

Augmentative and Alternative Communication (AAC) Scotland has online learning modules, posters, communication cards and guides to support people in communicating. https://www.aacscotland.org.uk/home/

MENCAP has a variety of resources including case studies to help support healthcare professionals in communicating with people with complex needs. http://www.mencap.org.uk

Blue Flag **Total Communication**

Total communication is an approach that supports people with complex communication needs. It was developed to empower people to help them express themselves and form connections (Sense 2019). Total communication was born from the concept that when communicating, we are not just a talking head, we use non-verbal communication through our bodies (Thomsen 2010). Total communication refers to all available means of communication, be this limited verbal speech, sounds, spontaneous non-verbal means and low technological devices (Rautakoski 2010). This approach is reliant on a partner to facilitate and clarify the meaning in a conversation. A study by Rautakoski (2010) in the training of people with severe to moderate aphasia and their communication partners in the use of total communication found that both the individuals and their partners recognised that they interpret the use of different communication means in relatively the same way. The study found that participants perceived the level of interaction increased during the study, as both were more familiar with different modes of communication (Rautakoski 2010).

One in four adults experiences a mental health condition in any given year (National Institute for Health and Care Excellence (NICE) 2019), many of whom also have comorbid obesity, asthma, diabetes mellitus, chronic obstructive pulmonary disease, chronic heart disease, stroke and heart failure (Public Health England (PHE) 2018). Nursing associates will encounter people with mental health problems throughout their nursing career, and they can enhance their communication encounters with people with mental health problems by:

- Having a fundamental knowledge of the main mental health problems
- Giving the person time with no distractions
- Letting the person share as much or as little as they want to
- Not making assumptions or try to diagnose
- Keeping questions open ended
- Talking about well-being, for example, exercise and diet
- Listening carefully and repeating what you have heard to check accurate understanding
- Being aware of stigma and the negative impact inaccurate prejudices can have on communication, for example, people with mental health problems are usually portrayed as violent and aggressive in the media, but this is not typical of the majority of people with mental health problems
- Knowing your limits and asking for help from other healthcare professionals if needed

Table 2.4 **The 7Cs of communication.**

TERM	MEANING
1. Clear	Avoid jargon and complex words. Focus on a specific message which makes the message understandable
2. Concise	Keep it brief, avoid repetition. Highlight the main message
3. Coherent	Ensure the message makes sense and is logical
4. Complete	The message must be complete and contain everything it needs to so that the receiver can respond or act
5. Concrete	Specific and clear, supported by facts and figures
6. Courteous	Considers both viewpoints (sender and receiver) and the feelings of the receiver. The message should be sincere and polite and delivered in a friendly and courteous manner
7. Correct	Uses appropriate and correct language. Check for mistakes. A correct use of language increases trustworthiness

Dementia can also affect an individual's ability to communicate. Dementia is not a condition in itself (Alzheimer's Research UK 2019). It is a term which describes the symptoms that occur when the brain is affected by certain conditions which cause the gradual death of brain cells. Dementia is a progressive condition. Examples of such conditions include Alzheimer's disease, vascular dementia, and Lewy body dementia. In the United Kingdom, there are currently around 850,000 people living with dementia (Alzheimer's Society 2017). The speed of which cognition declines can vary from person to person and may depend on which type of dementia they have (SCIE 2015). Symptoms of dementia can include loss of memory, reduced concentration, personality or behaviour changes, reduced ability to perform everyday tasks and problems with communication and reasoning skills. These changes in communication skills can be upsetting and frustrating for the person with dementia and those around them.

As people living with dementia experience changes in communication, they may experience word finding difficulties, repeat words or phrases, have naming difficulties, for example, not being able to name a watch but knowing it is something related to time and speech and grammar may become mixed up, making conversation difficult to follow. As a result of cognitive changes, the person with dementia can experience difficulty in following, processing and comprehending what is being said to them (Alzheimer's Society 2016). As a person's dementia progresses, their ability to communicate by spoken word can become increasingly impaired; however, they will continue to communicate in other ways, such as gesture, body language and facial expressions. In these circumstances, a person's behaviour becomes a way of communicating.

The nursing associate needs to ensure that they consider the changes someone with dementia may be experiencing and modify their communication to match where the person is in their dementia journey. This can include getting the person's full attention before you start, using shorter sentences, making one point per sentence, giving the person additional time to respond, rephrasing rather than repeat and paying attention to the person's body language as it can support what a person may be trying to verbally express. Further tips for communicating with a person with dementia are provided by the Alzheimer's Society (2016).

The final element of the PER tool is for the healthcare professionals to reflect on whether they achieved what they set out to, if it went well and what they could have done differently (Richardson 2017). The nursing associate will be familiar with models of reflection from both their pre-registration education programmes and revalidation requirements of the NMC. Some questions the nursing associate may want to ask themselves when reflecting on their communication experiences include:

- What did I like best about my use of communication skills?
- What did I like least about my use of communication skills?
- If I were to do this interaction again, what would I do differently and why?
- What have I learnt from this interaction?

To aid effective communication further, the nursing associate should consider the 7Cs of effective communication, which are applicable to both written and oral communication (Table 2.4). The 7Cs are used in business communication and media communications to ensure that the message is accurate for the target audience, and they are applicable to the nursing associate when interacting with patients.

Barriers to Effective Communication

Nursing associates who are aware of the common barriers to effective communication will be able to anticipate and react to ensure optimal communication and patient care. There are many factors that can create communication barriers, and some of the common ones are listed here:

Environmental barriers can arise due to issues with the setting in which care is provided, be it at home, close to home or in hospital; all can impact communication due to factors such as noise, lack of privacy and lack of control over who is present.

Personal barriers can be created by healthcare professionals, including nursing associates, working in areas where staff conflict and workloads are high, resulting in lack of time or support for patients. Communication can also be impacted when the nursing associate lacks skills or strategies for coping with difficult emotions, reactions or questions.

Physiological barriers: People can experience difficulty in hearing or speech following conditions such as stroke or brain injury. Hearing and eyesight problems become more common as we age, and as the population is living longer, these issues may become more prevalent in years to come. The nursing associate needs to develop an awareness of the challenges these barriers create for effective communication and work collaboratively with the patient, their family/carers and other healthcare providers such as speech and language therapists.

Psychological barriers such as fear and anxiety can impact a person's ability to listen to what the nursing associate is saying. Patients may worry about being judged or becoming emotional. The patient may struggle to explain their feelings and attempt to appear strong for someone else's benefit.

Cultural barriers can impede communication especially when the nursing associate is unable to demonstrate cultural competence. Lack of understanding, or lack of curiosity, about different cultures can result in negative patient experiences. Different cultures have different beliefs about personal space, understanding of illness and acceptable treatment options. It is important for nursing associates to think about their own experiences when considering cultural differences in communication and how these can challenge patients and healthcare professionals. It is important for the nursing associates to demonstrate cultural awareness when caring for people and to ensure that their needs, priorities, expertise and preferences are always valued and taken into account (Nursing and Midwifery Council 2018b).

Yellow Flag Cultural Beliefs and Values Associated with Non-verbal Communication

In some eastern European cultures, a smile denotes happiness and would be seen as inappropriate in a situation of when caring for someone who is seriously ill (Leifer 2019). Whereas in other cultures, a smile is used to reassure. Similarly, with the use of eye contact – some cultures interpret direct eye contact as a sign of engagement, and others consider this to be disrespectful. In western cultures, nodding of the head can be seen as understanding or agreement, while an inclined head can indicate that the person is listening (Richardson 2017). Nursing associates need to have an awareness of personal space, as the nurse who frequently invades someone's personal space can be seen as rude, whereas someone who is deemed reluctant to enter that personal space to offer comfort may be seen as 'cold' (Leifer 2019).

Language differences between the nursing associate and patient can cause communication errors. The nursing associate will need to work with families, colleagues and interpretation services to assist when language barriers exist. The use of jargon, acronyms and abbreviations (there are over 700 acronyms and abbreviations used by the NHS) can have a significant impact on communication, as it often results in misunderstanding. Literacy level can also significantly impact communication, and the nursing associate needs to be aware of the patient's ability to read and write when providing written patient information.

Conflict can arise for a variety of reasons and be positive when it offers an alternative viewpoint. It becomes a barrier when it detracts from the purpose of the communication. Nursing associates aim for collaborative relationships with patients but caring for people when they are at their most vulnerable can lead to heightened emotion, and patients can react out of character, appearing rude or aggressive. Having good communication skills can help the nursing associate de-escalate or even prevent such responses and build patients' confidence and trust.

Difficult conversations should not in themselves be barriers to effective communication. A nursing associate can lack confidence and competence in dealing with such emotive conversations, such as complaints (see chapter 9), suicide, end-of-life or organ donation thereby creating communication barriers that impact the patients and their family/carers. Effective communication with relatives and caregivers can be important in determining what the patient would want. In any holistic care provision, it is important to consider the patient's family and include family members and engender an interprofessional approach. In order to work with family members as collaborators in care, we need to understand how to communicate with them (Haddad et al. 2019). Patients' relatives benefit from clear, accurate and consistent information about their relative's condition delivered in a timely way in an appropriate environment (Richards & Edwards 2019). Effective communication is vital for patients and relatives when a patient is receiving end-of-life care. The nursing associate would need to monitor the activities of living but also engage in challenging conversations the patient or relatives may want to have. By talking about death and dying, the nursing associate is acknowledging the patients' desire to plan and organise; it is also giving the family a clear expectation that their loved one is going to die. The nursing associate needs to consider the appropriate time and place to have the conversation, as a busy ward environment is not conducive to this type of conversation (Fitzsimons 2018). The family should be told about an anticipated death away from the patient's bedside in a room where there will be no disruptions. For privacy, the door of the room should be closed, but with a clear path to it, as distressed relatives may want to leave the room. Everyone will be asked to sit down, so that the healthcare professional delivering the bad news is not standing over the relatives, the healthcare professional's tone of voice will be calm and their posture open. The relatives should be allowed time to process the information and freely express their emotions; they would want to do this in private. The healthcare professional can then return to the relatives and answer any questions they may have or give them another opportunity to discuss the information they have received (Woodrow 2019).

Templeman (2019) talks about the reflective practice of healthcare professionals and how this leads to developing knowledge, skills and behaviours in effective communication. By reflecting on challenging conversations, the nursing associate can develop new perspectives on those conversations and identify in what areas they want to develop their communication skills. This process will build the nursing associate's self-awareness and listening skills which will, as a result, make them a more effective communicator. Templeman (2019) describes good communication as skills in common courtesy, comforting and empathy. It is the ability to listen, summarise and paraphrase, whilst recognising the appropriate use of touch and how to negotiate personal space.

The ability to communicate effectively, with sensitivity and compassion, is paramount to the provision of high-quality person-centred care (NMC 2018a, 2018b). The competencies, within the nursing associate standards, must be demonstrated in a wide range of health and social care settings and adapted to meet the needs of people across their lifespan. Nursing associate's need a diverse range of communication skills and strategies to ensure that individuals, their families and carers are kept informed and supported to be actively involved in their own care wherever possible. Other chapters in this text will consider in more detail specific communication skills for nursing associate's.

Orange Flag Communicating with Older People with Cognitive Impairment

Confusion or disorientation in older people can be caused by a variety of factors such as infection, delirium or dementia. Older people with cognitive impairment are more at risk of developing delirium. Delirium is characterised as restlessness, agitation or aggression (hyperactive delirium), or being sleepy, quiet or withdrawn (hypoactive delirium). People generally present with a mixture of hyperactive and hypoactive delirium (National Institute for Health and Care Excellence 2014). Communication with people who are disorientated or confused can be challenging. Haddad et al. (2019), suggest that a healthcare professional should not maintain the confusion, but they should re-orientate the person, unless doing so would result in deep agitation or violence. Politely listening with interest will enable the healthcare professional to determine how deep the confusion is and from this can decide the best course of communication. Richardson (2017) talks about a humanistic approach to communication, that is, being empathetic and non-judgemental. The nursing associate should remain professional when in challenging situations and allow a moment before responding to an angry or distressed person. It is important that the nursing associate responds in calm manner and ascertains what is causing that distress or anger. Moving on from this point, the nursing associate needs to demonstrate empathy. In order to demonstrate empathy, the nursing associate needs to utilise their skills in non-verbal communication and should respond to the patient's experiences, not their own (Richardson 2017).

Conclusion

At the point of registration, the nursing associate will to have demonstrate that have the knowledge, skills and behaviours to communicate effectively with people across the lifespan in a variety of healthcare and social care settings.

Effective communication and relationship management skills have to be learnt and honed in order to ensure that the patient is at the centre of all that is done. To be able to communicate effectively, with sensitivity and compassion, and to manage relationships with people is key to the provision of high-quality, person-centred care.

When those people being care for and offered support to have special communication needs or a disability, it is important that the nursing associate make reasonable adjustments. This will mean that they will be able to provide and share information in such a way that promotes good health and health outcomes and enables equal access to the highest quality of care.

References

Aggarwal, V.B. and Gupta, V.S. (2001) *Handbook of journalism and mass communication.* New Delhi: Concept Publishing Company.

Alzheimer's Society. (2016) *Communicating, Factsheet 500LP*, London: Alzheimer's Society.

Alzheimer's Society. (2017) *What is dementia, Factsheet 400LP. [online]* Available: https://www.alzheimers.org.uk/sites/default/files/migrate/downloads/what_is_dementia.pdf. Accessed 6 September 2020.

Alzheimer's Research UK. (2019) *11 things you need to know about dementia. [online]* Available: https://www.alzheimersresearchuk.org/about-dementia/facts-stats/11-things-you-need-to-know-about-dementia/. Accessed 6 September 2020.

Boggs, K. (2016) Communicating with children, in Arnold, E. & Boggs, K (eds.) *Interpersonal relationships: professional communication skills for nurses* (7th edn),. Philadelphia: Elsevier, 345–363. ISBN: 978-0-323-24281-3

Edwards, S. and Coyne, I. (2019) *A nurse's survival guide to children's nursing (updated)*, London: Elsevier.

Fitzsimons, B. (2018) *End-of-life care; when there is only one chance to get it right.* [online] Available: https://www.rcplondon.ac.uk/news/end-life-care-when-there-only-one-chance-get-it-right. Accessed 6 September 2020.

Grainger, C. (2018) Effective communication skills, in Peate, I. (ed.) *Learning to care; the nursing associate*, London: Elsevier, 83–95.

Haddad, A., Doherty, R. and Purtilo, R. (2019) *Health professional and patient interaction*, Missouri: Elsevier.

Lasswell, H. (1948) The structure and function of communication in society, in Bryson, L. (ed.) *The communication of ideas*, New York, NY: Institute for Religious and Social Studies, 117.

Leifer, G. (2019) *Introduction to maternity and pediatric nursing* (8th edn), London: Elsevier.

Mansell, J. (2010*) How to guide 3; communication for people with profound and multiple learning disabilities*, London: Mencap.

MENCAP. (n.d.) *Communicating with people with learning disability. [online]* Available: https://www.mencap.org.uk/learning-disability-explained/communicating-people-learning-disability. Accessed 6 September 2020.

Mental Health Foundation. (2019) *Learning disability statistics.* [online] Available: https://www.mentalhealth.org.uk/learning-disabilities/help-information/learning-disability-statistics. Accessed 6 September 2020.

National Institute for Health and Care Excellence. (2019) *NICEimpact mental health.* [online] Available: https://www.nice.org.uk/about/what-we-do/into-practice/measuring-the-uptake-of-nice-guidance/impact-of-guidance. Accessed 6 September 2020.

National Institute for Health and Care Excellence. (2014) *Delirium in adults; Quality standard [QS63].* [online] Available: https://www.nice.org.uk/guidance/qs63. Accessed 6 September 2020.

Nelson, J. (2012) *Introduction to counselling skills: text and activities* (4th edn), London: Sage.

Nursing and Midwifery Council. (2018a) *Standards of proficiencies for nursing associates.* [online] Available: https://www.nmc.org.uk/globalassets/sitedocuments/education-standards/nursing-associates-proficiency-standards.pdf. Accessed 3 October 2019.

Nursing and Midwifery Council. (2018b) *The code - professional standards of practice and behaviour for nurses, midwives and nursing associates.* [online] Available: https://www.nmc.org.uk/globalassets/sitedocuments/nmc-publications/nmc-code.pdf. Accessed 3 October 2019.

Parliamentary and Health Service Ombudsman. (2019) *Complaints about the NHS in England: quarter 2 2018–19.* [online] Available: https://www.ombudsman.org.uk/sites/default/files/2018-12/Complaints_about_the_NHS_in_England_Quarter_2_2018-19_Final_Accessible.pdf. Accessed 6 September 2020.

Parnell, T.A. (2015) *Health literacy in nursing: providing person centred care*, New York, NY: Springer Publishing Company.

Public Health England. (2018) *Severe mental illness (SMI) and physical health inequalities: briefing.* [online] Available: https://www.gov.uk/government/publications/severe-mental-illness-smi-physical-health-inequalities/severe-mental-illness-and-physical-health-inequalities-briefing. Accessed 6 September 2020.

Raphael-Grimm, T. (2015) *Art of communication in nursing and health care: an interdisciplinary approach*, New York, NY: Springer Publishing Company.

Rautakoski, P. (2011) Training total communication, *Aphasiology*, 25(3): 344–365. doi: 10.1080/02687038.2010.530671.

Richards, A. and Edwards, S. (2019) *A nurses survival guide to the ward* (3rd edn), London: Elsevier.

Richardson, B. (2017) Communication, in Moore, T. & Cunningham, S. (eds.) *Clinical skills for nursing practice, Abingdon*: Routledge, 23–46.

Roberts, J.F., Fenton, G. and Barnard, M.C. (2015) Developing effective therapeutic relationships with children, young people and their families, *Nursing children and Young People*, 27(4): 30–35. doi: 10.7748/ncyp.27.4.30.e566.

Royal College of Nursing. (2016) *Why communication is important.* [online] Available: https://rcni.com/hosted-content/rcn/first-steps/why-communication-important. Accessed 6 September 2020.

SCIE. (2015) *Dementia.* [online] Available: https://www.scie.org.uk/dementia/about/. Accessed 6 September 2020.

Sense. (2019) *Total communication.* Retrieved 9 November 2019. [online], Available: https://www.sense.org.uk/get-support/information-and-advice/communication/total-communication/. Accessed 9 November 2019.

Templeman, J. (2019) Communicating, in Holland, K. & Jenkins, J. (eds.) *Applying the roper Logan Tierney model in practice* (3rd edn), London: Elsevier, 105–142.

Thomsen, O.N. (2010) From talking heads to communicating bodies: cybersemiotics and total communication, *Entropy*, 12(3): 390–419. doi: 10.3390/e12030390.

Woodrow, P. (2019) *Intensive care nursing; a framework for practice* (4th edn), London: Routledge.

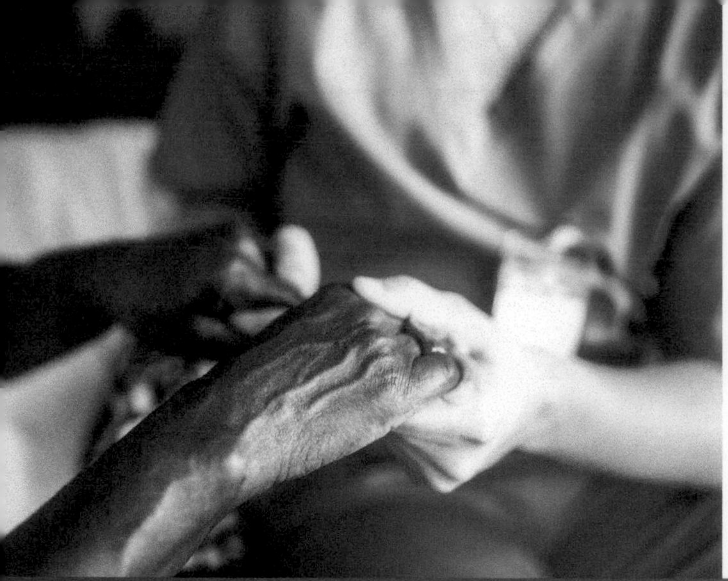

3

Interpersonal Skills and Therapeutic Relationship Skills

Joanna Regan[1] and Karen Wild[2]

[1] Leeds Teaching Hospitals Trust, UK
[2] Nurse, UK

Chapter Aim

- **This chapter aims to provide the reader with an insight into the special nature of interpersonal and therapeutic relationship skills in patient–nursing associate interactions.**

Learning Outcomes

By the end of this chapter, the reader will be able to:
- **Identify interpersonal and therapeutic relationship skills**
- **Understand the skills required to enable a therapeutic relationship**
- **Discuss the importance of the '6Cs' that underpin the (National Health Service) NHS's professional commitment to always deliver excellent care**

Test Yourself Multiple Choice Questions

1. **The Nursing and Midwifery Council (NMC) standards of proficiency for nursing associates were published in:**
   A) **1993**
   B) **2018**
   C) **2010**
   D) **2008**

The Nursing Associate's Handbook of Clinical Skills, First Edition. Edited by Ian Peate.

Companion website: www.wiley.com/nursingassociate

2. **The key elements of a therapeutic relationship can be described as:**
   A) **Respect for the person**
   B) **Receptivity which involves good listening skills**
   C) **Empathy and self-awareness of one's own skills and limitations**
   D) **All of the above**
3. **The Dignity Challenge Framework (Health and Social Care Advisory Service 2010) identifies respect as:**
   A) ***'Allowing people to freely access health care'***
   B) ***'The provision of free prescriptions to minority groups'***
   C) ***'The need to support people with the same respect you would want for yourself or a member of your family'***
   D) ***'The need to allow freedom of speech and reciprocity of care'***
4. **In 1961, Carl Rogers described respect in terms of *unconditional positive regard*:**
   A) **True**
   B) **False**
5. **The Code (NMC) was updated in:**
   A) **2003**
   B) **2008**
   C) **2000**
   D) **2018**

Introduction

Engaging in nursing implies that you have a commitment to caring for your patients and clients and to caring for yourself and that you possess a wider desire to care for the well-being of others and communities. Caring cannot exist without the sharing of information and feelings, and the very close relationship between the nursing associate and their patient is no different. To establish this close relationship requires that the nursing associate be able to confidently display interpersonal and relationship skills in all aspects of care. The Nursing and Midwifery Council (NMC) (2018a) standards state that 'The ability to communicate effectively, with sensitivity and compassion, and to manage relationships with people is central to the provision of high-quality person-centred care'.

A therapeutic relationship has been defined as one which is perceived by patients to be caring, supportive, non-judgemental and to offer a perception of safety from threatening events. The key elements of a therapeutic relationship can be described as respect for the person, receptivity which involves good listening skills, empathy and self-awareness of one's own skills and limitations. Figure 3.1 demonstrates the varied aspects of what is considered to encompass the therapeutic relationship.

Touch Point

The key elements of a therapeutic relationship can be described as respect for the person, receptivity which involves good listening skills, empathy and self-awareness of one's own skills and limitations.

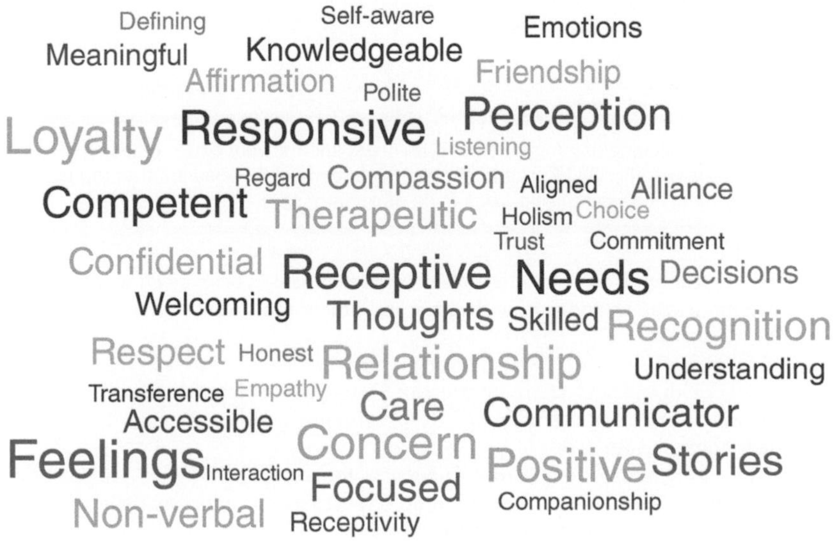

Figure 3.1 Aspects of the therapeutic relationship.

Once deemed to be a dangerous bond, therapeutic relationships between patients and nurses are now encouraged in order to provide the best support and care within the practice setting. Over the years, several nurse theorists have supported the idea of a nurse–patient relationship. As early as, Hildegard Peplau (1952) asserted that the nurse–patient relationship is the foundation of nursing practice. The experience of caring and being cared for creates a human dynamic where both parties encounter personal growth through that experience. She highlighted what she termed 'character roles' of the nurse, including the nurse as a resource, interpreting information and answering questions; the nurse as a technical expert, providing expert physical care through clinical skills and the nurse as a teacher, nurturing, understanding and providing instruction. Travellbee (1966) used the phrase 'therapeutic use of self' where the purpose of nursing is to establish human-to-human relationships. Watson (1979) asserted that therapeutic relationships are two-way reciprocal relationships, where each grows and learns from the other.

Nursing associate proficiencies and platforms of NMC (2018a) state:

The ability to communicate effectively, with sensitivity and compassion, and to manage relationships with people is central to the provision of high-quality person-centred care. These competencies must be demonstrated in practice settings and adapted to meet the needs of people across their lifespan.

Annex A is an overarching proficiency necessary to be achieved in all six platforms of the proficiencies.

Blue Flag Relationships

Case study

A woman visits the local centre of excellence for cancer treatment. In the outpatient department, she sees the same nursing team when she visits for regular chemotherapy treatment.

'All of the staff are warm and welcoming; they want to make you feel the best you can in a difficult situation. One staff member "goes the extra mile" if you know what I mean. I really like her; she makes me feel happy to see her, she listens intently and recognises when I am extra anxious. Once she took time out to introduce me to a volunteer makeup and style therapist, I had told her that I was anxious about an upcoming family wedding. She is knowledgeable and highly skilled in her work but is honest enough to say if she is unsure of anything that I ask'.

At this point, you might want to take a step sideways and reflect on what aspects you would want to see in a healthcare worker who is supporting you through a vulnerable health episode. Perhaps, many of the aspects highlighted in Figure 3.1 would have come into your mind: a sense of caring, a genuine interest in you, someone who is respectful and communicates well, someone who makes you feel like an individual and someone who feels that the time with you is as important as anything else that might be going on. Similar skills occur in several human relationships, for example, mentor–mentee, teacher–learner, doctor–patient and so on.

Green Flag Standards of proficiency for nursing associates, NMC

Communication and relationship management skills

At the point of registration, the nursing associate will be able to:

Identify the need for and use appropriate approaches to develop therapeutic relationships with people

A therapeutic nurse–patient relationship can be defined as a helping, nurturing and sensitive interaction, considering the individual's physical, emotional, mental, social, sexual and societal needs.

Take Note

Caring cannot exist without the sharing of information and feelings, and the very close relationship between the nursing associates and their patient is no different. To establish this close relationship requires that the nursing associate be able to confidently display interpersonal and relationship skills in all aspects of care.

The key components of a therapeutic relationship are unique, never time dependant (a brief meeting, or a relationship that extends through time) and are centred around the patient to support and enhance healing and functioning, what Peplau in 1991 described as 'professional closeness'. These components include the following:

- **Respect**

The Dignity Challenge Framework (Health and Social Care Information Centre 2010) identifies respect as '*the need to support people with the same respect you would want for yourself or a member of your family*'. Respect implies a recognition of the individual as they are, engaging in an open and non-judgemental attitude to those in your care.

The Essence of Care document (Department of Health 2010) benchmarks for respect and dignity provide best practice guidance to ensure people (clients, patients and carers) experience care that is focused upon respect and encompasses their values, beliefs and personal relationships. The 2015 National Health Service (NHS) Constitution for England states:

We value every person – whether patient, their families or carers, or staff – as an individual, respect their aspirations and commitments in life, and seek to understand their priorities, needs, abilities and limits. We take what others have to say seriously. We are honest and open about our point of view and what we can and cannot do. (National Health Service 2015)

Green Benchmarks for respect and dignity.

FACTOR	BEST PRACTICE
Attitudes and behaviours	Individuals feel that they matter all the time
Personal world and personal identity	Patients experience care in an environment that actively encompasses individual values, beliefs and personal relationships
Personal boundaries and space	Staff protect people's personal space
Communication	Individuals experience communication with staff that respects their individuality
Privacy – confidentiality	Individuals experience care that maintains their confidentiality
Privacy, dignity and modesty	Individuals receive care which protects their privacy, dignity and modesty
Privacy – private area	Individuals can have access to areas that safely maintain privacy

Source: Based on Department of Health (2015).

Rogers (1961) described respect in terms of *unconditional positive regard*. This approach to respecting another relies on the ability to accept an individual's personal beliefs despite one's own feelings. Rogers' approach recognises the abundance of experiences and exposures individuals have experienced in their lifetime, making their beliefs and behaviours unique. Acceptance does not imply approval or agreement, rather a non-judging approach to the person as an individual.

Touch Point

Respect implies a recognition of the individual as they are, engaging in an open and non-judgemental attitude to those in your care.

- **Genuineness**
  Being oneself within the context of a professional healthcare role is referred to as genuineness. Rogers (1961) describes this approach as *congruence*, where the carer does not hide behind a professional veneer but rather promotes an open and genuine contact. In a nurse–patient relationship, the nursing associates' perceptions are underpinned by their values and beliefs and their own culture; these inevitably play a role in how they facilitate genuineness (Van den Heever et al. 2015).

It can be difficult to adapt our behaviours to be genuine within the context of the care setting; we are taught to be polite, pleasing, socially and professionally appropriate which can detract from a true demonstration of genuineness. Consider the approach of the nurse in the two scenarios in the Blue flag example, in the sexual health clinic below:

Blue Flag Brief patient encounter. Sexual Health Clinic

Scenario 1
Patient: *'this is really embarrassing, last night I had unprotected sex and I don't really know what to do, what if I am pregnant'*
Nursing associate: *'OK, (smiles) I need to first take some details, then I'll get the clinic doctor to come and sort you out. Please wait there'*

Scenario 2
Patient: *'this is really embarrassing, last night I had unprotected sex and I don't really know what to do, what if I am pregnant'*
Nursing associate: *'I am glad that you have come today, please, don't feel embarrassed. I can tell that you are anxious, and that's perfectly understandable. Let's just take some time to find out a little more about your experiences yesterday. Are you comfortable to share this with me?'*
(Patient nods and shares her experience.)
Nursing associate: *'Thank you for sharing what happened with me, I understand how difficult this can be. OK, there are several options that we can explore together, and you need to know that at some point, the clinic doctor will be here to see you. I hope that you will feel comfortable enough to ask me anything along the way that you are unsure of…'*

Red Flag

When the nursing associate learns and develops their skills in incorporating sexual health issues during a consultation or discussion and the patient feels the nursing associate is genuine, then this has the real potential to highlight issues that the patient may feel they would otherwise be unable to discuss.

- **Empathy**

Empathy is the ability to understand and envision another's experience; to *walk in another's shoes* enables us to feel how others go through everyday life.

Supporting Evidence

Empathy and compassion

http://listen.health.org.uk/ *Walk in another's shoes*

This website enables you to gain an insight into the experiences of people who engage with healthcare and social care provision. You can choose whose story you wish to engage with. It invites you to 'walk in another's shoes' as a means of empathising with an individual's experiences of healthcare and social care.

When we empathise, we actively express an awareness of what healthcare and social care feels like from the patient's perspective. This includes validating those feelings and experiences, communicating that you are aware and do understand and that you 'connect' with the individual (Dougherty et al. 2015). In nursing, empathy includes maintaining an appropriate emotional distance from the patient to ensure objectivity. In order to express true empathy, the nursing associates must be able to put aside their own opinions so that these do not influence the perceptions of their patients' experience (Jones 2019). It also requires that they emotionally distance themselves from others' experiences; they need to see the world from their patients' perspective without experiencing the same level of emotional response.

Yellow Flag Beliefs and values

'Patients are not objects, and nurses are not robots'

Frances Riley is a ward sister for an acute general medicine ward in John Radcliffe Hospital in Oxford. She is a part of a project working on improving end-of-life care on the ward, focused on four areas: earlier recognition that patients are approaching end of life, prioritising comfort, understanding the needs of family members and improving the use of end-of-life care medication.

'I think empathy is closely linked with compassion and dignity and it's a fundamental part of our job. It's about seeing each patient as an individual. Patients are not objects, and nurses are not robots – it's about personal interaction. To be a good nurse, you need to have more than technical skills. There's got to be empathy there to make it a positive hospital experience for patients and families'.

Source: The Health Foundation (2016).

Touch Point

When we empathise, we actively express an awareness of what healthcare and social care feels like from the patient's perspective.

- **Trust**

Caring requires nurses to establish trusting relationships with patients and to be trustworthy professionals. Trust is critical in the nurse–patient relationship because, often, the individual is in a vulnerable position. Imagine being totally dependent on another in a healthcare crisis. To give oneself over into the trusting care of another is an enormous act. Trust is overarching in these types of scenarios. Even in routine clinical situations, trust is a cornerstone of the therapeutic relationship. The practice nurse at your local health centre is entrusted with your private

Supporting Evidence

Therapeutic relationships in day surgery: A grounded theory study

http://usir.salford.ac.uk/id/eprint/8820/2/Acr3F.pdf

This study interprets the narrative from patients who experience care in a day surgery unit to identify significant therapeutic interventions as perceived by those patients.

'I got great comfort from the staff. The entire experience (day surgery) is about entrusting your body and well-being to people whom you have never met before. I think some of the ways in which this trust was engendered in me was, well, by a few things really … explanations of what to expect … general chit chat with the nurses … being in a ward with other people and seeing them go through the same process'. (Mary, age 42 years)

Source: Mottram (2009)

> **Touch Point**
> Trust is critical in the nurse–patient relationship because often the individual is in a vulnerable position.

information, and you trust that nurse to check the shelf life of your travel vaccines. Patients need to believe that nurses are honest, knowledgeable, can be depended on and will not judge.

- **Rapport**
  Rapport is an essential component of the nurse–patient relationship and is established from the first encounter with the patient. This can be challenging, to say the least, and some healthcare professionals struggle to relax into an easy rapport on first meeting. All the aspects of the therapeutic relationship discussed in this chapter so far come into play when we develop a rapport with an individual. Clear attention to the individual and a genuine interest will help to establish a rapport. Body language and non-verbal communication come into their own; smile, calmness, interpersonal warmth, a desire to make the person feel at ease, comfort, privacy and safety all play a role. (More detailed information about non-verbal communication is available in Chapter 2 of this text.)

Initially, the nursing associate can establish a rapport with the patient through the questions they ask; this helps the nurse to understand the person's frame of reference, how they are feeling and what they understand about their situation. Both verbal and non-verbal prompts facilitate the process, alongside open-ended questioning. Figure 3.2 shows the stages of motivational interviewing identified by Miller & Rollnick (2002). The so-called OARS model highlights the key skills of motivational interviewing:

- **O – Open-ended questioning** invites the person to talk freely, for example, 'how are you today?'
- **A – Affirmations** provide a positive regard for what the person is saying, for example, 'you have a real insight into why you are here today, and I can help you to understand more about your time in hospital'.
- **R – Reflective listening** conveys through feedback that you are listening and taking note of what is said; often, the discussion will reflect the person's own words, for example, 'you say that you are anxious about having an anaesthetic?'
- **S – Summarising** helps to establish that what was said is understood and agreed between you both, bringing together all the points made as a conclusion.

More formal and structured interviews, such as nursing assessment, are built on the initial rapport that you establish in a non-emergency situation.

Tips for establishing a rapport with your patient:

- Introduce yourself, say 'hello' and ask the person's name. Use that name in conversation.
- If appropriate, use touch to establish warmth and genuineness.
- Employ effective non-verbals such as maintaining a respectful distance, using eye contact, nod to show you understand, adopt an open stance and sit with the person if they are sitting
- Be aware of the environment and privacy
- Be aware of distractions such as pain or discomfort
- Be culturally sensitive and aware
- Actively listen and reflect feelings back to the individual
- Speak calmly and slowly and avoid technical language
- Maintain professional boundaries

> **Touch Point**
> Clear attention to the individual and a genuine interest will help to establish a rapport.

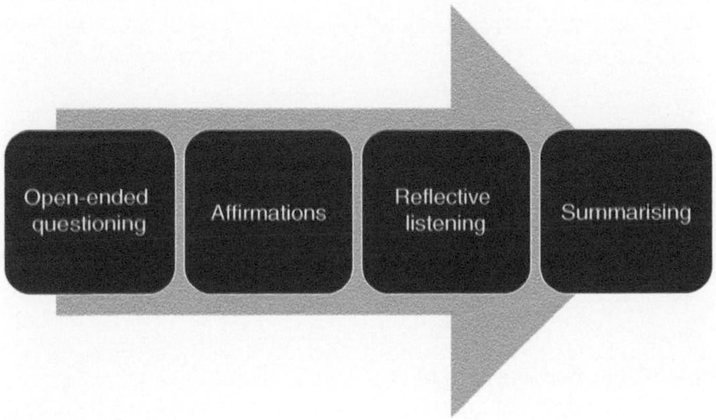

Figure 3.2 The OARS model of motivational interviewing.

Take Note

The key elements of a therapeutic relationship can be described as respect for the person, receptivity which involves good listening skills, empathy and self-awareness of one's own skills and limitations.

Maintaining Professional Boundaries

Maintaining professional boundaries is essential in the nurse–patient relationship. The lines of professional behaviour can be easily blurred. Crossing professional boundaries can be subtle and not easily recognised. Care is so varied, and the nursing associate will at some point perform intimate tasks or procedures on patients, spending time to develop trust and a therapeutic relationship. The nursing associate must always consider the boundaries of a professional and therapeutic relationship in terms of being underinvolved or overinvolved with their patient's care. The nursing associate must recognise if they are building a personal relationship with a patient and should understand the implications of doing so. The nursing associate must always ensure their patient's care, treatment and needs, which are paramount. Should the nursing associate find it difficult to maintain a therapeutic and professional relationship, they must request help and support and step away from the situation. The following are examples to assist the nursing associate in understanding if they are at risk of breaching a professional boundary:

- Agreeing to contact or meet a patient out of the working environment
- Discussing other colleagues or your working environment negatively
- Engaging in discussions regarding your personal life in detail
- Giving one patient more time than another unnecessarily
- Agreeing to keep secrets with a patient
- Accepting a friend request on social media
- Receiving gifts (Nursing and Midwifery Council 2018b)

The 6Cs

Healthcare and social care in the United Kingdom are constantly changing and evolving. Government policy, technological advancement, demographics, patterns of disease and life expectancy all play a part in the everchanging demands on healthcare and social care. These demands are faced by the professionals who support individuals and groups in healthcare and social care settings. What is constant amongst all this change is the commitment to always deliver excellent care.

Yellow Flag Beliefs and values

Though the world has changed, our values haven't. As nursing, midwifery and care staff we know that compassionate care delivered with courage, commitment and skill is our highest priority. It is the rock on which our efforts to promote health and well-being, support the vulnerable, care for the sick and look after the dying is built.

Source: National Health Service (2016). Public Domain

The 6Cs of nursing arose out of a need to ensure that high standards of care were consistently delivered. This was in the wake of damming reports of care from the Frances Report (Mid Staffordshire NHS Foundation Trust 2013) and the Cavendish Review in the same year, which highlighted failings in the delivery of care and the subsequent lack of public confidence in the services (Department of Health 2013). The Chief Nursing Officer for England and the Director of Nursing for the Department of Health, Public Health England, identified the core values that underpin nursing care:

- Care
- Compassion
- Competence
- Communication
- Courage
- Commitment

Each value is equal, not one is more important than the other. They focus on putting the person being cared for at the heart of the care they are given. Figure 3.2 shows the person at the heart of the 6Cs. Nurses have been praised for their application and leadership in applying the 6Cs in their everyday encounters with patients, and the inherent values have been rolled out to all staff who engage in healthcare and social care. Figure 3.3 highlights the person at the heart of the 6Cs.

Supporting Evidence Clinical Leaders Network 2014

The 6Cs belong to everyone working in the healthcare and social care services. They belong to all health and care staff from nurses, midwives, doctors, porters, care staff, physiotherapists, dieticians and managers, both clinical and non-clinical, to executive Boards and commissioning Board.

Source: http://www.cln.nhs.uk/6csforeveryone/ (accessed September 2019)

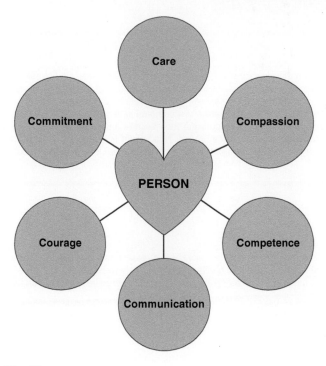

Figure 3.3 **The person is at the heart of the 6Cs.**

Care

Often described as the core activity in healthcare and social care, the concept of care can be difficult to pinpoint. When asked to define what nurses do, for example, the response is often that they care for people. While this is true, it is a very narrow idea of what caring is. In this text, there is a unit which focuses on the 'care and support with hygiene and the maintenance of skin integrity'. This implies that caring is related to physical aspect of hands-on support; however, if one acknowledges the therapeutic nature of care, as described earlier in this chapter, there is a suggestion of the unique bond that nurses and individuals have in the delivery of care. Indeed, when supporting hygiene and skin integrity needs, the nurse is delivering support within all the domains of health: physical, psychological, social, spiritual, mental, sexual and societal health. Care is overarching in this sense and cannot work in isolation without input from the other Cs. People should be able to trust in the care that is delivered, and care should be timely, respectful, and competently delivered, with the person at the core of all interactions.

Orange Flag

When the nursing associate provides care that is non-judgemental, then the risk of stigmatising a person is reduced. Some people with mental health problems have reported that the social stigma that is attached to mental ill health and the discrimination that they experience can make their difficulties worse, and this can also make it harder to recover. The nursing associate is ideally placed to reduce the damaging effects of stigma.

Touch point

People should be able to trust in the care that is delivered, and care should be timely, respectful, and competently delivered, with the person at the core of all interactions.

Compassion

When we show compassion, we are demonstrating not only empathy, respect and dignity but also an overwhelming desire to relieve or intervene in another's distress or suffering. Ballett and Campling in 2011 discussed the idea of compassion as emotional kindness. They assert that kindness is a natural response that drives people to pay attention to each other, to understand another's needs and to do well for others. This idea was supported by Meredith et al. (2018) who studied the emotional needs of patients following heart attack. The study eloquently draws from the narrative of patients and members of the multidisciplinary team to highlight examples of emotional kindness to support emotional healing. Healing in this respect is focused on the psychosocial aspects of care. Emphasis is put on the role of emotional intelligence (EI) in healthcare and social care staff. They state that '*a fundamental aspect promoting enhanced social support was the emotional intelligence of health professionals*'.

Developing EI helps the nursing associate to have a more positive attitude to care, and those with a high level of EI demonstrate more ease in establishing relationships and a higher level of adaptability. Healthcare and social care workers who recognise subtle changes in a person's behaviour, stress levels or demeanour can intervene with compassion to emotionally support patients in their care.

Blue Flag Relationships

Case study

Compassionate care

An elderly patient admitted to an elderly care ward at 2 a.m. for end-of-life care sadly passes away within hours of admission. The family do not speak English and are understandably distressed. The nursing associate caring for the patient is unable to access an interpreter to help him understand the family's wishes. He contacts the senior nurse on call to ask for support and advice. The senior nurse makes several phone calls to other departments to locate a professional who can converse with the family. A nurse on another ward who is finishing her shift who can communicate with the family ascertains their wishes and organises the appropriate documentation to be completed, allowing the family to take their relative to their preferred place of rest. This meant her staying 2 hours after the end of her shift.

The member of staff was later praised by the family through the Trust's Patient and Liaison Advisory Service for the care and compassion shown to the family.

Yellow Flag Values

NHS Constitution for England 2014

We ensure that compassion is central to the care we provide and respond with humanity and kindness to each person's pain, distress, anxiety or need. We search for the things we can do, however small, to give comfort and relieve suffering. We find time for patients, their families and carers, as well as those we work alongside. We do not wait to be asked, because we care.

Source: The NHS Constitution for England, Updated 14 October 2015. Retrieved from: https://www.gov.uk/government/publications/the-nhs-constitution-for-england/the-nhs-constitution-for-england#nhs-values. Public Domain

Take Note

When we show compassion, we are demonstrating not only empathy, respect and dignity but also an overwhelming desire to relieve or intervene in another's distress or suffering.

Competence

Nursing requires constant updating of knowledge and skills in order to keep up to date with the latest practices and to understand an individual's health and social needs. Patients have a wide range of needs and treatment requirements, and they also come from a variety of walks of life. Lots of training and time spent on personal development ensures that professionals in healthcare and social care settings possess the expertise, clinical and technical skill needed to effectively care, based on research and evidence, to a high standard.

Green Flag Standards of proficiency for nursing associates

'Nursing associates are a new profession, accountable for their practice. Once they are practising, nursing associates can undertake further education and training and demonstrate additional knowledge and skills, enhancing their competence as other registered professionals routinely do. The roles played by nursing associates will vary from setting to setting, depending on local clinical frameworks, and it may also be shaped by national guidance'.

Source: Nursing and Midwifery Council (2018a)

Being aware and knowledgeable about a subject or care pathway will enable the nursing associate to make appropriate, evidence-led decisions. Any clinical decisions made by the nursing associate must be defendable and justifiable. Nursing associates must be self-aware and know the limitations of their skills and abilities and must only engage in care delivery that they are competent to carry out. Self and peer appraisal can help the nursing associate to identify gaps in learning. The use of portfolios and progress reports can be effective in supporting the development of skills and knowledge and the application of care. The NMC has a role in regulating the profession to ensure ongoing learning and development to support competence; it does this by ensuring:

- Students and trainees gain skills and knowledge to be safe and effective
- Standards of education and training are mapped with NMC standards
- Once registered, practitioners remain professionally up to date.

Green Flag Standards of proficiency for nursing associates

'It will be important for nursing associates to demonstrate cultural awareness when caring for people and to ensure that the needs, priorities, expertise and preferences of people are always valued and taken into account'.

Source: Nursing and Midwifery Council (2018a)

Cultural competence is the ability to provide care to patients with diverse values, beliefs and behaviours. Nursing associates must tailor the delivery of healthcare and social care to meet patients' social, cultural and linguistic needs. Cultural competence is the ability to interact effectively with people of different cultures and address health inequalities. Being culturally competent is not just about respecting and appreciating the cultural contexts of patients' lives, neither is it a one-size-fits-all approach – it is about understanding the way we deliver healthcare and responding to the needs of our diverse population (National Health Service 2019).

Violet Flag Social issues

Case study

A female patient who is a member of the Traveller Gypsy community is being assessed in the Emergency Assessment Unit. She has presented with severe abdominal pain. Her husband refuses to allow her to be seen by any male members of the healthcare team. According to 'Fairhealth. Health Equity Action and Learning':

- *'There are often strict rules around gender with some Gypsy and Traveller communities, meaning that women will only agree to see female doctors .... When communicating with members of Gypsy and Traveller communities, it may be useful to keep in mind that many will have experienced discrimination or stigmatisation from mainstream services. This may affect how they act or feel when accessing care. Therefore, it is important to ensure staff are welcoming, patient and understanding'.*

Source: https://fairhealthlearning.s3.eu-west-2.amazonaws.com/Women's+Health/index.html#/lessons/kRQPUOEAYdCYqp3HmFKirg3jwTiuNe_t (accessed August 2020)

Supporting Evidence

The cultural competence programme. NHS Health Education England and The Royal College of Midwives

https://www.e-lfh.org.uk/programmes/cultural-competence/ (accessed August 2020)

This link invites you to access the Cultural Competence – e-Learning for Healthcare programme to help you to enhance your cultural competence within the healthcare and social care setting.

Take Note

Any clinical decisions made by the nursing associate must be defendable and justifiable. Nursing associates must be self-aware and know the limitations of their skills and abilities and must only engage in care delivery that they are competent to carry out.

Communication

Communication is vital in any human interaction and is fundamental in all areas of healthcare and social care. Nursing associates must be good listeners, as this is the key to good communication. Chapter 2 in this text explores communication in great depth. Simple and concise communication with colleagues is all vital as is legible writing of patient records, handling feedback, recording, reporting and monitoring care. Nursing associates work within an interdisciplinary and multi-agency environment. They work in teams and must be effective communicators to provide continuity of care. What's more, because we live in a multicultural society, it is essential that patients are communicated with in a language that they understand.

Touch Point

Simple and concise communication with colleagues is all vital as is legible writing of patient records, handling feedback, recording, reporting and monitoring care.

Courage

It has been said that courage is the most admired of the virtues, that cowardice is despised and that bravery is esteemed (Comte-Sponville 2002). Courage represents an essential nursing vision of the 6Cs developed by Cummings & Bennet (2012). Subsequently, in the Leading Change, Adding Value framework, Cummings (2016) states, 'we know that compassionate care delivered with courage, commitment and skill is our highest priority'. Nursing associates are accountable for their actions and have a duty of care to their patients. Nurses must be courageous and do what they think is right and must be bold enough to confront the fear of difficulties. They often must stand by what they believe, even if others do not like it. Peate (2015) advises that healthcare and social care staff should be courageous and:

- *Do the right thing*
- *When things are wrong, speak up and question*
- *Be influential: when cynics are around, face up to them*
- *Be open to those who may challenge you*
- *Be brave and make things happen, be innovative*
- *Lead by example*
- *Do not give up*

(Peate 2015, p. 218)

Commitment

Nursing associates should possess a high level of commitment to their role. The role is highly demanding, and a commitment to patients and populations is the foundation of what healthcare and social care professionals do. Alongside this, a commitment to colleagues through a unified direction to uphold quality care. Working in teams can be challenging, but teams need a commitment to work together across disciplines in order to reach an integrated goal.

The public expectation is that healthcare and social care professionals can be relied on, trusted to do the right thing. Upholding professional standards and conduct outside of the workplace, being role models and maintaining one's own health and well-being all require a high degree of commitment. Alongside this, nursing associates must also demonstrate a commitment to the profession, upholding the many aspects of The Code (2018b).

Green Flag **The code NMC**

'When joining our register, and then renewing their registration, nurses, midwives and nursing associates commit to upholding these standards. This commitment to professional standards is fundamental to being part of a profession. We can take action if those on our register fail to uphold the Code. In serious cases, this can include removing them from the register'.

Supporting Evidence

The 6Cs, NHS leadership academy

https://www.leadershipacademy.nhs.uk/6cs/

This website highlights Doctor Claire Price-Dowd's blog. As senior lead for evaluation and patient experience at the NHS Leadership Academy, she talks about the importance of the 6Cs in healthcare and social care.

Touch Points Revisited

- The key elements of a therapeutic relationship can be described as respect for the person, receptivity which involves good listening skills, empathy and self-awareness of one's own skills and limitations.
- Respect implies a recognition of the individual as they are, engaging in an open and non-judgemental attitude to those in your care.
- When we empathise, we actively express an awareness of what healthcare and social care feels like from the patient's perspective.
- Trust is critical in the nurse–patient relationship because often the individual is in a vulnerable position.
- Clear attention to the individual and a genuine interest will help to establish a rapport.
- People should be able to trust in the care that is delivered, and care should be timely, respectful and competently delivered, with the person at the core of all interactions.
- Simple and concise communication with colleagues is all vital as is legible writing of patient records, handling feedback, recording, reporting and monitoring care.

References

Ballett, J. and Campling, P. (2011) *Intelligent kindness: reforming the culture of healthcare*, Glasgow: Bell and Brain LTD.

Comte-Sponville, A. (2002) *A short treatise on the great virtues: the uses of philosophy in everyday life*, London: William Heineman.

Cummings, J. (2016) *Leading change, adding value. A framework for nursing, midwifery and care staff*, Leeds, UK: NHS England publications gateway approval number: 05247.

Cummings, J. and Bennett, V. (2012) *Developing the culture of compassionate care: creating a new vision for nurses, midwives and care-givers*, Leeds, UK: NHS Commissioning Board, Department of Health, Crown copyright.

Department of Health. (2013) *The Cavendish review: an independent review into healthcare and support workers in the NHS and social care settings*, London: TSO.

Department of Health. (2015) *Essence of care (2010) benchmarks for respect and dignity*, London: DH. HMSO.

Dougherty, L., Lister, S. and West-Oram, A. (2015) *The Royal Marsden manual of clinical nursing procedures* (9th edn), Chichester: Wiley Blackwell.

Health and Social Care Information Centre. (2010) *Dignity through action (vulnerable adults) resource 2: dignity workshop pack*, London: Health and Social care Advisory Service.

Jones, N. (2019) The 6Cs, in Peate, I. (ed.) *Learning to care. The nursing associate*, London: Elsevier.

Meredith, S.J., Wagstaff, C.R.D. and Dicks, M. (2018) Getting to the heart of the matter: an ethnography of emotions and emotion regulation in cardiac rehabilitation, *Qualitative Research in Sport, Exercise and Health*, 11(3): 364–381. doi: 10.1080/2159676X.2018.1548373.

Mid Staffordshire NHS Foundation Trust. (2013) *Report of the mid Staffordshire NHS foundation trust public enquiry*, London: TSO.

Miller, W.R. and Rollnick, S. (2002) Motivational interviewing, *Preparing people to change addictive behaviour* (2nd edn), New York, NY: Guilford Press.

Mottram, A. (2009) *Therapeutic relationships in day surgery: a grounded theory study.* [online] Available: http://usir.salford.ac.uk/id/eprint/8820/2/Acr3F.pdf. Accessed September 2019.

NHS. (2014) *Five year forward view.* [online] Available: https://www.england.nhs.uk/wp-content/uploads/2014/10/5yfv-web.pdf. Accessed September 2019.

NHS. (2015) *The NHS constitution for England.* [online] Available: https://www.gov.uk/government/publications/the-nhs-constitution-for-england/the-nhs-constitution-for-england#nhs-values. Accessed September 2019.

NHS. (2019) *About the cultural competence programme.* [online] Available: https://www.e-lfh.org.uk/programmes/cultural-competence/. Accessed September 2019.

Nursing and Midwifery Council (2018a) *Future nurse: Standards of proficiency for registered nurses*, London. MNC.

Nursing and Midwifery Council. (2018b) *The code, Professional standards of behaviour for nurses, midwives and nursing associates*, London: NMC.

Peate, I. (2015) Without courage, the other C's will crumble, *British Journal of Healthcare Assistants*, 9(5): 218.

The Health Foundation. (2016) *What empathy means to me, newsletter.* [online] Available: https://www.health.org.uk/newsletter-feature/what-empathy-means-me. Accessed September 2019.

Travellbee, J. (1966) *Interpersonal aspects of nursing*, Philadelphia: F.A. Davis.

Peplau, H.E. (1952) *Interpersonal relations in nursing: a conceptual framework of reference for psychodynamic nursing*, New York, NY: Putnam.

Rogers, C. (1961) *On becoming a person*, Boston: Houghton Mifflin.

Van den Heever, A.M., Poggenpoel, M. and Myburgh, C.P.H. (2015) *Nurses' perceptions of facilitating genuineness in a nurse–patient relationship.* [online] Available: https://www.sciencedirect.com/science/article/pii/S1025984815000095?via%3Dihub. Accessed September 2019.

Watson, J. (1979) *Nursing: the philosophy and science of caring*, Colorado: University of Colorado Press.

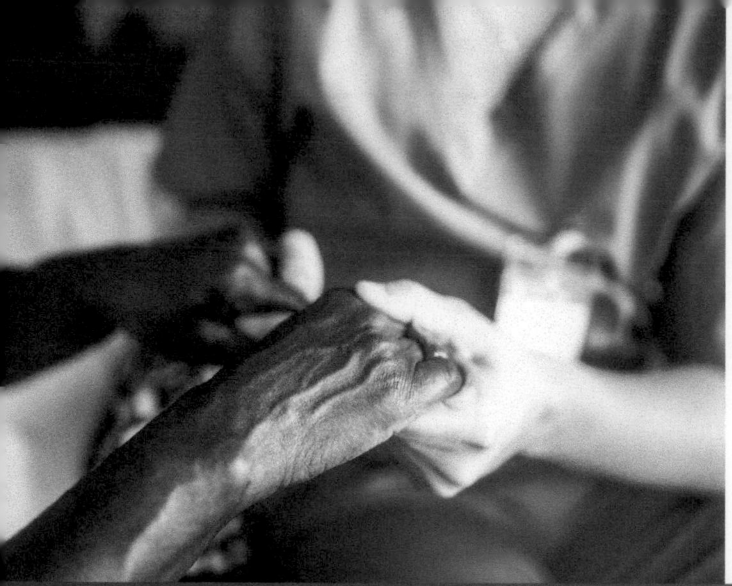

4

Working in a Team

Jacqueline Chang

Kingston University and St George's University of London, UK

Chapter Aim

- This chapter aims to introduce the reader to the different elements of team working and the importance of effective leadership.

Learning Outcomes

By the end of this chapter, the reader will be able to:

- Understand the importance of working as a team in healthcare
- Develop an understanding of your own role in a team
- Look at different types of teams and the importance of leadership

Test Yourself Multiple Choice Questions

1. Which of the following describes a team accurately?
   A) People doing the same task
   B) People working together
   C) People working in the same place
2. Which Nursing & Midwifery Council (NMC) publication outlines the role of the nursing associate as part of a team?
   A) The Nursing & Midwifery Council (2018b) standards of proficiency for the nursing associate
   B) The Code (Nursing & Midwifery Council 2018a)
   C) Both of the above
3. Which team member is the most important?
   A) The leader
   B) The person there the longest
   C) No one

The Nursing Associate's Handbook of Clinical Skills, First Edition. Edited by Ian Peate.

Companion website: www.wiley.com/nursingassociate

4. **What is an essential leadership skill?**
   A) To be motivational
   B) To be persuasive
   C) To be confident
5. **Which of the following describes a good team?**
   A) A group of people working together towards a common goal
   B) A group of people working towards a common goal, motivating and supporting each other
   C) A group of people with a goal

Introduction

Team work is an essential activity for healthcare and social care providers to perform in an effective manner. The nursing associate has a key role to play in leading teams as well as working within teams. The NMC's (Nursing & Midwifery Council 2018a) standards of proficiency for the nursing associate require you to be able to demonstrate an awareness of the roles, responsibilities and scope of practice of different members of the nursing and interdisciplinary team as well as your own role within it. You are also required to support and motivate other members of the care team and to interact with them in a confident manner and apply the principles of human factors and also environmental factors when working in teams.

This chapter provides you with a fundamental understanding of effective team working so you are able to effectively and responsibly access, input and apply information and data by using a range of methods including digital technologies and share them appropriately within the interdisciplinary teams. Another key aspect of effective team working is to support, supervise and act as a role model to nursing associate students, healthcare support workers as well as those who are new to care roles, review the quality of the care they provide, promote reflection and offer constructive feedback.

When required to, you should contribute to team reflection activities, as this can help to promote improvements in practice and services and to discuss the influence of policy and political drivers that have the potential impact on health and care provision.

Teams and Groups

All teams are groups, but not all groups are teams. A group is a collection of people who have something in common, such as a common interest or culture. Generally, a person may be in a variety of groups (friendship, sporting, religious, hobbies, social, and so forth), and these informal groups do not need to have a goal or a specific intention; they are simply people enjoying being together. In contrast, a team is defined by the National Health Service (NHS) Leadership Academy (2013) as a group of people who work together towards a common goal. When people run in a race, for example, they are a group, and when they work together to achieve a certain finish time, they are a team. A team can be of any size depending on the task required. To be functional, a team needs to utilise the best qualities of each member, and in order to do that, it is essential that these qualities are recognised.

Working in a team is a complex process and it is important to understand the details of this (Salas et al. 2018). There are many different roles within a team, and it is important to understand these. If everyone did the same thing at the same time, the end goal would not be achieved. Different people with different strengths are needed to make sure a goal can be achieved. Keeping with the running example, some runners are stronger in the first part of the race, some are good finishers and some are good on hills. If their different strengths are utilised at different times, the goal for the team is more likely to be met. For effective teamwork, understanding these strengths and utilising them is essential. It is therefore helpful to look at the different personality types and how their strengths can be utilised best.

Touch Point

There are several types of teams and groups

1. How many teams are you in?
2. How many groups are you in?
3. What is the difference between a team and a group?

Take note

What do you think are your personal strengths when working in a team? Do you think you fall naturally into a certain role?

Personality Types

Belbin (1981) stated that an effective team needs nine different roles in order to be successful (see Table 4.1). This does not mean that each team needs nine members as one person could perform two or three roles. Each role is of equal importance to the other ones, and the different roles are needed at different points in achieving the task. What is essential is that people are comfortable in the roles they are given, and this will allow them to perform well.

Take Note

There is a lot of information on www.Belbin.com
Which role(s) do you think you fit into?

Carl Jung (1921) was a psychoanalyst who believed that people were either an introvert or an extrovert and that they acted instinctively on feelings or thoughts. He stated that in a team it is best to have a variety of personality types and to understand that no one type is better than any other. It is important to understand the team members and use their natural strengths. Knowing a preferred working style and being able to utilise it will strengthen the team. The colour types are outlined in Table 4.2.

This theory was expanded upon by Myers and Briggs in 1926 to make it more accessible to individuals. They created a short questionnaire to help discover a person's personality type.

Table 4.1 The roles.

ACTION	PEOPLE	CEREBRAL
Shaper: keeps momentum +challenging +dynamic -can offend people -aggressive	**Coordinator**: delegates work load +mature +confident -over delegates -manipulative	**Plant**: highly creative problem solver +creative +generates ideas -absent minded -poor communicator
Implementer: planner +practical +reliable -inflexible -stubborn	**Team worker** +co-operative +diplomatic -can be indecisive -avoids confrontation	**Monitor**: makes logical judgements +strategic +discerning -overly critical -indecisive
Completer: scrutinises at the end +conscientious +perfectionist -worrier -controlling	**Investigator**: idea finder +outgoing +enthusiastic -might be overoptimistic -can lose interest	**Specialist**: in-depth knowledge +dedicated +single minded -too much information -narrow expertise field

Source: Based on Belbin (1981).

Table 4.2 Introverts and extroverts.

INTROVERT THINKERS 'LET'S DO IT RIGHT'	EXTROVERT THINKERS 'LET'S DO IT NOW'
Cool Blue	Fiery Red
cautious precise deliberate questioning formal	competitive demanding determined strong-willed purposeful
INTROVERT FEELERS 'LET'S DO IT IN A CARING WAY'	EXTROVERT FEELERS 'LET'S DO IT TOGETHER'
Earth Green	*Sunshine Yellow*
caring encouraging sharing patient relaxed	sociable dynamic demonstrative enthusiastic persuasive

Source: Based on Jung (1921).

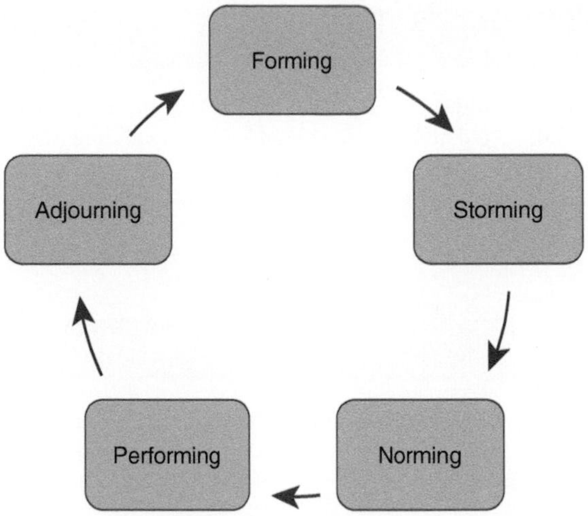

Figure 4.1 The team cycle. *Source:* **Based on Tuckman & Jenson (1977) in Bonebright (2010).**

Take Note

www.myerbriggs.org has a free online questionnaire to complete which will give a brief outline and explanation of your personality type.

Touch Point

Regardless of where you work in any scenario that calls for teamwork to accomplish specific tasks, this will bring out the best and also the worst of the personalities in those who are participating. Competitive energies, communication skills as well as the respective levels of commitment to the project are all factors that will affect how effectively team members can work together.

We have seen that there are many different personality types, and a mixture of them is ideal for a successful team. In an ideal situation, if a team can be selected to ensure that the different roles are accounted for, then it will be a successful team. However, this is not how healthcare teams are selected. In the workplace, a variety of people are put together, often with no prior knowledge of each other, and they are expected to work together, as a team, to produce certain outcomes. As there are many different personality types, plus the fact that people work differently, when a team is formed, there are various phases that it must go through to become a functioning team. Tuckman (1965) (see Figure 4.1) devised a model to explain the life cycle of a team, and this is still referred to today.

Forming: At this stage, the group do not know each other. They need to orientate themselves to each other and to the task itself. Ground rules need to be made, and relationships within the group need to be established.

Storming: This is the period of unrest and conflict where the group is still finding its way and getting to know each other. At this stage, relationships can become strained whilst people are still finding their way.

Norming: In this phase, the group know each other better and understand each other and how everyone works. The strengths and weaknesses of each team member are understood and utilised in a productive way.

Performing: This is the most productive phase of the cycle. The group are working well together in their respective roles and are focused on the task.

Adjourning: This was added in 1977 to demonstrate the importance and inevitability of all groups separating.

Note that this cycle is not always one way. Some groups get stuck at the storming or norming stage and do not get to perform as a team. Some groups go through the stages very slowly, and the ability to perform well as a team is postponed. Also, team membership can change mid-cycle which can put a norming or performing team back into the storming phase.

Leadership

As well balanced and dynamic as a team may be, it cannot function without a leader. There are many different leadership styles and models, and each leader will find their own natural style (Marquis & Huston 2012). This next section of this chapter considers three different leadership styles.

Touch Point

Think about the leaders you have worked well with. What did you like about the way that they worked and their leadership style? Did they work in a particular way that inspired and motivated you?

Are there managers you did not enjoy working with? What was it that caused this?

If you were to become a leader, what type of leader would you like to be?

Transactional Leadership

Transactional leadership is a traditional leadership model of one person instructing another person to do a task in exchange for a reward, for example, their pay. While this appears like a rather cold and formal style of leadership, if done well with good communication and delegation skills, the team member will find reward in completing the task and feeling like a valued member of the team, as well as through their pay. In healthcare, tasks are allocated by the nurse in charge of that area to the rest of the team, but ideally, the team want to work together to provide high-quality holistic care for the patients.

Transformational Leadership

This leadership model requires a leader to work towards a vision they really believe in. This vision also needs to be realistic and achievable (Ellis & Bach 2015). For healthcare, the vision should be a high level of safe and effective patient care, and by believing in this vision and inspiring their colleagues, they will lead their team to delivering this.

The Servant Leader

When people think of a leader, they tend to picture one identified person out in front with a group of followers behind them. Often, this person is allocated directly into that role. In healthcare, many of the leaders are people who have worked in the environment for a number of years and have progressed within their role. They have served first and worked their way up to leading as their experience and confidence grew. They are known as servant leaders (Howatson-Jones 2004), as they both perform the tasks and lead the teams as they continue to do the tasks in their leadership role. They lead by example and are a good role model for their teams, providing motivation and inspiration through working together.

NHS Leadership Model

The importance of good leadership and team working is not new to the NHS. The Francis report of 2013 commented on the management and leadership within the NHS and made recommendations for practice including arguing that managers should not be locked in their offices but should be supervising the care being delivered. Following this, the NHS Healthcare Leadership Model was launched in 2013 and proposed that the leader affects the behaviour of their team and ultimately the care given. Barr and Dowding (2019) highlight that poor leadership leads to poor care. A model was created with nine dimensions which are outlined in Table 4.3. The NHS Healthcare Leadership Model of 2013 tasks aspiring leaders to assess themselves in each one using the probes provided on their website. The Leadership Academy states that if the leaders can meet the nine dimensions, then they will inspire their team to focus and work together to deliver high-quality care.

In 1973, a theory called *action-centred leadership* was developed to help demonstrate how to achieve the best level of teamwork (Adair 1973) (see Figure 4.2). An effective leader needs to focus on achieving the task by developing each individual person to be able to work well in the team. This is done through motivation, evaluation, organisation and good communication. The task needs to be approached in an organised focused manner. Each individual needs to be praised and recognised for their natural abilities and their contributions with training offered if needed. The team needs effective communication skills and the maintenance of good morale.

The three circles in Adair's model (Figure 4.2) overlap because:

1. The task needs a team as one person alone cannot accomplish it.
2. If the team needs are not met, the task will suffer and the individuals will not be satisfied.
3. If the individual needs are not met, the team will suffer and the performance of the task will be impaired.

If all three of these circles are addressed and maintained, then the team will work happily and be productive which is what the goal for all teams should be.

Team working in healthcare is identified as important in both The Code (Nursing & Midwifery Council 2018b) and the nursing associate platforms. Platform 4 of the standards of proficiency for the nursing associates (Nursing & Midwifery Council 2018a) is devoted to working in teams and to the nursing associate embedding their role into the interdisciplinary team.

Table 4.3 The Nine Dimensions.

1. Inspiring shared purpose
2. Leading with care
3. Evaluating information
4. Connecting our service
5. Sharing the vision
6. Engagin g the team
7. Holding to account
8. Developing capability
9. Influencing for results

Source: Based on Lynas (2013).

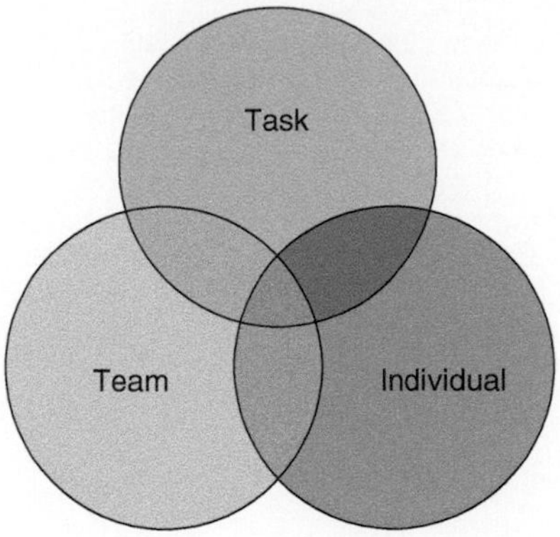

Figure 4.2 Action-centred leadership. *Source:* Based on Adair (2010).

The Code (Nursing & Midwifery Council 2018b) discusses the importance of working cooperatively and of displaying leadership qualities in order to provide the best care possible at all times.

Green Flag

Throughout a nursing associate's career, all registrants will have opportunities to demonstrate leadership qualities, regardless of whether or not they occupy formal leadership positions.

Working cooperatively is part of Practicing Effectively, and all registrants are required to:

8.1 Respect the skills, expertise and contributions of your colleagues, referring matters to them when appropriate
8.2 Maintain effective communication with colleagues
8.3 Keep colleagues informed when you are sharing the care of individuals with other health and care professionals and staff
8.4 Work with colleagues to evaluate the quality of your work and that of the team
8.5 Work with colleagues to preserve the safety of those receiving care
8.6 Share information to identify and reduce risk
8.7 Be supportive of colleagues who are encountering health or performance problems. However, this support must never compromise or be at the expense of patient or public safety

Source: based on Nursing & Midwifery Council (2018a)

Both the Code and the Proficiencies (Nursing & Midwifery Council 2018a, 2018b, respectively) share various elements of team working, including effective communication, supporting colleagues and respecting the scope of practice of colleagues and of yourself. These qualities are essential for good teamwork, and every nursing associate should consider them when delivering care.

All healthcare interventions have an interdisciplinary approach. In community care settings, the nursing team work together as a team of healthcare assistants, nursing associates, staff nurses and district nurses. They work utilising the strengths of each individual and their scope of practice. They work in collaboration with general practitioner (GP) services and community specialist nurses. There may also be involvement from specialist medical teams. Should a patient then need to go to hospital, they are cared for by the inpatient services including healthcare assistants, nursing associates, staff nurses, ward sisters, matrons, specialist nurses, the medical team and allied health professionals such as physiotherapists, occupational therapists, speech and language therapists, pharmacists and many others. The importance of effective team working cannot be overemphasised to ensure that the patient's needs are met fully from all members of the team. The complications that can arise by having so many different professionals involved are high, and the more complex the needs of patients and service users, the more complex are the health services provided. This multi-agency working means that effective team working is essential. In order to ensure that a patient is cared for effectively in every part of their journey, each individual team must work in collaboration with each other. This requires effective communication, candour, openness and having the common goal of good patient care. Adair's model of 1973 clearly demonstrates how these elements work together to provide the highest quality and safest care.

Case Study

Jane, a 28-year-old lady struggles with lower abdominal pain for three days. As the pain is becoming increasingly worse, she goes to see her GP. The GP diagnoses appendicitis and recommends that Jane goes to Accident and Emergency (A&E) department. As Jane's friend can drive her there, the GP does not call an ambulance but stresses the importance of attending that day and gives Jane a letter to present on arrival. The GP advises Jane to take an overnight bag with her should she be admitted.

Jane goes to A&E 2 hours later and is seen by a triage nurse who takes a history and does some clinical observations. The nurse associate takes the required blood tests, performs an electrocardiogram and cannulates Jane.

Jane is reviewed by the A&E specialist registrar and referred for surgery. In theatre, Jane is looked after by the theatre team of healthcare professionals, including the nurse associate, the associate practitioner, the nurse, the operating department practitioner, the anaesthetist, the surgeon and then the recovery team.

Post-surgery, Jane is admitted to a surgical ward where she stays for one night. While there, she receives care from the ward nursing team consisting of the healthcare assistant, the nurse associate, the nurse and the ward sister. The pharmacology team reviews her medication. She is also reviewed by the surgical team consisting of the junior doctor, the specialist registrar and the consultant.

The next day, Jane is discharged home under the care of her GP. As she is mobile, she sees her practice nurse to monitor her wound the next day.

Consider

In the space of three days, Jane was under the care of eight different healthcare teams.
Where could errors in care provision have occurred?
What was important for ensuring no errors in care provision occurred?
How can a nurse associate act to ensure no errors in care provision occur?

Conclusion

This chapter has provided the reader with insight and understanding concerning the various elements of team working and the importance of effective leadership. A team is synergistic when there is a mixture of strengths and abilities working together. Nursing associates bring with them a range of skills, strengths and abilities, and no one team role is more important than any other. The nursing associate must understand their own skills and strengths to help find their place in a team. A team will not survive without a leader who motivates and inspires.

References

Adair, J. (2010) *Develop your leadership skills*, London: Kogan Page.

Barr, J. and Dowding, L. (2019) *Leadership in health care* (4th edn), London: Sage.

Belbin, R.M. (1981) *Management teams*, Oxford: Elsevier

Bonebright, D. (2010) 40 Years of storming: a historical review of Tuckman's model of small group development, *Human Resource Development International*, 13(1): 111–120.

Ellis, P. and Bach, S. (2015) *Leadership, management & team working in nursing* (2nd edn), London: Sage.

Francis, R. (2013) *Report of the mid Staffordshire NHS foundation trust public inquiry*, London: The Stationery office.

Howatson-Jones. (2004) The Servant leader, *Nursing Management*, 11(3): 20–24.

Jung, C. (1921) *Psychological types, The collected works of CG Jung*, Vol 6 Bollingen Series XX.

Lynas, K. (2013) *NHS leadership academy. [online]* Available: www.leadershipacademy.nhs.uk

Marquis, B. and Huston, C. (2012) *Leadership roles and management functions in nursing* (7th edn), Philadelphia: Lippincott Williams & Wilkins.

NHS Leadership Academy. (2013) *The healthcare leadership model*, London: NHS.

Nursing & Midwifery Council. (2018a) *Standards of proficiency for nursing associates*, London: Nursing & Midwifery Council.

Nursing & Midwifery Council. (2018b). *The code: professional standards of practice and behaviour for nurses, midwives and nursing associates*, London: Nursing & Midwifery Council.

Salas, E., Reyes, D. and McDaniel, S. (2018) The science of teamwork: progress, reflections, and the road ahead, *American Psychologist*, 73(4): 593–600.

Tuckman, B. (1965) Developmental sequence in small groups, *Psychological Bulletin*, 63(6): 384–399.

Tuckman, B. and Jenson, M. (1977) Stages of small group development revisited, *Group and Organisation Studies*, 2(4): 419–427.

www.belbin.com

www.myerbriggs.org

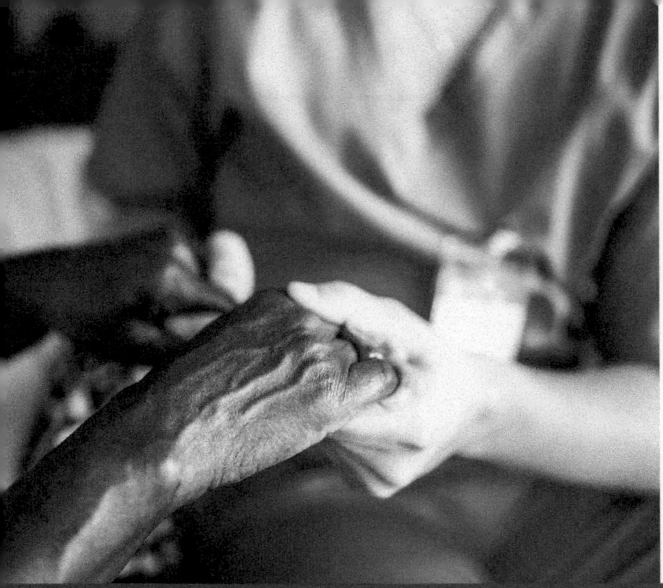

5

Listening Actively

Jacqueline Chang

Kingston University and St George's University of London, UK

Chapter Aim

- This chapter aims to assist the reader in developing an understanding of the art of listening actively.

Learning Outcomes

By the end of this chapter, the reader will be able to:

- Consider the relevance of a therapeutic relationship in healthcare and social care.
- Explore the importance of active listening in healthcare and social care delivery and the barriers to active listening
- Introduce methods of active listening

Test Yourself Multiple Choice Questions

1. Which part of the standards of proficiency for nursing associates (Nursing & Midwifery Council 2018a) highlights the importance of clear communication?
   A) Platform 1
   B) Platform 5
   C) Annexe A
2. Which are the best types of questions to use when communicating with a patient?
   A) Open questions
   B) Closed questions
   C) Leading questions
3. When do healthcare professionals need to communicate effectively with patients?
   A) When doing an assessment
   B) When planning care
   C) All the time

The Nursing Associate's Handbook of Clinical Skills, First Edition. Edited by Ian Peate.

Companion website: www.wiley.com/nursingassociate

4. **The Code (Nursing & Midwifery Council 2018b) instructs nurses and nursing associates to:**
   A) **Actively listen to people**
   B) **Use a range of verbal and non-verbal communication methods**
   C) **Use written communication as well as verbal communication to ensure understanding**
5. **In the Code (Nursing & Midwifery Council 2018b), which section is devoted to communication?**
   A) **Section 7**
   B) **Section 4**
   C) **Section 9**

Introduction

Communication skill is something that is taught in all nursing associate training programmes. The role of the nursing associate is to provide face-to-face care to the patient (and, where appropriate, to the family), and effective communication is a key part of that. This chapter will provide you with an understanding of the importance of listening actively and how that helps to develop a therapeutic relationship. Some of the techniques of active listening will be explained, and there will also be a discussion of some of the barriers faced in healthcare to provide a therapeutic communication interaction.

Take Note

Consider a time when you are with a patient. How focused are you on what they are saying? Are you able to be in that moment with them, or are there points when your mind is distracted by other things?

Blue Flag

When working closely with patients, they will often tell you important things, and they may tell you these things because they have got to know you, they like you, they trust you and they can relate to you.

Hearing what patients are saying and truly listening and attending to what it is that they are saying is a key skill.

Communication is an essential element of healthcare. Without communication between the healthcare professional and the patient, care cannot be negotiated, and therefore, it cannot be delivered. The Nursing & Midwifery Council (NMC) documents the Standards of Proficiency (2018a) and The Code (2018b); both have communication as a requirement for registered professionals. The Standards (Nursing & Midwifery Council 2018b) go into detail about how best to communicate. If a healthcare professional were to meet these communication standards all of the time, their communication skills would be excellent. The relevant elements of the professional documents can be found below.

Despite these clear guidelines and requirements, communication is still an issue in healthcare, and there are regular complaints regarding how healthcare staff fail to communicate effectively. The data collected by The National Statistics for National Health Service (NHS) Digital in 2017–2018 found that 15.2% of complaints made about hospital and community health services were related to the communication skills of the healthcare team. This is clearly an issue that needs to be addressed, and effective communication skills cannot be assumed; they need to be learned. The Code (2018b) mentions communication throughout highlighting communication skills under the theme of Practise Effectively and states that the nursing associate must communicate clearly, and in order to achieve this, the nursing associate must:

- Use terms that people in your care, colleagues and the public can understand
- Take reasonable steps to meet people's language and communication needs, providing, wherever possible, assistance to those who need help to communicate their own or other people's needs
- Use a range of verbal and non-verbal communication methods and consider cultural sensitivities to better understand and respond to people's personal and health needs
- Check people's understanding from time to time to keep misunderstanding or mistakes to a minimum
- Be able to communicate clearly and effectively in English.

Green Flag

The NMC Standards of Proficiency for Nursing Associates (2018b) states that nursing associates must be able to safely demonstrate the following:

1. Underpinning communication skills for providing and monitoring care:
   1.1 actively listen, recognise and respond to verbal and non-verbal cues
   1.2 use prompts and positive verbal and non-verbal reinforcement
   1.3 use appropriate non-verbal communication including touch, eye contact and personal space
   1.4 make appropriate use of open and closed questioning
   1.5 speak clearly and accurately
   1.6 use caring conversation techniques
   1.7 check understanding and use clarification techniques

1.8 be aware of the possibility of own unconscious bias in communication encounters
1.9 write accurate, clear, legible records and documentation
1.10 clearly record digital information and data
1.11 provide clear verbal, digital or written information and instructions when sharing information, delegating or handing over responsibility for care
1.12 recognise the need for translator services and material
1.13 use age appropriate communication techniques

Source: Based on Nursing & Midwifery Council (2018b)

The explanation provided by the Standards regarding what the nursing associate must demonstrate safely (Nursing & Midwifery Council 2018b) is a description of a therapeutic conversation as part of a therapeutic relationship.

The Therapeutic Relationship

A therapeutic relationship is a relationship between a patient and a healthcare professional which is built on mutual trust and respect. There must be honesty, but clear professional boundaries, and the healthcare professional must show understanding, care and empathy.

In 1952, Hildegard Peplau devised a model for therapeutic relationships and interactions. In this model, Peplau focused on psychology and communication and produced a four-stage model which is illustrated in Figure 5.1.

The first stage of Peplau's model is the orientation phase. This, in healthcare, is when the practitioner and patient first meet. At this point, the patient has needs, and the healthcare professional is the person to address these needs. This is the stage where the felt need is expressed by the patient. It is here where questions are asked and information is given in order to understand each other and the situation, where boundaries are identified, and at this stage, trust starts to develop.

The second stage is the identification phase. This is where the patient and the healthcare professional work together to formulate goals and to implement the care. This is largely led by the healthcare professional, and in this phase, the healthcare professional may take on many roles including that of a care giver, an emotional supporter and educator amongst others.

The third stage is the exploitation phase; the patient is becoming more independent and more confident. They are starting to look after themselves and can start to look at being discharged from care. They have learnt from the healthcare professional and are no longer as dependent on them.

The final stage is the resolution phase. This is where the relationship ends because the patient is discharged home and is no longer in need of the therapeutic relationship. The interaction ends, and the relationship is terminated.

A direct correlation between Peplau's model and the nursing process has been identified in literature over time as illustrated in Box 5.1. The major difference between the two is that Peplau's model is linear, whereas the nursing process is cyclical. The key similarity is the mutual respect required for this relationship to work and the implemented care to be successful.

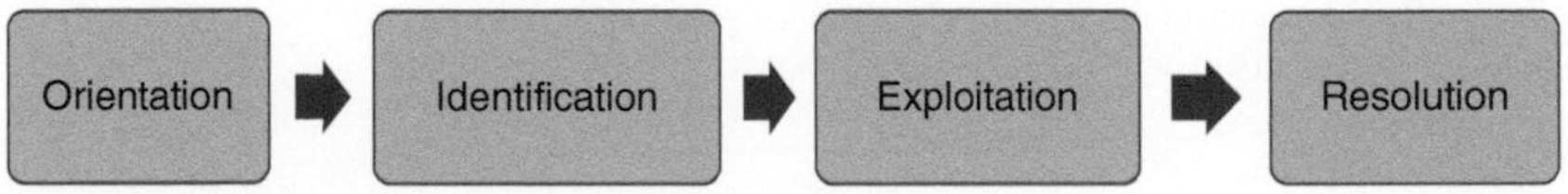

Figure 5.1 Peplau's model of interpersonal relations. ***Source:*** **Based on Peplau (1952).**

Box 5.1 Peplau's Model Compared with the Nursing Process

PEPLAU'S MODEL	THE NURSING PROCESS
Orientation Information gathering	**Assessment** Information gathering
Felt need expressed Patient identifies their needs.	**Nursing diagnosis** The nurse and the patient identify the current issues.
Identification Care required is identified by the patient and is implemented largely by the healthcare professional with involvement from the patient.	**Care planning (implementation)** The nurse (with the patient) plans how the care will be administered by the team.
Exploitation The patient becomes more independent and requires less input from the healthcare team.	**Implementation** The negotiated care is performed with the patient.
Resolution The patient is discharged, and the therapeutic relationship comes to an end.	**Evaluation** The nurse and patient assess the care given to determine what changes are required, if any. This may be the end of the relationship, or further needs are identified, and the cycle starts again.

The Importance of Active Listening

In order to build that therapeutic relationship, the healthcare professional must communicate with the patient and, furthermore, communicate effectively. A key aspect of communication includes listening. Of course, everyone would claim to listen to people, but in a therapeutic relationship, the healthcare professional must listen actively. This is different from listening passively to someone speak; the technique of engaging in active listening requires much effort and skill. Haley et al. (2017) identify that the skill of active listening demonstrates a higher level of empathy than demonstrated through passive listening; active listening can help the healthcare worker to become more empathetic.

Communication is an essential element of healthcare, and Alsawy et al. (2019) found that meaningful conversations can reduce feeling of isolation and depression. They also found that when the patients felt their healthcare professionals were actively listening to them, the communication interaction was more enjoyable and meaningful for them. True active listening requires practice and reflection, and Nemec et al. (2017) state that besides training to learn the skills, a therapeutic interaction requires both physical and mental preparation.

Red Flag

Listening is a key component of communication, and a part of this involves being quiet. When the nursing associate fails to listen, vital information can be missed, and this can have a detrimental effect on a person's physical and mental health.

How to Listen Actively

There are two specific elements of communication that a healthcare professional needs to be aware of in order to demonstrate that they are hearing the person they are listening to. They are verbal and non-verbal communication. Webb & Mille (2011) describe these as attending *verbally*, *vocally* and *non-verbally*. These will be explained, in turn, starting with non-verbal communication, also referred to as *non-verbal attending*.

Firstly, it is important to physically demonstrate that there is time for this interaction (Sally & Dallas 2010). This can be achieved by closing the door, drawing curtains and providing privacy. It is also important to ensure there are no interruptions during the interaction. Sitting with the patient, as opposed to standing over them, also shows that there is time for this interaction.

Avoiding physical barriers is very important. It is tempting to take notes to ensure nothing is forgotten, but this is an immediate barrier to effective communication (Ali 2018). Therapeutic communication should be a conversation, so taking notes is not appropriate and may make the patient feel uncomfortable. Taking notes can create pauses and breaks, and should this happen, then natural communication is stilted. The use of furniture can also be an issue. If a table is in between the healthcare professional and the patient, then there is a physical barrier which may hinder the interaction, so this should be avoided. How the healthcare professional physically presents themselves is also important, as this is another element of non-verbal communication.

Take Note

There are many factors (human and material) that can impact active listening negatively. The nursing associate, when aware of these issues, can take steps to help alleviate the impact.

One way to remember how to optimise communication through body posture is the pneumonic SOLER (Egan 2010). Table 5.1 provides an explanation of the mnemonic SOLER.

It is important to note that silence is a very important part of communication, and not everyone will be comfortable with that. Silence allows a person time to gather their thoughts and time to find the confidence to say what it is that they needs to say. Allowing silence will also demonstrate that the interaction is not going to be rushed and that the importance of the interaction is understood. Prince-Paul & Kelley (2017) explain that silence can be considered as a part of mindful listening and a powerful type of non-verbal communication.

Table 5.1 SOLER.

S	Sitting squarely
O	Open posture (arms not crossed)
L	Lean forward toward the other person
E	Maintain appropriate Eye contact
R	Relax

Source: Based on Egan (2010).

Box 5.2 Examples of Different Question Types Focusing on Pain

Closed	Do you have any pain right now?
Leading	You have pain right now, yes?
Open	Tell me about your pain.

Verbal communication is an important part of active listening, and there are two different elements to this. Verbally attending is one of these elements. As discussed earlier, the communication interaction should be a conversation; in order to aid this, the use of open questions is imperative. Closed questions – where a yes or no answer is expected – allow people to give one-word answers which are a barrier to communication; these types of questions do not encourage patients to communicate. Leading questions – where a patient is given the answer within the question – can result in patients not stating their own feelings but what they are led to agree with. These questions do not encourage communication. Open questions allow the patients to speak from their perspective with no prior expectations from the healthcare professional. Box 5.2 illustrates how the same question can be asked in three different ways to elicit more information.

The other element of verbal communication is referred to as vocally attending by Webb & Mille (2011). It is important to make noises to demonstrate listening at appropriate points. These give the patient reassurance and cue them to continue. These noises may include the use of small words such as 'a-ha', 'hmm' and 'yes'. Another option is using reflective statements including 'I understand', 'I see what you mean' and 'that sounds like it was difficult for you'. These demonstrate understanding which also gives reassurance and encouragement to continue. A further element of verbal communication in active listening is paraphrasing what has been said. By repeating back what has been said and paraphrasing it, it is clear that the patient has been heard and that can create a good level of trust between the patient and the healthcare professional. It also shows that the healthcare professional has understood the patient.

Orange Flag

As you actively listen, try to identify any key words that might be used to sum up how the person may be feeling, such as:

- frightened, or scared
- lonely
- fed up, or 'a bit down'
- pain, or discomfort
- worried
- anxious

Another way of ensuring that open questions are used is remembering the 5WH model:
What?
When?
Who?
Where?
Why?
How?
See also Chapter 2 of this text for further discussion of the 5WH model.

These 5WH questions have their origins in Aristotle's work or even earlier (Sloan 2010) and are an excellent way of finding out information, as none of these questions can be answered with a yes or a no. This gives the patients the opportunity to use their own words to explain their situation.

Barriers to Active Listening

There are many barriers to effective communication and active listening, and healthcare does present very specific challenges. It is important to recognise these barriers and try to find a way to minimise their effect on a therapeutic relationship.

One barrier to open communication is information giving (Ali 2017). As healthcare professionals with expert knowledge, it can be tempting to want to help the person and reassure them but by interrupting and not allowing them to speak, communication is stopped. Active listening is about listening, not giving information.

Listening actively with a person who speaks a different language requires some consideration. The non-verbal actions – body language and time – remain the same, but due to the use of an interpreter, the conversation will not flow in the same way. When using an interpreter, it is

> **Touch Point**
>
> What do you think is the biggest barrier to effective communication in healthcare?

essential to maintain eye contact with the service user and not with the interpreter. The use of silence is more challenging when using an interpreter, but it is important to remember the technique of active listening and try to use it. Using an interpreter also has implications on both confidentiality and privacy (Nursing & Midwifery Council 2018a). Sully & Dallas (2010) explore the implications of using a family member as an interpreter and the way in which that can affect communication. Using a family member provides a conflict of interest as they are not trained in translating medical terminology; they are also emotionally involved so may not translate exactly what they should; furthermore, the patient may not answer certain questions truthfully or openly in front of certain family members. By using a family member as an interpreter, the patient is not being allowed the time and space to be honest and open with the healthcare professional.

It is also important to consider who is in the room (or the area where the interaction is taking place) during the interaction; some patients may be comfortable discussing their concerns and fears in front of other people; however, others need more privacy. It is important to establish who, if anybody, the patient is happy to have in the room during the interaction. If a wrong person is in the room, then it may hinder the communication episode entirely, and this needs to be understood and respected.

Strong accents can be difficult to understand, and this therefore can hinder communication (Sully & Dallas 2010). The accent may be from the patient or from the healthcare professional. If a patient is struggling to understand what it is that the healthcare professional is saying, they may not feel confident enough to be open and honest with them. A therapeutic relationship cannot be assumed or forced. The patients will develop this relationship and will communicate with the healthcare professional whom they feel they are able to do this with.

Open and honest communication requires privacy. An inpatient hospital environment is not always the most private place. Curtains are not soundproof, and for someone to feel comfortable enough to be open and honest, privacy is a requirement. Unfortunately, there is not a lot that can be done about this, but being aware can help. Occasionally, depending on the environment, it is possible to go to a quiet room, but that is not always the case; speaking quietly and discreetly is sometimes the best that can be done. It is important to acknowledge this limitation with the patient should it occur, and it is also essential to maintain confidentiality (Nursing & Midwifery Council 2018a).

Violet Flag

Active listening is an act of care. It is an outward display of genuine interest in what another person has to say, and this is regardless of where that person is being cared for (the care setting).

The nursing associate needs to understand that the act of listening requires us to avoid imitation and, instead of this, to rely on our humanity as we strike a balance between openness and interpretation. When using this humanistic approach, this has so much potential to permit us to appropriately respond to those who speak to us, be this in a hospital, in the person's own home, in a place of detention or with those who have no homes – the homeless.

> **Touch Point**
>
> Active listening is an essential element of creating a therapeutic relationship. When a therapeutic relationship is created, a better healthcare experience can be enjoyed by everyone involved. Active listening takes time and experience, but it is important to invest in this essential communication skill.

Conclusion

One of the biggest challenges in healthcare is that of time. To be able to find time in a busy working day with a long list of patients who need care is very difficult. There is no solution to this, but if patients are not listened to and heard, then their healthcare needs cannot be met. By actively listening, the healthcare professional can foster relationships and be the right person for that patient to talk with – the development of a therapeutic environment. An interaction does not need to be long; if the healthcare professional can listen actively, hear what they are being told and act on it; then time need not be an issue.

References

Ali, M. (2017) Communication skills 2: overcoming barriers to effective communication, *Nursing Times*, 114(1): 40–42.

Ali, M. (2018) Communication skills 5: effective listening and observation, *Nursing Times*, 114(4): 60–61.

Alsawy, S., Tai, S., McEvoy, P. and Mansell, W. (2019) 'It's nice to think somebody's listening to me instead of saying "oh shut up"'. People with dementia reflect on what makes communication good and meaningful, *Journal of Psychiatric Mental Health Nursing*, 27(2): 1–11.

Egan, G. (2010) *The skilled helper: a problem management and opportunity development approach to helping* (9th edn), Pacific Grove, CA: Brooks/Cole.

Haley, B., Seongkum, H., Wright, P., Barone, C., Rettinganti, M. and Anders, M. (2017) Relationships among active listening, self-awareness, empathy, and patient centered care in associate and baccalaureate degree nursing students, *Nursing Plus Open*, 3: 11–16.

Nemec, P., Spagnolo, A. and Soydan, A. (2017) Can you hear me now? Teaching listening skills, *Psychiatric Rehabilitation Journal*, 40(4): 415–417.

NHS Digital. (2018) *Data on written complaints in the NHS*, England: Health and Social Care Information Centre.

Nursing & Midwifery Council. (2018a) *The code: professional standards of practice and behaviour for nurses, midwives and nursing associates*, London: Nursing & Midwifery Council.

Nursing & Midwifery Council. (2018b) *Standards of proficiency for nursing associates*, London: Nursing & Midwifery Council.

Peplau, H.E. (1952) *Interpersonal relations in nursing*, New York: Putnams Sons and (1988) London: MacMillan Education Ltd (reprinted).

Prince-Paul, M. and Kelley, C. (2017) Mindful communication: being present, *Seminars in Oncology Nursing*, 33(5): 475–482.

Sloan, M.C. (2010) Aristotle's Nicomachean ethics as the original locus for the Septem circumstantiae, *Classical Philology*, 105 (3): 236–251.

Sully, P. and Dallas, J. (2010) *Essential communication skills for nursing and midwifery (2nd edn)*, London: Elsevier Ltd.

Webb, L. and Miller, E. (2011) *Nursing: communication skills in practice*, Oxford: Oxford University Press.

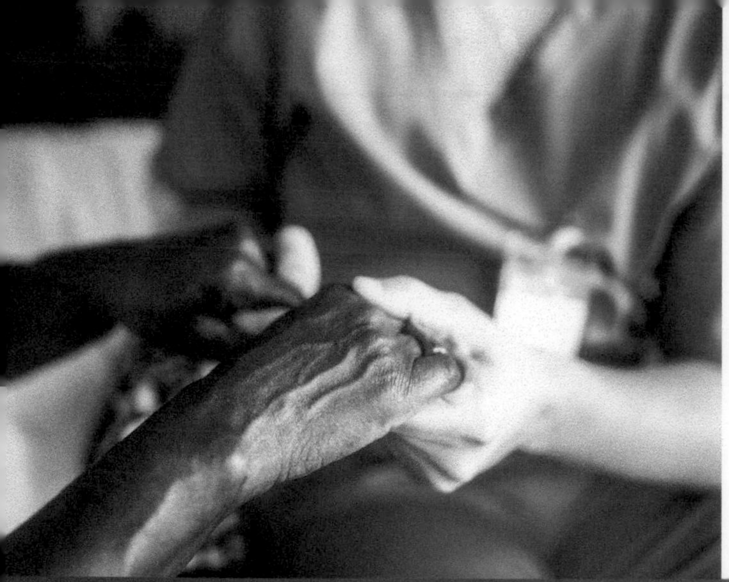

6

Information Gathering

Julia Williams

Bucks New University (Uxbridge Campus), UK

Chapter Aim

- **This chapter aims to provide the reader with an understanding of how information can be gathered and used to inform practice.**

Learning Objectives

At the end of the chapter, the reader will be able to:

- **Understand how evidence-based practice requires the nursing associate to listen, inform and involve patients in decision-making with regards to their care and treatment**
- **Demonstrate an awareness of the two types of knowing**
- **Appreciate the value of gathering information in the development of the therapeutic nurse–patient relationship**
- **Understand the advantages of being physically and mentally present in every interaction and the ability to prioritise relationship building**

Test Yourself Multiple Choice Questions

1. Hierarchy of evidence refers to:
   A) Legal data only
   B) A ranking system whereby a range of different methodologies are graded according to the validity of their findings
   C) A system that is based on objective data only
   D) All of the above
2. How many types of knowing are there?
   A) 1
   B) 2
   C) 3

The Nursing Associate's Handbook of Clinical Skills, First Edition. Edited by Ian Peate.

Companion website: www.wiley.com/nursingassociate

3. **Physical knowing relates to the patient's:**
   A) **Responses, psychological function and body type**
   B) **Responses and physical function**
   C) **Responses, physical function and body type**
4. **Psychological knowing relates to the patient's:**
   A) **Feelings, perceptions, expectations and beliefs**
   B) **Perceptions, expectations and beliefs**
   C) **Expectations and beliefs**
5. **The nursing associate is required to:**
   A) **Involve the patient in the decision-making of his/her care and treatment**
   B) **Advise and involve the family in the decision-making of their care and treatment**
   C) **Listen, inform and involve the patient in the decision-making of their care and treatment**

Introduction

One of the main roles expected of the nursing associate is to deliver hands-on, evidence-based patient-centred care as a part of the nursing team (Health Education England 2019; Nursing & Midwifery Council 2018a). The concept of patient-centred care refers to the caring of patients in a meaningful and valuable way that is entirely individual to that patient (McCormack & McCance 2010). The Nursing & Midwifery Council's (2018b) Code is clear in informing the nursing associates that they must act in partnership with those receiving care, and in order to do this effectively, they are required to gather relevant information from the patients and, if appropriate, their family.

The nursing associate has to listen, inform and involve the patient in the decision-making of his/her care and treatment. Evidence-based practice refers to the application of appropriate research findings to underpin practice, such as identifying the most effective treatment and management or having a deeper appreciation of the experiences of being a patient. In order to deliver such patient-centred care, both concepts need to work in harmony, requiring the nursing associate to sift through and gather the relevant information to support any given clinical situation. This chapter looks at how the nursing associate may gather information from a variety of sources. It will consider the theoretical features that allow nursing associates to do this, as ultimately, how and what information we gather will provide the knowledge to support clinical judgements and decision-making in the delivery of individualised patient care.

Green Flag

The Code (Nursing & Midwifery Council 2018b) requires the nursing associate to always practise in line with the best available evidence to make sure that any information or advice given is evidence-based, including information relating to using any healthcare products or services.

Therapeutic Nurse–Patient Relationship

Establishing positive and trusting therapeutic relationships with patients has long been recognised as an essential component of nursing practice and is important for effective care (Freshwater 2007; Mirhaghi et al. 2017). A therapeutic relationship such as this is defined by Feo et al. (2016) as a helping relationship that is based on mutual trust and respect; the nurturing of faith and hope; being sensitive to self and others and assisting with the satisfaction of the patient's physical, emotional and spiritual needs. This type of nursing involves understanding the true meaning of a situation, especially when it is not obvious or expected (Freshwater 2007). Successful interaction of focusing, knowing, anticipating and evaluating are skills used to build and maintain a trusting relationship (Feo et al. 2017).

Blue Flag

Maintaining trust and confidence with the patient is an ongoing process that ensures the preservation of humanity during the delivery of care (Mirhaghi et al. 2017) which is viewed as an important prerequisite to facilitating a patient-centred approach (Feo et al. 2016).

Knowing the Patient

Getting to know the patient within the context of his/her specific illness and the context of his/her lives is considered by Dewing et al. (2014) as two types of knowing: the physical and psychological knowing. The physical knowing relates to the patient's responses, physical function and body type, whereas the psychological knowing reflects the patient's feelings, perceptions, expectations and beliefs. These will determine the patients' own health beliefs, including their responses to illness, future life events and experiences.

Knowing the patient is vital in nursing; the nursing associate might state that we 'know the patient very well', but what does this really mean? What do we know and how do we know it? Several theories within the literature (Carper 1978; Watson 1985; Swanson 1991) have explored this knowledge for nursing practice, and it is reported that as such a situation as this 'knowing' cannot be based on formal scientific knowledge alone. Therefore, knowledge must be seen in another dimension associated with action and decision-making and is referred to as 'patterns of knowing' (Carper 1978). Carper's (1978) work sets out to bring together all the ways of knowing that are pertinent to nursing, integrating both practical and theoretical knowledge. Conducting a seminal piece of work, Carper (1978) explores the sources that nurses use to develop knowledge and beliefs about their practice and patient care by describing four patterns of knowing: empirical, aesthetic, personal and moral.

The first of Carper's (1978) four patterns, empirics, refers to the science of nursing, and it is empirical, factual and descriptive in nature. This type of knowing allows the nursing associate to acquire both objective information regarding the patient's condition and personal information concerning thoughts, feelings and experiences. The second is aesthetics; this refers to the art of nursing. Here, Carper (1978) reflects upon empathy as an important element of aesthetic knowing, suggesting that when a nursing associate learns to empathise, the different perspective of the patient life becomes apparent. The third relates to personal knowledge, and this is concerned with knowing, encountering and actualising of the individual self and in some respects relates to emotional intelligence and can be acquired through the therapeutic use of self (Currid & Pennington 2010).

Yellow Flag

Knowing the patient in relation to their specific illness and the context of their lives is essential; 'knowing' will reflect the patient's feelings, their perceptions, expectations and also their beliefs. This will establish the patient's own health beliefs as well as how they may respond to illness, future life events and experiences.

Defined as the 'ability to recognise the meaning of emotions and their relationships and to use them as a basis of reasoning and problem-solving' (Mayer et al. 2001, p. 234), emotional intelligence is not always easy to translate. To be emotionally intelligent is generally described as a core aptitude related to one's ability and capacity to reason with one's emotions, especially in relation to others (Freshwater & Stickley 2004, cited in Williams 2015), which might suggest that nursing associates may possess the knowledge and skills but lack the ability to transmit them, and for a successful nurse–patient relationship, a balance of both would seem essential. This will be discussed further within this chapter.

The final of Carper's (1978) four patterns of knowing is concerned with ethics. This focuses on the moral knowledge of the nurse, more specifically, a sense of knowing what is right and wrong for the patient. Every nursing associate will possess their own set of personal ethics and morals which they live by. Within healthcare practices, nursing associates should recognise healthcare dilemmas and make good judgements and decisions based on their values whilst keeping within the laws that govern them (Östman et al. 2019). Carper (1978) acknowledges that these patterns of knowing are not mutually exclusive, and nurses are seen to use attributes of all four patterns to successfully deliver patient-centred care.

Incorporating Carper's (1978) patterns of knowing, Johns (2000) suggests guided reflection as an addition pattern of knowing. The use of reflecting on experience as a means of enhancing clinical practice stems from the work of Schön (1983). Reflective and critical thought can help reason prejudices ensuring a growing awareness through reflective critical thought with regards to the nature of knowledge so not to assume things are true when they simply are not (Rolston et al. 2016). Benner (1984) points out that not all knowledge embedded in expertise can be captured in theory and furthermore believes that nurses need emotional space to think and feel about their practice. Reflective practice allows the nursing associate to explore the emotions that engaged or involved them in the situation, in the first place. Reflection can be described as the ability to explore one's own actions, thoughts and feelings and think purposefully to gain new insights, ideas and understanding (Rolston et al. 2016).

Following Carper (1978), further theories have focused on how nurses go about gathering information to get to know the patient. In brief, Watson's (1985) Transpersonal Caring theory indicated that nurses gain insight into a patient's response to illness through a relationship exemplified by respect, compassion and support, pointing out the critical link between a deep connection with the patient and the nurse's knowing, mirroring features of the therapeutic nurse–patient relationship. This is reinforced in Swanson's (1991) theory of caring, where the dimensions of knowing are defined further to include avoiding assumptions, cue seeking and engagement of self, alluding to features of emotional intelligence.

Touch Point

Carper's (1978) four patterns of nursing knowledge:

Personal knowing

Refers to the knowledge of ourselves, what we have seen and experienced. This type of knowledge comes through the process of observation, reflection and self-actualisation. As we know ourselves, we are able to establish authentic, therapeutic relationships.

Empirical knowing

Empirical knowledge is gained from research and objective facts. This knowledge is systematically organised into general laws and theories. This way of knowing is often referred to as the science of nursing.

Ethical knowing
This way of knowing helps develop our own moral code and our sense of knowing what is right and wrong. Nursing associates' personal ethics are based on their obligation to protect and respect human life.

Aesthetic knowing
Aesthetic knowing makes nursing an art. All the other ways of knowing are considered and through it aesthetic knowing.

Source: Based on Carper (1978)

Interestingly, Munhall (1993, cited in Stevens 2018) identified 'unknowing' as a further component of knowing, suggesting this is an awareness that the nurse does not and cannot know or understand of the patient when they initially meet. The skill of recognising this unknowing ensures that the nursing associate remains alert to the patients' perception of need. This echoes Mayer & Salovey's (1997) theoretical framework of emotional intelligence, where on initial meeting with the patient, the nurse perceives the situation by tuning in to his/her own self and emotional awareness and that of the patient in order to gauge the need of the situation. Part of this awareness is sometimes referred to as intuitive or tacit knowledge, just knowing and understanding common thoughts. Such knowledge adds to the gathering of information in the development of the therapeutic nurse–patient relationship.

Take Note

You never get another chance to make a first impression; a bad first impression is hard to change. Patients feel more relaxed and communicate more freely with someone they feel is professional.

To summarise these theories (Carper 1978; Watson 1985; Swanson 1991; Johns 2000), it is evident that the concept of knowing emerges from a deep and meaningful relationship between the nurse and the patient. Through the delivery of care, the nursing associate continuously strives to understand and interpret the needs of the patient. The ability to gather relevant information and use a variety of sources demonstrates a strong conceptual foundation of the meaning of knowing; however, it should be acknowledged that the level of information gathered will depend on the nursing associates' previous clinical experiences and interactions.

Violet Flag

Understanding and integrating the needs of patients is key to the provision of safe, high-quality care. Gathering information occurs in many ways and in many venues.

Health screening in the prison service occurs upon reception into custody and provides an ideal opportunity to detect and treat previously unmet healthcare needs. When assessment during reception is effective, this has real potential to identify health problems, especially serious mental illness.

Emotional Intelligence

Emotional intelligence is defined as the 'ability to recognise the meaning of emotions and their relationships and to use them as a basis of reasoning and problem-solving' (Mayer et al. 2001, p. 234).

Mayer & Salovey (1997) believed that emotional intelligence is related to thinking, through the ability to use reasoning, by way of information, to find meaning. This model is composed of four branches (see Table 6.1). Each branch has specific characteristics to meet the criteria of emotional intelligence. Each level or branch builds upon the previous one, and awareness of what each branch offers is individual. Enhancing relationships with others is a key component of healthy emotional interactions. The following is a brief description of the four branches. The first branch is the perception of emotion, which is the skill of accurately distinguishing emotion within oneself and others. Using emotion to facilitate thinking is the second branch. This branch enhances an individual's ability to assimilate emotion to facilitate thinking and to prioritise thinking and judgements.

Understanding emotion follows as the third branch, which allows application of the emotional knowledge gained in the first two levels of skills to translate emotions to meaning within the context of events. The highest level of the skills of emotional intelligence is the conscious regulation and management of emotion. This level of the model allows the nursing associate to remain receptive to emotional information while reflecting on the usefulness of it. This reflective skill provides the ability to evaluate emotional reactions not only within self but also those conveyed by others.

Touch Point

Emotional intelligence can be described as the ability to monitor or control own emotions, as well to the emotions of those around you. This involves recognising feelings, self-awareness, how emotions affect relationships and also how this can be managed.

Table 6.1 Branches and characteristics of emotional intelligence theoretical framework.

BRANCH 1	BRANCH 2	BRANCH 3	BRANCH 4
Perceiving emotions (PE)	Facilitating thought with emotions (FE)	Understanding emotions (UE)	Managing emotions (ME)
Characteristics	Characteristics	Characteristics	Characteristics
• Self-awareness • Emotional self-awareness • Accurate self-assessment • Self-confidence • Gauging the mood • Tuning into your sense	• Emotional self-control • Cognitive process – comprehension of language, learning, reasoning, problem-solving, decision-making • Intuition • Initiative • Adaptability • Conscientiousness • Trustworthiness	• Empathy • Recognition • Clinical reasoning • Critical thinking • Clinical judgement	• Communication • Working as a team – working towards similar goals • Nurturing relationships – buildings rapport • Change agent • Leadership • Developing self and others – personal growth • Influences • Conflicts

Source: Based on Mayer & Salovey (1997).

Eraut (2000) purposes two distinct elements of knowledge from which information is gathered; knowledge embedded in routines and protocols and knowledge that is explicitly needed at the time – intuition. Such knowledge may influence how the patient is assessed, what decisions are made and/or how the nursing associate interacts with the patient. Intuition is often proposed as one of the defining characteristics of expertise and has been the topic of considerable debate. Some believe that it does not exist (English 1993, cited in den Hertog & Niessen 2019), while others advocate intuition in nursing as a genuine phenomenon (Benner 1984).

Intuition is characterised has 'having a gut feeling' about something which might impress 'a bystander of the suddenness and nearly magical nature of these behaviours' (Gobet & Chassy 2008, p. 130). In general, intuition involves a rapid perception, lack of awareness of the process engaged, associated presence of emotions and holistic understanding of the problem situation (Benner 1984; Gobet & Chassy 2008). Mayer & Salovey (1997) proposed that some individuals possess greater ability than others to reason about and use emotionally intense information to enhance both cognitive activity and social functioning.

Our ability to perceive, process and manage emotional information varies greatly. Nursing is an emotionally demanding healthcare practice, and nursing associates need to understand their own emotions and perceptions in order to understand a patient's needs and hence develop a therapeutic relationship; by using our emotions, judgements are formed, and decisions are acted upon (James et al. 2010).

Tools for Gathering Relevant Information

Gathering relevant information is an important aspect of knowing the patient, and it can be challenging to determine exactly what information is needed to be appropriately informed in any given clinical situation. On occasions, it is also difficult to determine how to gather such information effectively. Some of this information is gathered through the development of what is known as the therapeutic nurse–patient relationship (Wiechula et al. 2016). Establishing such a relationship begins the moment the nursing associate meets the patient (Feo et al. 2017), and at this point, the nursing associate is required to draw upon their verbal and non-verbal communication skills and use of the senses and physical touch.

Supporting Evidence

Person-centred care and fundamental care are two interconnected areas in which nursing policy and healthcare reform are focusing on. Both initiatives highlight a positive nurse–patient relationship. For these initiatives to work, nurses need guidance with regards to how they can best develop and maintain relationships with patients. This study explains a novel methodological approach, known as holistic interpretive synthesis, for interpreting empirical research findings to create practice-relevant recommendations for nurses. The recommendations for the nurse–patient relationship created through this approach can be used by nurses to establish, maintain and evaluate therapeutic relationships with patients as they strive to deliver person-centred fundamental care.

Source: Feo et al. (2017)

A study by Bundgaard et al. (2012) illustrates through an investigation of what knowing the patient meant in an endoscopy clinic. These authors identified two themes: what to know and how to get to know. Nurse's information focused on practical issues related to the endoscopic procedure. Categories of necessary knowledge included anxiety, medication and previous experience. Nurses were reported to have uncovered the necessary information to 'get to know' their patient by using their senses and communication skills. These reflect the characteristics of emotional intelligence as stipulated by Mayer & Salovey (1997) (see Table 6.1), whereby skills and abilities such as self and emotional awareness, emotional self-control, empathy, comprehensive interpretation of language, active listening, tuning into and picking up on patient cues, verbal and non-verbal behaviours, intuition, clinical reasoning, clinical judgements, problem-solving and reflection all play an important role in getting to know the patient.

When greeting a patient or in any nurse–patient encounter, the nursing associates' goal is to set aside distractions and to give the patient their undivided attention. This requires the nursing associates to demonstrate the ability to be physically and mentally present in every interaction and the ability to prioritise relationship building. This focused attention may also help the nursing associate to shield the patient from the commotion and activity of the setting. Moreover, it may assist the nursing associate in what to anticipate and even in detecting small changes in the patient's condition (Kitson et al. 2013; Feo et al. 2017).

Orange Flag

The nursing associates has to be physically and mentally present in all interactions. This requires skill and attention to self and others as well as the environment.

The nursing associate should strive for conditions that support and promote privacy in nurse–patient encounters and a working environment that acknowledges the important contribution of the nursing associate's focus on the patient. This can be achieved, for example, by having guidelines or recommendations for disturbance during the nurse–patient encounter and having interior design that promotes and enables the nursing associates to place themselves face to face with the patient (Leary et al. 2014).

Gathering information about the patient's needs occurs by visual cues, such as by observing, for example, during an assessment on admission to the ward, the nursing associate might note how the patient is engaging in conversation: are they focused or do they have expression of concern or worry? Another contribution comes from listening to the words that are spoken, pauses and the strength of the patient's voice. Physical touch provides information through the patient's reactions and serves to communicate information about their condition (Koutsopoulou et al. 2010). Getting to know the patient is a continuous process that does not stop, even when verbal communication is impossible due to the nature of a procedure (Kitson et al. 2013).

Red Flag

When the nursing associates gather information regarding the needs of the patient, they need to observe and take note of how the patient is engaging in conversation, determine if the patient is focused or is there and expression of concern or worry? Take note of words expressed, silences as well as the strength of the patient's voice.

The nurse–patient interactions and conversations should serve to help the nursing associate identify and address any of the patient's needs. The nursing associates should draw on the knowledge they obtain of the patients' feelings of nervousness/anxiety and their desire to maintain aspects of control. Because using this knowledge as a starting point may help them to foresee, understand and read patients' reactions and responses to the situation, it can also help them to individualise nursing care (Bundgaard et al. 2012). If open to it, the patient's response may instantly guide the nursing associate's course of action.

In every encounter, the nursing associate continuously responds to the patient's reactions and decides which course of action will best help guide the patient. These decisions are built on the nursing associate's general knowledge of typical reactions of patients who have undergone similar medical procedures and on knowledge of the individual patient in each situation (see Table 6.2).

Within the clinical setting, nursing associates have several key information sources that they can use to support knowing the patient (Pearson 2013). In addition to verbal interactions with the patient and family, nursing associates also obtain information through verbal interactions with other members of the healthcare team. Components of the patient's medical record are also sources of patient information, and nursing associates use nursing documentation as the primary mechanism to collect and communicate patient information. Interestingly, Olsen et al. (2013) discussed the importance of medical record documents for knowing the patient but found that nurses had limited time to refer back to the documents for information, indicating this was a barrier to gathering clinical information.

Take Note

Skills the nursing associate can use to gather information:

- Get to know the patient and be focused
- Gather clues and be observant for cues
- Establish a rapport and demonstrate empathy
- Gain trust and be non-judgemental
- Determine the patients' readiness to learn and their aspirations?
- Learn the patient's perspective and their concerns
- Ask the right questions
- Learn about the patient's skills and what does the patient already know?
- Involve and collaborate with others

Table 6.2 Skills to enhance information gathering.

NEED	SKILLS
Get to know the patient	• Introduce yourself and explain your role in the delivery of their care • Refer to #hellomynameis campaign • Utilise documentation including healthcare records • Observing the patient both physically and psychologically • Remember this is a continuous process • Demonstrate self and emotional awareness • Be attentive to every sign or signal from the patient • Transform the information gathered
Gather clues	Talk to the healthcare team members and observe the patient • Be careful not to make assumptions • Talk to the patient • Observe the patient's actions • Tuning into and picking up on patient cues • Take care not to misinterpret patients' reaction • Read and interrupt the patient's non-verbal cues
Establish a rapport	Make eye contact when appropriate, helping the patient to feel comfortable with you Notice and acknowledge the patient Actively listen to the patient's thoughts, feelings and concerns (and their families) • Undertake a comprehensive assessment • Recall something the patient has already told you about himself/herself Talk to the patient little and often depending on their need Demonstrate empathy • Evaluate and review progress of the nurse–patient relationship • Remain attentive • Appropriate use of physical touch
Gain trust	Show respect and treat each patient with compassion Remain non-judgemental Offer explanations using terminology that the patient understands • Paraphrase what the patient has told so that you acknowledge what has been said • Be receptive and responsive to patients' non-verbal communication Display high standard of professional knowledge, self-confidence and concern to gain the patients' trust Show concern Act as the patients' advocate
Determine the patient's readiness to learn	• Ask the patient about their goals, attitudes and motivations
Learn the patient's perspective	• Talk to the patient about worries, fears and possible misconceptions
Ask the right questions	• Use open-ended questions that require the patient to reveal more details • Listen carefully • The patient's answers will help you learn their core beliefs
Learn about the patient's skills	• Find out what the patient already knows and build on this knowledge
Involve others	Identify the significant people in the patients' life Identify what support they have and what they might need Collaborate with other healthcare professionals as needed

Gathering Credible Literature

Evidenced-based practice is reflected in and underpins the proficiencies for nursing associates (Nursing & Midwifery Council 2018). Within this chapter, it has previously been acknowledged that research in clinical practice allows the nursing associate to acquire both objective and subjective information regarding the patients' condition and their experiences of living with it. Gathering this type of information will guide and enhance what is gathered through the therapeutic nurse–patient relationship. While research plays an important factor in supporting the decision-making process without acknowledging the credibility of the research, the question of whether the findings can be trusted needs to be addressed. Two ways to determine this refer to critical appraisal and hierarchy of evidence.

Poorly conducted research seriously compromises the integrity of the research process; therefore, critical appraisal of the quality of clinical research is central to inform decision-making in healthcare. Critical appraisal is the process of carefully and systematically examining research evidence to judge its trustworthiness, its value and relevance in a particular context (Caldwell et al. 2011). It allows clinicians to use research

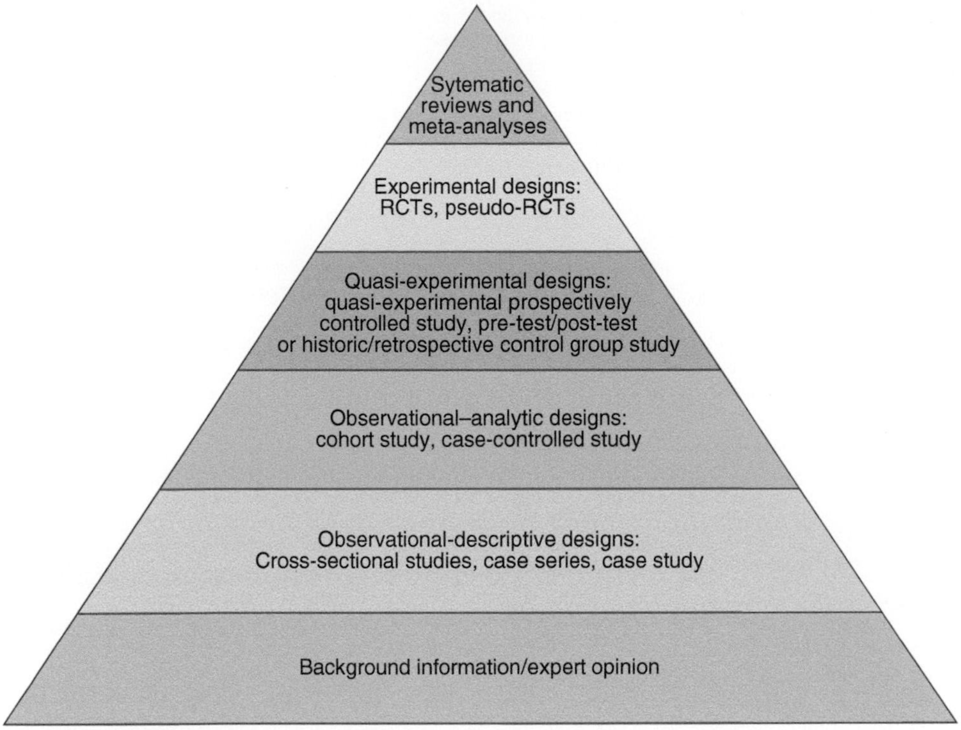

Figure 6.1 Hierarchy of evidence. ***Source:*** **Based on Evans (2003).**

evidence reliably and efficiently. Critical appraisal is intended to enhance the healthcare professionals' skill to determine whether the research evidence is true and relevant to their patients (Burls 2009). Critiquing tools such as Caldwell et al.'s (2011) Critical Appraisal Skills Programme (2011) and Joanna Briggs Institute's Critical appraisal tools (2017) are commonly used within nursing to critically appraise research.

Particularly, in medicine, there is a requirement to seek the best available evidence, and in order to understand this, knowledge of the hierarchy of evidence is required. Figure 6.1 illustrates how the hierarchy of evidence refers to a ranking system whereby a range of different methodologies are graded according to the validity of their findings (Evans 2003).

A number of hierarchies of evidence have been developed to enable different research methods to be ranked according to the validity of their findings. However, most have focused on the evaluation of the effectiveness of interventions.

Conclusion

This chapter has considered the importance of gathering relevant information so as to ensure the delivery of evidence-based patient-centred care. The therapeutic nurse–patient relationship has been acknowledged, indicating this is pivotal to patient-centred care. It has been acknowledged that the nursing associate will gather information to inform nursing practice from a variety of sources; however, it would seem that the effectiveness of this information gathering is somewhat reliant on the emotional intelligence skills of the nursing associate as well as underpinning an appreciation of the research process. Previous experience and expertise appear to develop these skills, as the less experienced nursing associate may not be as in tune with the patient in order to pick up the non-verbal cues of the patient, having not been exposed to similar clinical situations previously.

References

Benner, P. (1984) *Novice to expert: excellence and power in clinical nursing practice*, California: Addison Wesley.

Bundgaard, K., Nielson, K.B., Delmar, C. and Sørensen, E.E. (2012) What to know and how to get to know? A fieldwork study outlining the understanding of knowing the patient in facilities for short term care, *Journal of Advanced Nursing*, 68(10): 2280–2288.

Burls, A. (2009) *What is critical appraisal?*, Oxford, UK: University of Oxford.

Caldwell, K., Henshaw, L. and Taylor, G. (2011) Developing a framework for critiquing health research: an early evaluation, *Nurse Education Today*, 31(8): e1–e7. doi: 0.1016/j.nedt.2010.11.025.

Carper, B. (1978) Fundamental patterns of knowing in nursing, *Advances in Nursing Science*, 1(1): 13–23.

Currid, T. and Pennington, J. (2010) Continuing professional development: therapeutic use of self, *British Journal of Wellbeing*, 1(3): 35–42.

den Hertog, R. and Niessen, T. (2019) The role of patient preferences in nursing decision-making in evidence-based practice: excellent nurses communication tools, *Journal of Advanced Nursing*, 75(9): 1987–1995. doi: 10.1111/jan.14083.

Dewing, J., McCormack, B. and Titchen, A. (2014) *Practice development workbook: for nursing, health and social care*, Hoboken, NJ: Wiley Blackwell, Chapter 2.
Eraut, M. (2000) Non-formal learning and tacit knowledge in professional work. *British Journal of Educational Psychology*, 70: 113–136.
Evans, D. (2003) Hierarchy of evidence: a framework for ranking evidence evaluating healthcare interventions, *Journal of Clinical Nursing*, 12(1): 77–84. doi: 10.1046/j.1365-2702.2003.00662.x.
Feo, R., Conroy, T., Marshall, RJ., Rasmussen, P., Wiechula, R. and Kitson, AL. (2017) Using holistic interpretive synthesis to create practice relevant guidance for person-centred fundamental care delivered by nurses, *Nursing Inquiry*, 24(2): e121152. doi: 10.111/nin.12152.
Feo, R., Rasmussen, P., Wiechula, R., Conroy, T. and Kitson, A. (2016) Developing effective and caring nurse-patient relationships, *Nursing Standard*, 31(28): 54–63. doi: 10.778/ns.2017.e.10735.
Freshwater, D. (2007) The therapeutic use of self, in Freshwater, D. (ed.), *Therapeutic nursing: improving patient care through self-awareness and reflection*, London: Sage.
Freshwater, D. and Stickley, T. (2004) The heart of the art: emotional intelligence in nurse education. *Nursing Inquiry*, 11(2): 91–98.
Gobet, F. and Chassy, P. (2008) Towards an alternative to Benner's theory of expert intuition in nursing: a discussion paper, *International Journal of Nursing Studies*, 45(1): 129–139.
Health Education England. (2019) *Nursing associate and new support role in health care*, Health Education England. [online] Available: https://www.hee.nhs.uk/our-work/nursing-associates. Accessed September 2019.
James, I., Andershed, B., Gustavsson, B. and Ternestedt, B.-M. (2010) Emotional knowing in nursing practice: in the encounter between life and death, *International Journal of Qualitative Studies of Health and Well-being*, 5(5367): 1–15.
Johns, C. (2000) *Becoming a reflective practitioner*, London: Blackwell Science Ltd.
Kitson, A., Harvey, G. and McCormack, B. (1998) Enabling the implementation of evidence based practice: a conceptual framework. *Quality in Healthcare*, 7: 149–158.
Koutsopoulou, S., Papathanassoglou, E.D.E., Katapodi, M.C. and Patiraki, E.I. (2010) A critical review of the evidence for nurses as information providers to cancer patients, *Journal of Clinical Nursing*, 19(5–6): 749–765.
Leary, A., White, J. and Yarnell, L. (2014) The work left undone. Understanding the challenge of providing holistic lung cancer nursing care in the UK, *European Journal of Oncology Nursing*, 18(1): 23–28.
Mayer, J.D. and Salovey, P. (1997) What is emotional intelligence? in Salovey, P. & Sluyter, D.J. (eds.) *Emotional development and emotional intelligence. Educational implications*. New York, NY: Basic Books, 3–34.
Mayer, J.D., Salovey, P., Caruso, D.R. and Sitarenious, G. (2001) Emotional intelligence as a standard intelligence, *Emotion*, 3(1): 232–242.
McCormack, B. and McCance, T. (2010) *Person-centred nursing: theory and practice*, London: Wiley.
Mirhaghi, A., Sharafi, S., Bazzi, A. and Hasanzadeh, F. (2017) Therapeutic relationship: is it still heart of nursing? *Nursing Reports*, 7(1). doi: 10.4081/nursep.2017.6129.
Morley, D. (2016) Applying Wenger's communities of practice theory to placement learning, *Nurse Education Today*, 39: 161–162.
Nursing & Midwifery Council. (2018a) *Standards of proficiency for nursing associates*. [online] Available: https://www.nmc.org.uk. Accessed October 2019.
Nursing & Midwifery Council. (2018b) *Code professional standards of practice and behaviour for nurses, midwives and nursing associates*. [online] Available: https://www.nmc.org.uk/globalassets/sitedocuments/nmc-publications/nmc-code.pdf. Accessed December 2019.
Olsen, R.M., Østnor, B.H., Enmarker, I. and Hellzén, O. (2013) Barriers to information exchange during older patients' transfer: nurses' experiences, *Journal of Clinical Nursing*, 22(19–20): 2964–2973.
Östman, L., Näsman, Y., Eriksson, K. and Nyström, L. (2019) Ethos: the heart of ethics and health, *Nursing Ethics*, 26(1): 26–36.
Pearson, H. (2013) Science and intuition: do both have a place in clinical decision making? *British Journal of Nursing*, 22(4): 212–215.
Rolston, E.J., Karsten, K., Auditore, A., Gimber, P. and McMillan-Coddington, D. (2016) Transforming the clinical experience for associate degree nursing students, *Teaching and Learning in Nursing*, 12(1): 35–38. doi: 10/1016/j.teln.2016.08.007.
Schön, D. (1983) *The reflective practitioner: how professionals think in action*, Aldershot: Arena.
Stevens, S. (2018) Ways of knowing and unknowing in psychotherapy and clinical practice, *Journal of Trauma and Treatment*, 7(1): 418. doi: 10.4172/2167-1222.1000418.
Swanson, K.M. (1991) Empirical development of a middle range theory of caring, *Nursing Research*, 40(3): 161–166.
Watson, J. (1985) *The philosophy and science of caring: an essential resource*, Colorado, USA: Colorado Association.
Wiechula, R., Conroy, T., Kitson, A.L., Marshall, R.J., Whitaker, N. and Rasmussen, P. (2016) Umbrella review of the evidence: what factors influence the caring relationship between a nurse and patient? *Journal of Advanced Nursing*, 72(4): 723–734. doi: 10.1111/jan.12862.
Williams, B. (2015) Enhancing teaching relationships through therapeutic use of self, *The Journal of Mental Health Training, Education and Practice*, 10(1): 61–70. doi: 10.1108/jmhtep-04-2014-008.

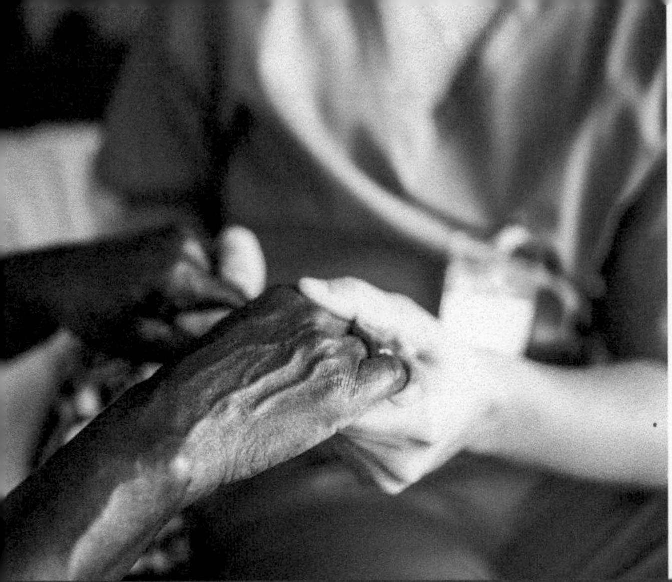

7

Escalating Concerns

Tom Walvin

University of Plymouth, UK

Chapter Aim

- **The aim of this chapter is to introduce the reader to the methods that may be used when escalating concerns about a patient.**

Learning Outcomes

By the end of this chapter, the reader will be able to:

- **Describe the role of the nursing associate in escalating concerns about a patient**
- **Use a structured method to escalate concerns**
- **Discuss the challenges of communication when escalating concerns about a patient**

Test Yourself Multiple Choice Questions

1. **What does 'SBAR' stand for?**
   A) **Situation, Background, Assessment, Reaction**
   B) **Safety, Background, Assessment, Ring for Help**
   C) **Scene, Background, Assessment, Respond**
   D) **Situation, Background, Assessment, Recommendation**
2. **In an acute hospital in the United Kingdom, which number can be called to summon emergency medical help for a patient?**
   A) **9999**
   B) **2222**
   C) **999**
   D) **3333**

The Nursing Associate's Handbook of Clinical Skills, First Edition. Edited by Ian Peate.

Companion website: www.wiley.com/nursingassociate

3. If concerned about a patient after completing an assessment, which healthcare professional could the nursing associate first escalate concerns to for clinical decision-making and advice?
A) Junior doctor
B) Speciality registrar
C) Registered nurse
D) Continue to manage the patient yourself

4. What does ABCDE stand for in the context of deteriorating patient care?
A) Airway, Breathing, Circulation, Deformity, Escalate
B) Airway, Breathing, Circulation, Disability, Escalate
C) Airway, Breathing, Circulation, Deformity, Examine
D) Airway, Breathing, Circulation, Disability, Exposure

5. Where can *detailed* information about the patient's admission assessment, tests and initial diagnosis be found?
A) Medical notes
B) Nursing handover sheet
C) Nursing care record summary
D) Ambulance clinical record

Introduction

The Nursing and Midwifery Council (NMC) educational standards require nursing associates to both understand how to escalate concerns to other appropriate healthcare professionals for expert help and how to recognise when a person's health has deteriorated and escalate as needed (Nursing & Midwifery Council 2018a).

This chapter will develop understanding of both of these by introducing different methods for escalating concerns about patients, discussing how to escalate effectively and describing the pitfalls in communication so that these can be avoided. The NMC Code (Nursing & Midwifery Council 2018b) also contains requirements with regards to deteriorating patients and escalation. The nursing associate is required to maintain effective communication with colleagues, to make a timely referral to another practitioner when any action, care or treatment is required and to arrange, wherever possible, for emergency care to be accessed and provided promptly.

Green Flag

The NMC Code contains requirement which are relevant to escalating concerns:

- 8.1 Respect the skills, expertise and contributions of your colleagues, referring matters to them where appropriate
- 13.2 Make a timely referral to another practitioner when any action, care or treatment is required
- 13.3 Ask for help from an appropriately qualified and experienced professional to carry out any action or procedure which is beyond the limits of your competence
- 15.2 Arrange, wherever possible, for emergency care to be accessed and provided promptly

The most common root cause of serious errors clinically and organisationally is related to inadequate verbal and written communication. The Institute for Innovation and Improvement (2010) notes that there are some important barriers to communication that occur across different disciplines and levels of staff. These barriers include:

- Hierarchy
- Gender
- Ethnic background
- Differences in communication styles between disciplines and individuals

Communication is more effective (and therefore patient safety) in teams where there are standard communication structures in place; Situation, Background, Assessment, Recommendation (SBAR) and Reason, Story, Vital Signs, Plan (RSVP) are examples of these standard communication structures.

Assessment and Planning Ahead

Healthcare professionals face constantly changing priorities. Consequently, when escalating a concern about a patient's health, it is important to consider carefully the information that needs to be given and how that information can be structured into a format which conveys the intended message: that the patient needs the immediate attention of the person receiving the escalation.

It is known that 'handover' of information is often cognitively taxing and complex due to the amount of information and data that is known about the patient. This can lead to handovers which are unclear or miscommunicate the nursing associate's desired outcome for the patient (Hill & Nyce 2010).

It is therefore important that when escalating concerns, the handover is planned and prepared. The focus should be on giving the essential information required to prompt the desired response and omit unnecessary information which may distract or overload the decision-making of the recipient.

In a situation where taking a few moments to plan the escalation is not possible, it is likely that the patient requires a more immediate response where a structured communication tool is not immediately required to get help. Within an acute hospital in the United Kingdom, this will be by summoning the medical emergency team (MET) or a cardiac arrest team by calling 2222. In the patient's own homes, general practitioner (GP) surgeries and non-acute or community hospitals, calling 999 for an ambulance is normally required.

There are two main structures which are recommended for escalating patient care (see Table 7.1). These are the SBAR or RSVP tools.

SBAR:	RSVP:
Situation	**R**eason
Background	**S**tory
Assessment	**V**ital Signs
Recommendation	**P**lan

Source: Resuscitation Council UK (2015).

The understanding of each term and examples of how to use each are found later in the chapter.

Planning your escalation and using one of the escalation tools are essential for ensuring an effective handover of patient information and concerns; reviewing all the information known about the patient by looking at the medical and nursing notes will enable you to plan each section of the escalation tool. It is likely that the reason escalation is required is because an assessment of the patient has already been completed; if not, utilising an Airway, Breathing, Circulation, Disability, Exposure (ABCDE) assessment will enable a systematic assessment of the patient and obtains the most up-to-date information about the patient's vital signs and clinical presentation.

Red Flag

Airway
Breathing
Circulation
Disability
Exposure

The ABCDE assessment is a systematic assessment of the body systems. The systematic approach ensures that all body systems are assessed in decreasing importance to the patient's deterioration. An intervention is required for each abnormal finding before moving onto the next element.

Completing an ABCDE assessment enables the practitioner to complete a comprehensive assessment of not only the clinical observations but also the signs and symptoms which can be found using:

- Look
- Listen
- Feel

A great deal of patient information is held and should be used as a part of the patient assessment, as well as planning for escalation:

- The medical notes – Inpatients in hospitals are 'clerked' at their start of their admission to hospital. This is where the admitting doctors (or other admitting clinicians) write information obtained from their first assessment of the patient, such as initial presentation, investigation findings and provisional diagnoses. The clerking is particularly useful as it will list the patient's past medical history, their medications at the time of arrival, allergies, a social history and other information which may be useful. Review the last few entries from ward rounds and other visits from other healthcare professionals – what is the patient's current condition? What plan of treatment is currently in place for this patient?
- The observation and fluid chart – The trend of the patient's observations is just as important as the latest single set of observations. Has the patient been declining slowly or has there been a sudden deterioration in their vital signs? Has there been any change in their urine output?

Orange Flag

Observations charts may not include neurological changes in observations. Be aware that new confusion, drowsiness or being unresponsive is indicative of patient deterioration and should be escalated quickly.

- The drug chart (prescription chart) – Review the medications that the patient has been receiving. Are any of these related to the concern you have about the patient? If so, this should be mentioned in the escalation.

- The nursing assessment – An essential source of information about the patient's past medical history, current diagnosis, allergies, nursing requirements and often patient preferences or concerns.
- Your assessment of the patient – Think about not only the clinical observations but what the patient looks like, sounds like, feels like and smells like. Sometimes, a patient can appear well in terms of their clinical observations but look very unwell. Signs and symptoms can often be more telling of deterioration than the clinical observations on their own.

Take Note

Clinical observations refer to the recording of the patient respiratory rate, pulse rate, blood pressure, oxygen saturations, temperature, blood glucose and level of consciousness. These are colloquially known as 'vital signs'.

- Resuscitation form/treatment escalation plan (TEP) – These documents will detail the decision-making regarding the appropriateness of resuscitation for a patient or the maximum ceiling of intervention that a patient may receive and thus should be considered as a part of escalation and communicated to the recipient.

Take Note

Planning your escalation is important to ensure that the information given during escalation is relevant and concise and prompts the receiver of the escalation to act immediately.

SBAR – A Structured Communication Tool

The SBAR method was originally designed as a communication tool by the US Navy, ensuring that important communications were concise and focused (Stonehouse 2019); this is the cornerstone of good patient escalation.

Randmaa et al. (2014) and Müller et al. (2018) demonstrated that the use of the SBAR method for handover improved escalation communication and patient safety. The SBAR method is now a well-known communication tool between healthcare professionals, ensuring that the person receiving the escalation is familiar with the structure of information being given; it improves accuracy and efficiency of handover which is important in cases of escalation of deteriorating patients.

The SBAR tool increases confidence of the speaker which in turn obtains the confidence of the healthcare professional receiving the escalation in the person giving it (Stewart & Hand 2017).

In Table 7.1, the elements of a complete handover are provided.

With regards to Table 7.1, this must also be documented, and the nursing associate must adhere to local policy and procedure.

Blue Flag

The 'Hello my name is. . . .' campaign, introduced by Dr Kate Grainger, encourages all staff, irrespective of their role, to introduce themselves when they are with patients and visitors. By simply introducing yourself with 'Hello my name is . . . .' is a simple gesture that can go a long way to helping reduce patient's anxiety.

Take Note

It is important to remember that all elements of the SBAR must be communicated. Consequently, an assessment must have taken place, and the person escalating must have knowledge of the situation and background of the patient before calling.

Touch Points

The prevailing gold standard handover structure, Situation, Background, Assessment, Recommendation (SBAR), was originally developed and effectively used by the US Navy.

The SBAR Communication Technique:

Situation: What is the situation; why are you calling the physician?
Background: What is the background information?
Assessment: What is your assessment of the problem?
Recommendation: How should the problem be corrected?

In a healthcare setting, the SBAR protocol is used as a framework for structuring conversations between healthcare professionals with the intent of improving communication in various care situations.

The SBAR is a reliable and validated communication tool and has been implemented in a hospital-based practice for sharing information among healthcare providers. For the tool to be used effectively, it does however require training (initial and ongoing) for all clinical staff to

Table 7.1 The elements of a complete handover.

SBAR ELEMENT	ACTIONS	EXAMPLE
Situation	Firstly identify yourself, your role and your location. Confirm the identity of the person you are handing over to. Explain the reason for your phone call and the immediate situation.	'My name is Renu Gupta; I'm a nursing associate on Ward 1. I'm calling about a patient who is experiencing chest pain currently'.
Background	State who the patient is, their age and other relevant identity information. Describe the reasons for their admission, the current medical and treatment plans, relevant past medical history, relevant medications, allergies, if relevant, and any other medical or nursing information that you consider important.	'I'm calling about Jane Doe, aged 85. She was admitted with chest pain two days ago and was diagnosed as having a non-ST elevation myocardial infarction in the emergency department with a raised troponin test, and she is currently awaiting an inpatient angiogram. She has hypertension and angina'.
Assessment	Give the findings of your assessment of the patient. You may find it helpful to use the ABCDE structure (see Red Flag, p. 55). Include observations which are abnormal or trends that are concerning and give the overall NEWS score afterward describing the observations. Do not forget to give non-numerical information such as the how the patient looks, how they feel and what they feel like to touch and other senses.	The chest pain started 10 minutes ago; she describes it as a crushing pain radiating to the left arm. She appears pale, and her skin is clammy. She is tachypnoeic with a respiration rate of 28, tachycardic with a heart rate of 112 and has a weak palpable radial pulse. She is hypotensive with a blood pressure of 92/56. Her total NEWS score is 7. We have performed a 12-lead electrocardiogram (ECG) which needs assessment.
Recommendation	This is where you explain your desired outcome and in many escalation situations will be focused on asking the other healthcare professional to attend and assess your patient, but you may have other requests in other situations that SBAR is useful for. Set boundaries and expectations to be met. Be courteous.	I would like you to come and assess this deteriorating patient immediately please.

ensure that communication is well understood. There is a lack of high-quality research on this widely used communication tool, and continued research is necessary to demonstrate the efficacy of applying SBAR in care areas.

RSVP

The RSVP escalation method was initially introduced by the Acute Life-threatening Events – Recognition and Treatment (ALERT) course (Featherstone et al. 2008). Table 7.2 provides an overview of the RSVP escalation method.

With regards to the discussion in Table 7.2, this must also be documented, and the nursing associate must adhere to local policy and procedure.

Touch Point

There are some differences between the SBAR and RSVP tool. Many organisations will instruct clinical staff on which one to use within the organisation. It is important, however, to remember that whichever tool you use, its purpose is planning and delivering escalation effectively and advocating for your patient's need for immediate help.

Who to Escalate To?

The routes of escalation will vary depending on your workplace, internal protocols and policies. Routes to escalation may change throughout the 24-hour shift. A list of options is provided, but you must familiarise yourself with the options available in your clinical area.

Yellow Flag

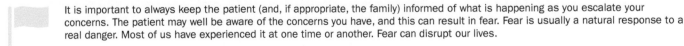

It is important to always keep the patient (and, if appropriate, the family) informed of what is happening as you escalate your concerns. The patient may well be aware of the concerns you have, and this can result in fear. Fear is usually a natural response to a real danger. Most of us have experienced it at one time or another. Fear can disrupt our lives.

Table 7.2 **An overview of the RSVP escalation method.**

RSVP ELEMENT	ACTIONS	EXAMPLE
Reason	State your name and role and confirm who you are talking to. Give the patient's name and location. Give the reason for the call.	My name is Janusz Nowak; I'm a nursing associate. I'm calling about a patient, Jane Doe, on Ward 1, who is experiencing chest pain currently.
Story	Give the background information about the patient, reason for admission, relevant past medical history and resuscitation status.	Jane is an 85-year-old female admitted two days ago with raised troponin test leading to a diagnosis of non-ST elevation myocardial infarction. She is awaiting an inpatient angiogram. Her past medical history is hypertension and angina. Her resuscitation status was assessed yesterday and she is for resuscitation.
Vital Signs	Give abnormal vital signs as well as sign/symptoms and a description of your visual assessment of the patient.	She appears pale and her skin is clammy. She is tachypnoeic with a respiration rate of 28, tachycardic with a heart rate of 112, with a weak, palpable radial pulse. She is hypotensive with a blood pressure of 92/56. All other observations are within normal parameters. Her total NEWS score is 7.
Plan	Give your current plan and ask for a further plan from the recipient. Ask now for anything you want them to do.	We are going to connect to a monitor and complete serial ECGs. Please come and assess this patient immediately.

Registered Nurse

A registered nurse is a healthcare professional who has expertise in the delivery of professional nursing care to patients. It is important to remember that registered nurses possess a number of assessment, evaluation and clinical decision-making skills as well as specific knowledge of disease pathology, pharmacology/medicines management and non-medical treatments and therapies within the context of compassionate and caring nursing skills.

Registered nurses also maintain accountability for patients under their care, and consequently, a registered nurse should be notified of your assessment of the patient.

The registered nurse may have the ability to manage a patient by putting into place a plan of care which may not necessarily require the patient to be escalated to a physician or other healthcare professional. Registered nurses may have significant experience in the specialism and have developed additional specialist skills and knowledge; they may have access to patient group directives or be non-medical prescribers, allowing them to administer medications without a direct prescription and as such, and they can be consulted for advice and intervention.

Nurse Practitioners (NPs)/Advanced Clinical Practitioners (ACPs)

These are registered nurses and sometimes practitioners from other healthcare professions who have advanced training, skills and knowledge which may overlap that of medical practitioners. NPs and ACPs may be able to provide advice, intervene and provide monitoring beyond that of other registered nurses and healthcare professionals.

Foundation Year 1 (FY1) and Foundation Year 2 (FY2) Doctors

FY1 doctors are 'newly qualified' doctors undergoing a pre-registration year of experience under very close supervision of a consultant or GP. FY2 doctors have completed the FY1 year and have obtained full registration as a doctor but remain under the supervision of a consultant. When working in a hospital, these are often the first point of contact for concerns about patients.

Core Trainee Or Specialist Trainee Doctors

These are doctors who have completed their foundation training and are now developing in their specialist field of medicine. These doctors are more experienced, and in the later years of training, they are often still referred to as an older term 'Specialist Registrars', meaning they are in the final stages of their training to become a consultant.

Consultant

A consultant is a doctor who has completed speciality training in their specialist medical field. It is rare that consultants provide immediate response to patient concerns; but many are approachable and will often be contacted by more junior doctors for advice and guidance.

Critical Care Outreach Team

Acute hospitals may have a critical care outreach team comprised normally of registered nurses (and sometimes other roles) with significant clinical experience in intensive care or the emergency department and therefore expert at assessing, monitoring and treating unwell and deteriorating patients.

Critical care outreach teams may also provide ongoing monitoring for unwell patients on wards and provide advice and support to nursing and medical staff.

Outreach teams may also carry out other technical roles too, for example, monitoring patient-controlled analgesia.

Medical Emergency Team (MET)/Crash Team

A medical emergency team (MET) or 'Crash Team' can be contacted on 2222 in an emergency in an acute hospital in the United Kingdom. This team comprises selected on-call clinicians normally from the on-call medical team, intensive care teams and critical care outreach teams who respond when called to a medical emergency. The Crash Team is also summoned by calling 2222 and is normally the same clinicians from the MET, although other staff such as resuscitation officers and anaesthetists may also respond to a crash call.

999 Emergency Services

In patient homes, GP surgeries, community hospitals and other community settings, the most appropriate response to a deteriorating patient is the ambulance service; within the United Kingdom, an emergency ambulance is arranged by calling 999.

The first person you speak to will be an operator who will ask you which emergency service you require and will connect you to the ambulance service when asked to. The next person you speak to will be an ambulance service call taker who is not a healthcare professional; therefore, it is important to give clear information about the patient, and this will enable them to complete a triage pathway and arrange the most appropriate response.

They will ask you a set of questions from a protocol which you must answer, even if they seem inappropriate, given your professional role. On arrival of the ambulance, you will normally handover to a clinician such as a paramedic, emergency care practitioner, ambulance technician or registered nurse all of whom have expertise in the management of unwell patients.

Violet Flag

The task of passing on important information related to an escalation of concern occurs in every care setting and between care settings (transfers of care) every day, for example, in a person's own home, the back of ambulances when transferring a patient for place of detention a hospital, community clinics, GP surgeries, to name a few. It is just as important in any of these care settings to ensure that the handover, the escalation of concern, is timely and performed in a systematic manner.

In acute and community inpatient hospitals in the United Kingdom, the use of the National Early Warning Score (NEWS) is now embedded into policies regarding identifying and escalating concerns about patient's clinical observations, with a scoring system used to identify who should be contacted to provide further assessment of the patient. NEWS is discussed later in the chapter.

Challenges of Communication

Patient safety is a key priority in patient care, and communication errors are the most common cause of adverse events during episodes of patient care. Nursing associates and other healthcare providers endeavour to avoid communication errors during patient handover. SBAR and RSVP communication tools can reduce adverse events in a hospital setting.

Loss of information in verbal handover between different staff groups is known to be a contributing factor in clinical incidents (Rabøl et al. 2011; Müller et al. 2018), and consequently, the development and use of escalation tools allow us to reduce the chance of error by utilising a standardised approach across all professions.

Poor communication is identified as being a factor in 35% of hospital complaints; noted particularly is the quality and accuracy of the information (Ford 2015). The quality and accuracy of information is very much determined by the person escalating concerns; therefore, utilising the earlier suggestions to prepare the handover beforehand and utilising a 'template form' or SBAR stickers (often required by some National Health Service (NHS) Trusts) can help increase the likelihood of good communication.

Delayed communication of escalation concerns has previously been a concern and is regarded as being just as serious as other failures of communication (Taran 2011). The development of the NEWS system indicates where patient observations are abnormal and prompts the need to escalate concerns; however, the clinical judgement remains paramount in regards to timely escalation and prioritising it above other conflicting care activities.

Touch Point

The NEWS was introduced around 2007, in recognition of episodes of failed care where healthcare professionals had not recognised or failed to escalate patient deterioration, or did not escalate appropriately.

The NEWS attributes point to each observation taken and collectively gives an indication of the patient's deterioration. The total score then identifies the type and route of escalation required (National Patient Safety Agency 2007). This is often embedded and adapted to fit with the hospital's policy and available staff and teams to escalate to.

It is important to remember that this a 'safety net' tool. It is not necessary to wait for a 'trigger' to escalate when concern about a patient is justified by assessment and clinical decision-making.

NEWS is becoming more popular outside of hospital environments, with adaptations starting to arise in nursing homes, GP surgeries and ambulance services. The evidence-base underpinning NEWS was developed in and for inpatient hospitals; therefore, further research is required to build evidence-base in using NEWS outside of a hospital environment.

Supporting Evidence

The following references supported the fundamental changes to the NHS approach to deteriorating patient care:

National Institute for Health and Care Excellence (2007) *Acutely Ill Adults: Recognising and Responding to Deterioration*. National Institute for Health and Care Excellence, London.

National Patient Safety Agency (2007) *Recognising and responding appropriately to early signs of deterioration in hospitalised patients*, London: National Patient Safety Agency.

Royal College of Physicians (2017) *National early warning score (NEWS) 2: standardising the assessment of acute-illness severity in the NHS*, London: Royal College of Physicians.

Conclusion

SBAR and RSVP are tools that can be used to communicate or escalate concerns about a patient's health. Continuity of patient care is achieved by the clear and concise transfer of patient clinical information from one healthcare provider to another during handover.

Effective communication is key in providing safe patient care. Communication failure in a healthcare setting has the potential to lead to serious medical errors.

Sharing patient-specific healthcare information during handover requires situational awareness. In the hospital setting, most of the communication related to patient care occurs between nurses and physicians.

References

Featherstone, P., Chalmers, T. and Smith, G. (2008) RSVP: a system for communication of deterioration in hospital patients, *British Journal of Nursing*, 17(8): 860–864.

Ford, S. (2015) *Communication errors behind third of hospital complaints*. [online] Available: https://www.nursingtimes.net/roles/nurse-managers/communication-errors-behind-third-of-hospital-complaints-22-09-2015/. Accessed 2 October 2019.

Hill, W. and Nyce, J. (2010) Human factors in clinical shift handover communication, *Canadian Journal of Respiratory Therapy*, 46(1): 44–51.

Institute for Innovation and Improvement. (2010) *Safer care SBAR implementation and training guide*, Coventry: Institute for Innovation and Improvement.

Müller, M., Jürgens, J., Redaèlli, M., Klingberg, K., Hautz, W. and Stock, S. (2018) Impact of the communication and patient hand-off tool SBAR on patient safety: a systematic review, *BMJ Open*, 8(8): e022202.

National Patient Safety Agency. (2007) *Recognising and responding to early signs of deterioration in hospitalised patients*, London: The National Patient Safety Agency.

Rabøl, L., Andersen, M., Østergaard, D., Bjørn, B., Lilja, B. and Mogensen, T. (2011) Descriptions of verbal communication errors between staff. An analysis of 84 root cause analysis-reports from Danish hospitals, *BMJ Quality and Safety*, 2011(20): 268–274.

Randmaa, M., Mårtensson, G., Swenne, C. and Engström, M. (2014) SBAR improves communication and decreases incident reports due to communication errors in an anesthetic clinic: a prospective intervention study, *BMJ Open*, 4(1): e004268.

Resuscitation Council (UK). (2015) *Immediate life support*, London: Resuscitation Council UK.

Stewart, K. and Hand, K. (2017) SBAR, communication, and patient safety: an integrated literature review, *MedSurg Nursing*, 26(5): 297+.

Stonehouse, D. (2018) The SBAR communication framework: for when you need action, *British Journal of Healthcare Assistants*, 12(9): 450–453.

Taran, S. (2011) An examination of the factors contributing to poor communication outside the physician-patient sphere, *McGill Journal of Medicine*, 13(1): 86.

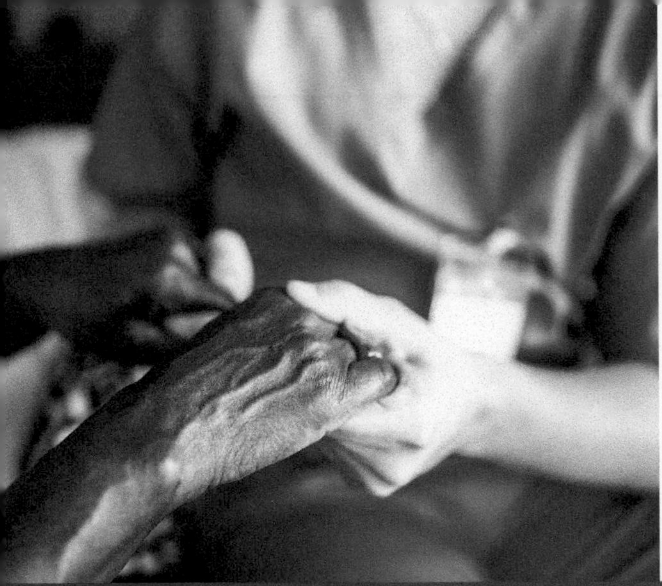

8

Written Communication

Stuart Baker

University of South Wales, UK

Chapter Aim

- The aim of this chapter is to support the readers in their understanding of their obligations when record-keeping.

Learning Outcomes

By the end of this chapter, the reader will be able to:

- Understand the purpose of records
- Have an understanding of the professional expectations on the practitioner with regards to record-keeping
- Understand the importance of maintaining clear and accurate records

Test Yourself Multiple Choice Questions

1. Who can access a health record?
   A) The patient, healthcare professionals and the police
   B) Lawyers, allied healthcare professionals and advocates
   C) Both A and B
2. Which of these pieces of legislation does not relate to record-keeping in health?
   A) The Communication in Nursing Act 2003
   B) Computer Misuse Act 1990
   C) Access to Health Records Act 1990
3. How does The Code (Nursing and Midwifery Council 2018a) relate to record-keeping?
   A) It underpins the need for records that are ambiguous and can hide multiple meanings
   B) It underpins the need for clear and accurate records
   C) It does not mention record-keeping at all

The Nursing Associate's Handbook of Clinical Skills, First Edition. Edited by Ian Peate.

Companion website: www.wiley.com/nursingassociate

4. **Is it important to sign a record, and if it is, then why is it?**
   A) It is not important, as everyone's handwriting is unique to them so it is easy to see who has made the record in question
   B) It is essential so that it is clear who has made a record
   C) It is not important as the off-duty records which staff are on duty at any time
5. **Which of these abbreviations could be confused as it could commonly have more than one meaning?**
   A) DOA
   B) NHS
   C) TPR

Introduction

The saying 'If it is not written it did not happen' has been the focus of record-keeping texts and lectures for many years. This simple statement contains many more complex truths that will be addressed throughout this chapter.

The Nursing and Midwifery Council (NMC) standards of proficiency (2018b) for nursing associates indicate that there are many aspects of communication that must be considered by the nursing associate, and this is explored within this chapter and other chapters of this text. This chapter explores the essential aspects of communication that pertain to the need to communicate both effectively and efficiently through written records and refers to the six platforms found within the Standards of Proficiency (2018b) as well as the NMC Code (2018a). This chapter explores the subject of record-keeping from both professional and legal viewpoints. A good starting point is to consider the purpose of a written record.

The Nursing and Midwifery Council (2018b) standards of proficiency for nursing associates represent the standards of knowledge and skills that a nursing associate must meet to be registered by the NMC as a safe and effective nursing associate. The following proficiencies apply to this chapter:

1.10 write accurate, clear, legible records and documentation
1.10 clearly record digital information and data
1.11 provide clear verbal, digital or written information and instructions when sharing information, delegating or handing over responsibility for care
1.14 demonstrate the ability to keep complete, clear, accurate and timely records
3.18 demonstrate the ability to monitor the effectiveness of care in partnership with people, families and carers. Document progress and report outcomes

The NMC updated its Code (Nursing and Midwifery Council 2018a) to ensure that nursing associates were also equally provided for by the NMC with a set of standards to ensure the protection of the public. In this chapter, this publication will be simply referred to as *The Code*.

The Written Record

A written record could be used for a number of purposes (examples of what may be considered as written records are listed in Box 8.1). Perhaps, the first thing that springs to mind is to record what has happened to a patient during a shift or care episode. This record needs to be of a certain standard which will be discussed later in this chapter. It could be reviewed firstly by colleagues using this as a means of communication to fully understand the events of the day when they are talking to the patient or relatives of the patient. It could be used in the same way by an allied health professional such as an occupational therapist who is treating the patient to have a better understanding of the patient's abilities and condition before providing treatment and care.

Patients can have access to their record by law (this will be discussed later), and this also puts a professional onus onto the nursing associate's record-keeping ability. Patients may want to see their records for clarification of the care that they have received or because they feel that there has been negligence; if they lack capacity according to the Mental Capacity Act (2005), they may have an advocate who can read their records so that they are in a better position to assist the multidisciplinary team to make decisions in the patients' best interest.

Box 8.1 Some Types of Record Used by the Nursing Associate

- Nursing assessment records
- Nursing care plans
- Observation charts
- Fluid balance charts
- Risk assessments
- Medication charts
- Incident forms
- Communication pages

Green Flag Legislation

Mental Capacity Act (2005)
This Act was created in 2005 to protect all adults who do not have the capacity to make decisions, either temporarily or more permanently. Capacity is decision specific and can relate to a small decision such as what colour dress to wear or a larger decision such as resuscitation in the event of death. A full description of the Mental Capacity Act (2005) can be found online.

The police may request access to a patient's notes in certain circumstances, and they may use a court order to do so. The person in charge of the patient's care is known as the 'data controller' and may share the records informally without the order being sought. Certainly, this applies where the access is in the public interest such as when a patient has a communicable disease and the public health department requires the police's assistance in finding a patient and preventing the transmission of the disease.

Finally, a solicitor or legal professional may request access to records. The records that they may request may be the medical records only, but they may also want to examine nursing records as well. Potentially, therefore, nursing records could be used in court of law.

Touch Point

There are a number of organisations and individuals that can access nursing and medical records. As nursing associates, it is necessary to ensure that all records that are made are in a format that can be followed and understood by others. The remainder of this chapter is dedicated to making record-keeping clear and compliant with policies and procedures.

Now that it has been established that a variety of people may access records for an equally varied number of reasons, the remainder of this chapter has been divided into two sections. First, the professional requirements from the NMC will be discussed in depth. The second part of this chapter includes a brief discussion on some legislative background to record-keeping.

Violet Flag

The records that the nursing associate writes (regardless of format) can be used by other agencies to help them make decisions regarding a person's needs, for example, the housing department and the local council. The housing department may request to see documentation regarding the patient's ability to carry out the activities of living (can they walk up a flight of stairs unaided), and the local council may use the data in the nursing associate's documentation to help determine if the person is entitled to certain benefits. By implementing the following, the nursing associate may be able to avoid issues related to record-keeping:

- Always use factual, reliable, accurate, objective and unambiguous patient information.
- Employ your senses in order to record what you did, for example, 'I heard', 'felt' and 'saw'.

Where necessary, use quotation marks when you are recording what has been said to you.

- Be sure there is evidence provided for any decision recorded, for example, denying access to a visit from parents.
- Notes must be accurately dated, timed and signed, with your name printed alongside the entry, and avoid the use of initials.
- Make a note of any objections you may have to the care that has been given.

Do not include jargon, meaningless phrases, such as 'patient had a good day', irrelevant speculation and offensive subjective statements.

- When writing notes, where this is possible, do so with the involvement and understanding of the patient or carer.

Professional Requirements

When considering record-keeping, it is important to start with the Nursing and Midwifery Council's (2018a) standards of proficiency for nursing associates that concludes that all nursing associates must keep clear and accurate records which are relevant to their practice, but while there is no specific professional document on keeping records, nursing associates must refer to The Code for guidance. Section 10 states that all nursing associates are to 'keep clear and accurate records that are relevant to your practice'. The Code reminds the nursing associate that this applies to all records that are kept as part of the nursing associate's role and is not limited to just patients' records. The Code then lists a number of practical actions in subsections of Section 10.

The first subsection clarifies that every record must be made in a timely manner and as soon after the event as possible. This reminds the nursing associate that, as often as possible, records must be made at the time an event happens or as soon after it happens as possible. This is for several reasons but primarily as a record made while the sequence of events is fresh in the mind is probably going to be a more accurate record than one that is made later. This is just the same for a patient record as for an accident form or any other record. The second reason for making a timely record is a reminder that all records are made to improve patient safety. A record made in good time will help to prevent duplication of an episode of care. For example, if an action has been taken based on an old record rather than the latest episode of care, the patient could have the same drug administered twice or have the same referral made twice.

The next practical action listed in Section 10 is that the written record maintained by the nursing associate must ensure that all risks that have been identified or problems have been recorded along with the steps that have been taken to remedy these risks and problems. This action helps to ensure that other healthcare professionals who use the records have all the information that they need. One example of this is if the nursing associate identified that a patient was finding it difficult to mobilise with a walking stick, this would be recorded along with the fact that the patient had been referred to the physiotherapist. When the physiotherapist visits the patient, they can see clearly from the record what the problems were and why the referral had been made. Another application here that has to be considered is that if a patient was to make a claim of negligence regarding their care. The record relating to their care must clearly show that the nursing associate had identified the patient's care need and reported it to the registered nurse in charge before recording this in the nursing notes. This would then demonstrate that a risk had been identified and appropriate steps had been taken to alleviate this risk.

The third practical action requires that all records must be completed accurately and without any falsification. It is not realistic to maintain records without ever making a mistake either by misspelling a word or by using a word that you did not mean to use in that context. Therefore, it will be necessary to mark a mistake or delete a word within a written record. This must be done by scoring through the mistake with a single line rather than obliterating the mistake with scribbles or correction fluid (liquid paper).

Take Note

Mistakes must only be altered with a single line through the error and initials inserted. The nursing associate must not totally obliterate a word written in error.

Supporting Evidence

In the rare case of needing to alter a record, the original entry must remain visible (draw a single line through the record), and the new entry must be signed, timed and dated (RCN 2015).

It is essential that all nursing associates do not falsify records either by recording that something has occurred when it has not or by falsifying or forging a signature attributing a record to another person for whatever reason. You may come across a record made by another healthcare professional that has not been signed by them. In a situation like this, do not consider putting their signature adjacent to the record; the two choices which could be followed are:

1. Alert the individual as soon as possible so that they can add the necessary signature to the record or
2. Where there is going to be a considerable gap in time before this signature can be entered, a senior nurse on the ward (or care area) must be advised, and appropriate action can be taken.

Blue Flag

Nursing associate Lilly Myers is caring for a patient named Renuka in her own home. She had been off duty for three days; she looks at Renuka's care plan and the documentation written by staff nurse Willis who had been caring for her over the previous three days and notices that the staff nurse has forgotten to sign the various entries she has made in Renuka's nursing notes, in fact all of them. Lilly calls staff nurse Willis who is office based and explains the situation to her. Staff nurse Willis requests, 'please can you sign the entries for me and when I get back off leave in two weeks I will counter sign'. Lilly refuses, and staff nurse Willis says in a rather harsh tone, 'that is the last time I do you any favours, any way I am on leave now'. How do you think Lilly should proceed?

When the nursing associate is undertaking a programme of education leading to registration and is completing clinical learning outcomes during a clinical placement, it is important that only the allocated mentor or practice supervisor signs off the clinical learning outcomes as they are completed. The situation may arise where the student and the mentor discuss a clinical learning outcome, but then, the mentor forgets to sign. This is a form of record, as indicated by the NMC, which does not directly relate to patient care; however, this record does enable the student to progress to registration and then directly affect patient care. Therefore, it is essential that the student does not falsify this signature in this situation but requests the mentor to complete the record at their next meeting.

Section 10 requires that each nursing associate attribute any entry that they make in any paper or electronic records to themselves, in essence they own that entry. This is linked to the previous practical action very closely. If the record is paper based, then it is essential that the signature (or initials on certain records) is clearly identifiable and consistent. In many clinical areas, a register will need to be completed which allows the nursing associates to first clearly write their name and then adjacent to this enter a specimen of both their signature and their initials (see Figure 8.1).

This is a particularly useful approach to accountable record-keeping when looking at records historically and examining records that have been made by agency or bank staff that may have only made a limited number of entries and indeed their signatures alone are not familiar.

If the record is made electronically, then it is essential that it be 'signed' by the correct author. This will require healthcare professionals to log off a computer and then log in with their own identity before making an entry; otherwise, the entry will be attributed to the healthcare professionals who have already logged into that recording device. While this signature or identity may not be seen by the individual making the entry, the computer system will record who was logged in as the person making the entry. This reinforces the importance of logging off from any device after a record has been made and also that the login details are not shared with another nurse or nursing associate so that any record subsequently made is attributed directly to the nursing associate who is identified as being logged on to the recording device.

Signature register: The Hollies General Practice			
Name	Grade	Specimen signature	Specimen initials
Peter Carter	Practice nurse	Peter Carter	PCC
Blessings Aniowu	Healthcare assistant	Blessings K. Aniowu	BKA
Medwyn Bevan	Nursing associate	Medwyn Bevan	MB
Selina McGraw	Practice manager	Selina Mc Graw	SMG

Figure 8.1 An example of a specimen register used in a general practice.

One of the final subsections within Section 10 requires the nursing associate to make sure that all records are clearly written, dated and timed, and that they do not include unnecessary abbreviations, jargon or speculation. As this subsection contains detailed guidance for record-keeping, this will be now discussed in several sections. These requirements of the NMC Code are also echoed by the NMC proficiency standards (2018) that state that records are to be written accurately, clearly and legibly. Accuracy and clarity are quite inseparable. The nursing associates must also remember that there will be quality standards in their workplace that will govern how they are required to undertake documentation; they must not deviate from these standards.

Touch Point

Think about a record that you have written. Was this record both accurate and clear? How could this be improved?

Legible and Clearly Written

These are two terms used by the NMC which possibly have similar meaning, although clearly written could be interpreted as more than just legibility. To reiterate, the nursing associate must ensure that all records are made in such a way that they can be read by another healthcare and social care professional. Legibility is therefore very important to ensure that all records made communicate necessary information about the patient for whom the record has been made. As discussed previously, when looking at who has access to records, it was seen that a number of professionals, including the legal community, police as well as healthcare and social care professionals can also access records, and as such, content must not be ambiguous or difficult to read or decipher. Legibility requires that when a record is made by hand, black indelible ink is used, and pencil must not be used as this can be erased and rewritten at any time. Furthermore, many pencil leads fade with time; therefore, this does not make a permanent record. Often, local policy requires all record makers use black ink as this can be more permanent and photocopies and scans better than blue ink. If in doubt as to what a local policy is on record-keeping, then using black ink is always a safe default position; you must seek advice if you are unsure. Legibility is also concerned with the alteration of a record in a clear way. A record that has been clearly written will also consider other issues such as language.

Language

The language used in records must be unambiguous in its meaning. This requires that it is factual and not open to interpretation in any way which could lead to confusion and ultimately could result in a patient not receiving the care they need or care that may cause them harm. If a patient, for example, has had their vital signs measured and recorded every 15 minutes, then this frequency must be recorded rather than a simple entry to state that the patient's vital signs have been measured. The fact that the reader now knows that the vital signs have been recorded every 15 minutes conveys a message that the patient's needs are such that they require close monitoring.

Yellow Flag

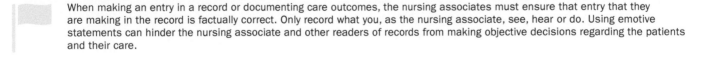

When making an entry in a record or documenting care outcomes, the nursing associates must ensure that entry that they are making in the record is factually correct. Only record what you, as the nursing associate, see, hear or do. Using emotive statements can hinder the nursing associate and other readers of records from making objective decisions regarding the patients and their care.

Another example would be if a patient is incontinent of urine and faeces, the written record should be identifying this rather than simply stating that the patient has been incontinent as this again does not fully and accurately convey or report on the needs of that patient. This would also have implications for future reviews to be completed; they may not be accurate as the information about the type of incontinence is not available to the next person undertaking a review. The subsequent reviews are also recorded, and as such, the principles of accuracy and clarity will also apply.

Red Flag

When the nursing associate fails to document care provision in the correct manner, this can result in serious harm to a patient's health and well-being. These failures are attributable to human errors. Harm can occur when there is a wrong or delayed response to care, and this can be a result of failure to capture documented signs and symptoms and laboratory tests and failure to undertake, document and report care findings. Poor documentation, failure to read and understand a patient's nursing and medical record, can put a patient at serious risk of harm.

Reducing the risk of patient harm during care delivery (and this includes documentation and record-keeping) must be at the forefront of policy and practice, and the nursing associates have to ensure that all they do are done in the best interest of those they have the privilege to care for.

Jargon and Abbreviations

Language that is used in record-keeping must also be jargon free. It is worth remembering that the language used in the record could be interpreted or misinterpreted by any of the previously mentioned groups, including families, patients, allied health professionals and external agencies such as the police. There are abbreviations that are commonly used in all walks of life such as National Health Service (NHS) which most people would know refers to the NHS; however, there are many times when jargon or abbreviations should not be used, for example, MI which could stand for myocardial infarction but could equally stand for motivational interview or DOD which could mean date of discharge or date of death.

This does not mean that medical terminology and abbreviations should not be used such as cerebrovascular accident (CVA) as opposed to writing stroke (note the convention of writing the term in full and then abbreviating the term afterwards. This gives clarity as to abbreviations and their meaning later in the record.) In this instance, it is the lay term stroke that has several meanings, whereas CVA is quite explicit.

Due to instances where a word used in a record has had different connotations and the appropriate or required action has subsequently not been forthcoming, the requirement for records to be made clear by being jargon free is apparent. Linked to this section, there has to be a consideration of spelling.

Spelling

Many computer programmes used for record-keeping contain spell checkers, although these should not be relied upon as when words are not spelt correctly but the misspelled word is still a word, the spell checker would overlook this. For example, if the word 'loose' was mistyped as 'lose', this would have a different meaning, but as it may be a proper word, the mistake would be undetected by the computer. This highlights the importance of proofreading the entries, as other healthcare and social care professionals reading this record would assume that the patient had lost their bowels completely rather than having diarrhoea which is the intended message.

In written records, there are no spell checkers that can be used. Few nursing associates or registered nurses would be able to ever say that they had never made a spelling mistake or typing error within a record; how these are managed and minimised can improve the accuracy and clarity of the record. In some instances where perhaps a drug name is being recorded or a diagnosis is being written, it is essential that the word is spelt correctly. In these instances, it is a good practice to use a good nursing or medical dictionary. Many of these dictionaries are available online and are easily accessible through apps on mobile devices. The earlier guidance regarding making corrections is important so that the reader can see that the misspelled word has been changed and that the crossed-out word was nothing more than a correction and not an attempt to alter or falsify a record. While discussing clarity of a record, it has to be considered that a record should be timed and not just dated to demonstrate that care has been provided and there is sequential logic to the entry.

Supporting Evidence

The Royal College of Nursing (2010) has produced some good suggestions in a tool kit, for nursing associates and other healthcare professionals with dyslexia, dyspraxia and dyscalculia.

Dated and Timed

The NMC requires that all records be dated and timed, and all records must be made in a timely fashion as soon as the event as is reasonably possible, and The Code emphasises this. All computer records will be automatically dated and time-stamped when the record is made; however, the computer will not recognise that a record may relate to an event that occurred two hours ago and the time attributed to the record will be the current time. Therefore, it is imperative that all nursing associates attribute the correct time. The same can occur during the night where a record is made after midnight relating to an episode of care that occurred before midnight. In this instance, the date as well as the time needs to be correctly identified. This applies equally in a written record, but the written record will make no automatic assumption or entry in relation to the date and time, and the nursing associate must make this a clear part of any record that they make. The timing of a record demonstrates the sequence of care events. Ideally, records are made at the time of the event and, therefore, will be in the correct chronological order; however, when this is not possible, it is a good practice to indicate the time that the record relates to so that anyone examining the records historically (in retrospect) can establish a time line of events. The format of the time must be considered; the 24-hour clock is much harder to confuse in a record that uses the 12-hour clock. For example, in the 12-hour clock, 1 o'clock appears twice, whereas in the 24-hour clock, these are clearly written as 01:00 h and 13:00 h. Recording 1 a.m. and 1 p.m. can be confusing, and the differentiation in the 24-hour clock is very clear. The final NMC element of The Code with regards to record-keeping is the issue of speculation.

Speculation

The subject of speculation in records made by nursing associates is an important requirement when considering clarity. Not making any speculation in record-keeping requires accuracy, and there must be no guessing, for example, recording that a person with a high temperature may be septic when the diagnosis has not been confirmed by a senior nurse or doctor demonstrates speculation. All records must be factual in nature.

Touch Point

How could these five records be documented so that they are not speculative?

Mrs Jones has a high temperature	
Mr Thomas has passed a large amount of urine this afternoon	
Mrs Kowalczyk's blood glucose is high, and she will probably have a stroke	
Mrs Evans has diarrhoea; she must have eaten something bad	
I think Mr Morgan is in pain	

Speculation could also be interpreted as an attempt to gamble. Putting this into the context of record-keeping, it would mean drawing conclusions with only part of the evidence; here, the nursing associate speculated and fails to consider facts. Gambling could mean that there is a 50% chance that the conclusion drawn is correct. This means that there is also a 50% chance that the conclusion drawn is incorrect; therefore, all records must be maintained factually and not speculatively. Similarly, speculation could mean 'to assume'. Just because a person appears a certain way, an assumption must not be drawn. Again, records must deal in facts only. The next requirement of the NMC Code that relates directly to record-keeping discusses secure storage.

Safe Storage

Section 10.5 of The Code states that all nursing associates must take all steps to make sure that records are kept securely. Whether a record is made and stored electronically or by hand, the requirement and expectation regarding storage is the same. Firstly, computerised records will generally be stored securely, and the backup of such documents will be automated by an IT department so that the final security and integrity of a record is maintained on the whole without the nursing associate having to be concerned with safe storage of the record. Safe storage also concerns access to records, and the nursing associate is accountable and responsible for any actions or omissions. With regards to safe storage, many computers have a lock screen which automatically engages after a set period of time that the computer is idle. This set time varies from computer to computer but could be as little as a couple of minutes to 15 minutes. In this time, anyone could access the computer if the lock screen has not been manually or automatically engaged and affect the safe storage and integrity of records. The process of manually engaging this lock screen is usually quite straightforward but will mean that the nursing associate will then need to log in to the device again, ensuring that the security of the records has been maintained by limiting access.

Orange Flag

A nursing associate in a very busy outpatient clinic had forgotten to manually log off from the workstation that he was working at. The next user (the ward clerk) sits down to access the computer and notices that the records that the nursing associate was using belong to his ex-wife; he reads the records and discovers that his ex-wife had, on more than three occasions, attempted suicide.

The content of the record was inflammatory and accusatory; the ward clerk was clearly upset by what she was reading.

The negligent action caused by the nursing associate in failing to log off from the workstation caused psychological harm to the ward clerk who was clearly distressed by what she had read. What action should be taken next?

When considering safe storage of manually made records, it is the nursing associate who is accountable for ensuring that the record that they are accessing and making an entry in is returned to its safely stored position that it was in before it was used. Some records will be stored at the patients' bedside or in their own home, but other records will be stored centrally in the clinical area. It is crucial that the nursing associate considers the record that is being accessed and stores it appropriately thinking again about how limited the access to the record needs to be.

Take Note

Further information on safe storage of manually generated records should be read locally as care providers will have requirements that each nursing associate must be aware of.

Finally, in Section 10, nursing associates are reminded to collect, treat and store all data and research findings appropriately. While many nursing associates may not consider themselves to be part of a research team, much of the data that is recorded during day-to-day work could be used as valuable data in a research project. When considering data being used as part of a research project, the project will have been granted ethical approval from the organisation overseeing the study. This ethical clearance will include clarification of how data will be gathered, collected, stored, analysed and reported. Whether acting in the capacity of a data collector or indeed the researcher, it is imperative that the nursing associate follows the guidelines set in the research proposal that has been analysed by the relevant ethical body. What is very important to consider in this section is that often data is accessed retrospectively. If a research study, for example, was being conducted into whether turn charts were effective in the prevention of pressure ulcers, the researcher may look at records relating to previous admissions where patient outcomes are already known. This puts an onus on nursing associates to ensure that all records are clear and accurate as all records could potentially form part of a research study. This final requirement has so many close relations with the other requirements of section 10 of The Code (2018a) that it clearly demonstrates how important record-keeping is professionally.

Having considered record-keeping from a professional perspective and addressed all the aspects described in The Code (2018a), it is clear to see that record-keeping should be fundamentally straightforward; however, there are many strands to record-keeping that are so intertwined that it is difficult to do one without the other. For example, to keep a clear record, it has to be legible, dated, timed and so on. In the next part of this chapter, the legal perspective will be addressed in an attempt to demonstrate that the reason nursing associates have to keep clear and accurate is that a number of different Acts and pieces of legislation may require records to be scrutinized.

From a Legal Perspective

This chapter cannot attempt to compete with the many texts that have been written on the legal duties of a nurse. See Table 8.1 for an overview of some elements of legislation that impact on record-keeping.

Table 8.1 Some aspects of legislation that impacts record-keeping.

ASPECT OF LEGISLATION	DISCUSSION
Access to Health Records Act (1990)	This relates to records of deceased patients since 1 November 1991; however, access is only allowed if the record would not cause harm to any living person.
Access to Medical Reports Act (1988)	Allows individuals to apply in writing to access their health records and then allows patients to disagree with a report or to correct any inaccuracies; however, access can be denied by a doctor if they feel that the record could harm the individual or that the record also has information relating to a third party who has consented to the release of the record.
Civil Evidence Act (1995)	This Act allows the use of records as evidence in civil legal proceedings
Computer Misuse Act (1990)	This Act created three separate offences. The first is the unlawful access of computer records, the second is access with the intent to commit further offences and the third is the unauthorised modification of computer materials.
Data Protection Act (1998) (updated in 2018)	The Data Protection Act regulates how personal data is processed regardless of how it is stored, i.e. manually or digitally. Processing data includes how a record is stored, obtained, recorded in the first instance, used (including disposal), disclosed and shared. Eight principles underpin this Act. The Data Protection Act was updated in 2018 to include General Data Protection Regulation (GDPR) standards from the European Union. The Act was updated to ensure that the law was fit for the digital age and the ever-increasing amount of personal data that is being generated and being processed. More about the Data Protection Act can be accessed through an internet search or nursing textbook.
Freedom of Information Act (2000)	This Act makes it a requirement for public bodies such as the NHS to make records available if asked for them. There are restrictions such as public interest whereby it may be judged that it is not in the public interest to have some records made public.
Public Interest Disclosure Act (1998)	This Act makes it clear that any record can be made public if the disclosure is in the public interest. This is often referred to as whistleblowing and can be described as the time that confidentiality can be broken in the instance of a 'qualifying disclosure'

Supporting Evidence

Griffith (2015) links the professional and legislative aspects of record-keeping very well.

To summarise, this brief overview of a selection of some Acts that relate to record-keeping have been included for a good reason. It is to emphasise that all records that are made during the daily work of the nursing associate are compliant with the professional standards discussed earlier in this chapter as many of these Acts require that the record could be accessed historically. This means that a record that has been made today could be scrutinized at any time in the future; therefore, maintenance of a clear and accurate record is an essential aspect of the nursing associate's role.

Touch Points Revisited

- Nursing associates must ensure that documentation is in a format that can be followed and understood by others
- All records made by a nursing associate must be clear, accurate and unambiguous
- Local policies on safe storage of records must be read, understood and adhered to

References

Access to Health Records Act. (1990) [online] Available: https://www.legislation.gov.uk/ukpga/1990/23/contents. Accessed 21 August 2019.

Access to Medical Reports Act. (1988) [online] Available: https://www.legislation.gov.uk/ukpga/1988/28/contents. Accessed 21 August 2019.

Civil Evidence Act. (1995) [online] Available: https://www.legislation.gov.uk/ukpga/1995/38/contents. Accessed 21 August 2019.

Computer Misuse Act. (1990) [online] Available: https://www.legislation.gov.uk/ukpga/1990/18/contents. Accessed 21 August 2019.

Data Protection Act. (1998) [online] Available: https://www.legislation.gov.uk/ukpga/1998/29/contents. Accessed 21 August 2019.

Data Protection Act. (2018) [online] Available: http://www.legislation.gov.uk/ukpga/2018/12/contents/enacted. Accessed 21 August 2019.

Freedom of Information Act. (2000 [online] Available: www.legislation.gov.uk/ukpga/2000/36/pdfs/ukpga_20000036_en.pdf. Accessed 21 August 2019.

Griffith, R. (2015) Understanding the code: keeping accurate records, British Journal of Community Nursing, 20(10): 511–514.

Nursing and Midwifery Council. (2018a) *The code: professional standards of practice and behaviour for nurse and midwives and nursing associates*, London: Nursing and Midwifery Council.

Nursing and Midwifery Council. (2018b) *Standards of proficiency for nursing associates*, London: Nursing and Midwifery Council.

Public Interest Disclosure Act. (1998) [online] Available: https://www.legislation.gov.uk/ukpga/1998/23/contents. Accessed 21 August 2019.

Royal College of Nursing. (2010) *Dyslexia, dyspraxia and dyscalculia: a toolkit fir nursing staff*, London: RCN.

Royal College of Nursing. (2015) *Record keeping: the facts*, London: RCN.

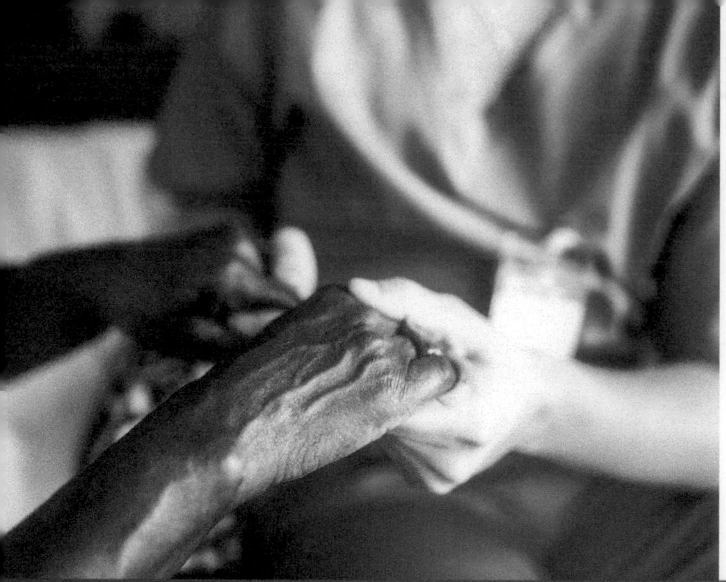

9

Addressing Compliments and Complaints

Ian Peate

School of Health Studies, Gibraltar

Chapter Aim

- **This chapter aims to provide the reader with an awareness of the National Health Service (NHS) complaints procedure and how to manage compliments and feedback.**

Learning Outcomes

By the end of this chapter, the reader will be able to:

- **Demonstrate an awareness of the NHS complaints procedure**
- **Discuss the stages of a complaint**
- **Outline the role of the Parliamentary Health Service Ombudsman**
- **Understand how receiving feedback regarding compliments as well as complaints has the potential to enhance care provision**

Test Yourself Multiple Choice Questions

1. **All complaints:**
   A) Must go through a formal process
   B) Have to be reported to the NMC
   C) Should be used as a form of feedback and an opportunity to learn
   D) Must be documented in a member of staff's personal file
2. **Revalidation is:**
   A) A requirement only impacting on the registered nurse and midwife
   B) The process that allows the nursing associate to maintain their registration
   C) Undertaken every year
   D) Also called CPD

The Nursing Associate's Handbook of Clinical Skills, First Edition. Edited by Ian Peate.

Companion website: www.wiley.com/nursingassociate

3. **If accepting a gift:**
   A) **This might be seen as an attempt for the patient to gain preferential treatment**
   B) **The nursing associate must report this to the NMC**
   C) **The nursing associate must report this to the NMC and the Chief Executive Officer**
   D) **The nursing associate must include this in their annual appraisal (annual review)**
4. **Feedback may come from:**
   A) **Colleagues and management**
   B) **Patients and service users**
   C) **Healthcare and social care students**
   D) **All of the above**
5. **Refusing to accept a gift:**
   A) **Will always enhance care provision**
   B) **Has the potential to damage relations with the patient**
   C) **Can cause corporate harm**
   D) **Is a hallmark of a profession**

Introduction

The nursing associate may receive feedback from a number of people in a number of formats, for example, through complaints and feedback in the form of compliments. The trainee nursing associate receives ongoing performance feedback about their progress throughout their nursing associate programme of study. There are specific procedures, local and national, that must be followed when a complaint has been made.

The Nursing and Midwifery Council's (NMC) (2018a) Code requires the nursing associate to respond to any complaints made against them professionally; in order to do this, they must never allow someone's complaint to affect the care that is provided to them; all complaints should be used as a form of feedback and an opportunity to learn from this through reflection so as to improve practice. In order to uphold your position as a nursing associate, you must refuse all but the most trivial gifts, favours or hospitality; if you accept them, this could be interpreted as an attempt for the patient to gain preferential treatment (Nursing and Midwifery Council 2018a). On admission to the register, the Nursing Associate Proficiencies (Nursing and Midwifery Council 2018b) require the trainee nursing associate to demonstrate they are able to respond to feedback to develop professional knowledge and skills.

Compliments

From time to time, a patient or a member of the patient's family may wish to express their gratitude to the nursing associate or the team to show that they care for what they have done. The gratitude can be expressed in many ways: verbally, a thank you card, a box of chocolates, a bowl of fruit or a packet of biscuits. All of these can be gratefully received with thanks and used as evidence to support the quality of care given, yet the NMC (2018a) compels you to refuse all but the most trivial gifts, favours or hospitality.

Green Flag

There may be organisational polices that require you to declare any gift you receive. This is done in part to ensure transparency and reducing potential conflicts of interest.

NHS England (2017a) has produced guidance for staff regarding managing conflicts of interest in the NHS.

Indeed, revalidation, the process that allows nursing associates to maintain their registration with the NMC, demands that you receive feedback, written or verbal, formal or informal. The feedback may come from patients and service users or colleagues and management (Nursing and Midwifery Council 2019).

Blue Flag

Refusing to accept a gift has the potential to damage relations with the patient. Accepting a patient's gift can be beneficial; it can strengthen the friendly relationship between the nursing associate and the patient by acknowledging the patient's autonomy, adding to the patient's self-worth and to reinforce trust.

Individuals might derive great pleasure from giving gifts, and if a gift is rejected, this has the potential to hurt or offend the person who is giving.

There is pleasure in both giving and receiving, and usually no harm is done; however, the nursing associate must always be cautious about accepting any gift. Organisational guidelines (local policy and procedure) may help to decide on the appropriateness or inappropriateness of receiving any kind of gift, monetary or otherwise. There are alternatives to gift giving, for example, the patients or their family could:

- Make a donation to a charity
- Make a contribution to the hospital, clinic, unit charity fund if there is one
- Complete an employee recognition form or write a letter
- Provide feedback via the Friend and Family Test

Touch Point

If you are given a gift (a tangible gift) regardless of value, you should politely refuse it. Always seek advice about accepting a gift from patients or their family.

Managing Complaints

Most of the time, the care that is provided to people in the NHS and by other care providers such as those in the independent and voluntary sectors is of a high standard with positive outcomes. However, things can and do go wrong from time to time and complaints are made.

The total number of all reported written complaints in 2017–2018 was 208,626. This is the equivalent to 4,012 written complaints a week or 572 complaints per day (NHS Digital 2018). The NHS has a single approach that deals with complaints allowing flexibility to respond and to learn from mistakes that may have been made.

The NHS Constitution (DHSC 2015) describes principles and values of the NHS in England and also provides information on how complaints can be made about NHS services. The Constitution has been updated and includes additions and developments associated with:

- Patient engagement
- Feedback
- Duty of candour
- End-of-life care
- Integrated care provision
- Complaints
- Patient information
- Staff rights, responsibilities and commitments
- Dignity, respect and compassion

When a person is unhappy with the services they receive, it is important for the nursing associate to inform them (and, if appropriate, their family) of their rights. People have the right to make a complaint about any aspect of NHS care, treatment or service. The Local Authority Social Services and NHS Complaints (England) Regulations 2009 is the legislation that governs NHS complaints. These regulations make provision for *complaints* made on or after 1 April 2009; they introduced a revised procedure for the handling of complaints by local authorities, in respect of complaints about adult social care and by NHS bodies, primary care providers and independent providers in respect of provision of NHS care. The regulations united adult social care and health complaints processes into a single set of arrangements.

Each organisation will have arrangements for people to raise concerns or make complaints. Referral to the Patient Advisory Liaison Service (PALS) can help people navigate the complaints process. The creation of PALS was as a result of the NHS Plan (Department of Health 2000). PALS are intended to enable patients and the public to access information and raise concerns with their Trust; they offer confidential advice, support and information on health-related matters. They provide a point of contact for patients, their families and their carers. PALS provides help in many ways, it can:

- help with health-related questions
- help resolve concerns or problems when using the NHS
- advise people how to get more involved in their own healthcare.

PALS are not a part of the complaint's procedure; they can provide information about:

- the NHS
- the NHS's complaints procedure, including how to get independent help if the person wishes to make a complaint
- support groups outside the NHS.

Touch Point

If patients are unhappy with the services that they receive, they have the right to make a complaint about any aspect of NHS care, treatment or service. There is legislation in place that govern the complaints process.

NHS Complaints

A complaint or concern is defined by NHS England (2017b) as an expression of dissatisfaction about an act, omission or decision of NHS England, either verbal or written and whether justified or not, that requires a response. NHS England is expected to treat complaints with sincerity and ensure that complaints, concerns and issues that are raised by patients, relatives and carers are investigated in an unbiased, non-judgmental, transparent, timely and appropriate way. The outcome of any investigation, with any resulting actions, has to be explained to the complainant by the investigating organisation.

Patients' rights include:

- Have their complaint acknowledged and properly investigated
- Discuss the manner in which the complaint is to be handled and know the period in which the complaint response is likely to be sent
- To be kept informed of progress and to know the outcome including an explanation of the conclusions and confirmation that any action needed has been taken on
- Take a complaint about data protection breaches to the independent Information Commissioners Office if not satisfied with the way the NHS has dealt with this.

A complaint can be made by the person who is affected by the action, or it may be made by a person who is acting on behalf of a patient in any case where that person:

- Is a child (under the age of 18 years):

In the case of a child, NHS England must be satisfied that there are reasonable grounds for the complaint being made by a representative of the child and, furthermore, that the representative is making the complaint in the child's best interests.

- Has died:

In the case of a person who has died, the complainant must be the personal representative of the deceased. NHS England has to be satisfied that the complainant is the personal representative.

- Has physical or mental incapacity:

In the case of a person who is unable by reason of physical capacity, or lacks capacity as defined by the Mental Capacity Act 2005, to make the complaint themselves, NHS England needs to be satisfied that the complaint is being made in the best interests of the person on whose behalf the complaint is made.

- Has given consent to a third party acting on their behalf:

In the case of a third party pursuing a complaint on behalf of the person affected, the following information needs to be collected:

  - Name and address of the person making the complaint
  - Name and either date of birth or address of the affected person
  - Contact details of the affected person so that they can be contacted for confirmation that they consent to the third party acting on their behalf.
  - Has delegated authority to act on their behalf, such as in the form of a registered Power of Attorney which must cover health affairs.
  - Is an MP acting on behalf of and by instruction from a constituent.

Violet Flag

People in prison should receive the same healthcare and treatment in prison as anyone outside of prison, for example, they can have medication and support from the prison healthcare team if they have a mental illness. Those in prison should also be able to see a doctor, dentist, optician or other healthcare professionals for their physical health.

All healthcare services for prisoners are funded by NHS England. Complaints should be made to NHS England about any problems experienced with the prison's healthcare service.

NHS England's Ask, Listen, Do project (2018) aims to make it easier for people with a learning disability, autism or both (and their families and carers) to give feedback, raise a concern or make a complaint about healthcare, social care or education.

Children and young people have the right to make a complaint about something that goes wrong or if they not happy about the way they have been treated. However, a child or young person may be worried about making a complaint because they may not want their parents to know about the issue or they might be worried that they will not be taken seriously. Complaints must be kept confidential except in very exceptional cases where the child or young person is deemed at risk of harm. The child or young person does not have to put their complaint in writing; they should be given the option, if they prefer, to talk it through with someone. If a child or young person does not want to make a complaint themselves, they can ask someone else to make a complaint for them. Parents, a friend or an advice worker can make the complaint if permission has been given.

Giving Feedback

NHS Friends and Family Test, launched in 2013, was designed to help those who provide services to have a better understanding of whether their patients are happy with the service provided, or if there are improvements required. The initiative is a quick and anonymous approach to giving views after receiving care or treatment across the NHS. The feedback, good or bad, can help to improve the quality of care.

Organisations who offer services can devise additional ways of receiving feedback, and these should be clearly displayed for patients and visitors to see. If a person is unhappy with an NHS service, they should be encouraged to discuss any concerns early on with the service provider, with the intention of addressing any issues quickly. A number of problems can be dealt with using this approach; in some cases, however, the person may feel more at ease speaking to someone who is not directly involved in the case.

Complaints can range in severity from unhappiness about food to concerns arising as a result of an allegation of professional misconduct or inappropriate or incorrect surgical intervention. Those who make a complaint about the care or treatment received have a right to expect a prompt, open, useful and honest response. This includes an explanation of what has occurred and an apology. The nursing associate must never prejudice the care or treatment provided for a patient because a complaint has been made.

The Local Authority Social Services and NHS Complaints (England) Regulations 2009 require each NHS body to make arrangements for the handling and consideration of complaints. These arrangements that have to be accessible, ensure that complaints are dealt with speedily and

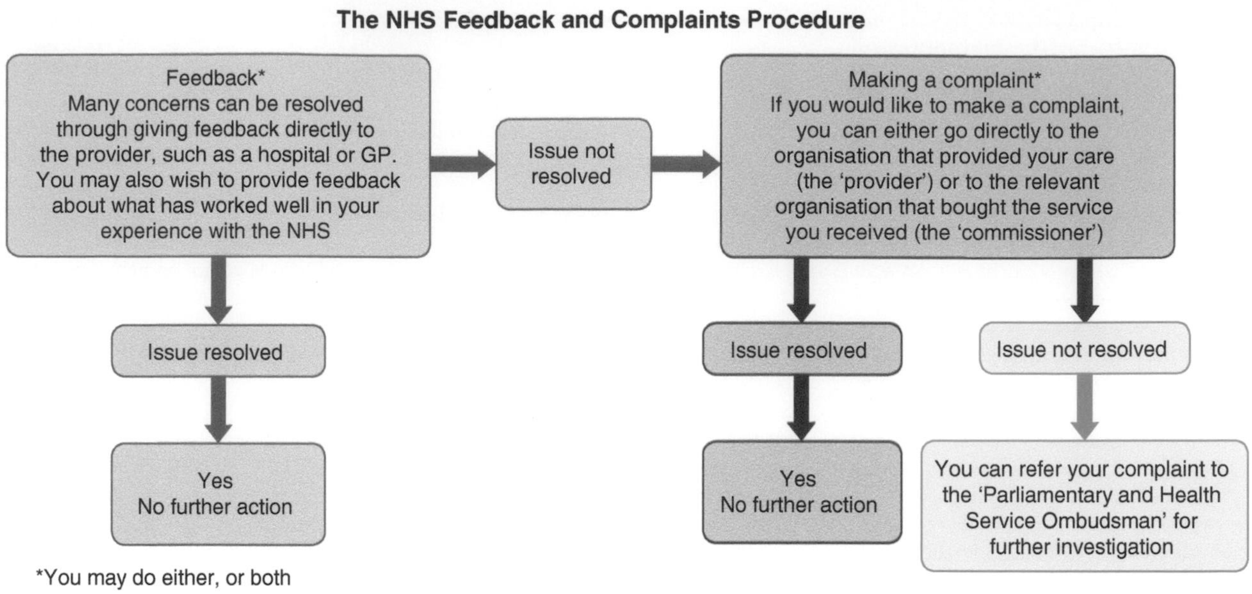

Figure 9.1 The NHS feedback and complaints procedure.

efficiently and that patients are treated courteously and sensitively as far as possible and are involved in decisions about how their complaints are handled and considered. There must be a copy of the arrangements available in writing, and when requested, a copy must be given, free of charge, to any person who requests one.

Figure 9.1 provides an overview of the NHS feedback and complaints procedure.

How to Make a Complaint

The Department of Health and Social Care does not manage individual complaints. Complaints are dealt with through the NHS complaints procedure. A complaint can be made:

- By telephone
- By email
- By post
- In British Sign Language (BSL)

Blue Flag

NHS England is required to make the necessary reasonable adjustments so as to receive, investigate and respond to any complaint. For those whose first language is not English, a translation and telephone interpreting service can be made available. Complaints can be accepted and respond to in alternative formats, for example, Braille.

There are timescales associated with making a complaint. Complaints must be made not later than 12 months after the date on which the matter which is the subject of the complaint occurred or 12 months after the date on which the matter which is the subject of the complaint came to the notice of the complainant. It is still possible to investigate the complaint effectively and fairly, if there are good reasons for not having made the complaint within the timeframe. NHS England may decide to still consider the complaint, for example, longer periods of complaint time-scales can apply to specific clinical areas.

Red Flag

Responding to patient complaints within the specified timescale is important. NHS patients have 12 months from the date of an incident, or the date they first became aware of a problem, to make a complaint. It is important to be aware of the limits set out by the NHS complaints procedure for acknowledging, investigating and responding to complaints.

The Process

All complaints will be acknowledged no later than 3 working days after the day the complaint is received. This will usually be in writing; however, it can be given verbally in some situations; this is usually the exception as opposed to the norm. An offer should be made to discuss the following with the complainant:

- The handling of the complaint
- Timescales for responding
- Expectations and desired outcome if unclear

If the complaint was given verbally, the complainant is given a copy of their verbal statement (this is considered the formal complaint) and asked to confirm that it represents the issues that they wish to raise.

The complainant is provided with a named contact with their contact details who will be their point of contact throughout the complaints process. A case officer will gather relevant information about the case, ensuring that this is accurately recorded. The complainant can expect that:

- They will be kept up to date with the progress of their complaint.
- If a case has passed the 40 working day target (or the timescale agreed with the complainant if different), the complainant (and, if relevant, the advocate) should receive an update every 10 working days thereafter the target has been surpassed. This may be by telephone, email or letter; the format, however, must be agreed with the complainant.
- They can expect to receive a quality response with assurance that action has been taken to prevent a recurrence.
- They will be informed of any learning.

On receipt of the investigation report, a response to the complaint will be prepared, and the case officer will include information on the next stages of the complaint's procedure should the complainant wish to take matters further.

If the complaint is about more than one NHS organisation, the person only need to send a letter to one of the organisations; they (the NHS) should contact the other organisation and work with them to deal with the complaint. Where complaints involve more than one body, discussions will take place between the bodies concerned about the most appropriate body to take the lead in coordinating the complaint and communicating with the complainant. The same procedure is used to complain about adult social services arranged, provided or commissioned by the local authority. If there is a complaint, for example, about both a hospital and adult social care services, the person need only write just the one letter explaining all the problems and whoever the letter is addressed to will contact the other organisation. If NHS England receives a complaint involving several bodies, permission is required from the complainant before sharing or forwarding a complaint to another body; consent will need to be obtained.

As soon as it is reasonably possible after completing the investigation, and within the timescale agreed with the complainant, a formal response in writing is sent to the complainant which will be signed by the National Director or Nominated regional Director for sign off. The response will include:

- An explanation of how the complaint has been considered
- If appropriate, an apology
- An explanation based on the facts
- Whether the complaint in full or in part is upheld
- The conclusions reached in relation to the complaint including any remedial action that the organisation considers to be appropriate
- Confirmation that the organisation is satisfied any action has been or will be actioned
- Where possible, the response will include details of any lessons learnt
- Information and contact details of the Parliamentary and Health Service Ombudsman as the next stage of the NHS complaints process

Parliamentary and Health Service Ombudsman

The Parliamentary and Health Service Ombudsman was set up by Parliament to provide an independent complaint handling service for complaints that have not been resolved by the NHS in England and the UK government departments. It is not part of government or the NHS in England. It is neither a regulator nor a consumer champion.

If a complaint has been made under the NHS complaints procedure and the person is not satisfied with how it was dealt with at the first stage which is known as local resolution, they have a right to request an independent review by the Parliamentary and Health Service Ombudsman. However, the Parliamentary and Health Service Ombudsman may not be able to look at the complaint if:

- legal action is already being taken
- the person is planning to take legal action
- there is a course of legal action open to the person that is reasonable or was reasonable to be followed

A request for an independent review must be made within 12 months of the incident occurring or when the person first became aware that something had gone wrong.

Many cases that are considered by the Parliamentary and Health Service Ombudsman can take some time, depending on the circumstances and complexity of the problem. If the Parliamentary and Health Service Ombudsman upholds the complaint, it can request the organisation to say sorry and provide an explanation of what went wrong. It may also call for changes to prevent the same incident happening again or request a review of procedures. The Parliamentary and Health Service Ombudsman can also order financial compensation; this, however, is normally lower than a court could award.

Yellow Flag

There are a number of factors that might prevent people from raising concerns or making complaints about the standard of care that they or a loved one have received. Fear of causing a fuss or being seen as a troublemaker is the most commonly cited reason.

Touch Point

Complaints made about services or the care provided by the NHS can be dealt with locally or, if appropriate, can go through various processes to ensure that the patient's complaint is addressed fairly and fully. The nursing associate should always seek advice when providing the patient with details concerned with making a complaint, as it can be a long and complex process for all parties.

Conclusion

Despite attempting to maintain open, honest and effective communication, complaints can and do occur. Many complaints are associated with poor communications. Complaints can vary in severity from displeasure about the cleanliness of toilets to allegations of professional misconduct. If complaints do occur, they are dealt with (when appropriate) at a local level adhering to local policy. The NHS complaints procedure can be used to help arrive at a satisfactory explanation of the cause of the complaint. The overall aim is to address the complaint speedily and efficiently, courteously and considerately. The nursing associate should always seek advice when a complaint has been made, as it can be a complex process for all concerned.

Compliments are also received by the nursing associate from patients and families. If gifts are given, the principle is not that the nurse must never receive gifts or favours; they should never be understood as being given by the patient to the nursing associate in return for preferential treatment.

References

Department of Health. (2000) *The NHS plan: a plan for investment, a plan for reform*, London: DH.

Department of Health and Social Care. (2015) *The NHS constitution, The NHS belongs to us all.* [online] Available: https://assets.publishing.service.gov.uk/government/uploads/system/uploads/attachment_data/file/480482/NHS_Constitution_WEB.pdf. Accessed August 2020.

NHS England. (2017a) Managing conflicts of interest in the NHS, *Guidance for staff and organisations.* [online] Available: https://www.england.nhs.uk/wp-content/uploads/2017/02/guidance-managing-conflicts-of-interest-nhs.pdf. Accessed August 2020.

NHS England. (2017b) *NHS England complaints policy.* [online] Available: https://www.england.nhs.uk/wp-content/uploads/2016/07/nhse-complaints-policy-june-2017.pdf. Accessed August 2020.

NHS England. (2018) *Ask, listen, do.* [online] Available: https://www.england.nhs.uk/learning-disabilities/about/ask-listen-do/. Accessed August 2020.

NHS Digital. (2018) *Data on written complaints in the NHS - 2017-18 [PAS].* [online] Available: https://digital.nhs.uk/data-and-information/publications/statistical/data-on-written-complaints-in-the-nhs/2017-18. Accessed August 2020.

Nursing and Midwifery Council. (2018a) The code, *Professional standards of practice and behaviour for nurses, midwives and nursing associates.* [online] Available: https://www.nmc.org.uk/globalassets/sitedocuments/nmc-publications/nmc-code.pdf. Accessed August 2020.

Nursing and Midwifery Council. (2018b) *Standards of proficiency for nursing associates.* [online] Available: https://www.nmc.org.uk/standards/standards-for-nursing-associates/standards-of-proficiency-for-nursing-associates/. Accessed August 2020.

Nursing and Midwifery Council. (2019) *Revalidation.* [online] Available: https://www.nmc.org.uk/globalassets/sitedocuments/revalidation/how-to-revalidate-booklet.pdf. Accessed August 2020.

Annexe B

Procedures

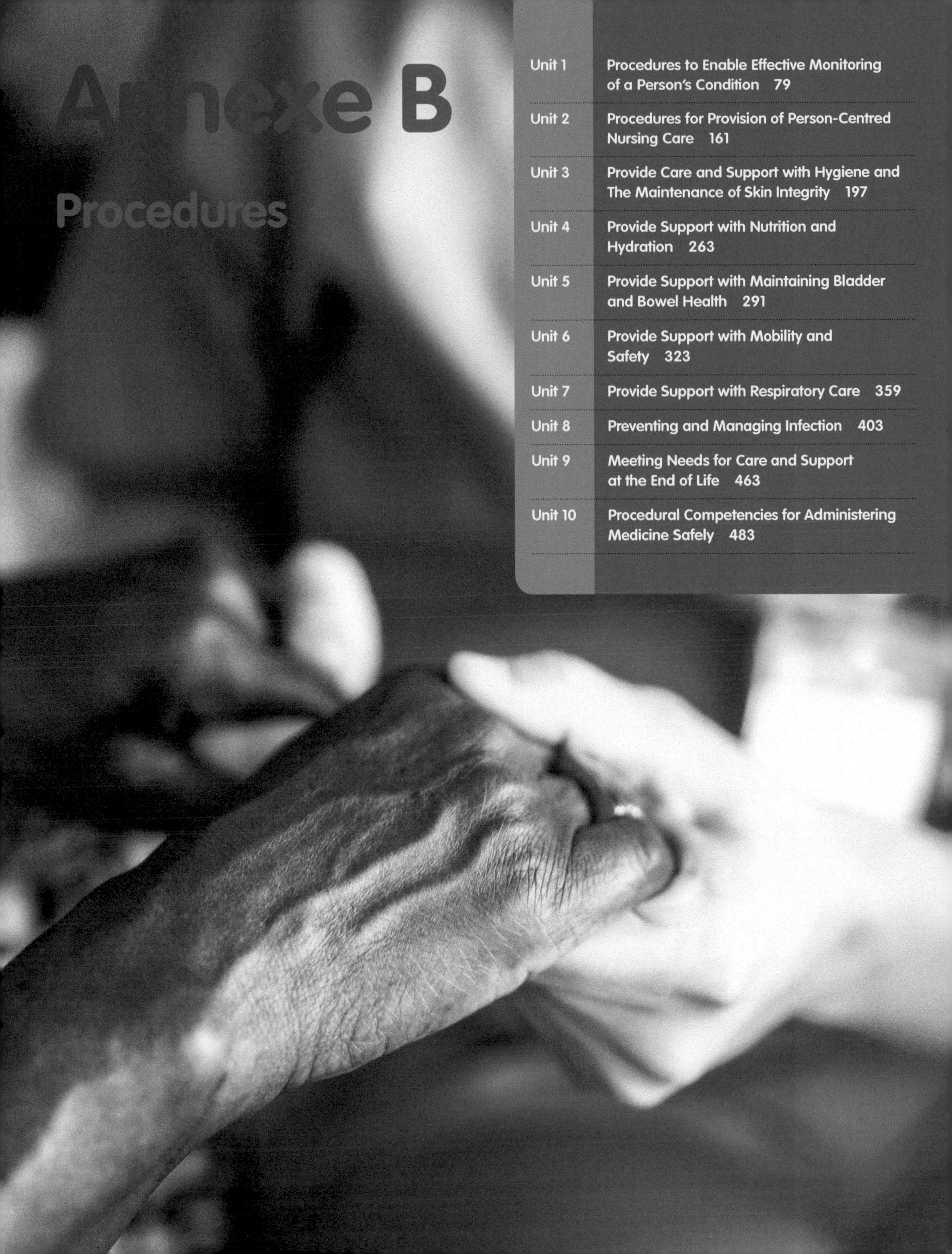

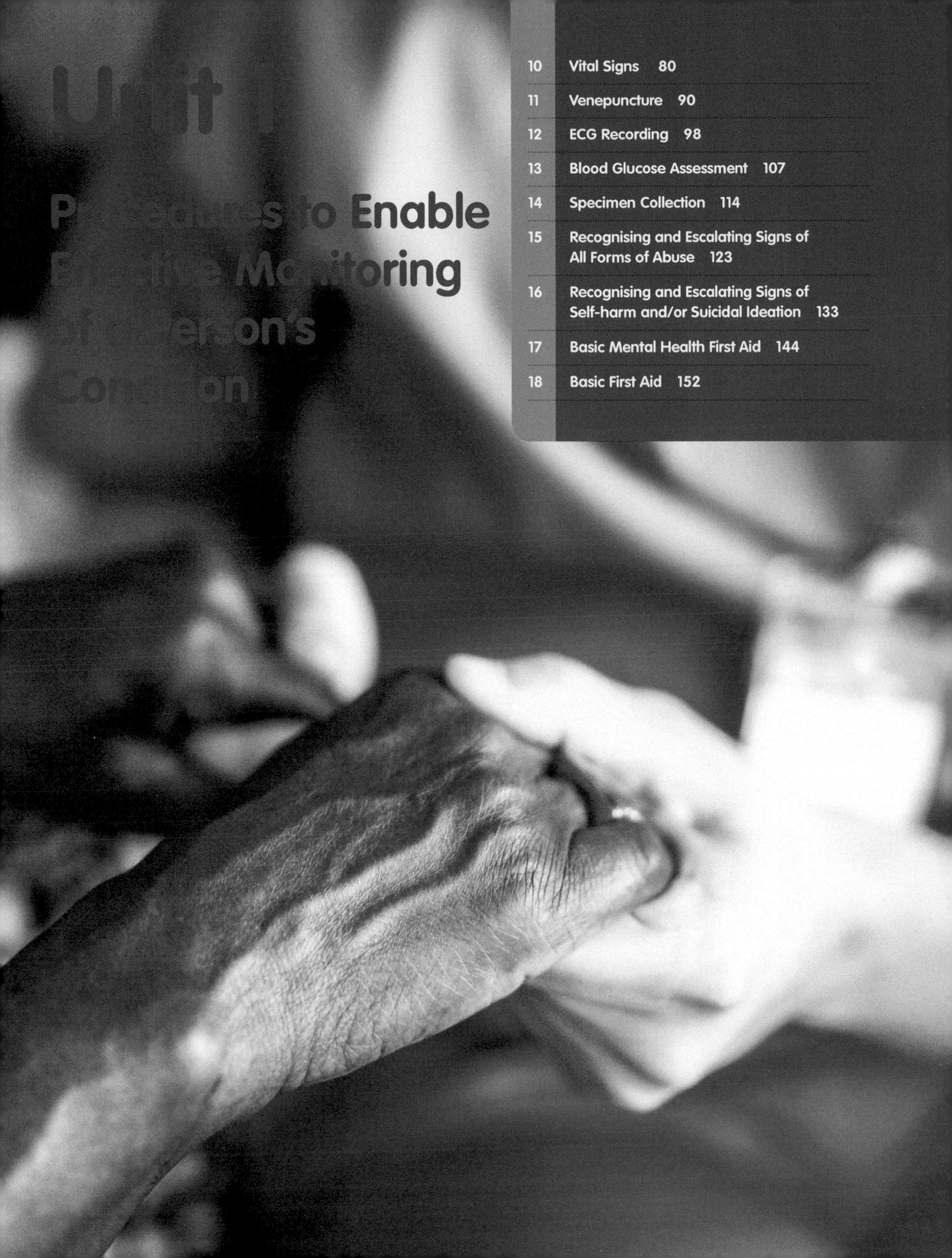

Unit 1

Procedures to Enable Effective Monitoring of a Person's Condition

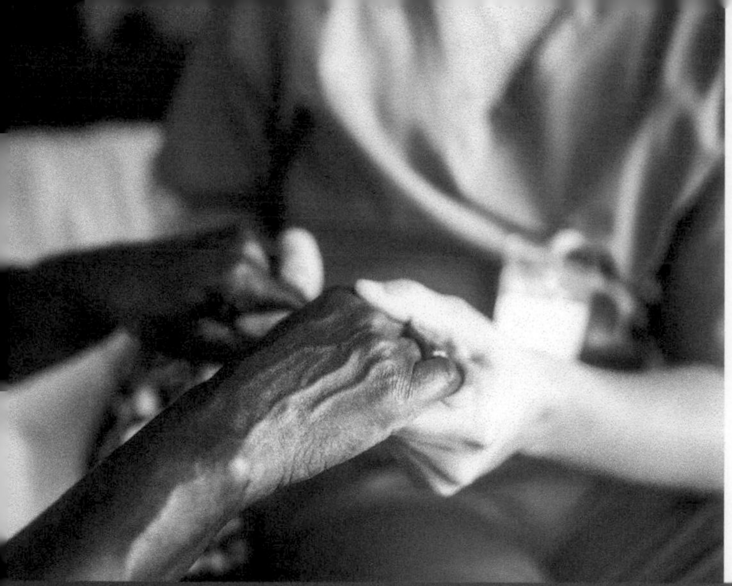

10

Vital Signs

Carl Clare

University of Hertfordshire, UK

Chapter Aim

- **This chapter aims to provide readers with an insight into measuring the vital signs (blood pressure, pulse, respirations and temperature) and the body mass index (BMI).**

Learning Outcomes

By the end of this chapter, the reader will be able to:
- **Understand the clinical relevance of the vital signs**
- **Demonstrate the correct measurement of blood pressure, pulse, respirations and temperature**
- **Understand the clinical relevance of BMI**
- **Demonstrate the correct techniques for measuring BMI in patients with different physical abilities**

Test Yourself Multiple Choice Questions

1. **When taking a client's pulse, it is best practice to count the heart rate for:**
   A) 15 seconds
   B) 30 seconds
   C) 45 seconds
   D) 60 seconds
2. **Before taking the blood pressure of a client, they should rest for:**
   A) 1 minute
   B) 5 minutes
   C) 10 minutes
   D) 15 minutes

The Nursing Associate's Handbook of Clinical Skills, First Edition. Edited by Ian Peate.

Companion website: www.wiley.com/nursingassociate

3. **The most common route for taking a client's temperature is:**
   A) Oral
   B) Rectal
   C) Tympanic
   D) Axilla
4. **The normal heart rate is between:**
   A) 40–100 beats per minute
   B) 50–100 beats per minute
   C) 60–100 beats per minute
   D) 70–100 beats per minute
5. **Hypertension is said to be present when the diastolic blood pressure is above:**
   A) 80 mmHg
   B) 90 mmHg
   C) 100 mmHg
   D) 110 mmHg

Introduction

In any healthcare situation, the ability to measure the following vital signs is an indispensable skill for ensuring patient safety and recognising patient deterioration:

- Pulse
- Blood pressure
- Respirations
- Temperature

Without the ability to measure, record and report these signs, it can be argued that the nursing associate is not adhering the Nursing and Midwifery Council (NMC) Code (2018a) in that they cannot meet the requirement to accurately identify, observe and assess signs of normal or worsening physical health in the person receiving care.

This chapter intends to help the student to understand how, and why, vital signs are measured. In accordance with the Code (2018a), it is essential to also appreciate that teamwork and communication are fundamental to good care. Thus, each skill should be undertaken with the understanding that results must be recorded accurately and, where required, communicated effectively to appropriate members of the healthcare team.

At the point of registration, the Nursing and Midwifery Council (2018b) requires the nursing associate to demonstrate effective approaches to monitoring signs and symptoms of physical, mental, cognitive, behavioural and emotional distress, deterioration and improvement; this includes accurately measuring the vital signs.

BMI is an important tool in the assessment of client health; both baseline BMI and any changes in BMI are clinically important assessments that may be indicators of changes in health status or indicators of disease. Therefore, the measurement of BMI is included in this chapter as an important tool for maintaining client safety.

It is assumed that before engaging in any assessment of the patient, you will:

- Wash your hands
- Introduce yourself to the patient
- Explain what you are going to do and gain consent
- Make the person comfortable

The discussions in this chapter relate to the adult. The principles described that underpin the techniques can be applied to other patient groups such as the child and young person. The various parameters described will need to be adapted to reflect the person's age. The Royal College of Nursing (RCN) (2017) has produced standards for assessing, measuring and monitoring vital signs in infants, children and young people.

Assessing the Pulse

Assessment of the pulse requires the patient to have been resting quietly before examination so that the results are not affected by exercise. While it is important in some cases to assess the effects of exercise on a client's pulse, it is most common in healthcare practice to measure the pulse in a resting state. Not only does resting heart rate give a baseline measurement, but the repeated use of resting heart rate ensures the measurement is made under the same circumstances each time allowing for the removal of confounding factors, such as exercise, which are known to affect heart rate.

Radial Pulse

Pulses can be found at many points on the body; see Figure 10.1 for a diagram showing the major pulse sites. When assessing the cardiovascular system, it is standard practice to begin with the radial pulse, and in many cases, this is the only pulse you will need to assess in a client. The radial pulse is found in the wrist on the same side as the thumb (see Figure 10.2). To assess the radial pulse, place two fingers on the point of pulsation, and using a watch with a second hand, count the number of beats in 60 seconds. It may be difficult to find the point of pulsation in a patient with a weak pulse or those with smaller arteries (for instance, smaller females), but it is essential that you are sure of your identification of the pulse before you begin to time the measurement. If the radial pulse is difficult to identify, then it may be necessary to assess the brachial pulse as an alternative to ensure accurate measurement (see Figure 10.1).

Once the pulse rate has been taken, then take time to assess the way the pulse feels:

- Is it thready and weak or strong and bounding?
- Is it regular or irregular?
- Is every pulsation the same strength?

The normal resting pulse rate will vary from patient to patient, and the resting pulse can be affected by many factors, including the physical fitness of the patient, the age of the patient and patient anxiety. The normal range for a patient's heart rate (pulse) is 60–100 beats per minute, but fitter clients may easily have a heart rate between 40 and 60 beats per minute. A weak and thready pulse may be suggestive of peripheral shut down in response to shock or a reduced pulse pressure. The regularity of the pulse and changes in pulse strength from beat to beat can be an important indicator of the presence of certain disturbances in heart rhythm such as atrial fibrillation. The pulse pressure is described in Box 10.1.

Blue Flag

White coat syndrome (also known as white coat hypertension or the white coat effect) describes a patient experiencing high blood pressure and anxiety when in a clinical situation.

A patient with white coat hypertension has high blood pressure levels in the clinical setting and normal blood pressure levels in their usual environment.

Box 10.1 The Pulse Pressure

The pulse pressure is the pressure created by the heart contraction (systole) over and above the resting pressure in the arteries.

To calculate the pulse pressure, you will need a blood pressure measurement. The calculation is then very simple:

Systolic Blood Pressure – Diastolic Blood Pressure = Pulse Pressure

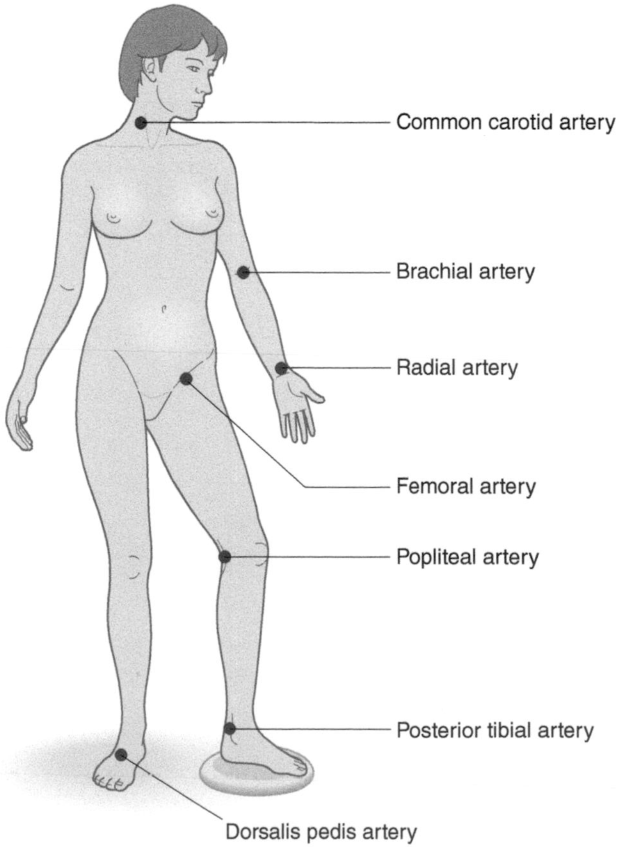

Figure 10.1 Sites of the major pulses. *Source:* Peate & Wild (2018). © 2018 John Wiley & Sons.

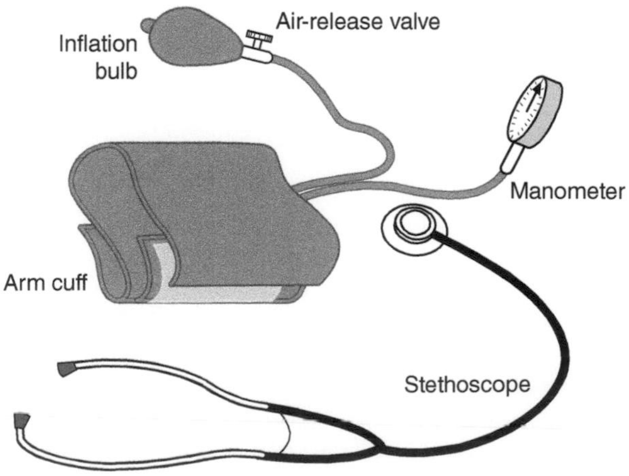

Figure 10.2 Radial pulse. *Source:* Peate & Wild (2018). © 2018 John Wiley & Sons.

Atrial Fibrillation

Atrial fibrillation is the most common altered heart rhythm in the United Kingdom (Adderley et al. 2019). The rhythm is normally associated with an irregularly irregular heart rate. The pulse will be irregular, and often pulse beats will vary in strength.

While it has become common in practice areas when taking repeated pulse measurements in a stable client to take the pulse over 30 seconds and double the number (to make beats per minute), it is important in atrial fibrillation to take the pulse for a full 60 seconds as the variability in rhythm can significantly affect the pulse rate.

When recording the heart rate (pulse) of a client with atrial fibrillation, it is important to record the fact that the pulse is irregular so that staff repeating the measurement are aware this is normal for the client. If the pulse has never been recorded as irregular before, it is important to inform senior staff of the change as the onset of atrial fibrillation is a significant clinical event.

Take Note

In atrial fibrillation, the rhythm normally accompanies an irregularly irregular heart rate. The pulse will be irregular, and often the pulse beats vary in strength.

Assessing the Blood Pressure

In order to take a patient's blood pressure, you will need (see Figure 10.3):

- Manual sphygmomanometer with a suitable size cuff
- Stethoscope

The patient should be seated and relaxed having rested for at least 5 minutes. As with the measurement of the pulse, the standard is to measure the resting blood pressure. Ensure that the patient is comfortable and that no tight clothing is restricting the arm and have the arm supported at the level of the heart, for instance, by a pillow.

1. Place the cuff of the sphygmomanometer around the arm with the centre of the bladder over the brachial artery. The bladder of the cuff should be large enough to circle 80% of the arm but not more than 100% (see Figure 10.4).
2. Estimate the systolic pressure by feeling the brachial pulse with two or three fingers and inflating the cuff until the pulse disappears. Remember to watch the reading on the sphygmomanometer so that you know at what point the pulse disappears. Release the pressure in the cuff. Estimating the systolic pressure ensures that you do not unnecessarily overinflate the cuff when measuring the blood pressure, thus avoiding unnecessary distress and potential harm.
3. Inflate the cuff again until the pressure is approximately 30 mmHg above the point that you estimated the systolic pressure to be. Inflating the cuff 30 mmHg above ensures a safe margin while avoiding unnecessary overinflation.
4. Place the diaphragm of the stethoscope on the place where the brachial pulse was palpated. Some people place the diaphragm before inflating the cuff – this is acceptable so long as no part of the stethoscope is underneath any part of the cuff.
5. Deflate the cuff at a rate of 2–3 mmHg per second until you hear a tapping sound (first Korotkoff sound). This is the systolic pressure – make a mental note of that number.

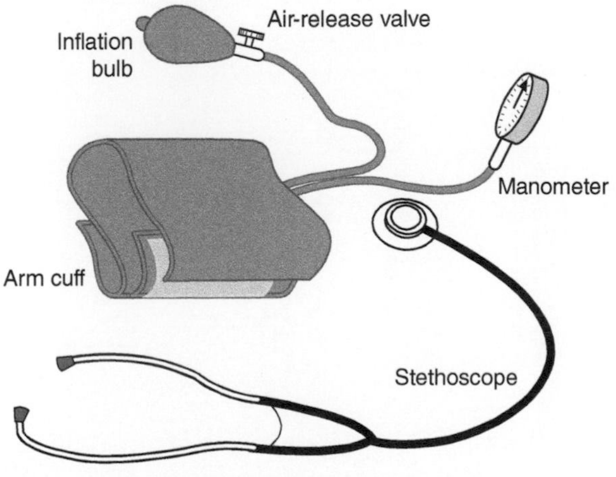

Figure 10.3 Sphygmomanometer and stethoscope.
Source: Gormley-Fleming & Martin (2018), p. 26.

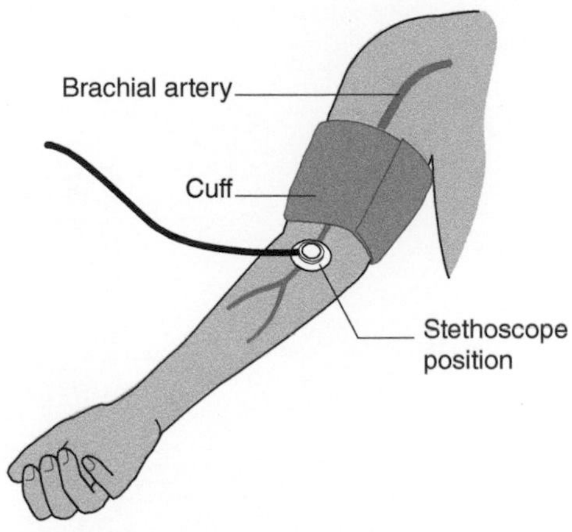

Figure 10.4 Correct positioning of cuff.
Source: Gormley-Fleming & Martin (2018), p. 26.

6. Continue to deflate the cuff at a rate of 2–3 mmHg per second until the tapping sound disappears (fifth Korotkoff sound). This is the diastolic pressure – make a mental note of that number.
7. Both the systolic and diastolic should be measured to the nearest 2 mmHg.
8. Deflate the cuff fully and record the systolic and diastolic on the appropriate documentation.

It is important to note that manual blood pressure measurement is a very technical skill that requires practice. It is best practice to measure blood pressures manually as often as you can. This ensures that you maintain the skill, and when you have a difficult blood pressure to record (for instance, someone with a low blood pressure), you are ready and able to undertake the assessment with competence and confidence.

Take Note What if the tapping sound never disappears?

Occasionally, when measuring the blood pressure, the tapping sound never disappears, leading to difficulties with recording the diastolic pressure. This can often be due to pressing too hard with the stethoscope. To begin with, reassess the blood pressure while trying to be gentler with the pressure on the stethoscope. If on repeating, the tapping noise does not disappear, then use the point that the sounds change as the measurement of diastolic blood pressure and record in the documentation that the fourth Korotkoff sound was used to measure diastolic blood pressure.

If using an electronic blood pressure monitor (Figure 10.5), the patient should be seated and relaxed having rested for at least 5 minutes. Ensure that no tight clothing is restricting the arm and have the arm supported at the level of the heart, for instance, by a pillow.

1. Place the cuff of the sphygmomanometer around the arm with the centre of the bladder over the brachial artery. The bladder of the cuff should be large enough to circle 80% of the arm but not more than 100%.
2. Read the systolic and diastolic blood pressures that are displayed and record on the appropriate documentation.

Violet Flag Home blood pressure monitor

If blood pressure is being monitored at home, the choice of home blood pressure monitor is essential:

- The general practitioner (GP) or hospital will provide an ambulatory blood pressure monitor that can be borrowed for a predetermined period of time.
- If purchasing a home blood pressure monitor, choose one that measures blood pressure at the upper arm, not at the wrist or finger.
- Ensure the right cuff size for the arm; it should wrap snugly around the upper arm, with enough space to slide two fingertips underneath. Most home blood pressure monitors come with a medium-sized cuff. If the upper arm is particularly larger or smaller than average, a different-sized cuff may be needed.
- A home-purchased blood pressure monitor should be approved for use in the United Kingdom.
- The blood pressure monitoring device should be serviced and calibrated to make sure it is accurate, at least once in every two years.

Supporting Evidence

Guidelines on taking blood pressures (including in pregnancy) can be found on the British Hypertension Society website: http://www.bhsoc.org/

This is a useful site that includes instructions (including videos) for taking blood pressures both manually and with an automatic monitor and a video quiz allowing you to practice listening to Korotkoff sounds and reading a sphygmomanometer.

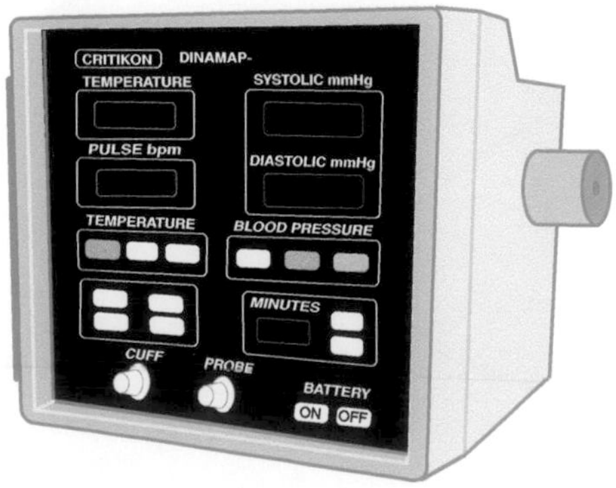

Figure 10.5 **Electronic blood pressure monitor.** *Source:* Gormley-Fleming & Martin (2018), p. 26. © 2018 John Wiley & Sons.

Normal blood pressure readings are considered to be between 90 and 140 mmHg systolic and 60 to 90 mmHg diastolic. However, patients should be reassured that one reading that is above these levels does not necessarily mean they have high blood pressure as blood pressure varies widely throughout the day, and unless they have symptoms (such as feeling dizzy), lower blood pressures in a client in the community are not necessarily an indication of a problem.

Touch Point

Pulse and blood pressure are the main methods for assessing the cardiovascular system in everyday practice. Alterations in either can be a signal of deteriorating health.

It is important (where possible) to know the 'normal' blood pressure and pulse for the client; this gives you a baseline to judge current readings against.

Whenever pulse and blood pressure are measured, the client should have been resting for at least 5 minutes. As blood pressure and pulse are physiologically dependent on each other, then they should be measured consecutively one after the other so the overall cardiovascular picture can be assessed.

Hypertension and Hypotension

Hypertension is the clinical term for high blood pressure. According to the National Institute for Health and Clinical Excellence (NICE) (2019), hypertension is present when the blood pressure reading exceeds 140/90 mmHg. If repeated measurements are recorded above either of these levels, then the client should be advised to visit their GP for appropriate assessment and treatment.

Hypotension is the clinical term for low blood pressure. Clinically, a systolic blood pressure of less than 90 mmHg may indicate a problem. However, this depends on the context and what is the client's normal blood pressure. A mobile client in the community who is not reporting symptoms such as dizziness may exhibit hypotension without it being a clinical problem (however, it is best to advise them to see their GP). A client in a hospital bed following acute surgery whose blood pressure drops to less than 90 mmHg from a higher pressure may be at risk (for instance, they may be bleeding) and should be reported to senior staff immediately (National Institute for Health and Clinical Excellence 2007).

Assessing Respirations

Assessing respirations is an important task of any healthcare professional; unfortunately, it is one that is regularly missed, estimated or even made up (Wong 2018). The importance of respiratory rate as a clinical indicator cannot be underestimated; it has been shown that respiratory rate is an important indicator of serious disease or deterioration (Cretikos et al. 2008).

In order to measure a client's respiratory rate accurately, it is important that the measurement is taken over 1 minute, the client is unaware and not talking. Understandably, this is very difficult to arrange; traditionally, nurses would measure respiratory rate while their patients had a thermometer in their mouth and thus could not talk! Unfortunately, the move to tympanic temperature measurement has taken that trick away. Increasingly, it is becoming necessary to be more 'devious' when taking respiratory rate. One potential trick is to pretend to be doing paperwork at the bedside while watching the client's chest from the corner of your eye; however, this does not stop the client from moving. Another common way is to take the client's pulse for 2 minutes but use the second minute to assess the respiratory rate. Ask your practice supervisors for any 'tricks' they may have for taking respiratory rate.

It is also helpful when measuring the respiratory rate to view the movement of the client's chest (while maintaining dignity) so that the respiratory movement of the chest can be seen and counted. Tactile measurement of the respiratory rate is possible (by placing your hand on the client's chest), but this makes the client aware of the fact you are assessing their respiratory rate.

The accuracy of the assessment is reliant on many factors outside your control, and the best we can do is to minimise these (Hill et al. 2018). One of the most important factors is to take the respiratory rate over 1 minute as measurements over a shorter period of time have been proved to be inaccurate (Rimbi et al. 2019).

The 'threshold' for an abnormal respiratory rate remains a difficult issue to define, and it is most useful to use the parameters set by the Royal College of Physicians (2017) in the National Early Warning Score 2 (NEWS2) track and trigger system. In NEWS2, a respiratory rate outside the parameters of 12 to 20 respirations per minute is given a higher 'score', and thus, it is safe to assume the 'normal' respiratory rate is 12 to 20 respirations per minute.

Green Flag

Estimating respiratory rate is both dangerous and a breach of the NMC Code (2018). Respiratory rates are an important indicator of patient deterioration and failing to measure them accurately may put the patient at risk.

Chapter 49 of this text considers the measurement of respiratory status, peak flow and pulse oximetry.

Orange Flag

Those with serious mental illness are over three times more likely to have a physical health problem, more likely to engage in health risk behaviours and may die up to 10–20 years earlier than the general population. Findings by Howard (2011) indicate the importance of undertaking vital signs monitoring to improve physical health outcomes for those with mental health issues.

Temperature

The final measurement in the standard suite of 'vital signs' is the client's temperature. Alterations in temperature can be indicative of a variety of clinical conditions, and measuring the client's temperature regularly allows healthcare providers to monitor for changes in a timely manner. Taking the client's temperature is also necessary when assessing the effect of an intervention to increase or decrease temperature. Table 10.1 details temperature measurement ranges.

Though there are many routes to take a temperature, it has become most common (in adults) to measure the temperature via a tympanic thermometer, and thus, this chapter will only discuss that route. Tympanic thermometers have become common in healthcare for a variety of reasons including the fact they are hygienic, fast and more acceptable to clients over other routes. However, if used inappropriately, a tympanic thermometer will deliver incorrect readings (normally lower than the actual body temperature); thus, it is important to ensure the correct technique is used, see Figure 10.6.

- Ensure a clean cover is attached to the probe and is secured appropriately in place
- Gently pull the client's ear up and back to gain access to and straighten the ear canal
- Insert the probe gently into the ear canal until you have a seal with the skin
- Activate the measurement
- Record the result
- Dispose of the cover.

Red Flag Sepsis

Traditionally, the role of temperature measurement in the risk for sepsis has focused on an increased temperature (over 38°C). However, the NICE guidelines (2017) make no mention of raised temperature as a risk indicator for sepsis (though it is a clear indicator for infection). The risk stratification notes that a temperature below 36°C is a moderate to high risk factor (when taken in consideration with other signs). Thus, it is of note that a low temperature (in the absence of known hypothermia due to environmental factors) is an indicator of a potentially life-threatening condition. Yet, it is not unknown for a high temperature to be present in sepsis, and thus, it is best practice not to rule out potential sepsis due to a high (or normal) temperature.

Table 10.1 Temperature measurement ranges.

Hypothermia	<35.0°C
Pyrexia	>38.0°C
Normal range	35.1°–37.9°C

Source: Robertson & Hill (2019). © 2019 Mark Allen Holdings Ltd.

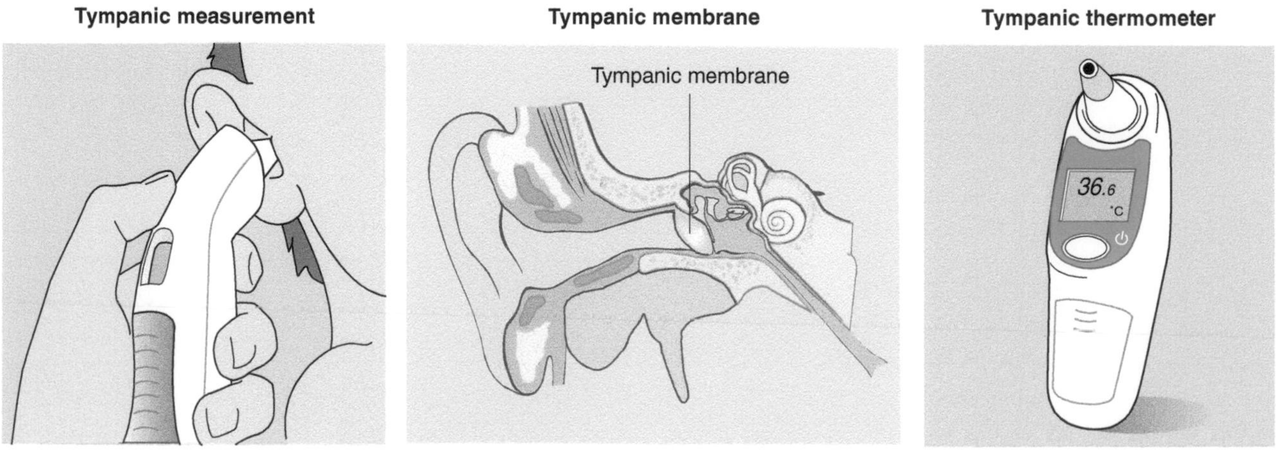

Figure 10.6 Taking the temperature with a tympanic thermometer. *Source:* Gormley-Fleming & Martin (2018), p. 32. © 2018 John Wiley & Sons.

Body Mass Index (BMI)

BMI is a measure of height to weight that is used to calculate if a person's weight is healthy. The popularity of the BMI as a tool for measuring a person's healthy weight has exploded in the last 10 years to the extent it is now calculated in most points of contact with healthcare services (GP, outpatient clinic and hospital ward). The vast majority of discussion around BMI is focused onto the obese client; however, it must be made clear that the BMI has an upper and lower range and that a BMI below the lower threshold is still an 'abnormal' finding and should be reported as such.

Yellow Flag **BMI Beliefs**

The 33rd British Social Attitudes report (Curtis et al. 2016) included the analysis of social attitudes to obesity.

The report noted that obesity has become a stigmatising condition in the United Kingdom, attitudes to people with obesity are often negative and in many cases is considered as a personal issue and associated with negative personality traits.

The perception of obesity also carries a gender bias; in the same research, people were shown a range of pictures, and it was found that the respondents were more likely to label the female pictures obese than the male pictures.

It is important that healthcare providers are aware of both the societal attitudes to obesity and their own. Studies have shown that not only do healthcare providers hold negative attitudes towards obese clients but that these attitudes may affect healthcare provision.

Source: Based on Swift et al. (2013)

The importance of the BMI as a health screening tool cannot be overstated. Patients who are obese are at increased risk of many diseases (including diabetes, heart disease and cancer), and there is a recognised increased risk for all-cause mortality (dying by any cause) in obese clients (Aune et al. 2016). Thus, recognising obesity and prompting treatment or action by the client is a major aspect of improving health in this client group.

Calculating BMI

There are many BMI calculators online, for instance, at https://www.nhs.uk/live-well/healthy-weight/bmi-calculator/, though, in a clinical setting, it is common to use a BMI chart such as the one in Figure 10.7.

Occasionally, it may be necessary to calculate the BMI yourself, and this is done by the equation:

$$\text{Weight in kilograms} \times \text{height in metres squared } (\text{kg} \times \text{m}^2)$$

BMI Chart

Underweight | Healthy | Overweight | Obese | Extremely obese

WEIGHT lbs	100	105	110	115	120	125	130	135	140	145	150	155	160	165	170	175	180	185	190	195	200	205	210	215
kgs	45.5	47.7	50.0	52.3	54.5	56.8	59.1	61.4	63.6	65.9	68.2	70.5	72.7	75.0	77.3	79.5	81.8	84.1	86.4	88.6	90.9	93.2	95.5	97.7
HEIGHT in/cm																								
5'0" - 152.4	19	20	21	22	23	24	25	26	27	28	29	30	31	32	33	34	35	36	37	38	39	40	41	42
5'1" - 154.9	18	19	20	21	22	23	24	25	26	27	28	29	30	31	32	33	34	35	36	36	37	38	39	40
5'2" - 157.4	18	19	20	21	22	22	23	24	25	26	27	28	29	30	31	32	33	33	34	35	36	37	38	39
5'3" - 160.0	17	18	19	20	21	22	23	24	24	25	26	27	28	29	30	31	32	32	33	34	35	36	37	38
5'4" - 162.5	17	18	18	19	20	21	22	23	24	24	25	26	27	28	29	30	31	31	32	33	34	35	36	37
5'5" - 165.1	16	17	18	19	20	20	21	22	23	24	25	25	26	27	28	29	30	30	31	32	33	34	35	35
5'6" - 167.6	16	17	17	18	19	20	21	21	22	23	24	25	25	26	27	28	29	29	30	31	32	33	34	34
5'7" - 170.1	15	16	17	18	18	19	20	21	22	22	23	24	25	25	26	27	28	29	29	30	31	32	33	33
5'8" - 172.7	15	16	16	17	18	19	19	20	21	22	22	23	24	25	25	26	27	28	28	29	30	31	32	32
5'9" - 175.2	14	15	16	17	17	18	19	20	20	21	22	22	23	24	25	25	26	27	28	28	29	30	31	31
5'10" - 177.8	14	15	15	16	17	18	18	19	20	20	21	22	23	23	24	25	25	26	27	28	28	29	30	30
5'11" - 180.3	14	14	15	16	16	17	18	18	19	20	21	21	22	23	23	24	25	25	26	27	28	28	29	30
6'0" - 182.8	13	14	14	15	16	17	17	18	19	19	20	21	21	22	23	23	24	25	25	26	27	27	28	29
6'1" - 185.4	13	13	14	15	15	16	17	17	18	19	19	20	21	21	22	23	23	24	25	25	26	27	27	28
6'2" - 187.9	12	13	14	14	15	16	16	17	18	18	19	19	20	21	21	22	23	23	24	25	25	26	27	27
6'3" - 190.5	12	13	13	14	15	15	16	16	17	18	18	19	20	20	21	21	22	23	23	24	25	25	26	26
6'4" - 193.0	12	12	13	14	14	15	15	16	17	17	18	18	19	20	20	21	22	22	23	23	24	25	25	26

Figure 10.7 **BMI chart.**

Once the BMI has been calculated, then it is necessary to compare the number with the ranges for BMI (National Institute for Health and Care Excellence 2014).

CLASSIFICATION	BMI (KG/M^2)
Healthy weight	18.5–24.9
Overweight	25–29.9
Obesity I	30–34.9
Obesity II	35–39.9
Obesity III	40 or more

Source: National Institute for Health and Care Excellence (NICE) (2014). © 2014 NICE

Discussions of whether the BMI is the most accurate measure of obesity are common; however, both the National Institute for Health and Care Excellence (2014) and clinical authors (see Adab et al. 2018) note that BMI is the most useful tool for general screening, but at times, other measures (such as waist circumference measurement) may be valuable.

There are occasions where it is not possible to measure a client's BMI (for instance, in the critically ill); in these circumstances, it is possible to estimate BMI by using the mid-upper arm circumference (MUAC). This measure is widely recognised as having limited accuracy but is still a useful tool for measuring BMI when other methods are not available (Brito et al. 2016).

To measure MUAC, the arm should be bent at the elbow to a 90° angle (Figure 10.8). Measure the distance between the bony protrusion of the shoulder and the point of the elbow. Mark the midpoint between the two; this is the mid-upper arm and the point where the measurement will be taken. To measure the circumference, use a non-stretch measuring tape and ask the patient to allow their arm to hang loose (thus avoiding arm muscle use), wrap the measuring tape around the arm so that it is snug (but not tight) and measure the circumference (Figure 10.9).

If MUAC is <23.5 cm, the BMI is likely to be <20 kg/m^2.

If MUAC is >32.0 cm, the BMI is likely to be >30 kg/m^2.

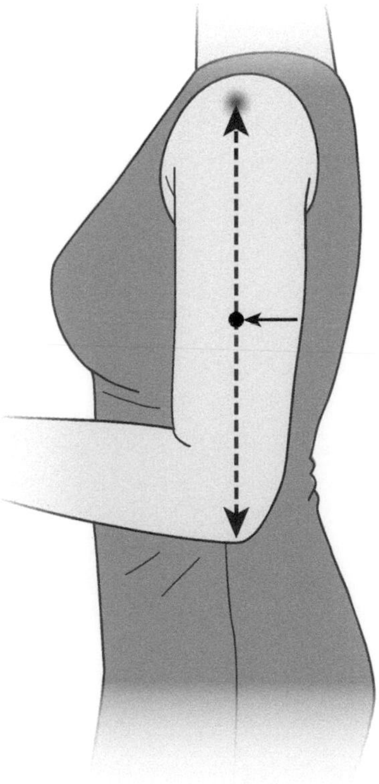

Figure 10.8 Measuring arm length. ***Source:*** **MUST Calculator (2003). © 2003 BAPEN reproduced with kind permission of BAPEN, British Association for Parenteral and Enteral Nutrition.**

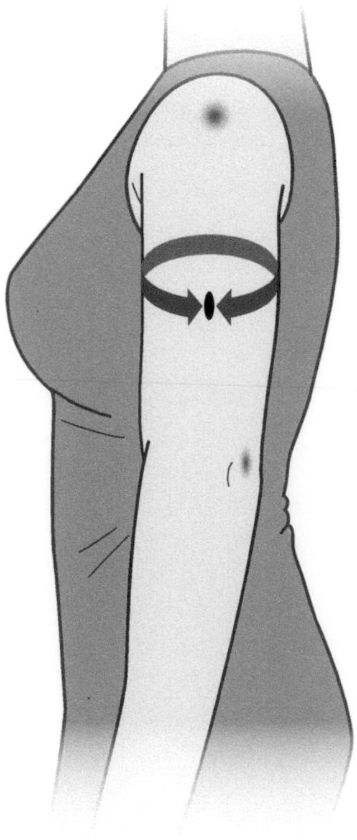

Figure 10.9 Measuring MUAC. ***Source:*** **MUST Calculator (2003). © 2003 BAPEN reproduced with kind permission of BAPEN, British Association for Parenteral and Enteral Nutrition.**

Touch Point

BMI is one of the few clinical measurements in use that carries a social stigma. When measuring and discussing BMI, it is necessary for the healthcare provider to be sensitive and to maintain privacy.

There are many ways to calculate BMI including online calculators, BMI charts and undertaking the calculation yourself. In some cases, it may not be possible to assess the client's height and weight, and in these circumstances, MUAC may be used.

McErlean, in Chapter 30 of this text, discusses BMI as a tool that can be used when assessing nutritional status. BMI is a starting point in identifying those people who are at risk of malnutrition and who may need a nutritional care plan.

Conclusion

A nursing associate needs to recognise and act appropriately when a patient's condition deteriorates. Monitoring vital signs is essential to identify and track changes in a patient's condition and recognise any symptoms of concern.

Vital signs are fundamental aspects of patient assessment providing a baseline and determining the patient's usual range. They assist in identifying deterioration or improvement in patient's condition and also help determine the level of care required.

Vital signs form part of an early warning scoring system and should be measured in response to the patient's condition; this is usually at least once in every 12 hours unless specified otherwise (National Institute for Health and Care Excellence 2007). Vital signs are recorded on admission and must be documented clearly and according to local policy and procedure.

References

Adab, P., Pallan, M. and Whincup, P.H. (2018) Is BMI the best measure of obesity? *BMJ* 2018, 360: k1274.

Adderley, N.J., Ryan, R., Nirantharakumar, K. and Marshall, T. (2019) Prevalence and treatment of atrial fibrillation in UK general practice from 2000 to 2016, *Heart*, 105(1): 27–33.

Aune, D., Sen, A., Prasad, M., Norat, T., Janszky, I., Tonstad, S., Romundstad, P. and Vatten, L.J. (2016) BMI and all cause mortality: systematic review and non-linear dose-response meta-analysis of 230 cohort studies with 3.74 million deaths among 30.3 million participants, *BMJ* 2016, 353: i2156.

Brito, N.B., Llanos, J.P.S., Ferrer, M.F., García, J.G.O., Brito, I.D., Castro, F.P.G., Caracena Castellanos, N., Acevedo Rodríguez, C.X. and Abizanda, E.P. (2016) Relationship between mid-upper arm circumference and body mass index in inpatients, *PLoS One*, 11(8): e0160480.

Cretikos, M.A., Bellomo, R., Hillman, K., Chen, J., Finfer, S. and Flabouris, A. (2008) Respiratory rate: the neglected vital sign, *Medical Journal of Australia*, 188(11): 657–659.

Curtis, J., Phillips, M. and Clery, E. (eds.). (2016) *British social attitudes: 33rd report*, London: National Centre for Social Statistics.

Gormley-Flemming, E. and Martin, D. (2018) *Children's nursing skills at a glance*. Wiley-Blackwell: Chichester.

Hill, A., Kelly, E., Horswill, M.S. and Watson, M.O. (2018) The effects of awareness and count duration on adult respiratory rate measurements: an experimental study, *Journal of Clinical Nursing*, 27(3–4): 546–554.

Howard, L. (2010) Supporting mental health nurses to address the physical health needs of people with serious mental illness in acute inpatient care settings, *Journal of Psychiatric Mental Health Nursing*, 18(2): 105–112.

MUST Calculator. (2003) Retrieved from: https://www.bapen.org.uk/screening-and-must/must-calculator. BAPEN, British Association for Parenteral and Enteral Nutrition.

National Institute for Health and Care Excellence (NICE). (2007) *CG50 Acutely ill adults in hospital: recognising and responding to deterioration*. [online] Available: https://www.nice.org.uk/guidance/cg50. Accessed 2 January 2020.

National Institute for Health and Care Excellence (NICE). (2014) *CG189 Obesity: identification, assessment and management*. [online] Available: https://www.nice.org.uk/guidance/cg189. Accessed 2 January 2020.

National Institute for Health and Care Excellence (NICE). (2017) *NG51 Sepsis: recognition, diagnosis and early management*. [online] Available: https://www.nice.org.uk/guidance/ng51. Accessed 2 January 2020.

National Institute for Health and Care Excellence (NICE). (2019) *NG 136 Hypertension in adults: diagnosis and management*. [online] Available: https://www.nice.org.uk/guidance/ng136/chapter/Recommendations#diagnosing-hypertension. Accessed 2 January 2020.

Nursing and Midwifery Council. (2018a) *The code. professional standards of practice and behaviour for nurses, midwives and nursing associates*. [online] Available: https://www.nmc.org.uk/globalassets/sitedocuments/nmc-publications/nmc-code.pdf. Accessed January 2020.

Nursing and Midwifery Council (2018a) *Standards of proficiency for nursing associates*. [online] Available: https://www.nmc.org.uk/standards/standards-for-nursing-associates/standards-of-proficiency-for-nursing-associates/. Accessed January 2020.

Peate, I. and Wild, K. (2018). *Nursing practice knowledge and care* (2nd edn). John Wiley & Sons: Chichester.

Rimbi, M., Dunsmuir, D., Ansermino, J.M., Nakitende, I., Namujwiga, T. and Kellett, J. (2019) Respiratory rates observed over 15 and 30 s compared with rates measured over 60 s: practice-based evidence from an observational study of acutely ill adult medical patients during hospital admission, *QJM: An International Journal of Medicine*, 112(7): 513–517.

Robertson, M. and Hill, B. (2019) Monitoring temperature, *British Journal of Nursing*, 28(6): 344–347. doi:10.12968/bjon.2019.28.6.344.

Royal College of Nursing (RCN) (2017) *Standards for assessing, measuring and monitoring vital signs in infants, children and young people*, London: RCN.

Royal College of Physicians. (2017) *National early warning score (NEWS) 2. Standardising the assessment of acute-illness severity in the NHS. Updated report of a working party*, London: RCN.

Swift, J.A., Hanlon, S., El-Redy, L., Puhl, R.M. and Glazebrook, C. (2013) Weight bias among UK trainee dietitians, doctors, nurses and nutritionists, *Journal of Human Nutrition and Dietetics*, 26(4): 395–402.

Wong, E.C.K. (2018) On being human: reflections on a daily error, *BMJ Quality & Safety*, 27(8): e4–e4. doi:10.1136/bmjqs-2017-007415.

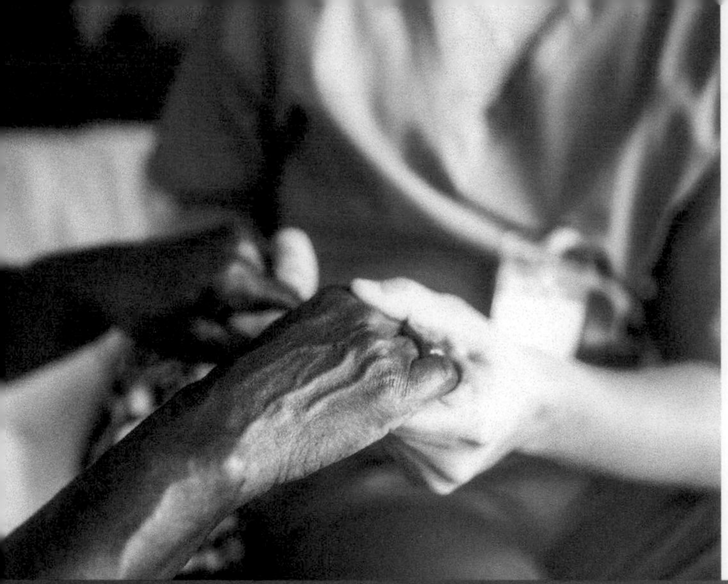

11

Venepuncture

Carl Clare

University of Hertfordshire, UK

Chapter Aim

- **This chapter aims to provide readers with an insight into the skill of performing venepuncture.**

Learning Outcomes

By the end of this chapter, the reader will be able to:

- **Understand the clinical indications for performing venepuncture to collect blood samples**
- **Explore the anatomy of the vein**
- **Describe the potential complications of venepuncture**
- **Explore the potential reasons for blood samples being rejected by the laboratory**
- **Demonstrate the correct technique for safely performing venepuncture**

Test Yourself Multiple Choice Questions

1. **Laboratory-based analysis of blood samples is involved in what percentage of hospital-based care decisions?**
   A) **50%–60%**
   B) **60%–70%**
   C) **70%–80%**
   D) **80%–90%**
2. **Veins are used for venepuncture because they are:**
   A) **Low-pressure vessels**
   B) **High-pressure vessels**
   C) **Variable pressure vessels**
   D) **None of the above**

The Nursing Associate's Handbook of Clinical Skills, First Edition. Edited by Ian Peate.

Companion website: www.wiley.com/nursingassociate

3. The types of veins used in venepuncture are:
   A) **Superficial veins**
   B) **Deep veins**
   C) **Perforator veins**
   D) **Communicating veins**

4. The purpose of valves in the veins are to:
   A) **Prevent bleeding**
   B) **Prevent backward flow**
   C) **Seal punctures in veins**
   D) **Prevent the veins being overloaded**

5. Venepuncture of an artery is treated by pressure on the puncture site for at least:
   A) **10 minutes**
   B) **15 minutes**
   C) **20 minutes**
   D) **25 minutes**

Introduction

The expansion of a number of skills beyond the medical profession and other staff has led to the need for a variety of healthcare workers to perform a wider variety of skills. The justification for the expansion of the skills has always been to improve client care and to smooth the client journey. This has never been more true than in the performance of venepuncture. Laboratory-based analysis of blood samples is involved in 60%–70% of hospital-based clinical decisions (Makhumula-Nkhoma et al. 2019), and the ability of a variety of healthcare workers to undertake venepuncture aids timely clinical decision-making. Previously, clients would have to wait for a doctor or a phlebotomist to perform venepuncture; the ability of appropriately prepared staff at the bedside to take blood samples will remove this wait and free up the time of others to concentrate on other activities.

This chapter aims to explore the anatomy of the vein to aid with visualising the procedure and help understand complications that may arise. The chapter also aims to explore the reasons for laboratory staff rejecting blood samples leading to the need for a repeat venepuncture and delaying the presentation of information from the blood analysis. Finally, the chapter will discuss the technique of safely performing venepuncture.

Take Note

Venepuncture is a psychomotor skill and must never be performed without adequate physical training and assessment. This chapter is meant as an aid to training and does not replace the need for that training.

It is assumed that before engaging in any intervention with a client, you will:

- Wash your hands
- Introduce yourself to the patient
- Explain what you are going to do and gain consent
- Ensure the person is comfortable.

The Nursing and Midwifery Council's (NMC) (2018a) standards of proficiency for nursing associates are the practice standards that provide the framework for ensuring that the nursing associate is fit for practice. These standards communicate to the public the standards that are expected from nursing associates. The standards are closely aligned to the Code of Conduct (Nursing and Midwifery Council 2018b).

The Anatomy of the Vein

Veins are the blood vessels that carry blood back to the heart from the bodily organs (and the lungs). They are the most useful blood vessels for taking blood samples because:

- They are low-pressure vessels and therefore will not bleed excessively once punctured.
- Some veins are close to the skin surface at many points, allowing fairly easy access.
- They have a relatively thin wall allowing for easier needle insertion.
- There are many veins that are large enough to allow the insertion of a needle without unnecessary trauma.

There are a number of different types of veins; however, for the purposes of this chapter, only the superficial veins will be discussed. Superficial veins, as the name suggests, are close to the surface of the skin (as opposed to deep veins), and they do not have an associated artery close by (reducing the possibility of puncturing an artery). The chapter will not discuss the physiology of veins as it is not necessary for the practice of venepuncture.

The structure of the wall of veins is similar to the structure of an artery in that both have:

- Inner layer (tunica intima) made up of a single cell layer (endothelium) on a thin basement layer of connective tissue
- Middle layer (tunica media) made of smooth muscle and elastic fibres
- Outer layer (tunica externa) which is a tough protective layer made of connective tissue and collagen

In veins, both the tunica media and tunica externa are significantly thinner than they are for an artery; the overall wall thickness is much thinner than that found in an artery. The benefit (from a healthcare perspective) of the much thinner muscle and protective layers is that veins are much easier to puncture with a needle.

There is another important difference between veins and arteries; this is the fact that veins have valves. The presence of valves in veins is to prevent 'backward flow' of blood in these low-pressure vessels. Valves are relatively delicate structures, and it is important to avoid damaging veins while performing venepuncture.

Site Selection for Venepuncture

The most common superficial veins to be used for venepuncture are the cephalic, basilic and median cubital veins (Figure 11.1). All of these veins can be found in the antecubital fossa (the front of the bend in the elbow).

Other sites for venepuncture include the forearm (using the cephalic, basilic or accessory cephalic veins) or the metacarpal veins in the hands (Shaw 2018).

Arm and site selection:

- Always avoid any arm affected by lymphoedema, as a result of mastectomy (especially with lymph node resection) or cerebrovascular accident
- Avoid sites affected by repeated or recent venepuncture
- Avoid sites near to fistulas or vascular grafts
- Avoid sites of psoriasis or eczema

Scarparis & Ford (2018)

Touch Point

- Arteries and veins have different structures.
- The most common point for venepuncture is the antecubital fossa (front of the elbow).
- Veins in the forearms or in the hands may be used.
- The veins in the hands are most often used in the venepuncture of older clients as they can be the most prominent in older age.

Complications of Venepuncture

The complications of venepuncture include:

Pain

Pain is subjective and always should be taken seriously when reported. Pain may be a response to the insertion of a needle into the skin, but severe pain or increasing pain may be the result of inserting the needle into a nerve. In the event of the patient reporting severe or increasing pain, the needle must be removed immediately to prevent further damage.

Pain perception in venepuncture may be affected by many factors, but personal experience is an important factor (McGowan 2014). Clients who have undergone repeated attempts at venepuncture or who have experienced complications (such as touching a nerve) will have a

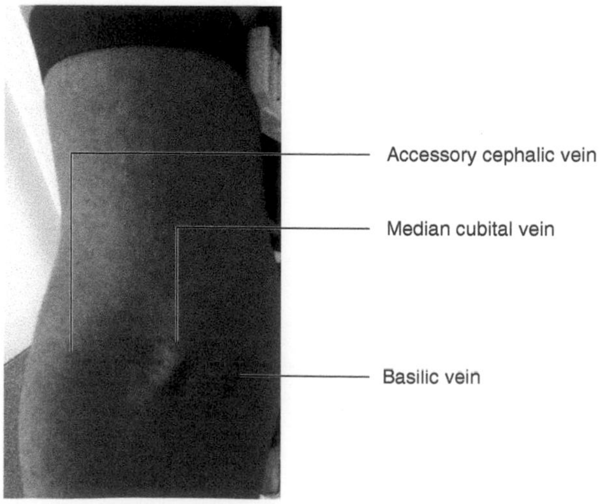

Figure 11.1 Accessory cephalic, median cubital and basilic veins. *Source:* From Lindsay et al. (2018), figure 47.1, p. 220.

heightened awareness of the impending procedure increasing their anticipation of the pain to follow. It is therefore important to discuss any fears a client may have with them to help allay any anxiety. Distraction techniques may also prove helpful in those with a heightened state of anxiety. It is never acceptable to lie to the client, and full consent must be gained before venepuncture. It is therefore useful to have a prepared script to use that utilises non-threatening words but does not ignore the actuality of venepuncture. Phrases such as 'sharp scratch' are often useful, and it may be helpful to discuss distraction techniques and phrases used with experienced personnel (especially your local phlebotomists).

Though venepuncture of the metacarpal veins (in the hands) is possible and may be useful in older clients, these should be used as a last resort as using these veins can be very painful.

Orange Flag

Needle phobia is an increasingly recognised difficulty for clients undergoing venepuncture. Estimates suggest that up to 1 in 10 of the population may experience needle phobia. The resulting fear and anxiety may activate the sympathetic nervous system to the extent that clients may experience nausea and vomiting or even pass out. Furthermore, the activation of the sympathetic nervous system due to needle phobia can also lead to venoconstriction (constriction of the veins) making venepuncture even harder.

The use of distraction techniques or meditation techniques (such as breathing exercises) may help these patients. The use of pain-relieving creams may also be considered to numb the skin; however, these creams require time to work, and the wait may be counterproductive in very anxious patients.

Blue Flag

When caring for children and young people, nursing associates must be able demonstrate proficiency. They are also required to identify when other health professionals such as a hospital play specialist or child psychologist may be required to be involved in preparation of the child or young person. They are also required to explain the potential for therapeutic holding, checking whether the child and/or parents are happy with this.

Venepuncture of an Artery

The venepuncture of an artery is easily noticed as the blood entering the tube will be under significant pressure. In these instances, it is important to remove the needle and apply pressure (to stop the subsequent bleeding) for at least 15 minutes. While applying pressure, observe the hand for blanching to make sure a blood supply is perfusing the tissues of the hand. Always record and report any insertion of a needle into an artery. Even after the person has stopped bleeding, arterial punctures can begin bleeding again, and thus, it will be necessary to ask the client to rest the arm and observe the site for any new bleeding. Significant bruising can appear following an arterial puncture, and the client should be informed of this.

Bleeding and Bruising

Even after venous puncture (inserting a needle into the vein), there is a possibility for bleeding to occur after pressure has been removed; this may be evidenced by further bleeding from the puncture site or the development of a bruise at the site. Inform the client not to use the arm for any heavy lifting or exercise for a few hours after venepuncture to allow the vein to heal sufficiently. If the arm begins to bleed again, then pressure will need to be reapplied for a further period of time.

Insertion of a Needle into a Nerve

This will almost certainly result in significant pain for the client. The needle must be removed immediately, the client informed of what happened and the incident recorded and reported.

Nerve injury will normally be obvious as the client will report one (or more) of the following symptoms:

- Electric shock in the arm
- Sharp, shooting pain in the arm
- Pain or discomfort in the hands (including pins and needles).

Damage to nerves by venepuncture is unusual but can happen, so recording the incident is important to aid future healthcare workers should the client return with symptoms of nerve damage.

Touch Point

The complications of venepuncture include:

- Pain
- Bleeding
- Bruising
- Nerve damage
- Inserting the needle into an artery.

Always listen to the patient before and during venepuncture as the information given can help you to make the procedure as safe and non-traumatic as possible.

Supporting Evidence

Guidelines for venepuncture are provided by the Blood Transfusion Services in the UK: Performance of the venepuncture (UK Blood Transfusion and Tissue Transplantation Services – UKBTS) https://www.transfusionguidelines.org/red-book/chapter-5-collection-of-a-blood-or-component-donation/5-6-performance-of-the-venepuncture

Undertaking Venepuncture

Venepuncture is an invasive procedure and should only be undertaken following appropriate training, education and assessment. When undertaking venepuncture, as with any procedure that breaks the skin, it is important that an aseptic no-touch technique is used.

- Confirm that you have the correct client. Ask them verbally and, where appropriate, check any wrist band; compare both the verbal response and the wrist band against the request form.
- Check the medical history of the client. Pay special attention to any sites of operation (surgical procedure) below the elbow and any mention of vascular disease.
- Where possible, and appropriate, ask the patient which arm they would prefer to have the blood taken from.
- Ask the patient if there is any reason they should not have blood taken from the chosen arm.
- Explain to the patient what you are going to do and gain explicit consent. Answer any questions the client may have.
- Ask the client to remove any clothing that is covering the site to be used. Offer assistance if required.
- Make sure the patient is in a comfortable, relaxed, position and their arm is supported.
- Check the sample request form for what samples are to be taken and check the policy for what order they should be drawn in.
- Assemble the equipment required. Checking equipment is in date and the seals are not broken.
- Always adhere to local policy and procedure.

Green Flag

Informed consent is essential when the nursing associate takes blood from a patient. All of the principles of gaining consent apply in this situation as in any other situation. Three requirements must be achieved in order to obtain informed consent:

1. Consent should be given by someone with the mental ability to do so.
2. Sufficient information should be given to the patient.
3. Consent must be freely given.

Box 11.1 provides information regarding equipment required and the procedure for venepuncture. Local policy and procedure must be adhered to at all times.

Red Flag Inserting a needle into a valve

Occasionally, despite best practice, you may insert the needle into a valve. This will be clear from the splash of blood into the collection tube, and then, blood will stop flowing as the valve closes over the needle. If this happens, it may be possible to clear the valve by advancing or withdrawing the needle slightly until blood flows again. Otherwise, remove the tourniquet, withdraw the needle and apply suitable pressure. Explain what is happening to the patient; once bleeding has stopped, try another site.

Violet Flag

Custody nurses provide healthcare services in police custody suites. They are responsible for conducting clinical assessments, identifying and implementing appropriate interventions, collecting forensic samples and offering advice and guidance to detainees and police staff.

Custody nurses are also involved in the taking of samples (such as blood) for analysis and assessing the health of those who may be under the influence of drugs and/or alcohol.

Haemolysed Samples

Haemolysis is the breakdown of red blood cells, leaking the contents of the cells into the surrounding plasma. Haemolysis can be attributed to:

- the equipment used
- tourniquet time
- the collection site (the more distal, the more chance of haemolysis)
- blood transportation policies (Makhumula-Nkhoma et al. 2015)

Box 11.1 Equipment Required and the Procedure for Venepuncture.

Equipment required for venepuncture:

- Clean surface for the equipment.
- Sample request form.
- Specimen bag.
- Gloves.
- Disposable apron.
- Alcohol gel.
- Tourniquet (depending on local policy, this may be new, one patient disposable use, or one cleaned in accordance with policy).
- Skin cleansing wipe or equivalent (depending on local policy).
- Needle holder.
- Needle (21G is standard; use 22G for small or fragile veins).
- If the metacarpal veins are to be used, then a butterfly needle with wings is easier for you and more comfortable for the patient than a standard holder/needle system. The butterfly needle should have a connector for the collection system attached by a short, flexible tube.
- Blood collection tubes.
- Gauze swabs and tape (check that the patient is not allergic to the tape used).
- Sharps bin.
- Pen.

The procedure (sample collection):

- Wash hands.
- Put on a disposable apron, and cleanse your hands with alcohol gel.
- Carry out an initial visual inspection of the client's skin and veins. Look for signs of bruising, breaks in the skin, swelling or any other reason to avoid a particular area.
- Apply the tourniquet about 8 cm above the venepuncture site, making sure the tourniquet is not so tight as to compromise circulation.
- Assess and palpate the veins.
  - A suitable vein will be bouncy to touch, do not have a pulse and after being depressed will refill rapidly.
  - Hard veins indicate thrombosis, and the vein should be avoided.
  - Valves will feel like a hard point to the touch and should be avoided.
- Clean the site as per policy.
- Release the tourniquet.
- Make sure all the equipment is to hand and ready to use. Preferably, this will be closest to your non-dominant hand, thus preventing reaching over during the procedure.
- Cleanse your hands with gel and put on gloves.
- Reapply the tourniquet.
- Hold the needle holder in your dominant hand with the bezel of the needle face up and remove the needle cover.
- Anchor the vein by placing the thumb of your non-dominant hand below the vein and pulling gently on the skin.
- Warn the patient they will feel a 'sharp scratch'.
- Hold the needle at an angle of 15–30 degrees and advance it through the skin stopping when you no longer feel resistance or if you feel a 'pop' (the needle entering the vein) (Figure 11.2).
- Pick up a blood collection tube and hold the needle holder in place, insert the tube into the holder and push it home with your thumb.
- With your non-dominant hand, remove the tourniquet as soon as blood flows into the tube.
- Remove the collection tube and invert it several times (do not shake).
- Repeat with as many collection tubes as required.
- Once the required tubes have been filled, pick up a gauze swab with your non-dominant hand. Remove the needle and apply pressure to the site with the gauze swab until bleeding has stopped.
- If it is possible, ask the patients to straighten their arm and apply pressure to the gauze swab, being aware of patients with limited strength or conditions such as arthritis.
- Dispose of the needle according to local policy.
- Label the blood collection tubes, including time and date of collection. Never label collection tubes before collection, and never leave the patient's side until the tubes are labelled as both can lead to errors in labelling.
- Check the site has stopped bleeding and that no bruising has appeared. Remember that in those clients who are taking anticoagulant medication it may take longer for bleeding to stop.
- Once you are satisfied bleeding has stopped, use tape to secure a fresh swab to the puncture site and ask the client to remove it in a few hours.
- Seal the samples in the specimen bag.
- Dispose of clinical waste.
- Wash your hands.
- Document and report as per policy.

Source: Modified from Shaw (2018)

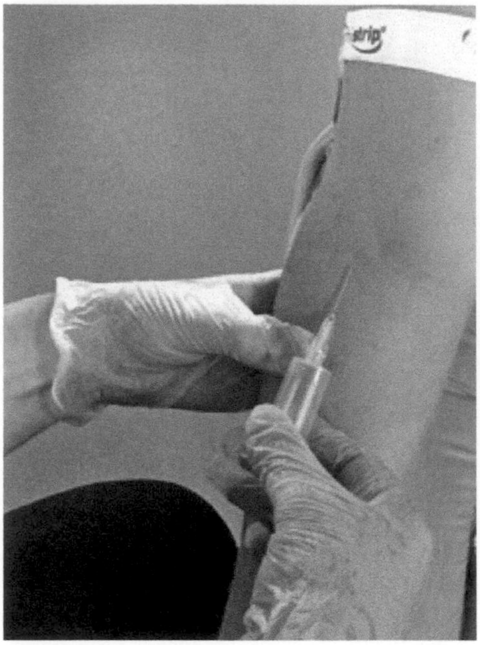

Figure 11.2 **Insertion of a needle at a 15–30° angle.** *Source:* from Lindsay et al. (2018), figure 47.1, p. 220.

Haemolysis leads to samples being rejected and thus the need for repeated venepuncture; this causes delays in patient data being available, increased pain from repeated venepuncture and has a cost implication in repeated tests.

Equipment Used

Samples collected via a cannula have a greater chance of being haemolysed, as opposed to those collected by a proprietary venepuncture system. Collecting samples into a syringe and then squirting the sample into a collection tube has an even higher rate of haemolysis. A proprietary collection system, even when using a butterfly needle, should be used to avoid complications.

Tourniquet Time

A tourniquet time of greater than 60 seconds appears to be related to haemolysis in the vein and venous stasis, leading to samples being haemolysed before collection. Minimise tourniquet time by releasing the tourniquet as soon as possible and never leaving it on for more than 60 seconds.

Collection Site

Samples collected from the antecubital fossa have a lower rate of haemolysis than those collected from a site distal to the antecubital fossa. Use the antecubital fossa where possible.

Blood Transportation Policies

Some hospitals use vacuum tube systems to transport blood samples which may lead to haemolysis. It is suggested that filling tubes to the recommended limit or above and mixing well reduces haemolysis. Ensure the tubes are filled to beyond the minimum level and invert several times (see manufacturer recommendations); do not shake the tubes.

Touch Point

Using the correct equipment, using the antecubital fossa, minimising tourniquet time and filling tubes appropriately all help to reduce the potential for the haemolysis of blood samples.

Conclusion

Venepuncture is a procedure that is performed by nursing associates and other healthcare staff in a wide variety of clinical areas as a clinical and diagnostic tool used to guide patient care.

Those nursing associates who undertake venepuncture must have received approved education and training and have been deemed competent to carry out the procedure. All nursing associates must practice within their scope of practice, adhering to local policy and procedure.

References

Lindsay, P., Bagness, C. and Peate, I. (Eds). (2018) *Midwifery skills at a glance*, Wiley-Blackwell: Chichester.

Makhumula-Nkhoma, N., Whittaker, V. and McSherry, R. (2015) Level of confidence in venepuncture and knowledge in determining causes of blood sample haemolysis among clinical staff and phlebotomists, *Journal of Clinical Nursing*, 24(3–4): 370–385.

Makhumula-Nkhoma, N., Weston, K.L., McSherry, R. and Atkinson, G. (2019) The impact of venepuncture training on the reduction of pre-analytical blood sample haemolysis rates: a systematic review, *Journal of Clinical Nursing*, 28(23–24): 4166–4176. doi:10.1111/jocn.14997.

McGowan, D. (2014) Peripheral intravenous cannulation: managing distress and anxiety, *British Journal of Nursing*, 23(Sup19): S4–S9.

Nursing and Midwifery Council. (2018a) *Standards of proficiency for nursing associates*. [online] Available: https://www.nmc.org.uk/standards/standards-for-nursing-associates/standards-of-proficiency-for-nursing-associates/. Accessed January 2020.

Nursing and Midwifery Council. (2018b) The code, *Professional standards of practice and behaviour for nurses, midwives and nursing associates*. [online] Available: https://www.nmc.org.uk/globalassets/sitedocuments/nmc-publications/nmc-code.pdf. Accessed January 2020.

Shaw, J.S. (2018) How to undertake venepuncture to obtain venous blood samples, *Nursing Standard*, 32(29): 41–47.

Scarparis, K. and Ford, C. (2018) Venepuncture in adults, *British Journal of Nursing*, 27(22): 1312–1315.

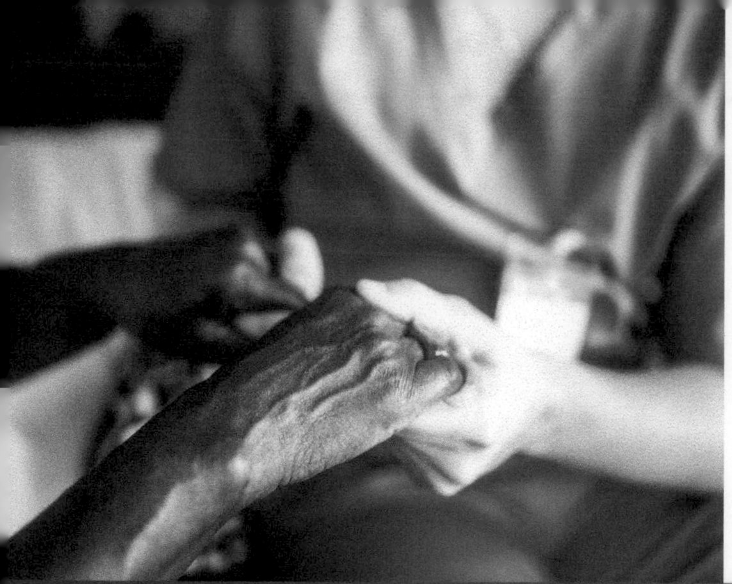

12

ECG Recording

Carl Clare

University of Hertfordshire, UK

Chapter Aim

- **This chapter aims to provide readers with the information necessary for recording a 12-lead electrocardiogram (ECG).**

Learning Outcomes

By the end of this chapter, the reader will be able to:
- **Understand the clinical importance of correct lead placement when recording a 12-lead ECG**
- **Demonstrate the correct lead placement when recording a 12-lead ECG**
- **Understand the clinical importance of recording a 12-lead ECG accurately**

Test Yourself Multiple Choice Questions

1. **Which condition is a 12-lead ECG not used to aid diagnose:**
   A) Myocardial infarction
   B) Unexplained fainting
   C) Chest pain
   D) Epilepsy
2. **In what position should a patient be placed for recording an ECG?**
   A) Flat
   B) Semi-recumbent
   C) Upright
   D) Recumbent

The Nursing Associate's Handbook of Clinical Skills, First Edition. Edited by Ian Peate.

Companion website: www.wiley.com/nursingassociate

3. The default paper speed for recording an ECG is:
- A) 10 mm/sec
- B) 15 mm/sec
- C) 20 mm/sec
- D) 25 mm/sec

4. Electromagnetic interference is very fast; on an ECG tracing, what frequency will the interference present?
- A) 50 Hz
- B) 60 Hz
- C) 70 Hz
- D) 80 Hz

5. The red lead is normally placed on:
- A) The right arm
- B) The left arm
- C) The right leg
- D) The left leg

Introduction

The 12-lead ECG is one of the skills in healthcare practice that appears simple but is in fact a skill that requires training, education, practice and knowledge. It is not a test that should be undertaken quickly or without due care, as even minor differences in the positioning of the ECG leads may affect the outcome of the test (Harrigan et al. 2012). As a patient's ECGs are often used in comparison with each other, over time, it is essential that all ECGs are taken using the correct technique each time an ECG is taken. The accuracy of the ECG that is recorded is dependent on many factors, and in this chapter, there will be a discussion of the correct technique for recording an ECG and how to deal with common issues that arise when making the recording.

Clinically, the 12-lead ECG is utilised in the diagnosis and monitoring of many conditions including:

- Myocardial infarction
- Angina
- Heart rhythm disturbances (arrhythmias)
- Chest pain
- Unexplained fainting
- As a screening test before surgery.

The interpretation of the 12-lead ECG is a diagnostic issue and remains the role of the medical staff; as such, all 12-lead ECGs must be reviewed by a member of medical staff at the earliest opportunity.

It is assumed that before engaging in any intervention with a patient, you will:

- Wash your hands
- Introduce yourself to the patient
- Explain what you are going to do and gain consent
- Ensure that the person is comfortable.

Green Flag

Recording a 12-lead ECG requires the patient to expose their chest completely. It is always therefore important to maintain privacy and dignity (Nursing and Midwifery Council 2018a).

- Ensure privacy is maintained by performing the procedure in a closed room or behind curtains
- The patients are required to remove all their upper clothes; the nursing associate should assist them if necessary; otherwise, maintain dignity by looking away/being busy while they do to avoid embarrassment
- Offer the presence of a chaperone
- Allow the patient to dress as soon as possible after the test
- If you need to have the ECG checked before removing the leads, cover the patient with a blanket

The Nursing and Midwifery Council (2018b) Standards of Proficiency for Nursing Associates require the nursing associate, at the point of registration, to be able to safely demonstrate routine ECG recording.

Machine Preparation

There are numerous 12-lead ECG machines in use in clinical practice, and it would be impractical to discuss the variations in models; however, before taking a 12-lead ECG, there are some checks to be made that are common to all machines.

- Ensure the machine is clean
- Ensure the battery is charged or there is access to mains electricity at the bedside
- All leads, cables and connectors should be intact with no evidence of fractures, faults or damage
- The machine is well stocked with electrodes, tissues, razors, skin preparation equipment and ECG paper
- Once you are at the client's bedside enter client's name and date of birth as a minimum. It is best practice to enter the hospital number as well.

Red Flag

Do not leave electrodes attached to the patient's cable or put neatly arranged rows of electrodes 'ready to go' on the trolley even if they are used on a daily basis. The electrode gel will dry out and the electrodes rendered unusable.

Electrodes should be stored in as airtight a condition as possible (for instance, resealing the packaging they came in), and expiry dates should be checked before use.

Area Preparation (Environment)

The environment/area in which the ECG recording is to take place must be:

- Private.
- Clean.
- Appropriately heated.
- Contain a bed or couch of sufficient size for the patient. The bed or couch should be height adjustable to enable the patient to get on and off easily while being able to be raised to a height suitable for you so that you do not have to crouch or bend over unnecessarily.

Patient Preparation

Communication

Communication is key to any healthcare intervention, and taking a 12-lead ECG is no different in this respect.

- Introduce yourself and explain the procedure you wish to undertake
- Ensure you have the correct patient by asking them to confirm their personal details
- Explain to the patient how the procedure is undertaken; include details such as the level of undress required, the use of adhesive electrodes and that the procedure is quick and painless
- Gain consent and ask the patient client if they wish a chaperone to be present (a carer or family member may also be present if the patient wishes)
- Clarify if the patient requires help with dressing and undressing.

Blue Flag

Explaining clearly and carefully to the patient about the ECG recording can help to alleviate fears and anxieties and enhance the patient–nursing associate relationships. Explain that an electrocardiogram – or ECG – is a simple and useful test which records the rhythm, rate and electrical activity of heart. Inform the patient that they do not need to do anything special to prepare for the test; they can eat and drink as normal beforehand.

The whole test takes a few minutes and is completely painless; the patient will be able to go home soon afterwards or return to the ward if already an inpatient. The results of the ECG may not be available immediately. The recordings may need to be looked at by a cardiologist to see if there are signs of a potential problem. There may be other tests required before it is possible to tell if there is a problem. The patient may need to visit the hospital, clinic or general practitioner a few days later to discuss the results.

Once consent has been gained, the patient is expected to undress their top half completely, and women will be required to remove tights to allow access to the ankles (socks may be rolled down if required). Ensure the area is private, and there is no risk of interruption to ensure their safety.

Once undressed, the patient will be required to lie on the bed or couch. Lower the bed/couch to an appropriate level to allow the patient to get on to the bed/couch; offer and provide assistance if required. It is important that the patient is comfortable and relaxed; otherwise, the recording may be affected. The patient is then placed in a semi-recumbent position of approximately 45° (Stevenson et al. 1989). Any variation from this (for instance, sitting up beyond 45°) must be recorded on the ECG.

Skin Preparation

Skin preparation is necessary before electrode placement to ensure good contact and to reduce artefact on the ECG recording (Clochesy et al. 1991). Care should be taken when preparing the skin of a patient with broken or frail skin.

- Chest hair may need to be removed (ensure consent before doing so)
- Skin may need cleaning due to dirt or greasy skin. There are several methods of doing this, but alcohol wipes are effective and reduce the need to dry the skin afterwards. Soap and water may be required if the client is especially dirty (for instance, blood from trauma)
- Exfoliation may be required; some electrodes come with proprietary abrasive material; otherwise, a paper towel will be good enough.

Lead Placement

The correct placement of leads is necessary to ensure a good-quality recording and to avoid errors in the recording due to incorrect lead placement (Harrigan et al. 2012).

Limb Lead Placement

The limb leads are generally colour coded to aid with identification (they are also often labelled with an abbreviation). The following colours are the standard colours used in Europe.

- Right arm limb lead (RA, red) – right forearm, proximal to wrist
- Left arm limb lead (LA, yellow) – left forearm, proximal to wrist
- Left leg limb lead (LL, green) – left lower leg, proximal to ankle
- Right leg limb lead (RL, black) – right lower leg, proximal to ankle

Some find it useful to use the mnemonic 'Ride your green bike' (Red yellow green black), starting with the right arm, to aid limb lead placement (Figure 12.1).

It has been shown that lead placement should be on the arms and legs and slightly closer to the centre (proximal) than the appropriate joint. Placing limb leads on the torso has been shown to change the ECG recording (Sheppard et al. 2011), and while this has been demonstrated to be a limited effect, standard practice statements require that any alteration to the limb lead position is recorded on the ECG (Campbell et al. 2017).

In the event of significant muscle tremor (causing artefact) or limb amputation, then limb placement may be moved to the upper thighs and upper arms, and this is noted on the ECG. It is important that if any limb lead is moved, then all leads are moved as mixed limb lead placement is contraindicated in recording 12-lead ECGs.

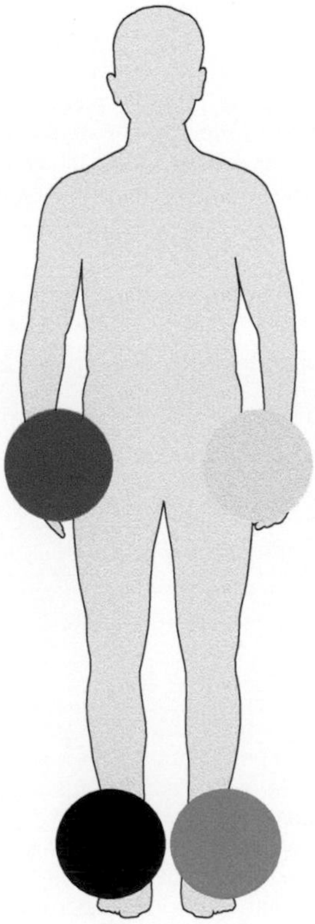

Figure 12.1 Limb lead position by colour.

Take Note

The lead placement discussed in this chapter refers only to recording a 12-lead ECG; lead placement for continuous monitoring and 24-hour ECG recordings uses the torso as the recordings are for different clinical reasons.

Chest Lead Placement

Chest lead placement takes time and concentration; the correct placement of chest leads is of vital importance, especially in situations where serial ECGs are being used to compare readings over a period of time. Chest leads are also known as precordial leads. Chest leads are traditionally labelled V1 to V6 (see Box 12.1) (though C1 to C6 can be seen in some texts).

When placing the chest leads, the most important lead position to find is V1; once V1 is placed, all other leads follow naturally from that, and if V1 is incorrectly placed, then all other leads will probably be incorrectly placed as well. To find the correct position for V1, run your fingers down the sternum, starting at the heads of the clavicles (collar bone), until you meet a bony horizontal ridge (the sternal angle or angle of Louis). With your finger on this ridge, slide it to the patient's right; your finger will drop into an intercostal space – this is the second intercostal space; now, move down to the third and then the fourth. Repeat this procedure on the opposite side of the sternum to locate V2.

Take Note

When locating chest lead positions (especially V1), do not palpate directly down from the clavicle as there is a possibility of counting the space before the first rib as the first intercostal space.

The next lead to be placed is V4. Moving down from the position of V2 to the next intercostal space (the fifth intercostal space) and the line of this space is traced until you have located the point corresponding to the mid-clavicular line. V3 is then placed between V2 and V4.

V5 is then placed in a horizontal line from V4 at the anterior axilla line (the 'start' of the armpit) and V6 horizontally from this point in the mid-axilla line. Do not 'curl' the placement of V5 and V6 to follow the intercostal space, as this changes their orientation to the heart (see Figures 12.3 and 12.4).

Yellow Flag

In female patients, electrodes are NEVER placed on top of the breast unless you cannot gain access to the normal position. If you do have to move onto the breast, write it on the recording. This may mean that when taking an ECG from a woman with large breasts, it may be necessary to lift the breast to gain access to the appropriate position. Where possible, ask the patient to lift the breast for you, and always be aware of cultural sensitivities towards touching intimate areas. If you must lift the breast for the patient, then use the back of your hand to reduce the chance of misinterpretation of the action. Remember to remove the electrodes after recording.

Recording the ECG

Confirm the settings have not been changed from the default:

- Speed 25 mm/sec
- Amplitude 10 mm/mV

Box 12.1 Chest Lead Placement

Precordial (chest) electrode positions (see Figure 12.2):
V1 (C1) – Fourth intercostal space at the right sternal edge
V2 (C2) – Fourth intercostal space at the left sternal edge
V3 (C3) – Midway between V2 and V4
V4 (C4) – Fifth intercostal space in the midclavicular line
V5 (C5) – Left anterior axillary line at the same horizontal level as V4
V6 (C6) – Left midaxillary line at the same horizontal level as V4 and V5.

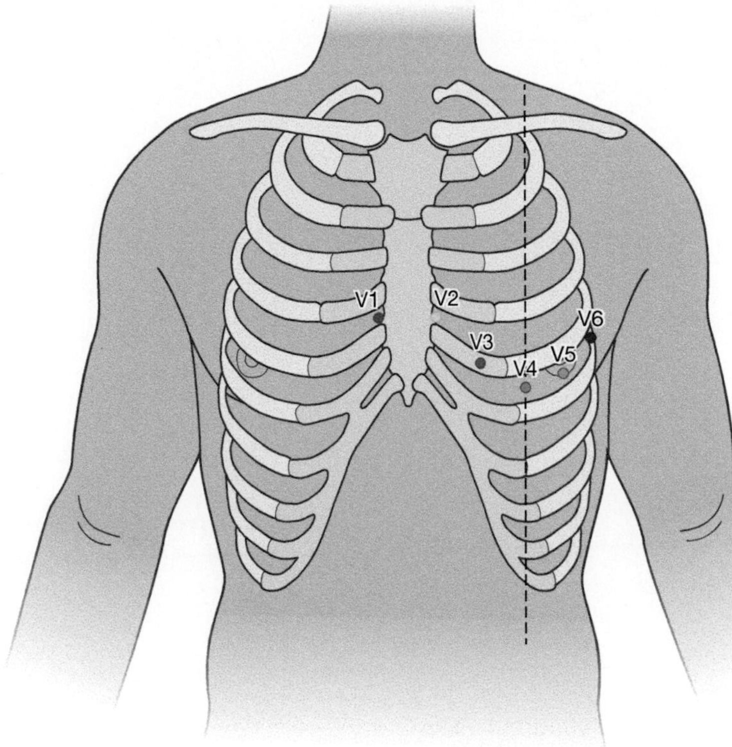

Figure 12.2 Chest (precordial) lead placement.

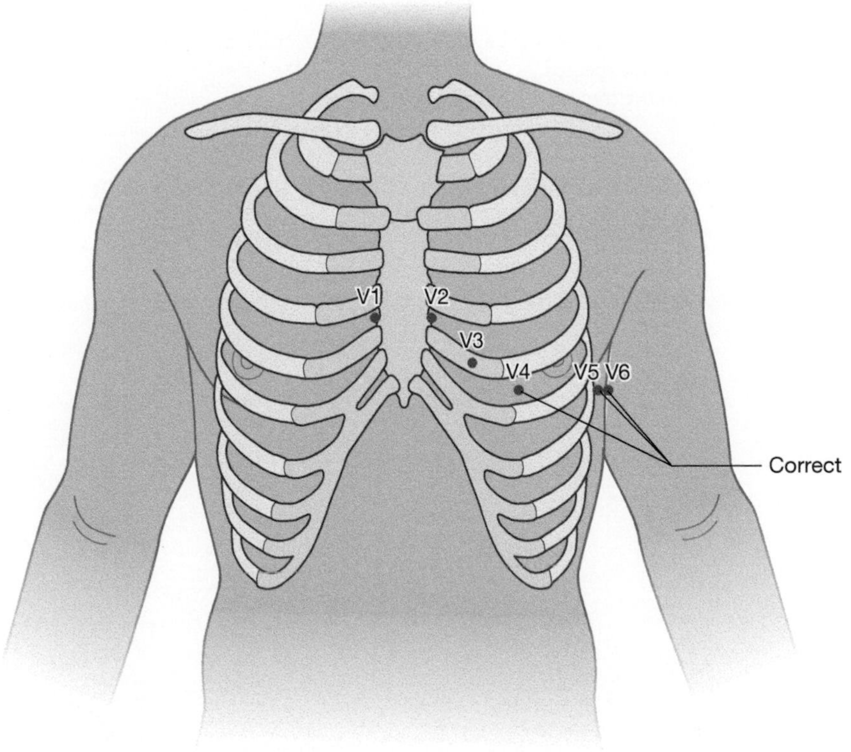

Figure 12.3 Correct placement of V5 and V6 (note the horizontal placement). *Source:* McStay (2019). © 2019 Mark Allen Holdings Ltd.

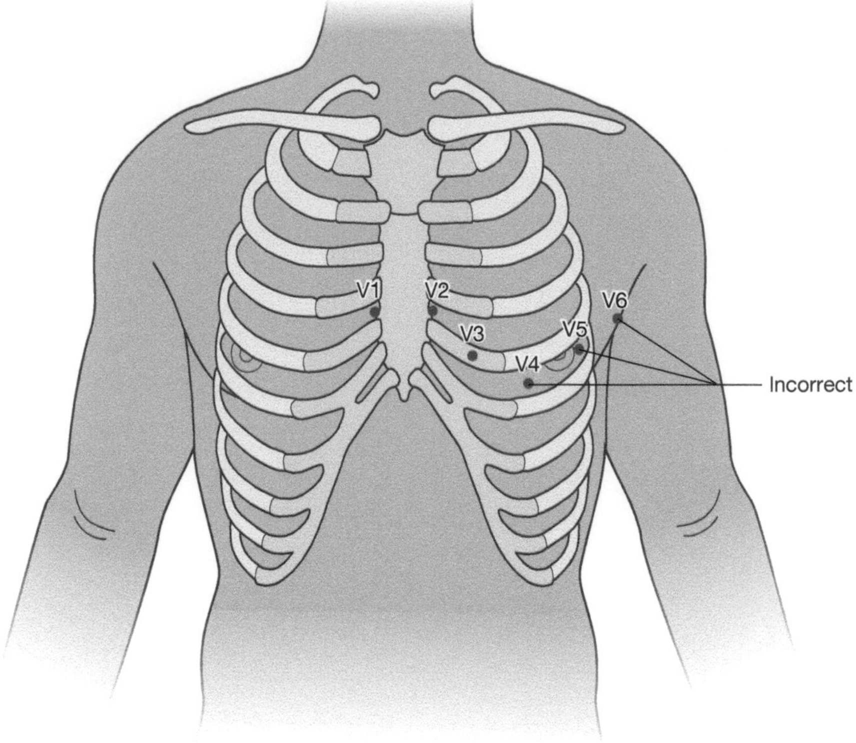

Figure 12.4 Incorrect placement of leads V5 and V6 (note the curvature of the placement). ***Source:*** **McStay (2019). © 2019 Mark Allen Holdings Ltd.**

ECG recording settings are not normally changed unless indicated by specific need; thus, it is unlikely the settings have been changed, but the best practice is to always confirm. Ask the patient to remain as still and relaxed as possible. Press the appropriate button to record the ECG. Once the tracing has been printed out, review it to confirm:

- The name and date are correct, as pressing the wrong button on the ECG machine may print out the ECG of the previous patient.
- The speed and amplitudes settings are as expected.
- There is no artefact or interference on the tracing.

Troubleshooting ECG Recordings

This section will look at some of the most common problems with 12-lead ECG tracings.

Most obvious in leads V4 and V6, the tracing is clearly not straight (see lead I for a mostly straight baseline). Causes of a wandering baseline (see Figure 12.5) include:

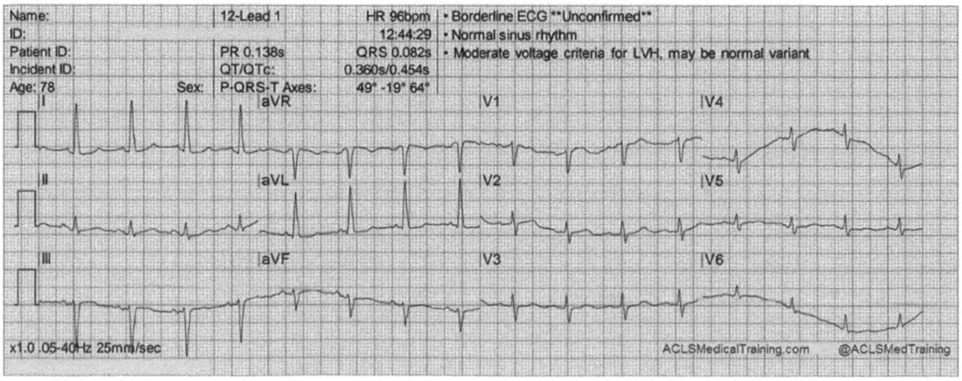

Figure 12.5 Wandering baseline.

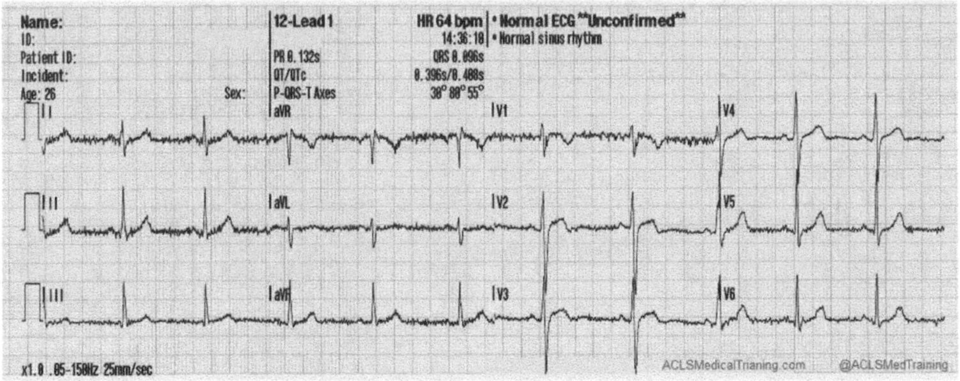

Figure 12.6 **Muscle tremor.**

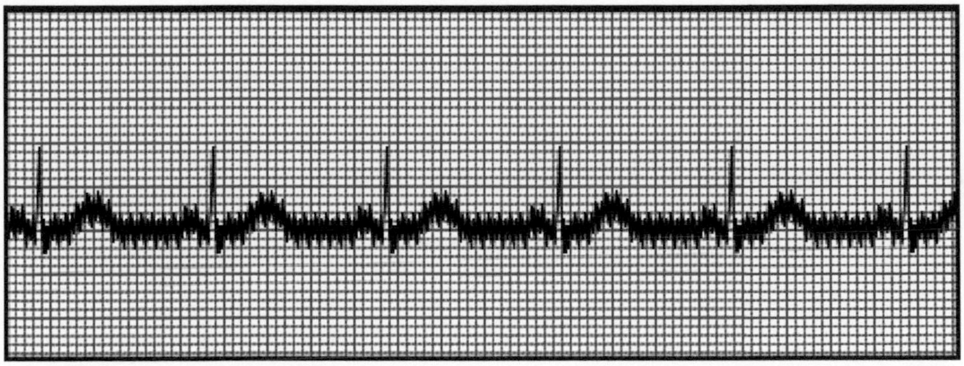

Figure 12.7 **Electromagnetic interference.** *Source:* ECG Artifact. Retrieved from: http://www.mauvila.com/ECG/ecg_artifact.htm. © 2004 Mauvila.

- Patients' movement: Ask them to relax and stay still.
- Dry or loose electrodes: Check all the electrodes and connections. Replace as necessary.

Causes of muscle tremor (see Figure 12.6) include:

- Primary tremor/Parkinson's disease: There is nothing that can be done about primary tremors and Parkinson's disease as they are medical conditions.
- Patients tensing their muscles (for instance, propping themselves up by their arms): Ask them to relax.
- Patient is shivering: Ensure an appropriate environmental temperature; cover the patient once the electrodes are connected.

The key to diagnosing electromagnetic interference (Figure 12.7) is that it is very fast (60 Hz), as it most often comes from machines using mains electricity. Modern ECG machines and electrical equipment in healthcare settings are usually shielded, but older equipment and equipment in the patients' homes may not be. Where safe to do so, turn off the mains electricity supply to any electrical equipment in the immediate area (for instance, electric beds), but be very careful not to turn off essential medical equipment such as monitors. In most cases, it is best to ask a colleague to identify what equipment can be disconnected from the mains electricity supply for a short period. Immediately after the ECG has been recorded, make sure to reconnect all equipment to the mains electricity.

Violet Flag

Telemonitoring is a medical practice that involves remotely monitoring patients who are not at the same location as the healthcare provider.

Home telemonitoring allows patients with long-term conditions, for example, heart failure to have their signs and symptoms assessed daily. In patients with heart failure, where the heart is failing to pump effectively, home telemonitoring may include the daily measurement of weight, blood pressure, heart rate and symptoms. These measurements are then transmitted to a clinician allowing a timely response to those whose condition is worsening, thereby helping to reduce unplanned hospital admissions.

After the recording has been made:

- Remove the electrodes and dispose of appropriately
- Lower the bed/couch to ensure the correct height for the patient
- If required, help the patient to redress

- Clean (adhering to local policy) and tidy the ECG machine and restock, if necessary
- Return the ECG machine to its appropriate storage space so other staff can find it and plug it in to maintain battery charge
- Ensure the ECG is reviewed by the appropriate staff
- Explain to the patient what the next steps are (i.e. when they will receive results).

Supporting Evidence

Stroobandt, R.X., Serge Barold, S. and Sinnaeve, A.L. (2016) *ECG from basics to essentials: step by step,* Chichester: Wiley.

This guide helps in developing a functional understanding of the setup, workings and interpretation of ECGs. It assists readers by providing step-by-step graphics and short, bite-sized explanations. The text comes complete with access to online practice tracings to help build confidence in interpretation once basic knowledge is acquired.

Conclusion

The ECG is simply a recording of the heart's electrical activity. Placing electrodes in the correct position on the skin and using an ECG machine can produce and record the electrical activity of the heart and the resulting waveforms. Depending on the type of machine used and the number of electrodes that are placed, several views of the heart's electrical activity can be recorded.

Recording an ECG is a complex task that should never be rushed; lead placement is especially important. If you are unsure if you are competent to undertake a 12-lead ECG recording, acknowledge your limitations and seek appropriate support.

References

Campbell, B., Richley, D., Ross, C. and Eggett, C.J. (2017) Clinical guidelines by consensus: recording a standard 12-lead electrocardiogram, *An approved method by the society for cardiological science and technology (SCST) 2017.* [online] Available: https://www.bmj.com/sites/default/files/response_attachments/2016/09/CAC_SCST_Recording_a_12-lead_ECG_final_version_2014_CS2v2.0.pdf. Accessed 3 January 2020.

Clochesy, J.M., Cifani, L. and Howe, K. (1991) Electrode site preparation techniques: a follow-up study, *Heart & Lung: The Journal of Critical Care*, 20(1): 27–30.

Harrigan, R.A., Chan, T.C. and Brady, W.J. (2012) Electrocardiographic electrode misplacement, misconnection, and artefact, *The Journal of Emergency Medicine*, 43(6): 1038–1044.

McStay, S. (2019). Recording a 12-lead electrocardiogram (ECG). *British Journal of Nursing*, 28(12): 756–760.

Nursing and Midwifery Council. (2018a) The code, *Professional standards of practice and behaviour for nurses, midwives and nursing associates.* [online] Available: https://www.nmc.org.uk/globalassets/sitedocuments/nmc-publications/nmc-code.pdf. Accessed January 2020.

Nursing and Midwifery Council. (2018b) *Standards of proficiency for nursing associates.* [online] Available: https://www.nmc.org.uk/standards/standards-for-nursing-associates/standards-of-proficiency-for-nursing-associates/. Accessed January 2020.

Sheppard, J.P., Barker, T.A., Ranasinghe, A.M., Clutton-Brock, T.H., Frenneaux, M.P. and Parkes, M.J. (2011) Does modifying electrode placement of the 12 lead ECG matter in healthy subjects? *International Journal of Cardiology*, 152(2): 184–191.

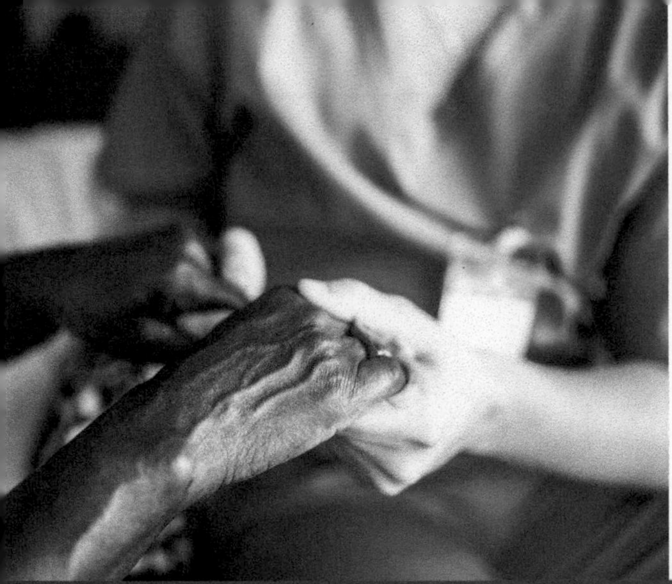

13

Blood Glucose Assessment

Carl Clare

University of Hertfordshire, UK

Chapter Aim

- **This chapter aims to provide readers with an insight into measuring the blood glucose of a patient using point-of-care blood testing or urinalysis.**

Learning Outcomes

By the end of this chapter, the reader will be able to:

- **Understand the clinical relevance of blood glucose**
- **Demonstrate the correct technique for measurement of blood glucose using urinalysis**
- **Demonstrate the correct technique for measurement of blood glucose using point-of-care blood testing (BM)**
- **Explore the strengths and weaknesses of both forms of blood glucose assessment**

Test Yourself Multiple Choice Questions

1. **HbA1c is used to measure:**
   A) **Glucose levels in real time**
   B) **Glucose levels over the preceding week**
   C) **Glucose levels over the preceding 2–3 months**
   D) **Glucose levels over the preceding 6 months**
2. **The most accurate form of glucose testing is:**
   A) **Urinalysis**
   B) **Capillary blood testing**
   C) **Laboratory analysis**
   D) **They are all equally accurate**

The Nursing Associate's Handbook of Clinical Skills, First Edition. Edited by Ian Peate.

Companion website: www.wiley.com/nursingassociate

3. **Capillary blood glucose should be tested in all patients**
   A) At the point of admission
   B) Daily
   C) Weekly
   D) Only if the patient is diabetic
4. **Factors affecting glucose levels in the urine include:**
   A) Age
   B) Pregnancy
   C) Time of day
   D) All of the above
5. **Patients on oral hypoglycaemic medicines should have their blood glucose tested**
   A) Four times a day
   B) Before meals
   C) Once a day
   D) Depending on the medicines prescribed

Introduction

The measurement of patient's blood glucose levels has become a common procedure for nursing associates and other healthcare workers, as well as for patients with diabetes. As with many practices and procedures, the procedures are only of value if the person carrying them out understands how to undertake the procedure, understands the value of the blood glucose assessment and records and reports the findings to senior staff. As noted by the Nursing and Midwifery Council (2018a, 2018b), it is a part of the role of the nursing associate to accurately identify, observe and assess signs of normal or worsening physical health in the person receiving care.

Violet Flag

Many people with diabetes have their own recording books; they will keep their blood glucose scores in these books (for example, those in the community); if a person you are offering care to has their own recording book and is having blood glucose measurements taken by you, ensure that the scores are recorded in the book as well as in your organisation's own observation chart. You should make sure you record your findings clearly and accurately so that they can be readily seen and understood. Always follow your organisation's policies and procedures on recording and reporting.

This chapter intends to help the student to understand how and why blood glucose is assessed and the strengths and weaknesses of the three main forms of blood glucose assessment. For the purposes of this chapter, the discussion will focus on the two most common ways to measure blood glucose:

1. Urinalysis
2. Point-of-care testing

   It will also touch on the third technique:

3. Laboratory testing of blood glucose.

As the laboratory testing of blood glucose requires the collection of a venous sample of blood via venepuncture, please refer to Chapter 11 'Venepuncture' for the correct procedure.

Reasons to Measure Blood Glucose

Testing for blood glucose may occur at several points in the day. Local policy for blood glucose testing should always take precedent over the recommendations of books or journal articles, but the most common times for blood glucose measurement are:

- At the point of admission to the hospital or care facility.
  - Many hospitals and hospital trusts require a random test at the point of entry to care as a simple screening tool. Undiagnosed diabetes remains a common condition in the United Kingdom with up to a million people having diabetes but being unaware of the fact (Holt 2014).
  - Especially in the Emergency Department, the care of a critically ill patient may be compromised by unrecognised (and therefore untreated) diabetes, and many patients who are aware they are diabetic do not wear any identification jewellery to identify the fact.
- All patients known to be insulin-dependent diabetics must be tested four times a day while in hospital.
  - The effects of illness, such as infection, are known to alter the blood glucose of patients with diabetes, as glucose may be released in response to trauma and illness. It is essential that blood glucose is controlled effectively during episodes of illness to aid recovery and prevent long-term complications.
  - The normal regimen is to test before meals (pre-prandial test) and before bedtime (hypoglycaemia during sleep is not uncommon).

- In some care facilities, all diabetic patients are tested four times a day for the first 2 days regardless of the treatment regimen for the diabetes.
  - This is to ensure the illness or trauma is not affecting blood glucose levels in the patient.
  - It may be the case that patients taking certain oral antidiabetic medicines (such as sulphonylureas) are tested four times a day for the entirety of their hospital stay. This is because some oral antidiabetic medicines are known to predispose patients to hypoglycaemia.
- Patients who have diabetes that is diet controlled or who are on oral antidiabetic medications may not need their blood glucose testing regularly after admission unless there are signs of infection.
  - In some organisations, a daily blood glucose measurement in these patients is required.
- All patients who commence acute steroid treatment should have a blood glucose on waking (before breakfast) and at one other time in the day.
- Acute steroid treatment is known to predispose patients to raised blood glucose, and this should be recognised as soon as possible.
  - Patients on long-term steroid medication should have blood glucose assessment at least once per year as they are predisposed to developing diabetes due to the steroid treatment.

In community care situations, blood glucose should be assessed:

- On admission for care to the service
  - As routine screening
- Prior to insulin injection
- If there is evidence of hypoglycaemia or hyperglycaemia
- If the patient is found unwell or confused
- If the patient has developed vomiting or diarrhoea
- If there are any changes made to the patient's diabetes medication
  - The frequency and duration of the testing is determined by the clinician in charge of the patient's care.

It is assumed that before engaging in any assessment of the patient, you will:

- Wash your hands
- Introduce yourself to the patient
- Explain what you are going to do and gain consent
- Make the person comfortable.

Blue Flag

There are many people with diabetes who have been taught how to check their own blood glucose levels and are very good at it. Others may be unable to do so because of illness or disability, so it may be the nursing associate who will be asked to undertake the procedure on their behalf.

Blood Glucose Levels

Appropriate blood glucose ranges depend on whether the patient is diabetic or not (see Table 13.1).

Urine Testing of Blood Glucose

While increasingly less common, the use of urinalysis remains widespread in the United Kingdom. Often, it is a measurement undertaken by patients who are diet controlled or on oral antidiabetic medication. The use of urinalysis in patients using insulin to control their diabetes is not recommended.

Table 13.1 Appropriate blood glucose levels.

TARGET LEVELS BY TYPE	UPON WAKING	BEFORE MEALS (PRE-PRANDIAL)	AT LEAST 90 MINUTES AFTER MEALS (POST-PRANDIAL)
Non-diabetic*		4.0–5.9 mmol/l	Under 7.8 mmol/l
Type 2 diabetes		4–7 mmol/L	under 8.5 mmol/L
Type 1 diabetes	5–7 mmol/L	4–7 mmol/L	5–9 mmol/L

* The non-diabetic figures are provided for information but are not part of the National Institute for Health and Care Excellence guidelines.
Source: Blood Sugar Level Ranges, 15 January 2019. Retrieved from: https://www.diabetes.co.uk/diabetes_care/blood-sugar-level-ranges.html (accessed 19 January 2020).

Urinalysis relies on the physiological fact that high blood glucose levels will lead to the 'overspill' of glucose into the urine via the kidneys. The level at which glucose will begin to appear in the urine is known as the renal threshold. The benefits of urinalysis are:

- It is a simple non-invasive test
- It is inexpensive

However, the weaknesses of urinalysis far outweigh its benefits (hence decreasing the use of it as a test).

- Urinalysis only identifies high blood glucose and cannot identify hypoglycaemia
- The renal threshold of patients varies:
- Between patients
- Across the day
- Is affected by ageing
- Is affected by kidney disease
- Is affected by pregnancy

Red Flag

If you find a patient has an abnormally high or low blood glucose level, report it to a more senior member of staff immediately and document your findings.

Thus, the renal threshold creates a variable baseline from which to measure blood glucose (Holt 2014).

- Without a machine to read the test stick, urinalysis relies on the subjective matching of colour between test strip and chart
- Urine tests tend to overestimate or underestimate blood glucose levels

And yet there are still occasions urine testing is undertaken.

Testing Urine for Glucose

- Collection of the urine specimen is covered in Chapter 14, and the procedure outline there should be followed for collection of urine for testing.
- Once the sample has been collected, confirm the patient's identity and gain consent to test the urine.
- Gather the equipment and sample (use a sterile container; contaminated samples must never be used). See Box 13.1 for the equipment for urine testing.
- Read the instructions on the testing strip container to confirm the time the strip must be immersed in the urine and the period of time after which the strip must be read (Bardsley 2015).
  - These times may vary across manufacturers, and thus, never assume that you know these timings, always confirm.
- Check the expiry date of the test strips.
- Decontaminate your hands with either sanitiser gel or by hand washing.
- Put on disposable gloves and apron.
- Decontaminate your working area and place clean paper towels on the surface. Place the specimen and the testing strips in the centre.
- Remove the test strip from the container.
  - Replace the lid immediately as test strips can be affected by exposure to air, and it prevents accidental spillage of the strips which would necessitate throwing them away.
- Immerse the strip in the container for the required amount of time ensuring that the test pads are fully immersed.
- Run the edge of the strip across the edge of the specimen container to remove excess urine.
- Place the strip flat on the paper towels and wait for the recommended amount of time.
- Hold the strip at an angle and compare the colour of the test pad with the reference chart on the container.
- Dispose of the specimen into the toilet; dispose of the other used equipment (specimen container, gloves, apron, test strip and paper towels) in the clinical waste bin and adhere to local policy.
- Decontaminate the testing area.
- Wash hands.
- Record and report the results.

Box 13.1 Equipment for Urine Testing

- Gloves
- Disposable apron
- Hand sanitiser
- Watch or clock with second hand
- Urine test strips (in their container)
- Paper towels

Point-Of-Care Blood Glucose Testing

Point-of-care testing for blood glucose (from now on known as a BM test or capillary blood glucose) has revolutionised the care of diabetic patients allowing both healthcare providers and patients to perform rapid and relatively accurate measurement of blood glucose levels. The onset of the point-of-care test decreases turnaround time to results (compared to a laboratory test) allowing for rapid testing and response to changes in blood glucose levels (Kiechle & Main 2000). For instance, management of a patient on a continuous insulin regimen where insulin levels may change every hour may not be possible using laboratory analysis of blood glucose sample as the time taken to gain the sample, transport it to the laboratory and have the laboratory test the sample and report the result will often exceed an hour.

Box 13.2 discusses the variables that can affect point of care testing.

Green Flag

Most people with diabetes can hold a driving licence and are able to carry on driving.

There are various regulations that have to be taken into consideration depending on what vehicle the person wants to drive, for example, a group 1 licence is needed to drive a car or motorbike. A group 2 licence is required if the person wishes to drive a lorry or larger vehicle. There are different rules for this type of licence, and they can be more complicated when the driver has diabetes.

Coded Versus Non-Coded Machines

The reasons for coding blood glucose machines is that the enzymes used in creating the test strips are created from microorganisms, and there is significant variability between them that can affect the electrical current required to test the sample. Strips are given a code that calibrates the machine for that batch of strips (Whitmore 2012).

Box 13.2 Variables That may Affect Point-of-care Testing

It is important to be aware of variables that can affect the results from point of care testing. Some factors cannot be avoided but should be taken into account when using the results; others are due to operator error, and once you are aware of them, they can be avoided.

Pre-analysis factors

- Arterial versus capillary blood samples
  - Arterial samples can give different results to capillary samples and should not be used, as this can alter trend data for a particular patient.
- Inadequate cleaning of the testing instrument
  - Always clean according to manufacturer's instructions.
- Incorrect quality control or testing procedures
  - Quality control is covered elsewhere in the quality control of blood glucose machines in this text.
- Sweat or body temperature extremes
  - Sweat can dilute and alter the blood sample.
  - Body temperature extremes can alter capillary blood flow in the extremities.
- Systolic blood pressure less than 80 mmHg
  - Low systolic blood pressure reduces blood flow to the fingertips; thus, capillary blood at the fingertips may not reflect the actual blood glucose in the central circulation.

Analytical factors

- Extremes of glucose
  - Most testing machines can only read glucose levels within a certain range. Check the manufacturers handbook for information.
- Improper technique
- Incorrect match between glucose monitor calibration and test strip calibration

Post-analytical factors

- Data entry errors

Audit of errors in blood glucose monitoring show the four most common errors to be:

1. Inadequate cleaning
2. Poor quality control procedures
3. Improper technique
4. Incorrect match between calibration of machine and test strip calibration

As can be seen from this, the four most common errors for blood glucose testing using capillary blood samples are due to human error. These are all factors under your control as much as any other member of the team and should never be considered someone else's responsibility.

Source: Based on Kiechle & Main (2000)

If not calibrated correctly, machines that require calibration can produce incorrect results. Newer generation blood glucose machines may have the calibration built into the test strip, and thus, calibration occurs automatically with each strip.

Quality Control of Blood Glucose Machines

All meters require their accuracy to be checked at regular intervals. This should be done according to the manufacturer's instructions using test solutions manufactured by them. Depending on the machine and manufacturer, testing solutions may be a single solution or a high and a low solution. You will be informed locally of how to and how often to perform quality control.

The procedure for testing blood glucose using a point of care (BM) machine is outlined in Box 13.3.

- Introduce yourself and explain what you wish to do
- Gain consent
- Check the patient identity
- Ask the patient to wash their hands or help them to clean their hands (as appropriate)
  - Sugar on the patient's finger may falsely elevate the reading
  - Do not use an alcohol wipe or sanitiser gel on the patient's hands, as this may affect the reading
- Wash your hands and put on the gloves
- Turn on the glucose meter
- Insert the test strip
- 'Load' the lancet (to prepare it for use)
  - Always use a new lancet
- Remove the cover of the lancet and hold it firmly to the side of the patient's finger
- Prick the patient's finger (see Figure 13.2)
- Squeeze the finger to produce a drop of blood (avoid squeezing too tightly)
- Place the drop of blood on to the test strip (see Figure 13.3)
  - The test strip may use a capillary action using a tube in the end of the strip, in which case, present the blood to the opening so it can draw up the blood.
- Ensure a sufficient sample has been collected (depending on the system used)

Box 13.3 Equipment Required for Capillary Glucose Measurement Using Point of Care (BM) Machine

- Glucose (BM) machine
  - Check if it has been calibrated for the test strips about to be used
  - Check if it has undergone quality control according to local policy
  - If one or neither of these have been carried out, then do them before testing
- Test strips
  - Check if they are in date
- Gloves
- Spring loaded lancet (see Figure 13.1)
- Gauze swab
- Sharps bin

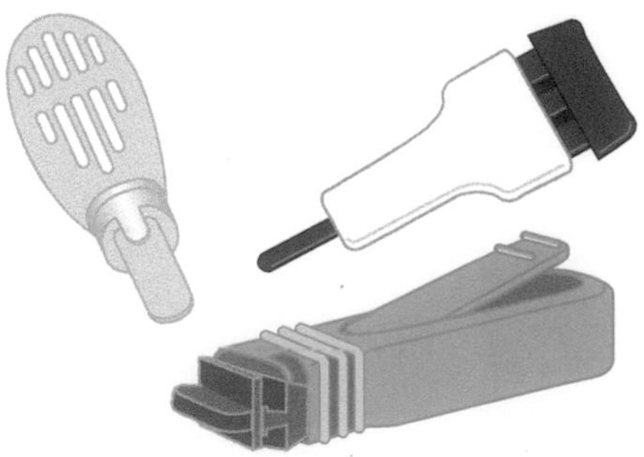

Figure 13.1 Lancets. ***Source:*** **Gormley-Fleming and Martin (2018), p. 36. © 2018 John Wiley & Sons.**

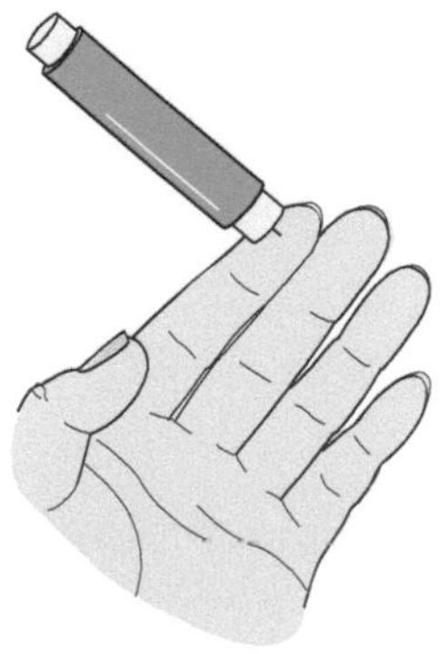

Figure 13.2 Finger prick. ***Source:*** **Gormley-Fleming and Martin (2018), p. 36. © 2018 John Wiley & Sons.**

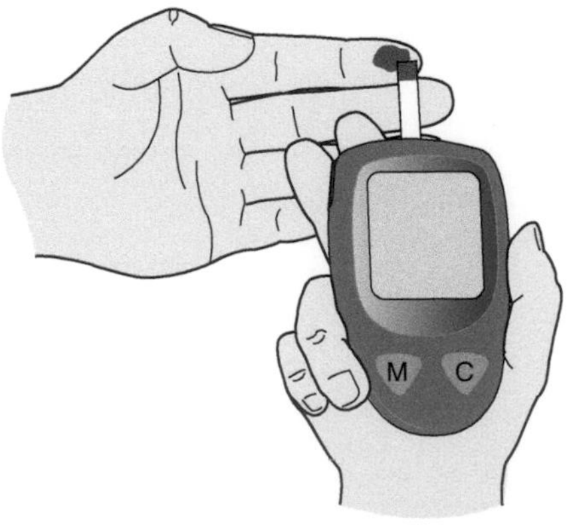

Figure 13.3 Dropping blood drop onto test strip. ***Source:*** **Gormley-Fleming and Martin (2018), p. 36. © 2018 John Wiley & Sons.**

- Give the patient a piece of gauze to stop the bleeding
- Read the value
- Dispose of the lancet in the sharps bin
- Dispose of all other clinical waste (gloves, test strip and gauze) into a clinical waste bin
- Record and report the results

Laboratory Testing of Blood Glucose

Considered the 'gold standard' of blood glucose testing (Holt 2014), laboratory analysis of blood glucose requires a venous sample of blood via venepuncture and can take two forms:

- Blood glucose
  A measure of blood glucose at the point in time the blood sample was taken
- HbA1c testing

Otherwise known as glycated haemoglobin, HbA1c provides information on the long-term blood glucose control of a patient. HbA1c is also known to be a good predictor of the long-term complications of diabetes due to poor blood glucose control. The test only measures the average blood glucose over a period of 2–3 months and is of no value in the immediate management of blood glucose.

Supporting Evidence

There are several places you may go to for evidence to support your study.

First and foremost, you must always make yourself familiar with the local policy of the healthcare organisation you are working in; policy is always evidence based, and following policy is a condition of your working contract or contract with the University.

Diabetes UK has a useful section on testing blood glucose, including a pictorial guide; this can be found at https://www.diabetes.org.uk/guide-to-diabetes/managing-your-diabetes/testing (accessed 16 January 2020).

Finally, the national standard for diabetes care and testing is provided by the National Institute for Health and Care Excellence (NICE). There are two useful sets of guidance:

NG17 (2016) Type 1 diabetes in adults: diagnosis and management which can be found at https://www.nice.org.uk/guidance/NG17 (accessed 16 January 2020) and NG28 (2019) Type 2 diabetes in adults: management which can be found at https://www.nice.org.uk/guidance/ng28 (accessed 16 January 2020).

All NICE guidance on diabetes can be found at https://www.nice.org.uk/guidance/conditions-and-diseases/diabetes-and-other-endocrinal-nutritional-and-metabolic-conditions/diabetes (accessed 16 January 2020).

Conclusion

Blood glucose testing can be performed in three ways:

- Urinalysis
- Point-of-care testing of capillary blood glucose (BM)
- Laboratory testing of glucose or HbA1c

Of the three point of care tests, testing using a capillary blood glucose (BM) machine is the one most likely to be carried out by a healthcare provider. Urinalysis can be inaccurate and limited in value; laboratory testing requires a venous blood sample and is relatively slow. Capillary testing is quick, relatively accurate and can give results for a wide range of blood glucose results.

There are four common errors in blood glucose testing using a BM machine, and all these are related to human factors. Only the healthcare provider performing the test can guarantee the accuracy of the test, and thus, correct the procedure is essential to patient safety.

References

Bardsley, A. (2015) How to perform a urinalysis, *Nursing Standard*, 30(2): 34–36.

Gormley-Fleming, E. and Martin, D. (2018) *Children's Nursing Skills at a Glance*. Wiley-Blackwell. © 2018 John Wiley & Sons.

Holt, P. (2014) Blood glucose monitoring in diabetes, *Nursing Standard (2014+)*, 28(27): 52.

Kiechle, F.L. and Main, R.I. (2000) Blood glucose: measurement in the point-of-care setting, *Laboratory Medicine*, 31(5): 276–282.

Nursing and Midwifery Council. (2018a) *The code: professional standards of practice and behaviour for nurses, midwives and nursing associates*, London: NMC.

Nursing and Midwifery Council. (2018b) *Standards for pre-registration nursing associate programmes*. [online] Available: https://www.nmc.org.uk/standards/standards-for-nursing-associates/standards-for-pre-registration-nursing-associate-programmes/. Accessed September 2020.

Whitmore, C. (2012) Blood glucose monitoring: an overview, *British Journal of Nursing*, 21(10): 583–587.

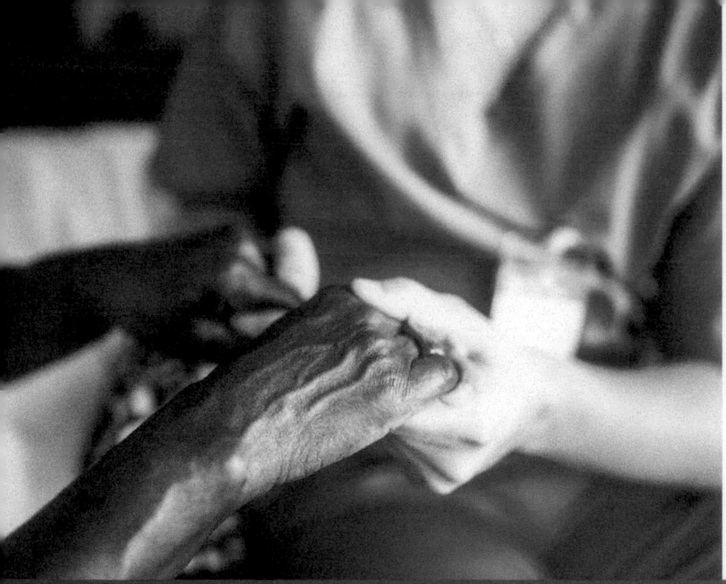

14

Specimen Collection

Carl Clare

University of Hertfordshire, UK

Chapter Aim

- **This chapter aims to provide readers with information and guidance for collecting specimens of urine, faeces, sputum and obtaining a nasal swab.**

Learning Outcomes

By the end of the chapter, the reader will be able to:

- **Understand the clinical importance of specimen collection**
- **Demonstrate the correct technique for the collection of urine, faeces or sputum specimens**
- **Demonstrate the correct technique for taking a nasal swab**
- **Explore the correct procedure for storage and transport of specimens**

Test Yourself Multiple Choice Questions

1. **Samples are used to do which of the following?**
   A) **Build a clinical picture**
   B) **Confirm a diagnosis**
   C) **Inform a treatment plan**
   D) **All of the above**
2. **Collecting a urine sample may involve taking a catheter sample of urine. Where should the sample be collected from?**
   A) **The end of the catheter (remove the collection bag)**
   B) **The tubing**
   C) **A port**
   D) **The bag**

The Nursing Associate's Handbook of Clinical Skills, First Edition. Edited by Ian Peate.

Companion website: www.wiley.com/nursingassociate

3. MSU is an abbreviation that stands for
 A) Mid-stream urine
 B) Multi-stream urine
 C) Medium stream urine
 D) Maximum stream urine

4. When collecting a faecal sample, you use:
 A) A sterile technique
 B) An aseptic technique
 C) A clean technique
 D) A dirty technique

5. Purulent sputum contains:
 A) Mucous
 B) Pus
 C) Blood
 D) Debris

Introduction

Collecting samples and taking swabs are, perhaps, some of the least glamorous (and, in some cases, most unpopular) roles a nursing associate may undertake in their career. Yet, the role that samples of urine, faeces or sputum play in the client journey can never be underestimated. Specimens are part of a holistic client assessment and can help to:

- Build a clinical picture
- Confirm a diagnosis
- Inform a treatment plan (Shepherd 2017a).

The correct collection and processing of samples aid in many aspects of healthcare and may make the difference in ensuring correct treatment. For instance, a sputum sample may aid with the identification of the pathogen causing pneumonia, allowing for a precisely targeted antibiotic regimen, shortening the required course of antibiotics and speeding recovery. A client with diarrhoea may be suffering from salmonella poisoning or a *Clostridium difficile* infection. The treatment for each is very different, and a client with *C. difficile* infection must be isolated from other clients to prevent spread. Finally, the screening of clients for meticillin-resistant Staphylococcus aureus (MRSA) on hospital admission is considered a vital part of the fight against this persistent pathogen, and the nose swab is one of the routine tests in this fight.

Nursing associates must be able to demonstrate proficiency in specimen collecting prior to having their name entered on the professional register (Nursing and Midwifery Council (NMC) (2018a). Once registered the nursing associate must ensure that they abide by the key themes underpinning the Code (Nursing and Midwifery Council 2018b):

- Prioritise people
- Practise effectively
- Preserve safety
- Promote professionalism and trust.

General Principles of Specimen Collection

Accurate specimen collection techniques are essential to reduce the risk of contamination (Shepherd 2017a). Specimens must be:

- collected at the correct time,
- using the correct technique and equipment and
- delivered to the laboratory as soon as practicable (Shepherd 2017a).

To ensure safety of all involved (from 'bedside' staff to porters, to laboratory staff), samples must be:

- collected in a way that minimises health and safety risks,
- collected using the correct equipment,
- documented correctly using the appropriate forms and
- stored and transported appropriately.

When handling samples, staff must:

- wear personal protective equipment (PPE) (see Chapter 45 of this text for a discussion of PPE),
- be aware of the risks involved with any sample collection or transportation and
- be deemed competent to undertake the task according to local policy.

Accurate documentation is essential when collecting any sample, storing and transporting. As such, request forms must be:

- filled in with the client's data (name, date of birth, hospital number),
- contain details of the specimen type and site,
- detail the investigation required,
- detail the reason for collection,
- be labelled with a high-risk label if required,

- identify who requested the test and how they can be contacted and
- detail the date and time the sample was collected.

Once collected, the sample label must contain, at the minimum:

- client's name and date of birth,
- ward or clinic, general practice,
- hospital or National Health Service (NHS) number,
- type and site of specimen and
- the date and time the specimen was collected.

Transportation of Specimens

While being transported, samples must be in a self-sealing polythene bag with two compartments, one for the specimen and a separate compartment for the request form (Shepherd 2017a).

Obtaining a Urine Specimen

Urine is a liquid created from the waste products filtered by the kidneys and passed to the bladder via the ureters. Under normal circumstances, urine is sterile and does not contain bacteria. One of the most common reasons for obtaining a urine specimen is to test for the presence of an infection, but this is not the only reason to obtain a urine specimen (Bishop 2008). Other reasons include:

- Pregnancy testing
- Dipstick testing (such as for glucose)
- Some sexually transmitted infections (such as Chlamydia)
- Protein in the urine (usually an early morning urine test)

Obtaining a urine specimen can be from either a catheterised or a non-catheterised client. Therefore, this section will discuss the two techniques separately beginning with obtaining a mid-stream urine (MSU) sample from a client without a catheter. At the end, a brief mention will be given to 24-hour urine collections.

Obtaining an MSU Sample

An MSU sample is the standard for urine sampling. Approximately 30% of urine samples are contaminated, and the mid-stream sample is intended to hopefully reduce the chances of this happening (Bishop 2008). The mid-stream allows for debris and cutaneous bacteria to be flushed away before the sample is taken, thus hopefully avoiding contamination.

The procedure for obtaining an MSU sample requires the full cooperation of the client (and is in fact normally carried out by the client). If a client is unable to follow instructions, then obtaining a mid-stream sample is not possible, and this should be noted on the sample form, so the laboratory is aware.

The following process is meant to be used to explain to the client how to take an MSU (see Figure 14.1).

- Give the client sterile urine specimen collection equipment and explain the procedure to them.
- Obtain consent for testing of the sample.
- Ensure that the client has a private place to undertake the collection. If not in a locked toilet cubicle, then ensure that the curtains are drawn around the bed and no one will enter.
- Ask the client to wash their hands.
- The client should then retract the foreskin (if present in males) or retract the labia (females) and wash the surrounding area with 0.9% saline or disinfectant-free soap and water. This is done to reduce the possibility of contamination by skin-dwelling bacteria. Products containing disinfectant should be avoided, as they may irritate the delicate skin (Dougherty & Lister 2015).

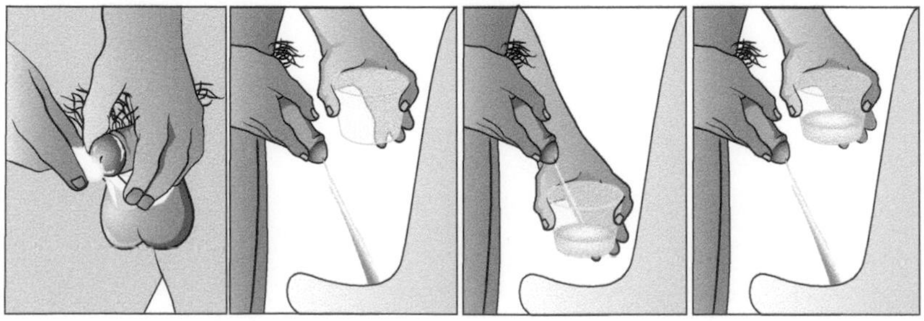

Figure 14.1 Obtaining an MSU from a male client. *Source:* Jevon and Joshi (2020), figure 13.1, p. 54. © 2020 John Wiley & Sons.

- The client should then pass the first third of the urine into the toilet or other receptacle. This is intended to 'flush' away any transient bacteria in the urethra.
- Without interrupting the flow, the client should introduce the wide necked collection equipment into the flow and collect a sample of approximately 15–30 mL.
- The remainder of the urine can then be passed into the toilet (or other receptacle).
- The client should then wash their hands.

Once the specimen has been obtained, the sample can then be sealed, labelled and placed into the appropriate specimen bag.

Early Morning Urine (EMU)

Occasionally, a client may be asked to take an early morning urine sample. The purpose of these samples is to collect urine that has been stored in the bladder overnight. Thus, the first urine of the morning should be collected. Even if the client gets up at 0500 hours to pass urine and then goes back to bed, it is this first urine of the morning that should be sampled. Except for the time of collection, early morning urine samples should be collected in the same manner as an MSU sample.

Catheter Specimen of Urine (CSU)

Often collected for the diagnosis of a catheter-acquired urinary tract infection (CAUTI), CSUs require the same diligence in avoiding contamination as MSU samples.

CSU should not be collected from the catheter bag; the urine in the bag is often not fresh, and collection via the tap used for emptying the bag will often lead to contamination. Catheter bag systems normally have a collection port built into the tubing to allow the clean collection of a fresh sample (Figure 14.2). To collect a CSU, sterile gloves are not required, but a no-touch technique must be used.

Box 14.1 provides a list of equipment required to collect a CSU.

- Explain the process to the client and gain consent.
- Ensure the privacy and dignity of the client at all times.
- Decontaminate your hands and put on the apron and gloves.
- Check if urine is present in the tube. If urine is not present, it may be necessary to clamp the tube a few centimetres below the sampling port and wait until sufficient urine has collected.
- Clean the collection port with an alcohol wipe and allow to dry. Not allowing the alcohol to dry may affect the sample collected.
- Stabilise the tubing by holding it below the collection port.
- Insert the syringe in the port (no needle should be required).
- Aspirate at least 10 mL of urine.
- Remove the syringe and put the urine into the collection container.

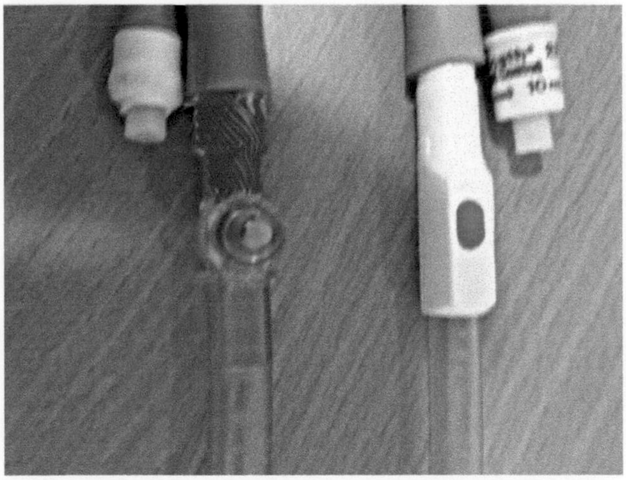

Figure 14.2 **Example specimen ports.** *Source:* Lindsay et al. (2018), figure 50.1, p. 234. © 2018 John Wiley & Sons.

Box 14.1 Equipment Required for a Collecting a Catheter Specimen of Urine

- Gloves
- Apron
- 10 mL syringe
- Alcohol wipes
- Sample collection container

- Close the container securely.
- Wipe sampling port again with a fresh wipe.
- If used, release the clamp.
- Dispose of the used wipes, apron, gloves and syringe in the clinical waste bin.
- Wash your hands.

Once the specimen has been obtained, the sample can then be sealed, labelled and placed into the appropriate specimen bag.

24-Hour Urine Collection

24-hour urine collections are sometimes used when the total amount of a product passed in the urine over 24 hours needs to be assessed. 24-hour collections are not used for microbiological testing and thus contamination, and all of the urine passed in a 24-hour period must be collected.

The urine will be stored in large containers provided by the laboratory and should be kept cool. Male clients must be warned not to pass urine directly into the containers, as they contain stabilising agents (such as boric acid) that would cause damage to the delicate skin of the meatus.

Ensure that the client has appropriate equipment to both collect the urine and pour it into the collection container without spillage.

Explain to the client that they should first pass urine into the toilet (emptying the bladder) and that at that point the 24-hour collection period begins. All urine passed after that time must be collected and stored in the supplied container. Just before the 24-hour period finishes, the client should try and empty their bladder one last time and collect that last amount of urine in the container. Once the 24-hour period is over, the urine should be delivered to the laboratory as soon as possible.

Touch Point

Urine samples are an important tool in the diagnosis and treatment of clients. At all times ensure that you maintain privacy and dignity when obtaining samples.

If samples are being collected for microbiological testing, the reduction of the potential for contamination is a primary concern and the procedures followed help to ensure this.

Supporting Evidence

The National Institute for Health and Care Excellence has a number of guidance pages about urinary tract infections (UTI). The main page can be found at https://pathways.nice.org.uk/pathways/urinary-tract-infections (accessed 17 January 2020) and contains pathways for UTIs in those under 16 years and those over 16 years.

Obtaining a Faeces Specimen

There are a number of reasons for collecting a sample of faeces (otherwise known as a stool specimen). These include testing for a variety of infectious agents (see Box 14.2).

Box 14.2 Infectious Agents Requiring the Collection of a Faecal Sample

Bacterial
Salmonella
Campylobacter
Helicobacter
Shigella
Escherichia coli (E. coli)
Clostridium difficile (C. difficile)
Parasites
Protozoa
Tapeworm
Entamoeba
Viruses
Norovirus
Rotavirus

Source: Shepherd (2017b)

Box 14.3 Equipment Required for Collecting a Sample of Faeces

- Disposable bedpan or receiver
- Sterile specimen pot with integral spoon (Figure 14.3)
- Gloves
- Apron
- Specimen form and bag

Yellow Flag

- While stool samples can help to diagnose conditions such as food poisoning, they can also help to identify to bowel cancer. The bowel cancer screening programme requires the patient to provide stool specimens.
- Many people are too embarrassed to provide a stool specimen for analysis, and this embarrassment can risk their health.

Faecal samples must be collected using a clean sampling technique (to avoid contamination with environmental bacteria). See Box 14.3 for the equipment needed to obtain a faecal sample.

Procedure

- Discuss the procedure with the client and gain consent.
- Maintain privacy and dignity at all times.
- Wash your hands and don disposable apron and gloves.
- Ask the client to pass urine before passing stool into the receptacle/bedpan so as to avoid contaminating the faeces with urine.
- Ask the client to defecate into the bedpan/receptacle.
- Where possible, collect toilet paper in a separate receptacle. This allows you to visually observe the stool more easily.
- Remove the bedpan/receptacle to the sluice/dirty room and visually inspect the stool. Observe the stool, noting consistency, the presence of blood or mucous and the presence of any tapeworm. Tapeworm will vary in size from a grain of rice to a ribbon shape.
- Use the spoon to collect enough faeces to quarter fill the specimen pot (Figures 14.3 and 14.4). If mucous or blood is present, ensure some is collected. If tapeworm is present, make sure some sections are included (Shepherd 2017b).
- Secure the top on the specimen pot.
- Dispose of the rest of the stool and the bedpan/receptacle.
- Remove gloves and apron. Wash your hands.
- Label the sample and put it in the sample bag.
- Send the sample to the laboratory as soon as possible.
  If there is going to be a delay in sending the sample, then it should be refrigerated.
- Record the findings of the visual inspection in the client notes and report any concerns.

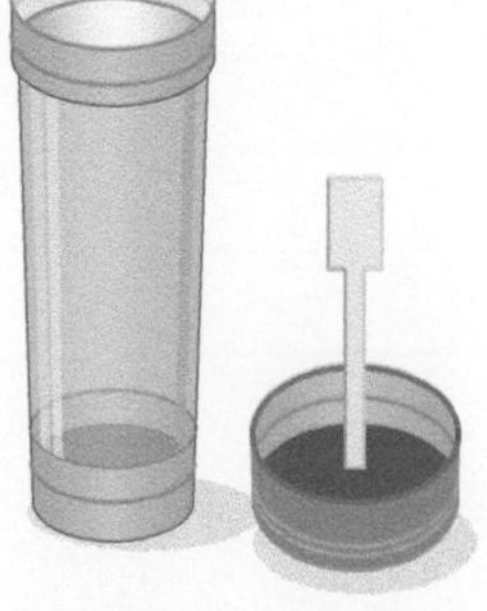

Figure 14.3 **Specimen pot with integral spoon.** *Source:* Lindsay et al. (2018), figure 50.1, p. 237. © 2018 John Wiley & Sons.

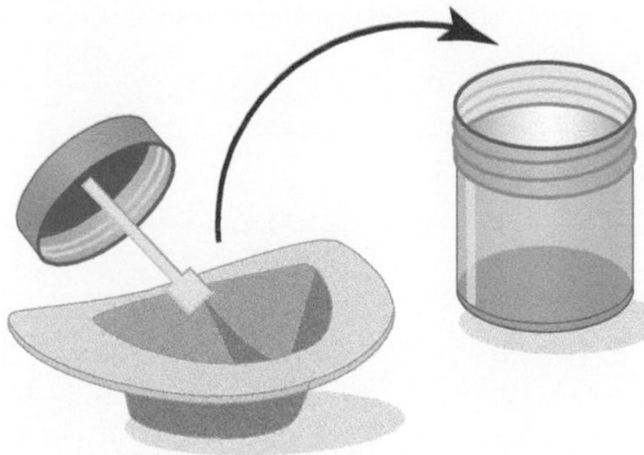

Figure 14.4 **Collecting specimen of faeces.** *Source:* Lindsay et al. (2018), figure 50.2, p. 237. © 2018 John Wiley & Sons.

Obtaining a Sputum Sample

The collection of sputum is one of the most common procedures in respiratory medicine (Blakeborough & Watson 2019). Sputum is a salivary matter mixed with mucus and pus from the respiratory system (Myatt 2017). Mucus is produced naturally by the trachea and bronchioles and traps dust, bacteria and other debris stopping them from reaching the lower parts of the respiratory system. In certain respiratory conditions, mucus production is increased, and the mucus-producing cells expand, limiting airflow and increasing symptoms such as cough. In clients with long-term respiratory diseases, such as chronic obstructive pulmonary disease (COPD), it can be difficult to detect the presence of a respiratory infection as the normal symptoms of mucus production, difficulty in breathing and cough are always present. A sputum sample not only allows microbiological testing for the presence of active infection but also helps identify the particular pathogen causing the symptoms and, therefore, aids the medical staff in prescribing the correct treatment (NICE 2019). Especially in clients with COPD, a sputum sample should be requested when the client shows an increased cough with the production of purulent sputum and signs of an infection, for instance, a raised temperature (Shepherd 2017c). Occasionally, if the client is finding it hard to cough up tenacious sputum, it may be helpful to have them inhale nebulised normal saline. This should only be done on the advice of medical or physiotherapy staff, and the nebuliser should be driven by compressed air unless directed otherwise. In Box 14.4, various types of sputum are described.

Sputum can be collected using invasive (suction) or non-invasive procedures; as the use of suction is covered in Chapter 41, this chapter will only cover the non-invasive collection of sputum.

Red Flag

Sputum collection can involve the production of aerosol particles, and thus, the nursing associate should wear appropriate PPE when collecting samples.

The exact equipment will depend on local policy and may include apron, gloves and face mask. In infectious respiratory diseases, such as active tuberculosis, COVID-19, filter masks will be required (see also Chapter 45). When wearing a mask, avoid the temptation to adjust it while wearing gloves until you have removed the gloves and washed your hands.

A list of equipment that is needed for the collection of a sputum specimen is presented in Box 14.5.

Procedure

- Explain the procedure to the patient and gain consent.
- Gather the required equipment.
- Wash hands and put on gloves, apron and mask (if required).
- Sit the patient up in a chair or bed and make sure they are comfortable.
- Ask the client to rinse their mouth with water to remove food debris; this water may be swallowed.
- Ask the client to take several deep breaths to help loosen the secretions. Some clients may find this difficult due to their respiratory condition, in which case do not insist they do this.
- Ask the client to force a deep cough. Try to obtain the sample from as deep in the respiratory system as possible. Again, some clients may find this difficult. Reassure them that whatever they can do is acceptable.

Box 14.4 Types of Sputum

- Mucoid – containing or resembling mucous
- Purulent – containing pus
- Mucopurulent – containing pus and mucous
- Frothy – visible froth
- Viscous – thick and sticky
- Blood-stained – visible blood present

Source: based on Richardson (2003)

Box 14.5 The Equipment Required for Sputum Sampling

- Sterile pot
- Gloves and apron
- If required, a face mask
- Glass of water
- Tissues

- The client should spit the sample into the collection pot, and the lid is then secured in place.
- Settle the client into a comfortable condition.
- Remove any PPE (for example, gloves and aprons) and wash your hands.
- Label the sample and bag for the laboratory.
- Send the sample as soon as possible, preferably within 4 hours (Shepherd 2017c).

Obtaining a Nasal Swab

Nasal swabs are a common practice in the NHS as they are one of the routine swabs used to detect MRSA when screening clients on admission (the others are axilla, groin and any wounds they may have) and more recently with regards to COVID-19. Simple to obtain, many clients prefer to undertake the swab of their nose themselves as it seems less unpleasant and less embarrassing. However, there will be times when it is the responsibility of the nursing associate to take the swab. In either situation, the procedure identified here should be followed or explained to the client. See Box 14.6 for the equipment needed for the taking of a nasal swab.

Procedure

- Explain the process to the client and gain consent.
- Wash your hands and put on gloves and apron.
- Ask the client to tilt their head backwards. This position is only necessary if the nursing associate is to perform the swab; it allows easier visualisation of the nasal passages.
- Moisten the swab with sterile saline, if advised (Figure 14.6) as the nasal mucosa is often dry, and a dry swab may be uncomfortable. Furthermore, bacteria may adhere better to a moist surface (Dougherty & Lister 2015).
- Insert the swab inside the nostril with the tip directed upwards (Figure 14.7) and rotate the swab gently to come into contact with the mucosa (Figure 14.8). It is not necessary to insert the swab too deeply into the nostril as this can be very unpleasant. Ensure that you can see the tip of the swab at all times.
- Using the same swab, repeat the procedure in the other nostril to ensure a good sample.
- Remove the cap from the transport tube and gently insert the swab all the way in until the handle of the swab and the tube fit together.
- Remove the gloves and apron and dispose of them with the saline vial.
- Wash your hands.
- Label the swab tube and complete the request form.
- Place the transport tube into a specimen bag and arrange for delivery to the laboratory.
- You must always follow local policy, adhering to the requirements that are pertinent to the individual test.

Box 14.6 Equipment Required for a Nasal Swab

- Gloves and apron
- Sterile bacterial swab (with transport medium) (Figure 14.5)
- 0.9% sterile saline

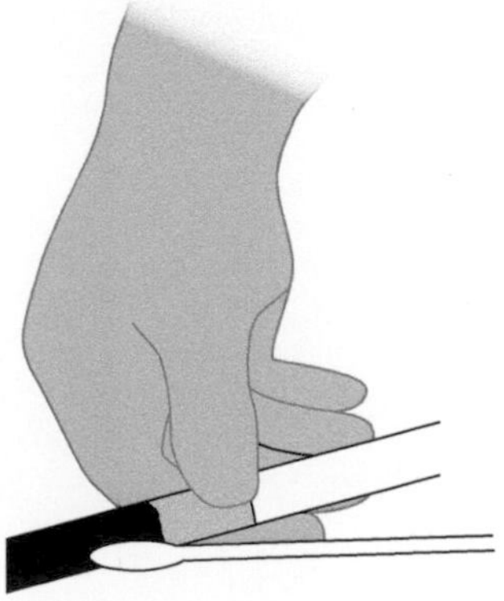

Figure 14.5 Swab with transport medium.

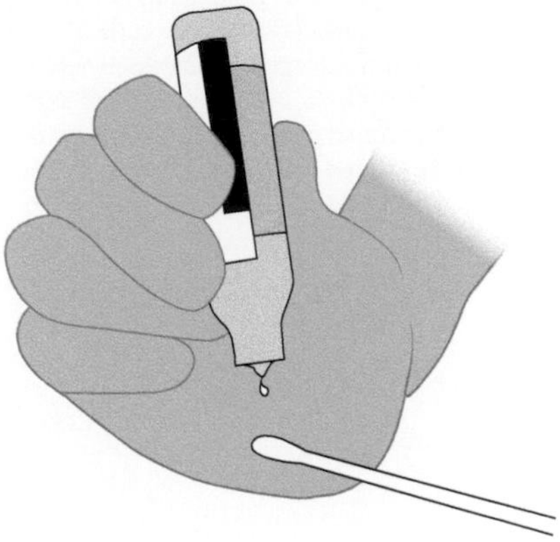

Figure 14.6 Moisten the swab with 0.9% saline.

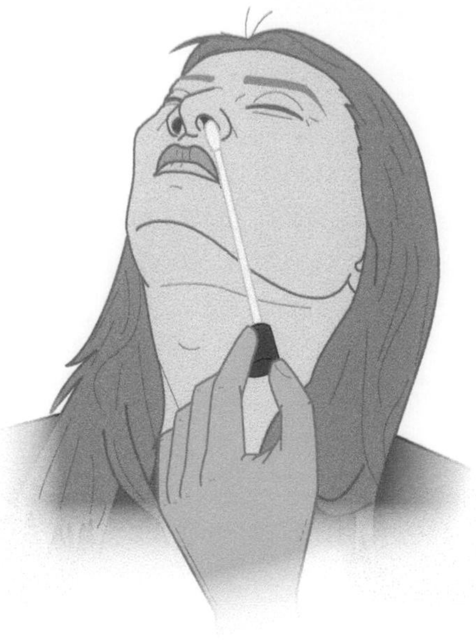

Figure 14.7 **Insert the swab into the anterior nostrils.**

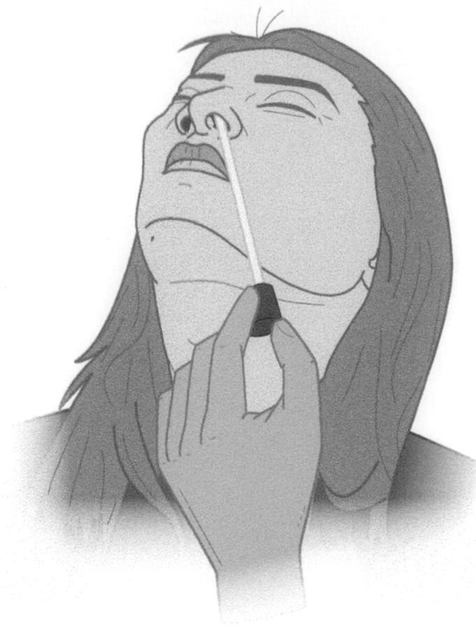

Figure 14.8 **Sweep the swab around the nares.**

Conclusion

Specimen collection, preparation and handling are common activities that are undertaken by nursing associates. Identifying pathogens and analysing specimens such as urine, faeces and sputum can assist with the assessment of a person's health status. The nursing associate is responsible for the collection, labelling and secure and safe transportation of specimens to the laboratory for analysis.

Nursing associates must have an understanding of how to gather specimens correctly so as to prevent risk to themselves and others and to prevent the potential transmission of disease.

References

Bishop, T. (2008) Urine testing, *Practice Nurse*, 35(12): 18–20.

Blakeborough, L. and Watson, J.S. (2019) The importance of obtaining a sputum sample and how it can aid diagnosis and treatment, *British Journal of Nursing*, 28(5): 295–298.

Dougherty, L. and Lister, S. (2015) *The Royal Marsden manual of clinical nursing procedures* (9th edn), Chichester: Wiley.

Higgins, D. (2008) Specimen collection: part 4 – obtaining a nasal swab. *Nursing Times*, 104(20): 26–27.

Jevon, P. and Joshi, J. (2020) *Medical Student Survival Skills: Procedural Skills*. Oxford: Wiley.

Lindsay, P., Bagness, C. and Peate, I. (Eds). (2018) *Midwifery skills at a glance*, UK: Wiley-Blackwell.

Myatt, R. (2017) Sputum collection and analysis: what the nurse needs to know, *Nursing Standard (2014+)*, 31(27): 40.

NICE. (2019) *NG115 Chronic obstructive pulmonary disease in over 16s: diagnosis and management*, London National Institute for Health and Care Excellence. [online] Available: https://www.nice.org.uk/guidance/ng115. Accessed 17 January 2020.

Nursing and Midwifery Council. (2018a) *Standards of proficiency for nursing associates*. [online] Available: https://www.nmc.org.uk/standards/standards-for-nursing-associates/standards-of-proficiency-for-nursing-associates/. Accessed January 2020.

Nursing and Midwifery Council. (2018b) The code, *Professional standards of practice and behaviour for nurses, midwives and nursing associates*. [online] Available: https://www.nmc.org.uk/globalassets/sitedocuments/nmc-publications/nmc-code.pdf. Accessed January 2020.

Richardson, M. (2003) The physiology of mucus and sputum production in the respiratory system, *Nursing Times*, 99(23): 63–64.

Shepherd, E. (2017a) Specimen collection 1: general principles and procedure for obtaining a midstream urine specimen, *Nursing Times*, 113(7): 45–47.

Shepherd, E. (2017b) Specimen collection 3: faecal specimen from a patient with diarrhoea. *Nursing Times*, 113(9): 27–29.

Shepherd, E. (2017c) Specimen collection 4: procedure for obtaining a sputum specimen, *Nursing Times*, 113(10): 49–51.

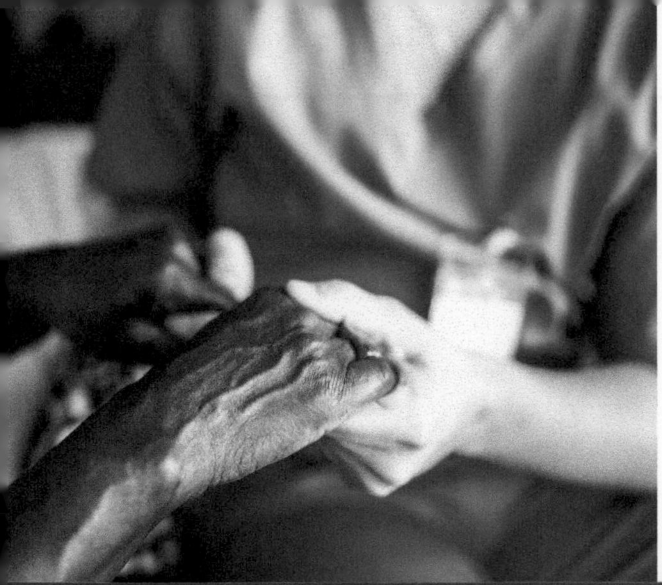

15

Recognising and Escalating Signs of All Forms Abuse

Jo Regan[1] and Karen Wild[2]

[1] Leeds Teaching Hospitals Trust, UK
[2] Nurse, UK

Chapter Aim

- **This chapter aims to provide the reader with an insight into recognising and acting upon all signs of abuse across the lifespan in the healthcare and social care setting.**

Learning Outcomes

By the end of this chapter, the reader will be able to:

- **Help the nursing associate identify types of abuse in children, young people and adults**
- **Demonstrate how to communicate and escalate all suspected episodes of abuse**
- **Be aware of the legislation that underpins the need to safeguard individuals in a health and social care setting**

Test Yourself Multiple Choice Questions

1. **Which platforms in the nursing associate proficiencies are associated with this chapter?**
   A) 1 and 2
   B) 4 and 5
   C) 1 and 5
   D) All of them

The Nursing Associate's Handbook of Clinical Skills, First Edition. Edited by Ian Peate.

Companion website: www.wiley.com/nursingassociate

2. **In what year was the Care Act enforced?**
   A) **1995**
   B) **2014**
   C) **2018**
   D) **1959**
3. **Modern slavery is not a form of abuse.**
   A) **True**
   B) **False**
4. **Which of the following statements is false?**
   A) **Safeguarding is about safety and well-being and about providing additional measures for those fully able to protect themselves from harm or abuse**
   B) **A fundamental human right for every person is to live a life that is free from harm and abuse**
   C) **All staff and workers working in healthcare and social care should be complying with safeguarding children, young people and adults at risk of harm or abuse**
   D) **Safeguarding teams and nominated safeguarding leads exist in National Health Service (NHS) and social care settings to support the ongoing training of staff and to provide help and guidance about vulnerable or 'at-risk' individuals**
5. **A person who is vulnerable and is being abused may show signs of:**
   A) **Increased body temperature**
   B) **Sudden changes in character, becoming distressed and tearful and appearing helpless**
   C) **Engaging in social activities**
   D) **Sleep apnoea**

Introduction

When individuals are in a vulnerable situation, all healthcare and social care professionals have a duty of care to protect them by ensuring that the best interests of individuals are met when they are recipients of care and ensuring the provision of support. This is a legal obligation and means that it is unconditional and applies not only to those in your direct care but also to others, for example, allied healthcare professionals, medical and ancillary staff and families and carers.

A fundamental human right for every person is to live a life that is free from harm and abuse and is considered an essential requirement for health and well-being. Safeguarding encompasses protection of the vulnerable, acting in their best interests, and acting on concerns that you may have within your practice setting. All staff and workers working in healthcare and social care should be complying with safeguarding children, young people and adults at risk of harm or abuse.

In applying safeguarding practices, the nursing associate is practising within Nursing and Midwifery Council (NMC) standards of proficiency (NMC 2018a) in relationship to platform 1 and being an accountable professional and also platform 5 in improving patient safety and quality of care.

Different legislation exists to support adults, young people and children in care settings. The Care Act (2014) sets out a legal framework as to how care systems should protect adults at risk from abuse or neglect. For children and young people, the Children and Families Act (2004) and the updated *Working Together to Safeguard Children (2018)* document outlines the duty that local authorities and their partners must improve the well-being of children in their localities.

Touch Point

The term safeguarding legislation refers to:
The Care Act 2014 (England)
The Safeguarding Vulnerable Groups (Northern Ireland) Order 2007
The Adult Support and Protection (Scotland) Act 2007
Social Services and Well-being (Wales) Act 2014

Supporting Evidence (Vulnerable Children) **Working together to safeguard children (Department of Health 2018)**

A full account of statutory provisions relating to children's safeguarding can be found in this document. It focuses on those which are relevant to the NHS.

There are some broad, fundamental safeguarding duties, namely:

- A duty of local authorities to 'safeguard and promote the welfare of children within their area who are in need'.
- A further duty to 'take reasonable steps . . . to prevent children within their area suffering ill-treatment or neglect'.
- All public sector agencies providing services to children, including local authorities and all NHS bodies, 'must make arrangements for ensuring that their functions are discharged having regard to the need to safeguard and promote the welfare of children'.
- A child-centred approach is required.
- A local authority must enquire whether it needs to take safeguarding action if it has reasonable cause to suspect a child in its area is suffering, or is at risk of, significant harm. This duty also covers any child in police protection or under an emergency protection

order.Safeguarding teams and nominated safeguarding leads exist in NHS and social care settings to support the ongoing education and training of staff and to provide help and guidance about vulnerable or 'at-risk' individuals. In a hospital setting, this is likely to be a registered nurse within the safeguarding team. In the community setting, this can be an individual such as a general practitioner (GP) or senior social services case worker.

- The term 'at risk' can refer to the vulnerability of individuals in care settings, and the risk of abuse or neglect can arise from several situations. These can include vulnerability because of age, cognitive impairment, mental health issues and/or physical disability. Several high-profile cases have emerged to highlight the issue of 'at-risk' situations, and two examples can be seen in the box below.

Violet Flag Psychosocial Flag

Examples of high-profile safeguarding/at-risk situations

Winterbourne View (Department of Health 2012): Six members of staff were convicted and sentenced to jail for the abuse and neglect of adults with learning difficulties at the Winterbourne View care home.

The Mid Staffordshire Enquiry: The Francis Report (2013) highlighted multiple failings of care and examples of widespread neglect at the Mid Staffordshire General Hospital.

Warton Hall: In May 2019, this private NHS-funded hospital for people with learning disabilities was exposed by undercover TV Panorama investigators for widespread abuse of patients (Peate 2019).

There are many types of abuse, these include:

- Physical
- Emotional or psychological
- Sexual and sexual exploitation
- Neglect
- Domestic abuse
- Modern slavery
- Discriminatory
- Institutional
- Financial
- Self-harm

Physical abuse can include assault, pushing, hitting (in children, this includes smacking and shaking), biting, pinching and scalding. There have been incidences of the use of cigarettes to physically burn. Poisoning and the misuse of medications can also be included within this category. Withholding food, warmth and depriving liberty by restraint are other examples.

Emotional or psychological abuse can harm an individual's emotional health. Such forms of mental cruelty can be as a result of mental stress, brought about by abuse aimed at denying basic rights to privacy, dignity, choice and self-expression. It includes acts that attack an individual's self-esteem or that isolate them or create an overdependence on an individual. Intimidation and bullying can be examples of emotional and psychological abuse. In children, a degree of emotional abuse is involved in any maltreatment. Emotional development can regress in children who are devalued socially or who are exposed to bullying and fear of those who are caring for them or being exposed to adverse danger. Overprotection and limited exposure to learning and development and preventing normal social interaction can also be considered within this category.

Orange Flag Psychological Problems

Bullying in the workplace, the nursing associate

The manager on my unit had been somebody I knew at school years before. She had asked me on several occasions to swap my shifts right at the last moment. I felt obliged to agree despite having dependants at home. On one occasion, I told her that I could no longer change shifts at such short notice and that it was making my work and home life difficult and upsetting. I asked her to at least give me fair warning of a change in my off-duty rotas.

She began to ridicule me in practice, in front of patients and my peers. On many occasions, she deliberately excluded me from discussions around the care and nursing interventions of my patients and then humiliated me for not following any changes that were needed. I felt that I was being pushed aside in favour of other staff members; they noticed it too. I felt demoralised and distressed.

A friend suggested I keep a diary of what was happening and how it made me feel.

Sexual and sexual exploitation can include direct and indirect involvement of an individual in acts or relationships of a sexual nature. Abuse in this category can include coercion or enforcement to take part in sexual activities. Activities may include physical contact that may or may not include sexual penetrative acts. Consent and mental capacity are important issues in this type of abuse. Children and those with impaired mental capacity may not understand the implications of sexual abuse. Examples might include oversexualisation of a child, the use of online pornographic images or being forced to watch sexual activity. As of October 2015, all healthcare professionals have a mandatory duty to report female genital mutilation (FGM) in girls under the age of 18 years (Department of Health 2015a, 2015b).

Green Flag Legislation

Department of Health (2015a, 2015b) FGM mandatory reporting duty

As of October 2015, all healthcare professionals have a mandatory duty to report FGM in girls under the age of 18 years.

Red Flag Serious Pathology

The types of FGM

The nursing associate needs to understand the physical presentation of FGM (infibulation).

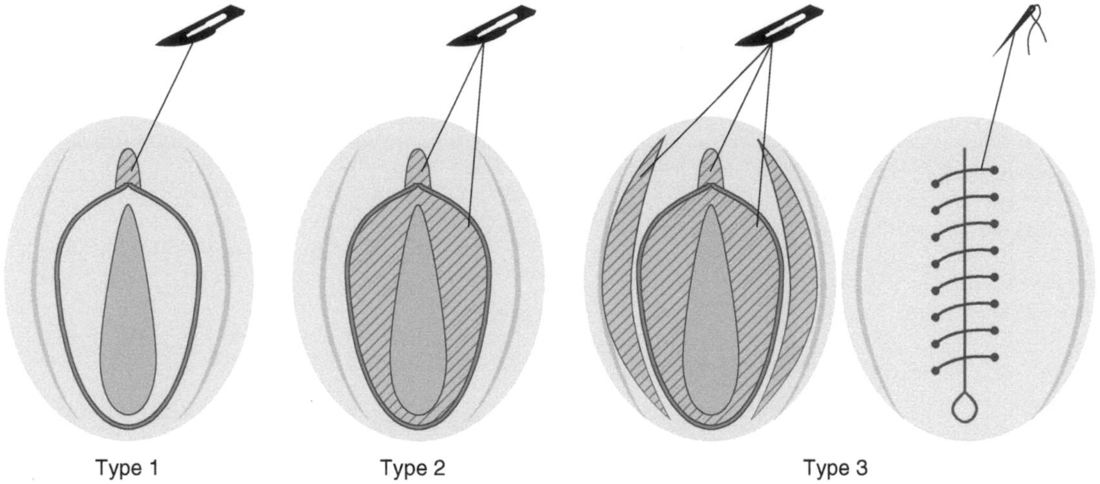

TYPE 1: The clitoris is removed.
TYPE 2: The labia minora is cut away.
TYPE 3: The labia majora is cut and sewn together to leave a small opening for the girl or woman to micturate and menstruate through.

Neglect can be described as intentional or unintentional. Intentional neglect is the wilful act of failing to provide care and/or basic needs such as nutrition, warmth, hydration and medication. It includes failure on the part of the carer to allow individuals access to healthcare and social care. In children and young adults, this can include withholding access to education. In pregnancy, neglect may occur as a result of maternal substance abuse.

Unintentional neglect may arise through lack of awareness and/or understanding of a person's needs. Informal carers may not know how to provide care or who to go to in times of need, or what the consequences of neglect may be.

Domestic abuse involves individuals aged 16 years and over who are victims of controlling, coercive or threatening behaviour, honour-based violence and violence between intimate partners or family members regardless of gender or sexuality (Gov.UK 2018). The Serious Crime Act of 2015 introduced the offence of coercive and threatening behaviour in intimate and familial relationships. Recognition of violence against women in domestic violence and abuse is part of the Social Services and Well-being (Wales) Act of 2014.

Despite the wider perception, women are not the only victims of domestic abuse; in 2018/19, 576,000 men (2.5%) and 1.2 million women (4.8%) were victims of partner abuse, equating to a ratio of two female victims to every one male victim. Nearly half of male victims fail to tell anyone they are a victim of domestic abuse (only 51% tell anyone). They are nearly three times less likely to tell anyone than a female victim.

Supporting Evidence Domestic Abuse

A Perfect Storm, Published August 2020 (c) Women's Aid

Domestic abuse has worsened during Covid-19 and frontline services expect rising demand

On Tuesday, 18 August 2020, Women's Aid released a new report: *A Perfect Storm – The impact of the Covid-19 pandemic on domestic abuse survivors and the services supporting them*.

The report shows how domestic abuse has worsened during the Covid-19 pandemic. It examines the impact on survivors and their children; how abusers use the pandemic as a tool of abuse; and how the services supporting survivors are affected.

You can access and read the document online with the following link:
https://1q7dqy2unor827bqjls0c4rn-wpengine.netdna-ssl.com/wp-content/uploads/2020/08/A-Perfect-Storm-August-2020-1.pdf

Modern slavery can be associated with forced labour and domestic servitude where individuals are isolated from the wider community, seemingly under the control of others. Other examples include human trafficking and sexual exploitation such as escort work, prostitution and pornography. Trafficked people commonly experience poor mental health with high prevalence of post-traumatic stress disorder, anxiety and depression (Public Health England 2017). Those being forced to pay off monies in the form of debt bondage may be coerced to work for nothing. Modern slavery is a crime under the Modern Slavery Act (2015).

Touch Point

Be aware of vulnerable groups such as those with disabilities, children living away from home, asylum seekers, children and young people in hospital, children in contact with the youth justice system, children and adults who are victims of domestic abuse and those vulnerable due to religion, ethnicity and so forth.

Also, be aware of those who may be exposed to violent extremism.

Discriminatory abuse results from unfair treatment based on such aspects as age, gender (including gender reassignment), religion, disability and sexual orientation. This includes negative behaviour, which is racist, ageist, sexist, homophobic or based on ethnic origin, disability and illness. The NHS Constitution of 2015 clearly states that individuals have the right not to be unlawfully discriminated against in the provision of NHS services (Department of Health 2015a, 2015b).

Institutional abuse occurs when there is a culture that restricts dignity, privacy, choice and fulfilment. Care workers may not deliberately be abusing individuals, but there may be subtle ways in which staff are used to doing things. Examples might include a lack of person-centred care with rigid care routines. The 'everybody has to have a bath' attitude might prevail. Disrespectful language and attitudes may be apparent; it also includes a lack of personal possessions and lack of consideration such as bedtimes and wake times, unsafe and unhygienic environments and non-protected mealtimes.

Financial abuse is the use of a person's property, assets, income, funds or any resources without their informed consent or authorisation. It includes:

- Theft
- Fraud
- Exploitation
- Undue pressure in connection with wills, property, inheritance or financial transactions
- The misuse or misappropriation of property, possessions or benefits
- The misuse of an enduring power of attorney or a lasting power of attorney, or appointee ship (NHS England 2015)

Self-harm: The Mental Health Foundation (2019) estimated that 400 in every 100,000 of the population self-harm. It is often seen as a cry for help or as a means of coping with stress or emotion that is overwhelming and out of control for individuals. This issue is dealt with in greater detail in Chapter 16.

Safeguarding is about safety and well-being and about providing additional measures for those least able to protect themselves from the types of harm or abuse described above.

Recognising Signs of Abuse

Witnessing direct abuse in action should always raise alarm bells. The nurse associate who sees, hears or is told of any act of abuse must act on it directly and immediately. The duty of care is on the individual who is being abused, and their safety and welfare are priority.

However, it is not always apparent that an individual is being abused. Those working with vulnerable adults in the community setting may be visiting individuals in isolation and not have an opportunity to witness abuse in action. In this scenario, there may be subtle signs that the nursing associate can pick up on.

Behavioural signs of abuse may include:

- Individuals becoming unusually quiet or withdrawn
- Unusual aggression or anger
- Looking unkempt or dirty, not self-caring
- Sudden changes in character, becoming distressed and tearful, appearing helpless
- Fear of being alone, not wanting to be left alone
- Physical signs such as bruising, cuts and unusual injuries with inconsistent explanation
- Repeated injuries
- Unusual overtly happy behaviour insisting that nothing is wrong.

You may notice alterations in the person's environment: the home may be dirty, cold or things may be missing, indicating financial abuse.

Supporting Evidence NSPCC learning

This website publishes a list of the executive summaries or full overview reports of serious case reviews related to children.

https://learning.nspcc.org.uk/case-reviews/recently-published-case-reviews/Children and young people, or those with a learning difficulty, can find it hard to express experiences of abuse due to confusion, shame, stigma or lack of recognition or understanding of abuse or neglect. The nature of the relationship with an abuser may make it more difficult to share experiences. Fears of not being believed, or of family breakup, of being put in care can influence how an individual communicates their experience. Language and learning difficulties, or the stage of a child's development, may make communication problematic.

> **Touch Point**
>
> An essential component of healthcare and social care is the recognition of safeguarding in practice. You must know how to raise concerns if you suspect or witness any types of abuse in your area of work.

Communicating and Escalating Abuse in Practice

In 2018, the Royal College of Nursing (RCN) produced an intercollegiate document that outlines the roles and competencies required by healthcare staff in their role in safeguarding adults. It identifies the following skills and attitudes that are paramount to the role:

- The ability to recognise signs of abuse, harm and neglect
- The ability to identify an adult at risk of harm, abuse or neglect
- The ability to seek appropriate advice and report concerns and be confident they have been understood
- An ability to listen to adults at risk, families and carers and to act on issues and concerns
- An ability to recognise how one's own beliefs, experiences and attitudes might influence involvement in safeguarding
- An ability to recognise how one's own action can impact on others

(Royal College of Nursing 2018)

Yellow Flag Emotions and Fears

In case of fear of not being believed or taken seriously as a member of healthcare staff, it is vital that you assure your patients that all reports of any type of abuse are taken seriously. It is important to gain their trust and that they understand you are there to help and support them.

Case study

An elderly patient was admitted to the Emergency Department, presenting with shortness of breath. The patient appeared unkempt on review, reporting his main carer as being his son. He had a plastic bag containing his medications, house keys and wallet. When asked if he had anything that he would like to be kept safe, he became agitated, insisting he didn't. The nurse was concerned not only regarding his well-being in terms of his appearance and apparent neglect but also of his increased agitation regarding his belongings. The nurse continued to 'chat' to the patient; after a short time, the patient claimed that his son was accessing his bank accounts taking money without his consent; hence, he had withdrawn a large sum of money and had it in his bag. The patient felt no one would believe him as he did give consent to his son to pay his bills and for his shopping from his bank account but not for his personal use. The nurse offered social work and safeguarding referrals; unfortunately, the patient declined. The situation was escalated to the nurse in charge who also spoke to the patient. Despite this, the patient continued to refuse any help stating repeatedly that no one would believe him. The patient was assessed to have capacity in making his own decisions by the medical team. The nurse spoke to the patient again, explaining that although he had declined any support, in view of what he had told the nurse, she did have a duty of care to refer him to the hospital safeguarding team.

The NMC provides the nursing associate with clarity on escalating concerns in practice. It quotes The Code (Nursing and Midwifery Council 2018b) which states the following:

Act without delay if you believe that there is a risk to patient safety or public protection.

To achieve this, you must:

- Raise and, if necessary, escalate (take further action on) any concerns you may have about patient or public safety, or the level of care people are receiving at your workplace or any other healthcare setting and use the channels available to you in line with our guidance and your local working practices.
- Raise your concerns immediately if you are being asked to practise beyond your role, experience and training.
- Tell someone in authority at the first reasonable opportunity if you experience problems that may prevent you working within the Code or other national standards, taking prompt action to tackle the causes of concern if you can.
- Acknowledge and act on all concerns raised to you, investigating, escalating or dealing with those concerns where it is appropriate for you to do so.
- Do not obstruct, intimidate, victimise or in any way hinder a colleague, member of staff, person you care for or member of the public who wants to raise a concern.
- Protect anyone you have management responsibility for from any harm, detriment, victimisation or unwarranted treatment after a concern is raised.

(Nursing and Midwifery Council 2018b Section 16) (See Figure 15.1)

> **Touch Point**
>
> *'If you witness or suspect there is a risk to the safety of people in your care and you consider that there is an immediate risk of harm, you should report your concerns straight away to the appropriate person or authority'.* (Nursing and Midwifery Council 2019)

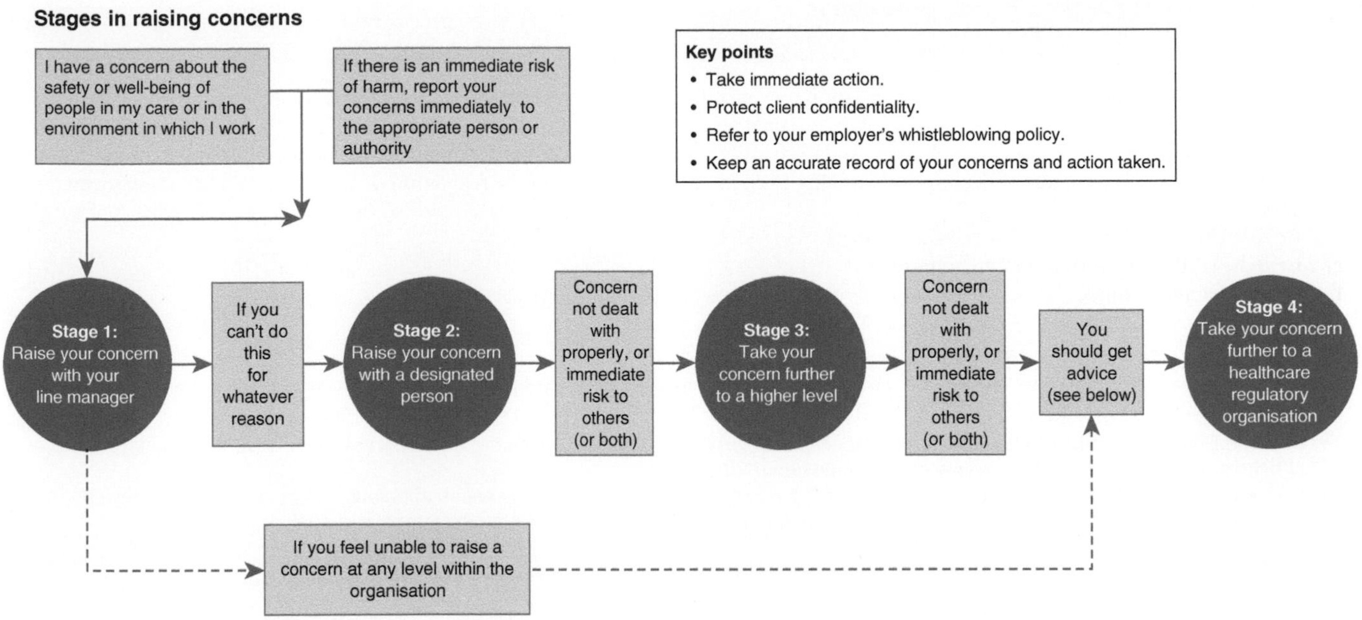

Figure 15.1 Raising concerns. ***Source:*** **Reproduced with permission of NMC.**

Supporting Evidence NMC, raising concerns

https://www.nmc.org.uk/standards/guidance/raising-concerns-guidance-for-nurses-and-midwives/case-studies-on-raising-concerns/

This NMC website provides four case studies on raising concerns in practice. The studies range from a GP setting, an acute setting, a rural setting and an example of a maternity care setting. You are invited to read the introductory description and to think about how you might act and raise concerns in each scenario. A brief overview is then provided for you to consider.

Communicating with the Abused Individual

I have concerns that someone may be suffering from abuse or neglect – how should I approach them, should I try to talk to them?

- If you feel confident in talking to the individual, broach your concerns in private. Explain your reason for concern, i.e. their appearance is not as it is normally, that they appear distant/withdrawn, that they are not participating in social activities as they normally would do and that you would like to help them.
- Give them time to talk but remember they may not feel able to 'open up'. They may feel by talking about it they could make the situation worse, feel as though everything is their fault, or feel threatened.
- The conversation will probably be upsetting for you too, but remain calm and listen. They need to feel safe and that they are not being judged and that they can put their trust in you.
- It is important that you find the person the right help at the right time. Give them time to talk about their situation, and if you feel able and confident, slowly introduce your suggestions for options of help that are available. It is important that you do not assure them that you will not tell anyone as you may have a duty to do so, depending on the level of abuse or neglect.
- During the conversation, you will be able to ask what help they think they need themselves. Assure them you can seek help on their behalf if they do not feel able to do so for themselves.
- If you feel the person is at risk of immediate harm, you must tell them of your concerns in a calm, supportive manner so you do not lose the trust you have gained. Explain how you can help in reporting and accessing the level of support they need.
- It is vital you listen to the person's wishes. You must remember that it will have been extremely difficult for them to tell you what has happened, and they will have put their trust in you to guide and support them in seeking the appropriate help.

Supportive Evidence Social care institute for excellence (SCIE)

Video: Safeguarding adults: looking out for each other to prevent abuse (11 minutes).

The video shows how effective communication can support safeguarding with the older person.

https://www.scie.org.uk/socialcaretv/video-player.asp?guid=d2966889-f552-4464-96d3-c22ebcf2a5ed

Being Open – Duty of Candour

The Care Quality Commission Duty of Candour regulation was introduced in November 2015, building on the 'being open' framework that was introduced in 2009. It is important that, as professionals, we are open and honest with patients and their families when a patient safety incident has happened. Being open simply means apologising and explaining what happened to the patient and their family. Communicating in a timely manner is a vital part of the process of dealing and learning from incidents. A breach of the regulation occurs when an element or elements of the process are not adhered to, including:

- Failure to promptly inform the patient of the incident
- Failure to be truthful with the patient and family
- Failure to offer an apology

Clinical Flag, Blue Flag **Relationship Issues**

Case study – Duty of Candour

The Duty of Candour applies when an unintended or unexpected incident happens when moderate harm, severe harm, psychological harm or death occurs. An example of this could be:

- Patient X is admitted to hospital with a chest infection and is treated with intravenous antibiotics. Patient X does not have any history of falls, but unfortunately, Patient X falls while mobilising to the toilet, sustaining a fractured neck of femur.

Following an incident, the care team must:

- Apologise to the patient and family
- Provide an explanation of what happened and why it happened
- Give the patient/family the opportunity to ask questions at this time, followed by an explanation of what immediate steps have been put in place to prevent or reduce the risk on the incident happening again
- Explain any treatment plans implemented at this time
- Make the patient/family aware that an investigation will be completed and feed this back either in writing or face to face
- Identify a Being Open Lead to be the main point of contact for the patient/family, who will support the patient/family following the incident and throughout the investigation
- Staff involved in the incident may also be distressed and must also be supported
- Send a letter (within 10 days) following the verbal apology, again explaining how the incident occurred, that it will be investigated and dates for completion of the investigation
- On completion of the investigation, a second letter should be sent summarising the key findings and offering a meeting to discuss further
- The incident should also be communicated to the patient's GP and social services to ensure that the patient receives the appropriate support when discharged
- Adhere to local policy and procedure

Touch Point **Being open – Duty of Candour**

In summary, the Being Open process has three key stages:

- Verbal apology/meeting
- Follow-up discussion to keep the patient and family updated on the investigation process
- Written explanation and discussion, depending on the patients'/families' wishes.

Whistleblowing

The Freedom to speak up: raising concerns (whistleblowing) policy for the NHS April 2016 NHS Improvement and NHS England states that speaking up about any concern you have at work is important. In fact, it is vital because it will help to improve services for all patients and healthcare staff. You may feel worried about raising a concern, but please do not be put off. In accordance with the Duty of Candour, senior leaders and healthcare organisations are committed to an open and honest culture.

How to raise a concern:

- You can raise a concern with your line manager or supervisor either verbally or in writing. This is usually the best way to raise your concerns.
- If you feel you are unable to do this, or you do not feel your concerns have been addressed or acted on, you should contact your organisation's whistleblowing guardian. Alternatively, there are other routes you can follow, e.g. your trade union representative, the NMC, your University Tutor, your clinical nurse educator, NHS and Social Care Whistleblowing Helpline.

As a healthcare professional, you have a duty to report a concern. If you are unsure about whether to report it, it is always best to do so. It does not matter if you have misinterpreted a situation if there is a reasonable explanation for your concerns. You can choose to raise your concerns anonymously; however, this may make the investigation more difficult and for you to be given feedback on the findings of the investigation. Organisations should be committed to an open and transparent culture where staff are encouraged and feel confident in raising concerns.

Clinical Flag, Blue Flag **Relationship Issues**

Case study: Whistleblowing

An agency member of staff raised a concern regarding 'unsafe' staffing levels on a ward with the Trusts Whistleblowing lead. This was investigated locally by a senior nurse. The reported shift was found to be extremely busy for several reasons including the sudden deterioration of a patient who required critical care support, a missing patient that had been reported to the police and several patients requiring one-to-one supervision. It was found that the nurse in charge had initially escalated the situation to the site manager who had sought support from another area for a short period. The investigation concluded that further support should have been sought at the time. This was fed back to the nurse in charge. The concern was recognised as being valid, and the outcome of the investigation was clearly explained to the nurse.

Examples of concerns you can raise:

- Lack of education/training
- Unsafe patient care
- Unsafe working conditions
- Lack of response to a reported incident
- Bullying
- Suspicions of fraud

All investigations should focus on lessons learnt and what can be done to improve on or prevent the same incident happening again. Lessons learnt should be anonymised and shared with the appropriate teams.

Touch Point **Freedom to speak up – Whistleblowing**

As a healthcare professional, you have a duty to report a concern. If you are unsure about whether to report it, it is always best to do so. It does not matter if you have misinterpreted a situation if there is a reasonable explanation for your concerns.

Touch Points Revisited

- The term safeguarding legislation refers to:
  - The Care Act 2014 (England)
  - The Safeguarding Vulnerable Groups (Northern Ireland) Order 2007
  - The Adult Support and Protection (Scotland) Act 2007
  - Social Services and Well-being (Wales) Act 2014
- Be aware of vulnerable groups such as those with disabilities, children living away from home, asylum seekers, children and young people in hospital, children in contact with the youth justice system, children and adults who are victims of domestic abuse and those vulnerable due to religion, ethnicity and so forth. Also, be aware of those who may be exposed to violent extremism.
- An essential component of healthcare and social care is the recognition of safeguarding in practice. You must know how to raise concerns if you suspect or witness any types of abuse in your area of work.
- *'If you witness or suspect there is a risk to the safety of people in your care and you consider that there is an immediate risk of harm, you should report your concerns straight away to the appropriate person or authority'*. (Nursing and Midwifery Council 2019)
- Being Open – Duty of Candour. In summary, the Being Open process has three key stages:
  - Verbal apology/meeting
  - Follow-up discussion to keep the patient and family updated on the investigation process
  - Written explanation and discussion, depending on the patients'/families' wishes.
- As a healthcare professional, you have a duty to report a concern. If you are unsure about whether to report it, it is always best to do so. It does not matter if you have misinterpreted a situation if there is a reasonable explanation for your concerns.

References

Care Act. (2014) *Chapter 23*. [online] Available: http:/www.legislation.gov.uk/ukpga/2014/23/pdfs/ukpga_20140023_en.pdf. Accessed September 2020.

Children and Families Act. (2004) Chapter 6. [online] Available: http://www.legislation.gov.uk/ukpga/2014/6/pdfs/ukpga_20140006_en.pdf. Accessed September 2020.

Care Quality Commission. (2015) *Regulation 20: duty of candour*, Newcastle Upon Tyne: CQC.

Department of Health. (2012) *Transforming care: a national response to Winterbourne view hospital final report*. [online] Available: https://assets.publishing.service.gov.uk/government/uploads/system/uploads/attachment_data/file/213215/final-report.pdf. Accessed September 2020.

Department of Health. (2015a) *Female genital mutilation (FGM) mandatory reporting duty*. [online] Available: https://assets.publishing.service.gov.uk/government/uploads/system/uploads/attachment_data/file/525405/FGM_mandatory_reporting_map_A.pdf. Accessed September 2020.

Department of Health. (2015b) *The NHS constitution. Section 3a*, London: Crown Copyright.

Department of Health. (2018) *Working together to safeguard children: a guide to inter-agency working to safeguard and promote the welfare of children*, London: Crown Copyright.

Francis, R. (2013) *Report of the mid Staffordshire NHS foundation trust public enquiry*, London: The Stationary Office.

GOV.UK. (2018, updated 2020) *Guidance: domestic violence and abuse*. [online] Available: www.gov.uk/guidance/domestic-violence-and-abuse#domesticviolence-and-abuse-new-definition, Accessed September 2020.

Mental Health Foundation. (2019) *[online] Available*: https://www.mentalhealth.org.uk/a-to-z/s/self-harm. Accessed September 2020.

Modern Slavery Act. (2015) [online] Available: https://www.legislation.gov.uk/ukpga/2015/30/contents. Accessed September 2020.

NHS England. (2015) *Safeguarding policy. [online] Available*: https://www.england.nhs.uk/publication/safeguarding-policy/. Accessed September 2020.

NHS Improvement. (2016) *Freedom to speak up: raising concerns (whistleblowing) policy for the NHS April 2016,* NHS England. [online] Available: https://improvement.nhs.uk/documents/27/whistleblowing_policy_final.pdf. Accessed September 2020.

Nursing and Midwifery Council. (2018a) *Standards of proficiency for nursing associates.* [online] Available: https://www.nmc.org.uk/standards/standards-for-nursing-associates/standards-of-proficiency-for-nursing-associates/. Accessed September 2019.

Nursing and Midwifery Council. (2018b) *The code: professional standards of practice and behaviour for nurses, midwives and nursing associates.* [online] Available: http://www.nmc.org.uk/globalassets/sitedocuments/nmc-publications/revised-new-nmc-code.pdf. Accessed September 2019.

Nursing and Midwifery Council. (2019) *Raising and escalating concerns for nurses, midwives and nurse associates*, London: NMC.

Peate, I. (2019) People deserve better. Editorial, *British Journal of Nursing*, 28(12): 745.

Public Health England (PHE). (2017) *Modern slavery and public health.* [online] Available: https://www.gov.uk/government/publications/modern-slavery-and-public-health/modern-slavery-and-public-health. Accessed September 2019.

Royal College of Nursing. (2018) Adult Safeguarding: roles and competencies for health care staff, *An intercollegiate document*, London: RCN.

Serious Crime Act. (2015) [online] Available: www.legislation.gov.uk/ukpga/2015/9/contents/enacted. Accessed September 2020.

Wales Social Services and Well-being (Wales) Act. (2014) anaw 4 [online] Available: www.legislation.gov.uk/anaw/2014/4/pdfs/anaw_20140004_en.pdf accessed September 2020

Women's Aid. (2020) *A perfect storm: the impact of the Covid-19 pandemic on domestic abuse survivors and the services supporting them.* Bristol: Women's Aid. [online] Available: https://1q7dqy2unor827bqjls0c4rn-wpengine.netdna-ssl.com/wp-content/uploads/2020/08/A-Perfect-Storm-August-2020-1.pdf. Accessed September 2020.

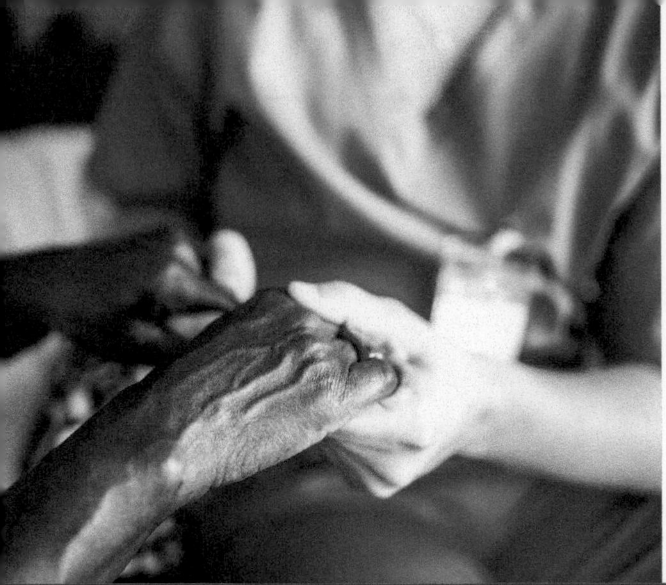

16

Recognising and Escalating Signs of Self-harm and/or Suicidal Ideation

Jo Regan[1] and Karen Wild[2]

[1] Leeds Teaching Hospitals Trust, UK
[2] Nurse, UK

Chapter Aim

- **This chapter aims to provide the reader with an insight into the reasons why individuals might self-harm or attempt to commit suicide and to aid understanding of how to best support these individuals within the practice setting.**

Learning Outcomes

By the end of this chapter, the reader will be able to:
- **Help the nursing associate identify types of self-harm and suicide in children, young people and adults**
- **Demonstrate how to communicate with and support those who present with self-harm or attempted suicide**
- **Be aware of the importance of triage and emergency management of those individuals who self-harm or attempt suicide**

Test Yourself Multiple Choice Questions

1. **Self-harm and suicide are the same issue.**
   A) **True**
   B) **False**
2. **Self-harm is not:**
   A) **A mental illness; it can be described as an indicator for internal stress or emotional distress**
   B) **Suicide, rather it is about staying alive**
   C) **Attention seeking or used to manipulate others**
   D) **All of the above**

The Nursing Associate's Handbook of Clinical Skills, First Edition. Edited by Ian Peate.

Companion website: www.wiley.com/nursingassociate

3. **Trichotillomania is:**
   A) Nail biting
   B) Scratching
   C) Hair pulling
   D) Cutting
4. **Members of the LGBT+ community are at risk of a range of mental health problems such as depression, suicidal thoughts, self-harm and alcohol and substance misuse.**
   A) True
   B) False
5. **The most common methods of suicide in both men and women of all ages are:**
   A) Drug overdose
   B) Hanging, suffocation and strangulation
   C) Carbon monoxide poisoning
   D) Stabbing

Introduction

Self-harm and suicide are very separate issues. If an individual attempts to hurt themselves, it does not mean that they necessarily want to die. However, suicide is when a person's aim is to end their life. For the purpose of this chapter, the two will be dealt with separately.

In applying practices to support and care for individuals who present with evidence of self-harm or suicide ideation, the nursing associate is practising within Nursing and Midwifery Council's (NMC) nursing associate proficiencies (Nursing and Midwifery Council 2018):

- Platform 1: Be an accountable professional
- Platform 2: Promoting health and preventing ill health
- Platform 3: Provide and monitor care
- Platform 6: Contributing to integrated care.

Self-Harm

Self-harm is the term used to describe when someone deliberately harms themselves as a way of dealing with their emotions. Self-harm is not:

- a mental illness; it can be described as an indicator for internal stress or emotional distress.
- suicide; rather, it is about staying alive.
- attention seeking or used to manipulate others.
- a trend or fashion thing.
- something that cannot be cured. People who self-harm can learn to manage emotions in different ways.
- done because individuals enjoy the pain; it is done for the relief gained from stress, emotional pain or self-loathing.

Self-harm is relatively common, according to Harmless (2019), the national voluntary organisation for people who self-harm (http://www.harmless.org.uk/). It is thought that around 13% of young people may try to hurt themselves on purpose at some point between the ages of 11 and 16 years, but the actual figure could be much higher (https://www.selfharm.co.uk). Figure 16.1 highlights some of the factors that can contribute to self-harm. Although it is not a direct attempt to take life, self-harm is a strong risk factor for suicide (Morgan et al. 2017). Individuals self-harm for a variety of reasons, and there is no common reason. What causes someone to self-harm may not be a trigger factor for another. We all manage inner emotions in a different way.

> **Touch Point**
>
> You may witness severe physical trauma as a result of self-harm in an individual. It is important to remember that the severity of an injury is not directly linked to the level of distress that the person is feeling. The act of harm is the important factor, not what a person has done or how severe the harm is.

Individuals who self-harm may do this in several ways, including:

- Cutting or scratching themselves
- Inserting objects into the body
- Burning themselves
- Starving or overeating
- Causing bruising to the body by hitting themselves
- Throwing their body against something that will harm the individual
- Taking overdoses or ingesting something harmful
- Hair pulling (also known as trichotillomania).

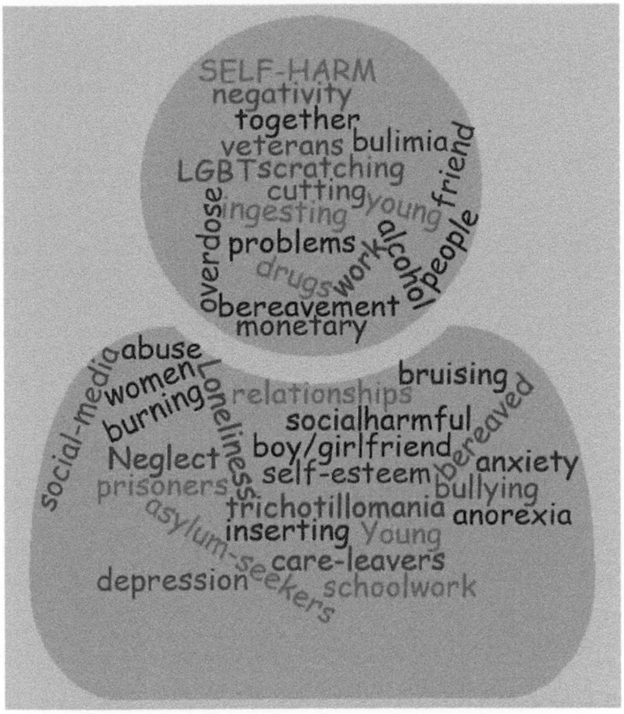

Figure 16.1 Examples of factors that can contribute to self-harm.

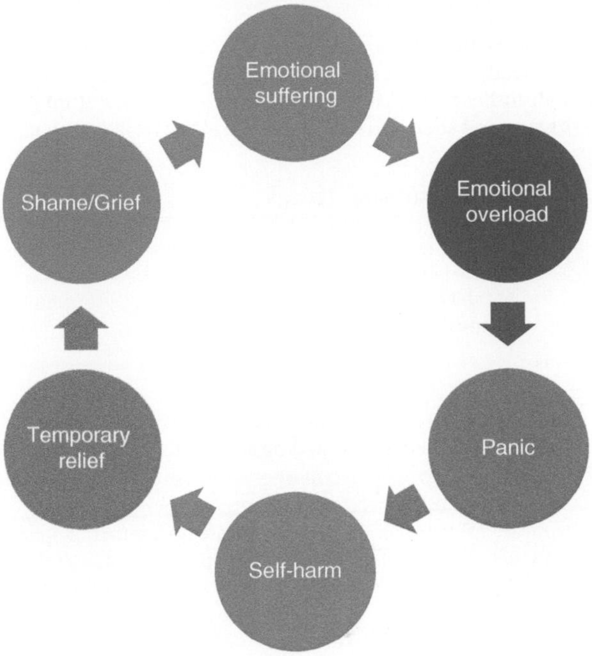

Figure 16.2 The cycle of self-harm. ***Source:*** **Adapted from Mental Health Foundation (2019a, 2019b, 2019c).**

There are many reasons that trigger self-harm. In young people, bullying, schoolwork pressures, negative perceptions of self and the pressure of social media are some of the most common factors that can lead to self-harm. Neglect and abuse, loneliness and dating problems may also contribute to self-harm. In young people, cutting is the most common form of self-harm (Nock 2009). In adults, work, social and monetary pressures, relationship problems, bereavement, drug and alcohol problems and poor self-esteem are just a few of the risk factors associated with self-harm.

More specific risk factors have been identified as:

- Experience of a mental health disorder which may include depression, anxiety, borderline personality disorder and eating disorders (Knightsmith 2015)
- Being a young person who is not under the care of their parents, or young people who have left a care home (Department of Health 2012)
- Being part of the LGBT+ community
- Having been bereaved by suicide
- Being a young woman
- Prisoners, asylum seekers and veterans of the armed forces (Wild & McGrath 2019)
- A group of young people who self-harm together: having a friend who self-harms may also increase the chance of self-harm (Royal College of Psychiatrists 2019).

Yellow Flag **Beliefs and Values**

Some members of the LGBT+ community are more likely to experience a range of mental health problems such as depression, suicidal thoughts, self-harm and alcohol and substance misuse (Mental Health Foundation 2019a, 2019b, 2019c).

This higher prevalence of mental ill health among members of the LGBT+ community seems, at least in part, due to the stress of prejudice and discrimination, isolation and homophobia, biphobia and transphobia. This can lead to some members of the LGBT+ community feeling unhappy with statutory services such as health services and can leave some of them with the perception that mental health services are discriminatory (Hughes et al. 2018).

Because individuals may experience some temporary relief at the start, self-harm can become someone's normal way of dealing with life's difficulties. Learning new coping strategies to deal with these difficulties can make it easier to break the cycle of self-harm in the long term (Mental Health Foundation 2019a, 2019b, 2019c). Figure 16.2 highlights this cycle.

It is important to acknowledge that self-harm is a coping strategy, and individuals find that they can gain relief from emotional pain or stress; they often feel a sense of being temporarily in control of their emotional hurt. Self-harm is about survival, and this is what sets it apart from acts of attempted suicide.

Communicating with an Individual About Self-Harm

Listening to individuals who are receiving care and support in the health and social care setting is such an important key skill (Silverman et al. 2013). Really listening to what someone is saying and recognising what is not said (such as non-verbal body language) require that we care enough to hear what is being conveyed even when it might make us shocked or feel uncomfortable. It can be difficult within often hectic healthcare and social care settings to find the time and space to truly listen to what a person wants to say – but these things are so important.

Blue Flag Relationship Issues

When supporting an individual in practice, it is important to use the correct language.

Avoid referring to the person who self-harms as a 'self-harmer'. This is a narrow and negative description and only defines the person in relation to that behaviour. It leaves little room to acknowledge and define individuals in relation to their broader personhood.

If a person is assessed as requiring help/support/treatment, the nursing associate must consider the environment in which the person is being looked after. A quiet area should be sort that can help the person feel safe, respecting their privacy and dignity. If a person is assessed as being high risk of self-harm, constant one-to-one supervision may be necessary. It is important that you:

- Create time for the person, in an environment where you will be free from interruption.
- Be aware of distractions such as mobile devices, office phones and computers.
- Convey to the individual that you are there to listen and give them your full attention.
- Show the person that you understand how difficult it is to be open and honest about their self-harm; ask them how they are feeling and the thoughts that are going through their mind.
- Try to focus and not show disgust or shock. Never judge.
- Reflect on your skills and be honest if you are out of your depth, and seek advice and guidance from your manager.
- Ensure that the individual's safety is paramount. You may need to seek medical help and support for the injured person.
- Allow the person to make informed choices, and support as far as you can any decisions that they make.
- Remain positive, but do not make false promises.

Take Note Communicating with an individual about self-harm

- Make time
- Listen
- Be open and honest
- Do not judge
- Offer support
- Maintain safety
- Remember the person behind the behaviour.

Green Flag Standards of Proficiency for Nursing Associates

At the point of registration, the nursing associate will be able to:

1.11 provide, promote, and where appropriate advocate for non-discriminatory, person-centred and sensitive care at all times. Reflect on people's values and beliefs, diverse backgrounds, cultural characteristics, language requirements, needs and preferences, taking account of any need for adjustments.

Source: Based on Nursing and Midwifery Council (2018)

Triage/Initial Assessment

Triage or initial assessment should always include an assessment of the person's underlying distress and whether the person is medically fit or requires medical attention.

Assessment should include:

- Physical state – Is the person physically well enough to engage in a medical assessment?
- Alcohol and drug use – Has the person used alcohol or drugs in the last 24 hours?
- Mental state – What mental health symptoms is the person presenting with?
- Mental health history – Is the person involved with mental health services?
- Current difficulties – What are the reasons for the person needing help?

Consent

A person presenting following self-harm may not always consent to treatment or further mental health assessment and support. If you are unsure of how to proceed, you must always ask a colleague for advice and guidance. No one situation is ever the same; the important thing to remember is to ensure that the person is given the appropriate information for them to make an informed decision if they can do so. A capacity and consent assessment must be made regularly throughout the person's assessment and or treatment (National Health Service 2019).

Mental Capacity

Having mental health capacity simply means the individuals have the ability to make their own decisions. The Mental Health Capacity Act 2005 states that a person is unable to make their own decisions if they cannot do one or more of the following things:

- Understand information given to them
- Retain information long enough to be able to make the decision
- Weigh up the information available to make the decision
- Communicate their decision

Touch Point

People must be offered support to make their own decisions before deciding they are unable to do so. The reason for determining if someone lacks mental health capacity is to be able to treat them even if they refuse and it is in their own best interests.

Reasons for a person not having capacity may be:

- A stroke or brain injury
- Substance misuse
- Unconsciousness, drowsiness or confusion.

(Mental Health Foundation 2019a, 2019b, 2019c)

If a person has the capacity to make a decision, then this decision must be respected, even if this is detrimental to their health and well-being, including further self-harm. This can be particularly difficult for healthcare professionals to accept. There is always help and support for you to access if you are struggling to manage or understand a situation.

If a patient is assessed as not having capacity, a professional is able to make a decision regarding treatment in the person's best interests. This person is known as the 'decision maker'. This person must be able to demonstrate the reasons why a decision has been taken and must document steps taken and factors considered to come to a decision. In life-threatening situations, it may be in the person's best interest to treat without any delay.

If the person is under the age of 16 years, and in some instances, up to 18 years, a referral to the Child and Adolescent Mental Health Services (CAMHS) should be made. This is a service that works with children who have emotional and behavioural difficulties including self-harm. CAMHS teams often include nurses, psychologists, psychiatrists, social workers, specialist substance misuse workers and psychological therapists.

Orange Flag **Mental Health and Psychological Issues**

Case study

A 22-year-old female presented to the Emergency Department with superficial cuts to her wrists and abdomen. She has no previous history of mental health issues or self-harm. The triage nurse immediately recognised she was not only extremely distressed but also very withdrawn. The nurse quickly took a set of baseline observations to assess how quickly she needed to be seen by a doctor. Clean dressings were offered and an opportunity to cover the superficial wounds was given. The nurse assessed her mental health as being a priority, so calmly took her to a cubicle and stayed with her until she was seen by a doctor. A referral was made to the liaison psychiatry team who assessed her mental health capacity and made a recommendation for urgent admission to an acute mental health facility.

Psychosocial Assessment Following Self-Harm

Psychosocial assessment is an integral part of a person's assessment and treatment following self-harm. A risk assessment and management plan should be reached and agreed with the person if possible. The assessment of risk and need are vital to determine the psychosocial issues that may explain reasons for self-harm and any further risks (Clements et al. 2019).

A psychosocial assessment following self-harm should include:

- The person's social situation
- Previous history of self-harm
- History of drug, alcohol and substance misuse
- Personal relationships
- Spiritual or religious needs
- Life events (this does not have to be recent).

Orange Flag Psychosocial Issues

Psychosocial risk assessment: self-harm

The purpose of the risk assessment is to identify if a person is at high risk of further harm, but it must be remembered that a person at low risk of further self-harm may still require further assessment, support and treatment. The assessment should be clearly documented in the person's notes and communicated with other healthcare and social care professionals involved in the person's care and treatment.

Self-harm can lead to suicide when it is no longer an effective coping mechanism, as it can cease to offset the feelings caused by stress or trauma. In a crisis, the person who self-harms repeatedly may find themselves desensitised to the effects of habitual physical pain through repeated harming episodes. The person may view a suicide attempt as less frightening (Stewart et al. 2014).

Red Flag Serious Pathology: Risk assessment

People who self-harm and present themselves at hospital are at increased risk of suicide, fatal alcohol or drug poisoning. Because self-harm may lead to suicide, individuals are assessed for their potential risk of suicide.

Supportive Evidence Online resources to support people who self-harm, their families and carers

National Self-Harm Network (NSHN) Forum http://www.nshn.co.uk/	Raises awareness and supports individuals, families and carers.
Self-Injury Support https://www.selfinjurysupport.org.uk/	Offers gender-specific support for women and girls.
LifeSIGNS http://www.lifesigns.org.uk/	User-led charity offering support and fact sheets.
The Mix https://www.themix.org.uk/	Offers targeted support to those who are under 25 years.
Sane http://www.sane.org.uk/	Charity aimed at meeting the challenge of mental health.
MindEd – www.minded.org.uk	MindEd has e-learning applicable across the health, social care, education, criminal justice and community settings. It is aimed at anyone from beginner through to specialist.
Place2Be – www.place2be.org.uk	Place2Be's services are acute and growing daily to provide early mental health support to children, parents and schools.
YoungMinds – www.youngminds.org.uk	Leading charity fighting for children and young people's mental health.

Suicide

In 2017, a total of 5,821 suicides were registered in the United Kingdom. According to the Office of National Statistics (ONS) 2017 saw the suicide rate for males in the United Kingdom at 15.5 deaths per 100,000 of the population. This equates to 4,382 deaths, the lowest rate since the time series began in 1981, and around a quarter of the total numbers recorded. There has been a general downward trend in suicide rates in men since 1981 (Office of National Statistics 2018). However, each year around 6,000 people take their lives in the United Kingdom, and many more people attempt suicide (National Suicide Prevention Alliance 2019).

Green Flag The Law

The Suicide Act 1961 (9 & 10 Eliz 2 c 60) is an Act of the Parliament of the United Kingdom. It decriminalised the act of suicide in England and Wales so that those who failed in the attempt to kill themselves would no longer be prosecuted.

Female suicide rates are always lower than males, and in 2017, the rate was 4.9 per 100,000 of the population. Again, there has been a downward trend since 1981, with a low point in 2007. Since then, the rate of suicide in females has been relatively consistent (Office of National Statistics 2018). Figure 16.3 displays the percentage difference between males and females who commit suicide.

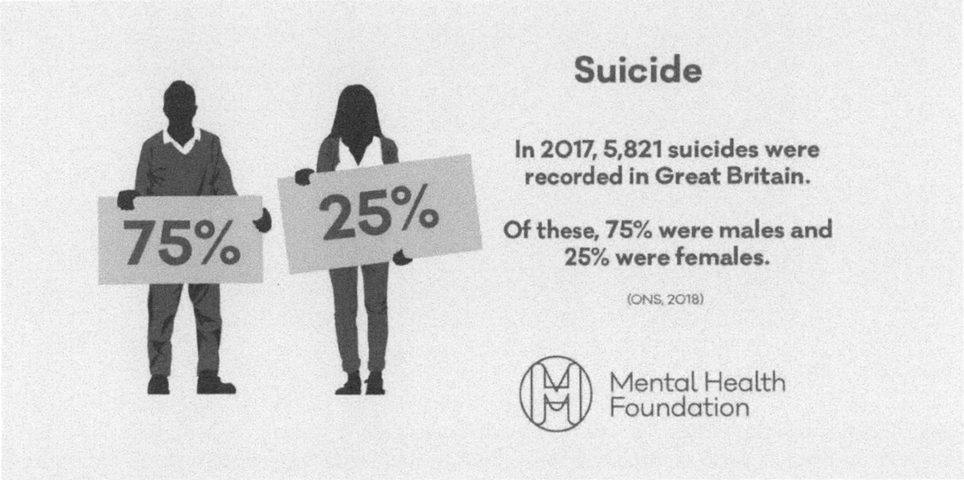

Figure 16.3 Percentage difference between males and females who commit suicide. *Source:* Suicide, Mental Health Foundation. © 2019 Mental Health Foundation.

- The most common methods of suicide in both men and women is hanging, suffocation and strangulation (59.7% male and 42.1% female).
- Poisoning is the second most common method and accounts for 18.2% in males and 38.3% in females.
  (Office of National Statistics 2018)

Touch Point

For males in England and Wales, hanging, suffocation or strangulation (all grouped together) has always been the most common method of suicide. The percentage of male hangings has shown a general upward trend from 2001 to 2017.

Recognising Suicidal Ideation in Practice

Patients with suicidal ideation who present in the healthcare and social care settings may not readily articulate their thoughts (Hawton & Van Heeringen 2000). Healthcare and social care practitioners should be aware of the risk factors associated with suicide to enable them to detect possible warning signs. Figure 16.4 showcases one of the aims of the National Suicide Prevention Alliance: reaching out. The National Suicide Prevention Alliance is a cross-sector, England-wide coalition committed to reducing the number of suicides in England and improving support to those bereaved or affected by suicide.

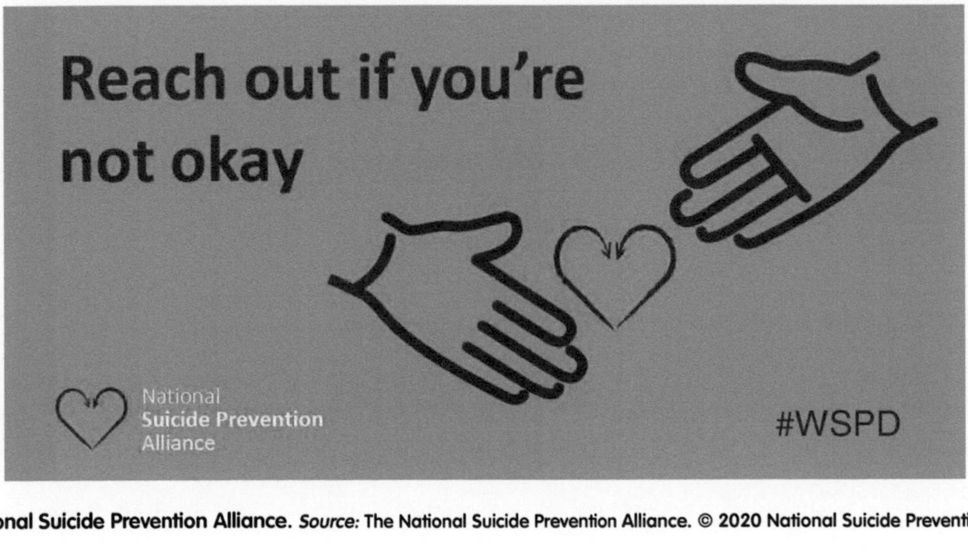
Reach out if you're not okay
National Suicide Prevention Alliance
#WSPD

Figure 16.4 The National Suicide Prevention Alliance. *Source:* The National Suicide Prevention Alliance. © 2020 National Suicide Prevention Alliance.

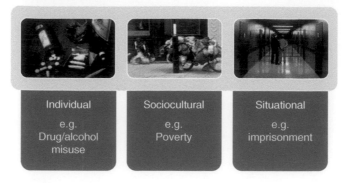

Figure 16.5 Risk factors associated with suicide.

According to the Mental Health Foundation (2018), several factors are known to be linked to an increased risk of suicide. These factors can fall into one of three categories: individual, socio-cultural and situational (World Health Organisation 2012). Figure 16.5 highlights the three categories – individual, sociocultural and situational factors – that are linked to a risk of suicide; these include:

- Drug and alcohol misuse
- History of trauma or abuse
- Unemployment
- Social isolation
- Poverty
- Poor social conditions
- Imprisonment
- Violence
- Family breakdown

Violet Flag Homeless People and Self-Harm/Suicide Risk

Traumatic childhood experiences such as abuse, neglect and homelessness are part of most street homeless people's life histories. In adulthood, the incidence of self-harm and suicide attempts is notable.

Source: McDonagh (2011)

People with a diagnosed mental health condition are shown to be at a higher risk of attempting and completing suicide, with more than 90% of suicides and suicide attempts having been found to be associated with a psychiatric disorder. Globally, the highest rates of suicide are associated with depressive disorders (World Health Organisation 2017).

Violet Flag Austerity and Suicide

'*There is a link between suicide rates and austerity – that has been clearly demonstrated*', says Siobhan O'Neill, the professor of mental health sciences at Ulster University. '*It's associated with being on benefits, with sanctions – there are plenty of case studies where that has been the last straw*'.

Source: Brandon (2017)

Touch Point

Patients who experience depression and anxiety often find healthcare professionals easier to talk to and so associate nurses are in a prime position to identify and support patients who may be at risk of suicide.

The experience of stressful life events appears to be linked with depressive symptoms and the onset of major depression in individuals, as well as suicide and suicidal thoughts. Previous suicide attempts and engagement in self-harming behaviours are also an indication of particular risk.

Take Note

Risk factors associated with suicide are complex, and although it is acknowledged that depression and self-harm are key risk indicators, many individuals who experience self-harm do not go on to take their lives, and not everyone who dies from suicide has a formal psychiatric or self-harm history.

Supporting Evidence

Video: U Can Cope (http://www.connectingwithpeople.org/ucancope)

This video spreads the message that it is possible to overcome suicidal thoughts and feelings and that there are many resources available to help those who are struggling to cope. Released on World Suicide Prevention Day – 10 September 2012.

Communicating with Those Who Feel Suicidal

Any voicing of suicidal ideation should be explored in a caring and concerned manner. Compassion is essential when interacting with an individual who may be suicidal. If the person discloses thoughts of suicide, it is important to find out as much information as possible. If you suspect that an individual is at risk, but suicidality is not disclosed by the person, it is important to be curious and seek more information about how the individual is feeling, including whether they have experienced thoughts of suicide. Asking about suicide will not put the idea into people's heads; in fact, it may reduce the risk; see also Chapter 17 of this text: Basic Mental Health First Aid.

Blue Flag Relationship Issues

'Help! I Don't Know What to Say to Somebody Who I Know Is At Risk of Suicide'

- Do not be afraid to use the word 'suicide'.
- Try to be direct, avoid confusing analogies like 'ending it all'.
- Say something direct but sincere like. . . *'Have you been having thoughts about harming yourself?'* The individual is more likely to give a more direct answer creating more clarity for you.
- If you feel comfortable with a gentler approach, try. . . *'You've mentioned you're feeling quite down and hopeless. Can you tell me if you've been thinking about suicide?'*
- Tell the patients they have done the right thing by seeking help and confiding in you. Let them know that you want to ensure their safety and help them get the support they need.
- Be honest with them and let them know you are concerned about their safety and want to share how they are feeling with other healthcare professionals to help decide the best plan of care.
- Ask them who they have at home or socially that they rely on, and how much support that person or people can realistically give.
- Explain what information you need to give to any carers and reassure the patient you do not need to disclose everything you have been told about what they are feeling.

It is important that individuals and carers are made aware of how to access support in a crisis (i.e. via general practitioner (GP), mental health services, 111, 999 and Emergency Department), and a shared care plan should be mutually agreed.

If an individual is assessed as being at risk of suicide, a risk assessment must be undertaken to determine the level of supervision required. This would usually require an individual having one-to-one supervision from a nursing associate, registered nurse or mental health unregistered or registered nurse. This can be referred to as 'enhanced care' which is an integral part of a therapeutic care plan to ensure the sensitive monitoring of the patient's behaviour and mental state (National Health Service Improvement 2018). Despite the cause, patients require safety, compassion and understanding at all times. The nurse should communicate with the patients in a quiet and sensitive manner, building their trust. If one-to-one care is required, the nurse providing the supervision must not leave the patient alone, including keeping bathroom and toilet doors ajar or unlocked to allow for constant uninterrupted supervision. Ongoing assessment of the patient's condition must be undertaken, and the level of supervision reviewed, for example, a patient may be allowed some degree of privacy if their risk has reduced, i.e. keeping the toilet door closed. This must be clearly documented in the plan of care. At all times, local policy and procedure must be followed.

Orange Flag Mental Health and Psychological Problems

When caring for someone at risk of taking their own life, the nurse must ensure the level of supervision is fully risk assessed and provided. If this is not available within existing staffing, the situation must be escalated to the matron/site manager and the issue documented.

The nurse must demonstrate compassion and understanding at all times.

Red Flag Physical Emergency

Case study

A 19-year-old male was brought to the Emergency Department following an attempt to take his own life by hanging. On admission, there were marks around the patient's neck, but he was fully alert and orientated. He was assessed by the medical team, deemed medically fit, but requiring mental health assessment. The patient was admitted to an acute assessment ward to await psychiatry input. A full risk assessment was undertaken by the psychiatry team, and the patient was assessed as needing continuous one-to-one care. It was agreed that a nursing associate would be best suited to care for him. This was swiftly arranged, ensuring the patient's safety was maintained, and one-to-one care remained until the patient was assessed by the mental health team and transferred to a mental health facility.

Touch Point

Dealing with suicide risk is stressful, and nursing associates should seek support and supervision in order to make sense of their feelings and to reflect on their management of suicide risk in practice.

Resource

'We need to talk about Suicide'
Health Education England and Public Health England
http://www.nwyhelearning.nhs.uk/elearning/HEE/SuicidePrevention/index.html(accessed July 2019).

This is a National Health Service (NHS)-based interactive course which takes between 60 and 90 minutes to complete (you won't be tested, just encouraged to interact!). Included in the presentation are videos and links to develop your knowledge and skills in talking and listening to people who are at risk, have attempted or are contemplating suicide.

Touch Points – Revisited

- You may witness severe physical trauma as a result of self-harm in an individual. It is important to remember that the severity of an injury is not directly linked to the level of distress that the person is feeling. The act of harm is the important factor, not what a person has done or how severe the harm is.
- People must be offered support to make their own decisions before deciding they are unable to do so. The reason for determining if someone lacks mental health capacity is to be able to treat them even if they refuse and it is in their own best interests.
- For males in England and Wales, hanging, suffocation or strangulation (all grouped together) has always been the most common method of suicide. The percentage of male hangings has shown a general upward trend from 2001 to 2017.
- Patients who experience depression and anxiety often find healthcare professionals easier to talk to and so nursing associates are in a prime position to identify and support patients who may be at risk of suicide.
- Dealing with suicide risk is stressful, and nursing associates should seek support and supervision in order to make sense of their feelings and to reflect on their management of suicide risk in practice.

References

Brandon, S. (2017) *Picking up the pieces: suicide prevention.* [online] Available: https://www.insidehousing.co.uk/insight/picking-up-the-pieces-suicide-prevention-51489. Accessed September 2019.

Clements, C., Hawton, K., Geulayov, G. and Waters, K. (2019) *Self-harm in midlife: analysis using data from the multicentre study of self-harm in England*, Cambridge, UK: Cambridge University Press.

Department of Health. (2012) *Preventing suicide in England: a cross-government outcomes strategy to save lives.* [online] Available : https://assets.publishing.service.gov.uk/government/uploads/system/uploads/attachment_data/file/267020/Preventing_suicide_equalities_impact-1.pdf. Accessed September 2020.

Harmless. (2019) [online] Available: http://www.harmless.org.uk/. Accessed July 2019.

Hawton, K. and van Heeringen, K. (eds.). (2000) *The international handbook of suicide and attempted suicide*, Chichester: John Wiley & Sons Ltd.

Hughes, E., Rawlings, V. and McDermott, E. (2018) Mental health staff perceptions and practice regarding self-harm, suicidality and help-seeking in LGBTQ youth: findings from a cross-sectional survey in the UK, *Issues in Mental Health Nursing*, 39(1): 30–36.

Knightsmith, P. (2015) *Self-harm and eating disorders in schools*, London: Jessica Kingsley Publishers.

McDonagh, T. (2011) *Tackling homelessness and exclusion: understanding complex lives, Joseph Rowntree foundation.* With contributions from all four projects of the Multiple Exclusion Homelessness Research Programme. [online] Available: https://www.homeless.org.uk/sites/default/files/site-attachments/Roundup_2715_Homelessness_aw.pdf. Accessed September 2019.

Mental Health Foundation. (2019a) *The truth about self-harm.* [online] Available: https://www.mentalhealth.org.uk/publications/truth-about-self-harm. Accessed July 2019.

Mental Health Foundation. (2019b) *Mental capacity.* [online] Available: https://www.mentalhealth.org.uk/a-to-z/m/mental-capacity. Accessed July 2019.

Mental Health Foundation. (2019c) *Mental health statistics: LGBT people.* [online] Available: https://www.mentalhealth.org.uk/statistics/mental-health-statistics-lgbt-people. Accessed July 2019.

Morgan, C., Webb, R.T., Carr, M.J., Kontopantolis, E., Green, J., Chew-Graham, C.A., Kapur, N. and Ashcroft, D.A. (2017) Incidence, clinical management, and mortality risk following self-harm among children and adolescents: cohort study in primary care, *BMJ*, (Oct 18 2017), 359: j4351. doi: 10.1136/bmj.j4351

National Suicide Prevention Alliance. (2019) *Strategic framework.* [online] Available: https://www.nspa.org.uk/wp-content/uploads/2019/02/NSPA-Strategic-framework-2019-2021_WEB.pdf. Accessed September 2019.

Nock, M.K. (2009) Why do people hurt themselves? New insights into the nature and functions of self-injury, *Current Directions in Psychological Science*, 18(2): 78–83.

Nursing and Midwifery Council. (2018) The code, *Professional standards of behaviour for nurses, midwives and nursing associates*, London: NMC.

Office of National Statistics. (2018) *Suicides in the UK: 2017 registrations.* [online] Available: https://www.ons.gov.uk/peoplepopulationandcommunity/birthsdeathsandmarriages/deaths/bulletins/suicidesintheunitedkingdom/2017registrations#suicides-in-the-uk. Accessed August 2019.

Royal College of Psychiatrists. (2019) [online] Available: https://www.rcpsych.ac.uk/mental-health/problems-disorders/self-harm. Accessed July 2019.

Selfharm. (2019) [online] Available: https://www.selfharm.co.uk/get-information/the-facts/self-harm-statistics. Accessed September 2019.

Silverman, J.D., Kurts, S.M. and Draper, J. (2013) *Skills for communicating with patients (3rd edn)*, London: Radcliffe.

Stewart, S., Baide, P. and Theall-Honey, L. (2014) Examining non-suicidal self-injury among adolescents with mental health needs in Ontario, Canada, *Archives of Suicide Research*, 18(4): 392–409.

Wild, K. and McGrath, M. (2019) *Public health and health promotion for nurses, At a glance*, Chichester: John Wiley and Sons Ltd.

World Health Organisation. (2012) *Public health action for the prevention of suicide*. [online] Available: http://apps.who.int/iris/bitstream/handle/10665/75166/?sequence=1. Accessed August 2019.

World Health Organisation. (2017) *Depression and other common mental disorders*. Available: http://apps.who.int/iris/bitstream/handle/10665/254610/WHOMSD?sequence=1. Accessed August 2018.

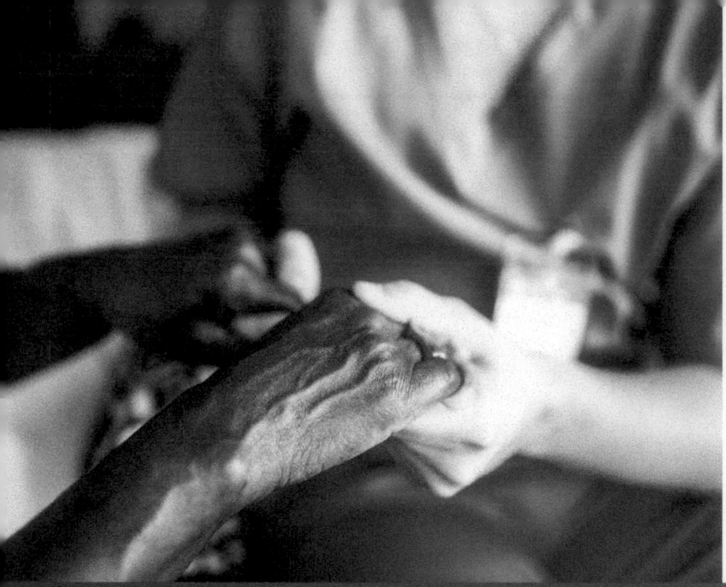

17

Basic Mental Health First Aid

Angelina L. Chadwick

University of Salford, UK

Chapter Aim

- **This chapter aims to explore the principles of basic mental health first aid.**

Learning Outcomes

By the end of this chapter, the reader will be able to:

- **Define basic mental health first aid**
- **Explore basic mental health first aid and the nursing associate's role**
- **Describe basic mental health first aid knowledge, skills and behaviours required by the nursing associate**

Test Yourself Multiple Choice Questions

1. **A key principle of basic mental health first aid is to:**
   A) **Provide counselling for someone with a mental health crisis**
   B) **Provide mental health promotion to someone with a mental health crisis**
   C) **Provide initial assistance to someone in a mental health crisis**
2. **What does the 'A' in ALGEE represent?**
   A) **Approach**
   B) **Ask**
   C) **Advise**
3. **What are nursing associates expected to do?**
   A) **Diagnose someone with a mental health problem**
   B) **Provide mental health-specific interventions**
   C) **Administer basic mental health first**

The Nursing Associate's Handbook of Clinical Skills, First Edition. Edited by Ian Peate.

Companion website: www.wiley.com/nursingassociate

4. 4. **Which of the following symptoms will someone experiencing a panic attack display?**
   A) **Bradycardia**
   B) **Tachycardia**
   C) **Hypotension**
5. **Which of the following behaviours might someone with a low mood display?**
   A) **Increased agitation**
   B) **Increased alertness**
   C) **Increased socialising**

Introduction

In this chapter, basic Mental Health First Aid (MHFA) principles will be defined and explored in the context of the nursing associate's role. The concept of MHFA was originally developed in Australia in 2001 and introduced in the United Kingdom in 2007. The need for MHFA has increased in recent years due to the demand for equal access and support for those with mental health needs, as is provided to those with physical needs. Parity of esteem is the term used frequently in government policies which seeks to place individuals with complex mental health needs on an equal footing as those with physical health needs (Royal College of Nursing 2019). Therefore, this chapter places equal emphasis for nursing associates to develop their knowledge and skills to support those with mental health problems in crisis, as they would someone with a physical health injury.

Basic MHFA

This can be defined as the initial assistance provided to a person who develops a mental health problem or someone in crisis (Kitchener & Jorm 2006).

Supporting Evidence

Betty Kitchener created the MHFA course in Australia in 2001. Visit the website for further information: https://mhfa.com.au.
The course was brought to the United Kingdom in 2007; further information can be located at https://mhfaengland.org.

Basic MHFA and the Nursing Associate

There are many licenced mental health first aiders within the United Kingdom due to the increase in mental health courses delivered nationally. While you may not be a licenced mental health first aider, as a nursing associate, you will be expected to recognise and support individuals who are developing mental health problems or those in crisis. The Nursing Midwifery Council (NMC) outlines in the standards of proficiency for nursing associates a number of competencies which support the need be able to recognise and respond to someone in mental distress. It has affirmed this need through the publication of the Skills Annexes A and B (Nursing Midwifery Council 2018a). Part 1 identifies that, at the point of registration, the nursing associate will be able to undertake the procedure to enable the effective monitoring of a person's condition. In 1.10, it is specified that the nursing associate will be able to administer basic MHFA.

Green Flag

The code of conduct (Nursing Midwifery Council 2018b, p. 14) 15.1 states that you can 'only act in an emergency within the limits of your knowledge and competence'.

This chapter will provide you with some basic MHFA knowledge to support your practice experience and further reading. It is important to remember that while you may be caring for patients within a non-mental health hospital inpatient setting or the community, those patients with physical health needs may develop mental health problems or be in crisis. Early recognition is required with support and, if necessary, signpost on for further professional specialist help.

As a nursing associate, you will need to have the knowledge and skills to be able to perform some basic MHFA until help arrives. This help may be in the form of the mental health liaison service within an inpatient area or the community mental health team. So before exploring the various basic MHFA scenarios and actions to undertake, you need to first understand how and what to look for. The knowledge and skills required to respond to MHFA situations can be linked to the following NMC platforms (Nursing Midwifery Council 2018b) in terms of the competencies you are expected to achieve.

- *Platform 1 – Being an accountable professional*
- 1.17 safely demonstrate evidence-based practice in all skills and procedures stated in Annexes A and B.

- 1.8 understand and explain the meaning of resilience and emotional intelligence, and their influence on an individual's ability to provide care.
- 1.9 communicate effectively using a range of skills and strategies with colleagues and people at all stages of life with a range of mental, physical cognitive and behavioural health challenges.
- *Platform 3 – Provide and monitor care*
- 3.3 recognise and apply knowledge of commonly encountered mental, physical, behavioural and cognitive health conditions when delivering care.
- 3.23 recognise people at risk of abuse, self-harm and/or suicidal ideation and the situations that may put them or others at risk.

Touch Point

As a nursing associate, you must always act in the patients' best interest, providing person-centred care while adhering to the NMC code of conduct. While you may not be a trained mental health first aider, there will be situations when you will be the person with someone who is in a mental health crisis or developing a mental health problem. You will be required to use the principles of basic MHFA. Always remember to work with the sphere of your practice.

Mental Health

Mental health is defined as a state of well-being in which every individual realises his or her own potential, can cope with the normal stresses of life, can work productively and fruitfully and is able to make a contribution to her or his community (World Health Organisation 2018). Therefore, people can have varying degrees of mental health. This can be viewed as a mental health continuum from mental well-being to mental disorder. Most of us have days when we feel good and yet others when we feel upset or sad but are still regarded as mentally well. As a nursing associate, some patients whom you care for within non-mental health settings may experience acute mental health problems in the form of acute psychological distress. This could be as a result of a treatment, illness, injury or undergoing a particular procedure. Some may even have diagnosed mental health problems such as depression or psychosis but are in your care due to their primary physical health need. It is important to understand that not all mental health or psychological crises require specialist mental health services, and that sometimes being supportive and listening to someone is all that is required. However, there are many mental health problems patients can experience, which include anxiety, depression, bipolar disorder, schizophrenia, dementia, drug and alcohol problems, eating disorders and self-harming behaviours. This chapter will focus on a few common ones with further reading recommended around the others.

Yellow Flag

Sometimes, people with different cultural and spiritual beliefs exhibit mental health crisis/problems through their physical pain/problems. This can happen because in their culture mental health problems are not recognised. Therefore, as a nursing associate, you need to be aware of both cultural and spiritual beliefs of those in your care and be aware of possible mental health problems.

Basic MHFA

The principles of basic MHFA include preserving life, preventing further mental distress, providing support and assistance to someone in crisis and promoting recovery. There are five basic steps of an MHFA action plan known as the acronym AGLEE that is similar to the first aid approach of check for **D**anger **R**esponse **A**irway **B**reathing and **C**irculation (DRABC). These are the initial steps need to be taken to assess, support and signpost on for further help as required.

Take Note

Use ALGEE as part of your MHFA action plan:
Approach, assess and assist with any crisis
Listen and communicate non-judgementally
Give assurance and information
Encourage appropriate professional help
Encourage other support
(Mental Health First Aid Australia 2019)

Approach, Assess and Assist

The first step is to approach someone. This can be difficult, but important, especially if someone is clearly distressed. Let the person know that you are there to help and support them. For example, if you are on the ward and you observe someone is distressed, you need to approach them, even if you are unsure of why they are distressed.

Orange Flag

Many people fear approaching someone who is in crisis or displays signs of mental health problems, due to stigma. Stigma develops when people lack knowledge and understanding of something or are prejudiced by negative media or other social influences. This can be potentially detrimental to those with mental health problems, through the lack of support they receive or a fear for their personal safety.

Always introduce yourself and approach adopting a reassuring tone. If you raise your voice, this could alarm the person, so speak calmly and slowly. While approaching a person, you have the opportunity, as a nursing associate, to assess them. This involves asking questions and making some observations by looking and listening to consider what is happening and what help is required. What the person tells you is crucial; however, their non-verbal behaviour can be equally significant. Their posture, verbal responses, eye contact, tone and pitch of their voice are all part of your observational assessment. For example, someone who is low in mood could present with a closed body posture. The person would appear slumped, head down, arms close to their body and may even sit away from you. Their eye contact will be poor, or they may avoid eye contact altogether. Verbal responses may be monosyllabic, using a low pitch in the tone of their voice, or alternatively, they may not have the energy to even speak to you due to their low mood.

Asking open questions is a good place to start to allow the person to tell you what the issue is in their own words, for example, 'How are you feeling?' or 'Can you tell me what has been happening today?' If someone is very distressed, then using closed questions allows them to simply answer yes or no by directing your questions specifically to what you need to know. So, an example would be 'Are you feeling low in your mood?' or 'I can see that you are clearly distressed, is it OK if I sit with you?' If you suspect the person is so distressed that they have suicidal ideas, then you will need to ask about this in a direct manner. This is because many people fear asking about suicide directly, yet it can be prevented if someone is encouraged to talk about how they are feeling. Sometimes, people may have thoughts of suicide because they are struggling with emotional pain, feelings of worthlessness or because they want to get help but do not know how.

Red Flag

While it is necessary to ask someone directly if they have any suicidal ideas, you need to observe for signs of self-harm as an indication of a suicide attempt. This could include signs such as self-inflicted incision wound(s) on their arms.

People with poor physical health to whom you provide care and support can be at risk of suicide; this could be due a recent life-changing diagnosis or a debilitating long-term condition. Moreover, some of those to whom you provide care for may have experienced traumatic events in the past, or certain groups of people such as men are more at risk. Suicide is the leading cause of death among men under the age of 50 years, with around three times as many men dying from suicide as women (Mental Health Foundation 2018). Therefore, asking someone directly is the only way to establish if they are experiencing suicidal thoughts.

Supporting Evidence

Mental Health Foundation is a UK charity for mental health, and it seeks to prevent and address sources of mental health problems. It invests in research and influences government policy. Visit its website for further information: https://www.mentalhealth.org.uk

Listen and Communicate

Listening non-judgementally can be difficult. However, to assist someone in a non-judgemental manner, you need to set aside whatever feelings or thoughts you have about them or their issues and listen to what they are actually saying. This includes your non-verbal communication such as your body language and non-verbal cues, which must correspond with what you are saying. For example, avoid looking disinterested as you reassure the person you are supporting. Listen to what the person says, and do not dismiss what they are experiencing. For example, if someone says that they are hearing voices but you do not, then you need to validate what they say they are hearing, but state that you are not experiencing what they are.

Give Support and Information

Giving support and information could involve reassuring a person verbally by informing them that you are there to help. If you think that they require further help, then be open and honest and inform the person that you intend to summon specialist help and why. Alternatively, this information may simply be who you are and what you can do to support them in their moment of crisis.

Encourage Appropriate Professional Help

This could include referring the individual to the mental health liaison service or contacting their general practitioner (GP). As a nursing associate, this will require you to be aware of the types of mental health services that are available and accessible in your area. This will help you to signpost the person to the right service. For example, if you have been visiting a patient in their home following surgery for an lower limb amputation and you assess their mood as low and tearful, then it will be important to contact the patient's GP in the first instance for further assessment and treatment. This could result in a home visit and the need for anti-depressant therapy, alongside counselling, to deal with the effects of this life-changing surgery.

Encourage Other Support

This can involve self-help strategies and signposting the person to where they can get additional support, or example, it could be using mindfulness as a strategy to help with anxiety or may be increasing their physical activity to help raise their mood.

Touch Point

When using the AGLEE action plan, you must adopt a non-judgemental approach and assess the person using both verbal questioning and non-verbal techniques. Listen and allow the person to tell you how they feel. Remain calm and reassure the person experiencing a mental health crisis. Ask the person if what they are experiencing has happened before and, if so, what strategies they have used or what support they require. Finally, be aware of the appropriate specialist professional services in your area to be able to signpost a person to if required.

Next, we will explore some common mental health problems, which, as a nursing associate, you need to be able to recognise, to be able to support the person in your care and if necessary signpost on for further help.

Anxiety, Panic Attacks and Post-Traumatic Stress Disorder

Anxiety can be described as a state of fear or apprehension of a real or imagined impending threat resulting in physiological changes. It can range from moderate to severe. Anxiety can be diagnosed as a common mental health problem if it impacts on an individual's ability to undertake their usual daily living activities. Someone with anxiety may experience the following symptoms, which have been categorised into four areas (see Table 17.1).

A panic attack results from an overwhelming experience of anxiety and intense fear that develops suddenly and usually peaks in 10 minutes. A panic attack is not a mental health disorder. Mental disorders derived from anxiety include phobias, generalised panic disorder (GAD), obsessive-compulsive disorder (OCD) and post-traumatic stress disorder (PTSD). As a nursing associate, you would be expected to recognise the

Table 17.1 Clinical features associated with anxiety.

PHYSIOLOGICAL		
Cardiovascular	Palpitations, tachycardia, hypertension, feeling faint	
Respiratory	Rapid shallow breathing, shortness of breath, choking feeling	
Neuromuscular	Increased reflexes, muscle spasm, tremor, restless, wobbly legs	
Gastrointestinal	Nausea, vomiting, abdominal discomfort	
Urinary tract	Frequency of micturition	
Integumentary	Flushed face, sweating, hot/cold spells	
BEHAVIOURAL	**EMOTIONAL**	**COGNITIVE**
Feels restless Avoids situations Hyperventilation Speech difficulties	Feelings of dread Apprehension Fear Impending doom	Negative thinking Catastrophising Rumination Poor memory Inability to concentrate

Source: Based on Norman & Ryrie (2018).

symptoms above and ask the patients if they know what is happening. Have they experienced anything like this before, if they have, ask them what help they need. Always introduce yourself to the person and reassure . It is crucial that you remain calm and speak slowly in a reassuring tone using short sentences, but be firm. Encourage them to do some slow deep breathing and to try and focus on something positive to distract them. Stay with them until they are out of crisis.

PTSD develops following a traumatic event and can affect those who witness it. They can continue to perceive an actual threat, which causes the body to respond in many ways. Physical arousal is caused by the associated anxiety, resulting in agitation and panic attacks. Emotionally, the person may feel anger, irritability, a low mood, guilt or shame. Behavioural changes include avoidance of situations. This can lead to other problems such as substance misuse, particularly alcohol (National Health Service 2017). Anybody can develop PTSD, including those involved in a road traffic accident, victims of violent crime, those with serious health problems, emergency service staff and those in the armed forces who witness traumatic incidents in their line of work. Veterans in particular experience PTSD, which is now being recognised; as a result, there are organisations that provide support for veterans including the National Health Service (2017).

Supporting Evidence

The National Health Service (NHS) now offers advice and support for veterans. This includes advice around PTSD as well as accessible services. Visit the website for further information: https://www.nhs.uk/using-the-nhs/military-healthcare/nhs-mental-health-services-for-veterans

Complex PTSD can arise from those who experience repeated traumatic events, for example, individuals subject to long-term sexual abuse. Supporting individuals with PSTD can require psychological therapies and possibly anti-depressant medication. However, if someone experiences a panic attack due to PTSD, then the actions discussed above in relation to anxiety should be utilised.

Violet Flag

Someone who has been assaulted in his or her own home and hospitalised as a result of it could develop PTSD. They could develop panic attacks when nearing discharge due to flashbacks and the fear of going back to their home where the assault occurred.

Depression

Depression is common and can be defined as a depressed or low mood with a loss of pleasure in most activities with many symptoms including functional impairment (National Institute for Health and Care Excellence 2018). As a nursing associate, you are not expected to diagnose someone with depression, but as part of your assessment, look for changes in their mood and behaviour. Patients who have physical health problems are more likely to develop a low mood, for example, pain can impact on a person's mood and their ability to tolerate pain.

Symptoms of depression include:

- Low mood
- Social withdrawal
- Difficulty in concentration/cognitive impairment
- Loss of enjoyment in interests and activities
- Irritable mood
- Feelings of sadness, despair, guilt or worthlessness
- Sleeping problems in either getting to sleep or early morning awakening
- Loss of appetite or overeating (comfort eating)
- Lethargy and lack of volition
- Slow movements or restlessness and agitation
- Thoughts about death or suicide

Other forms of depression include seasonal affective disorder, dysthymia and both prenatal and postnatal depression (MIND 2019).

Supporting Evidence

MIND is a charity that offers advice and support for those with mental health problems. They influence government policy to improve the care and services for those with mental health problems. Visit its website for further information: https://www.mind.org.uk

Following the application of the principles of AGLEE, you must treat the person with dignity and respect. Remember, everyone is unique and experiences psychological distress in different ways. Avoid blaming them for their illness or telling them to pull themselves together since this will not help them and probably make them feel worse. Offer emotional support and encourage them to talk about how they are feeling. If these feelings continue for a period of time, then specialist professional help will be required.

Psychosis

Recognising someone with a psychosis can be difficult, since there may be a gradual onset with behavioural changes. Symptoms of psychosis include the following:

- Changes in thoughts and perceptions
  - Seeing or hearing things that are not there
  - Difficulty in perceiving reality
  - Feeling disconnected
- Changes in behaviour
  - Social withdrawal
  - Isolation
- Changes in emotion and motivation
  - Emotional outbursts
  - Mood changes
  - Suspiciousness
  - Struggle with day-to-day tasks.

You need to treat the person with respect and dignity. Tailor your approach to what you observe in terms of the patients' behaviour and what they tell you. Avoid confrontation, direct eye contact and saying what they are experiencing is not real because you do not experience it. If the person is experiencing delusions or hallucinations, for example, they may express paranoid thoughts, that people are monitoring them, then reassurance is needed here, alongside open and honest and reality-based communication. This could be by saying 'I appreciate that you feel frightened because you believe that someone is watching you, but at this moment, I am the only person here and I would like to support you'. Be clear in your communication; speak using short concise sentences and at a steady pace. Adopt a non-threatening approach, always remain calm and maintain yours and the person's safety. Do not be alarmed or show fear; equally, do not aggravate the situation. Try to empathise with how the person is feeling in a non-judgemental manner, allowing the person to talk about how they feel. Using the example above, you could respond by saying, 'I can see how you would be frightened if you feel that someone is watching you, can you tell me why you feel this is?'

Take Note

As a nursing associate, alongside AGLEE, you need to always be open and honest in your communication. Adopt a calm and approachable manner, keep your discussions reality based and avoid challenging the person with a mental health problem or those in crisis. Be aware of the services to contact if you need to signpost someone onto further professional specialist support.

Professional Specialist Support

As a nursing associate, if someone requires further professional specialist support, then you need to be aware of the mental health services available within your local area. Services may include the mental health liaison service, community mental health team, GP services, counselling services, MIND and Improving Access to Psychological Therapies, to name but a few. However, sometimes, individuals can develop serious mental disorders which may require admission to a mental health unit. This can result in the detention of the patient if they are deemed to have a mental disorder and refuse or lack insight for the need of necessary treatment.

Green Flag

The Mental Health Act (1983 amended 2007) serves to protect the rights of the individual experiencing mental disorder as well as the public. There are many sections within the act, with some resulting in the involuntary detention of a person for assessment and or treatment.

Touch Points Revisited

- Nursing associates are required to always act in the patients' best interest while adhering to the NMC code of conduct.
- There may be situations where the nursing associate is required to perform basic MHFA if you are with someone who is in a mental health crisis or developing mental health problems.
- Always remember to work with the boundaries of your sphere of practice.
- Use the AGLEE action plan adopting a non-judgemental approach.
- Assess the person using both verbal questioning and non-verbal techniques.
- Listen and allow the person to tell you how they feel.
- Remain calm and reassure the person experiencing a mental health crisis.
- If required, refer on to appropriate specialist professional help as soon as possible.

References

Kitchener, B.A. and Jorm, A.F. (2006) Mental health first aid training: review of evaluation studies. *Australian and New Zealand Journal of Psychiatry* 40:6–8.

Mental Health First Aid Australia. (2019) *The MHFA action plan AGLEE.* [online] Available: https://mhfa.com.au/about/our-activities/what-we-do-mental-health-first-aid. Accessed 17 May 2019.

Mental Health Foundation. (2018) *Suicide.* [online] Available: https://www.mentalhealth.org.uk/a-to-z/s/suicide. Accessed 20 May 2019.

MIND. (2019) *Depression. [online]* Available: https://www.mind.org.uk. Accessed 20 May 2019.

National Health Service. (2017) *Veterans: NHS mental health services.* [online] Available: https://www.nhs.uk/using-the-nhs/military-healthcare/nhs-mental-health-services-for-veterans. Accessed 1 June 2019.

National Institute for Health and Care Excellence. (2018) *Depression in adults: recognition and management.* [online] Available: https://www.nice.org.uk/guidance/cg90. Accessed 20 May 2019.

Norman, I. and Ryrie, I. (2018) *The art and science of mental health nursing principles and practice*, London: Open University Press.

Nursing Midwifery Council. (2018a) *The code of conduct*, London: NMC.

Nursing Midwifery Council. (2018b) *Standards of proficiency for nursing associates*, NMC. [online] Available: https://www.nmc.org.uk/globalassets/sitedocuments/education-standards/nursing-associates-proficiency-standards.pdf. Accessed 7 May 2019.

Royal College of Nursing. (2019) *Parity of esteem – delivering physical health equality for those with serious mental health needs*, RCN: London.

World Health Organisation (2018) *Mental Health: Strenthening our response.* [online] Available: https://www.who.int/news-room/fact-sheets/detail/mental-health-strengthening-our-response. Accessed 15 January 2021.

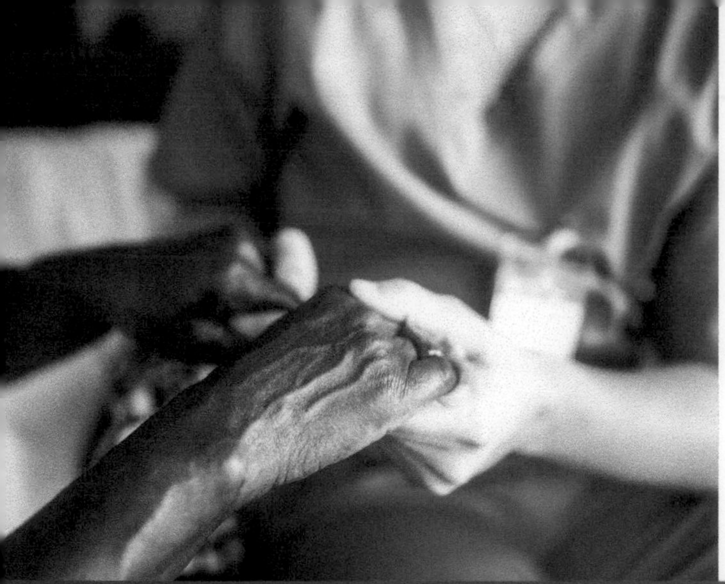

18

Basic First Aid

Angelina L. Chadwick

University of Salford, UK

Chapter Aim

- **This chapter aims to explore the principles of basic first aid.**

Learning Outcomes

By the end of this chapter, the reader will be able to:
- **Define first aid**
- **Explore first aid and the nursing associate role**
- **Describe first aid knowledge and skills required by the nursing associate**

Test Yourself Multiple Choice Questions

1. **In first aid, an initial assessment is known as a:**
   A) **Primary survey**
   B) **Tertiary survey**
   C) **Whole survey**
2. **If you find someone collapsed, you should:**
   A) **Undertake a primary survey**
   B) **Start basic life support**
   C) **Call for help**
3. **What does AVPU mean when assessing someone's conscious level?**
   A) **Alert, verbal, pain, unrecognisable**
   B) **Alert, verbal, pain, unresponsive**
   C) **Awake, verbal, pain, unresponsive**

The Nursing Associate's Handbook of Clinical Skills, First Edition. Edited by Ian Peate.

Companion website: www.wiley.com/nursingassociate

4. **How do you categorise burns?**
   A) **Superficial, partial thickness, full thickness**
   B) **Burn, scald, electrical, chemical**
   C) **In percentages**
5. **A severe loss of fluid is known as what type of shock?**
   A) **Cardiogenic**
   B) **Distributive**
   C) **Hypovolemic**

Introduction

In this chapter, *first aid* will be defined and explored in the context of the nursing associate role. This will be followed by a discussion around some situations that will require a first aid response, which you may encounter within your scope of practice and when not on duty. It will further identify the knowledge and skills required by you in order to be able to recognise and respond in these situations.

First Aid

'First aid is the initial assistance or treatment given to a person who is injured or taken ill' (St John Ambulance 2014, p. 12). The fundamental actions of first aid, aim to preserve life and prevent further deterioration.

Supporting Evidence

St John Ambulance (known as SJA) is a first aid charity that provides first aid cover using trained volunteers to communities and supports the emergency services at events. They also provide recognised training courses for individuals and organisations. Visit its website for further information: https://www.sja.org.uk/sja/default.aspx

A trained first aider, a volunteer or the person who arrives first on the scene can administer first aid. The United Kingdom has statutes in place governing first aid provision and responsibilities within the Health and Safety (First Aid) Regulations (1981).

Violet Flag

The nursing associate may be required to assist a range of people in a variety of settings. The SJA delivers tailored first aid courses to those who work with the homeless and drug and alcohol misusers. They also provide basic life support courses for homeless and vulnerably housed individuals. There are other organisations such as the Red Cross that support the homeless. The Red Cross provides free basic first aid courses for those who are homeless or at risk of homelessness.

Equipment required for first aid will be dependent on the area the nursing associate works in. Within an inpatient area, there may be a clinical room and a resuscitation trolley with all the necessary dressings and bandages to hand. Within a primary care environment, a first aid kit should be available. The contents of a first aid kit that is available for emergency use on an aeroplane, for example, will differ from what can be found in a household one; in Box 18.1, the contents of a standard first aid kit can be found. If you find yourself in a situation where you do not have any equipment to hand, then improvise. Use an item of clothing, for example, use a scarf, blanket or whatever you can find.

Box 18.1 First Aid Kit Contents

- Triangular bandages
- Assorted sized plasters
- Small-, medium- and large-sized sterile dressings
- Disposable gloves
- Sterile eye pads
- Hypo allergic tape

First Aid and Nursing Associates

It has been widely debated that nurses should have basic first aid skills and knowledge (Wilson 2005). The Nursing Midwifery Council (2018a) has affirmed this need through its publication of the Skills Annexe (Part B) within their standards of proficiency for nursing associates. Part 1 identifies that, at the point of registration, the nursing associate will be able to undertake the procedure to enable the effective monitoring of a person's condition. In Point 1.11, it specifies that the nursing associate will be able to recognise emergency situations and administer physical first aid, including basic life support (BLS).

Green Flag

The Code of Conduct (Nursing Midwifery Council 2018b, p. 14) 15.1 states that you can 'only act in an emergency within the limits of your knowledge and competence'.

This chapter will provide you with some basic first aid knowledge alongside your practice experience and further reading. In addition to this, your workplace will probably provide you with mandatory basic life support training. It is important to remember that while you may be caring for patients within hospital inpatient settings, it does not mean that patients cannot injure themselves, fall or suddenly deteriorate, in which case an assessment needs to be undertaken and help summoned. If you are working within the community, you may witness an accident when driving to a visit or arrive at a patient's home to find that they have suddenly become physically unwell. As a nursing associate, you will need to have the knowledge and skills to be able to perform some basic first aid until help arrives. This help may be in the form of the 'hospital resuscitation team' within an inpatient area or the paramedics in the community. Always remember to call for help either by pulling an emergency buzzer on the ward, telephoning for help or asking someone else to get help. You need to be aware of the emergency contact telephone numbers; for example, it could be 2222 for the hospital resuscitation team within inpatient areas and 999 for the ambulance service when in the community. So before exploring the various first aid scenarios and actions to undertake, you need to first understand how and what to look for. The knowledge and skills required to respond to emergency first aid situations can be linked to the following Nursing Midwifery Council (NMC) platforms (Nursing Midwifery Council 2018b) in terms of the competencies you are expected to achieve:

- *Platform 1 – Being an accountable professional*
  - 1.1 understand and act in accordance with the Code: Professional standards of practice and behaviour for nurses, midwives and nursing associates and fulfil all registration requirements
  - 1.17 safely demonstrate evidenced-based practice in all skills and procedures stated in Annexes A and B
- *Platform 3 – Provide and monitor care*
  - 3.6 demonstrate the knowledge, skills and ability to perform a range of nursing procedures and manage devices, to meet people's need for safe, effective and person-centred care
  - 3.11 demonstrate the ability to recognise when a person's condition has improved or deteriorated by undertaking health monitoring; Interpret, promptly respond, share findings and escalate as needed

Touch Point

As a nursing associate, you must always act in the patients' best interest, providing person-centred care while adhering to the NMC code of conduct. While you may not be a trained first aider, there will be situations where you will be the first person at the scene of an accident, injury or when a patient suddenly deteriorates, which will require to you to perform first aid. Always remember to work with the boundaries of your role.

Primary Survey

This is the first quick assessment and management of the patient and situation using the DR ABC approach. Use your senses in the assessment, look at the person, listen to them for any clues and feel where necessary. Remember to remain calm and always consider the patient's psychological welfare and offer reassurance.

Danger

This begins with checking the environment as you approach the patient for any signs of danger. Depending on where you are, this could include live electrical wiring, sharp or hazardous substances or other vehicles if attending at a road traffic collision. When checking the person, be aware of any bodily fluids and use gloves to protect yourself. Never put yourself at risk while trying to help someone else.

Orange Flag

While the focus in any first aid situation is the physical well-being of the patient, you need to consider their psychosocial health. Be supportive, always remain calm and offer reassurance using your interpersonal skills and remain with them until help arrives.

Response

Always check for any signs of response from the patient, ask them how they feel to elicit a response or gently shake their shoulders to gain a response being careful not to cause further injury. If there is no response, this means that they require urgent assistance and could be at severe risk, so make sure you have summoned help before you proceed to check the patient's airway.

Airway

To check a patient's airway, you need to use your senses. Listen to see if the patient can speak to you. If not, then the airway could be obstructed, so you need to look inside the mouth to see if there is anything obstructing the airway. Listen for any added noises from the airway, for example, snoring could indicate a partial obstruction. If the patient is unresponsive, they will not be able to maintain a patent airway. To open and clear the patient's airway, tilt the head and lift the chin (see Figure 18.1). Ensure that the patient's airway is clear before moving on to breathing.

Breathing

When assessing breathing, look to see if the chest is rising and falling and if the patient is breathing normally for 10 seconds. Listen for breath sounds indicating that the patient is breathing, and note the rate rhythm and depth of the breaths. Can the patient speak to you in full sentences, or are they struggling? Are there any added noises coming from the chest such as a wheeze which could indicate problems with breathing? Feel the chest to see if there is equal symmetry, if not, this could indicate some injury to the chest. If the patient is breathing but unresponsive, then place them carefully in the recovery position (Figure 18.2) and continue to monitor them until help arrives. If they are not breathing and unresponsive, then commence chest compressions as part of basic life support guidelines (Resuscitation Council 2015).

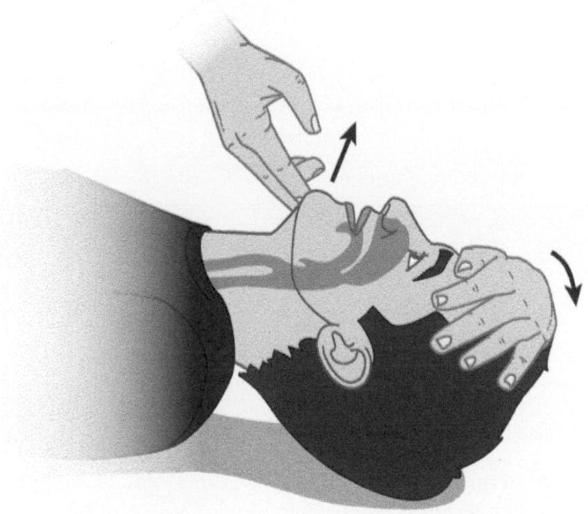

Figure 18.1 The head-tilt/chin technique.

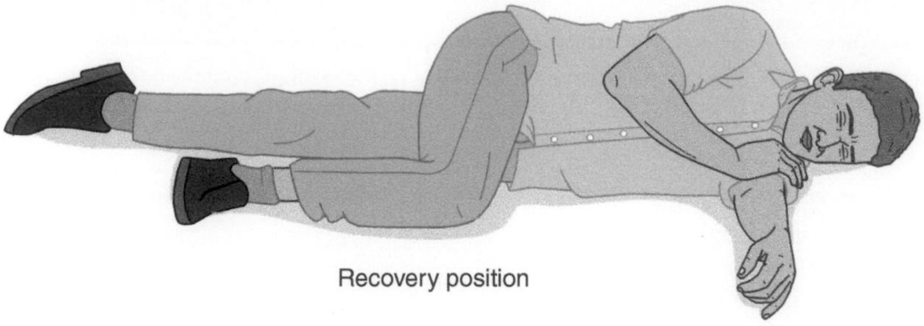

Figure 18.2 **The recovery position.**

Supporting Evidence

The United Kingdom Resuscitation Council develops and provides guidelines and training materials around resuscitation based on scientific evidence. It seeks to influence policy and practice through its research and production of standards. Visit its website: https://www.resus.org.uk

Circulation

When assessing circulation, look to see if there is any evidence of internal or external bleeding. Internal bleeding could be detected by bruising and or swelling. Look for signs of life, e.g. the patients' colour, are they a healthy colour, or is there evidence of cyanosis, either peripherally or centrally? Check if they feel warm or cold; if cold, it could indicate problems with their circulation, shock, due to injury or illness.

Yellow Flag

In light-skinned people, cyanosis presents as a dark bluish tint to the skin and mucous membranes. In dark-skinned people, however, cyanosis may present as grey or whitish (not bluish) skin around the mouth, and the conjunctivae can appear grey or bluish. In those with yellowish skin, cyanosis may cause a greyish-greenish skin tone.

Take Note

Use the DR ABC approach to assess the patient as part of your primary survey:
Danger
Response
Airway
Breathing
Circulation

Secondary Survey

This can be done following your primary assessment. Here, you need to assess the patient further following ABC with D and E.

Disability

Disability refers to the patients' conscious level. This needs to be assessed; a quick way of doing this is by using APVU. Are they able to readily talk to you? Are they **A**lert? Do they seem drowsy and only responding to your **V**oice and questions? Do they only respond to **P**ain with some stimuli, or are they **U**nresponsive? If they respond to pain or are unresponsive, they will not be able to maintain a patent airway, so this will need to be managed. It is important to be aware that an injury or illness can alter the patients' conscious level at any point; therefore, they must be closely monitored for any changes.

Red Flag

Your priority is to always maintain a patent airway. If you focus on dealing with an injury or do not assess the person's conscious level, the patient's airway is at risk of becoming compromised. They could be at risk of asphyxiation.

Head-to-Toe Examination

E refers to a head-to-toe examination of the patient, which includes checking them back to front, if they can move. Start at the head and slowly move down to their toes scanning for any signs of injury, abnormalities, skin colour changes, swellings, cuts and bleeding wounds and manage accordingly. Ask the patient to move their limbs and note any weakness.

History and Symptoms

Ask them what has happened, the history, leading up to this situation and any relevant medical history, medication and known allergies. Ask them about any symptoms they may have been experiencing, for example, pain; assess this further by asking about the type of pain, duration and location. If they are unresponsive, look for clues, medical card/bracelet or any medication. In any of the emergency first aid situations below, you must remember to always use the DR ABCDE approach first.

Take Note

The secondary survey includes:

- **D**isability using AVPU to assess level of consciousness
- **E** for a head-to-toe **E**xamination looking for any abnormalities or injuries
- Take a history including past medical history, medications and known allergies
- Ask about any symptoms the patient may have or be experiencing

Basic Life Support

Once you have undertaken the steps of DRABC and found the patient to be unconscious and not breathing, remember to call for help. Now, you need to perform basic life support (BLS) (see Figure 18.3). This involves commencing with 30 compressions to the centre of the chest. Using the heel of your palm and interlocking your fingers, with both hands and straight arms, press down on the patient's chest to a depth of 5–6 cm and at a rate of 100–120 compressions per minute. Following 30 compressions, you need to proceed with mouth-to-mouth resuscitation. Here, tilt the head back and lift the chin, placing your lips securely around the patient's, administering 2 breaths in 2 seconds. Continue to alternate 30 compressions to 2 rescue breaths until help arrives or until the patient is revived or you are unable to continue. Once help arrives, this could be the hospital resuscitation team or the paramedics, depending on where you are, the patient will probably require defibrillating. If you are trained (refer to your organisation's policy and guidance) and have an automated external defibrillator (AED), switch it on and follow the instructions. AEDs have been used by people who are untrained to save life. Clear, spoken instructions and visual illustrations will guide the user through the process. Lack of training (or refresher training) should not be a barrier to a person using one. If you are prepared to use the AED, then do not be put off from doing so.

Choking

This can occur anywhere and with anybody, usually when a foreign body becomes lodged within a person's throat. Depending on where you are, this could be food or medication, for example. Initially, the event may be mild where there is only partial obstruction, and the person may be able to clear it themselves. If severe, resulting in a total obstruction, then the situation can become life-threatening. First, ask the person to cough, and if you can see the obstruction, then remove it from their mouth. If the patient is unable to move the obstruction through coughing, then you may need to give them up to five back slaps, between the shoulder blades with your hand. Get them to sit or stand leaning forward when doing this so that, if the obstruction should dislodge, it can fall out of their mouth. If this action of back slaps fails, then stand behind the person placing both arms around them, placing your fist in your hand just under the person's diaphragm and sternum and thrust in and upwards up to five times. This action is known as abdominal thrusts and should clear the obstruction. Be careful to tilt your head to the side to avoid their head colliding with yours as you perform the abdominal thrusts. If the obstruction has still not moved, then revert to five further back slaps followed by another five abdominal thrusts. Ensure that you call for help early on in case the obstruction cannot be dislodged and the person loses consciousness. In this event, lie them down and commence basic life support while you wait for medical help.

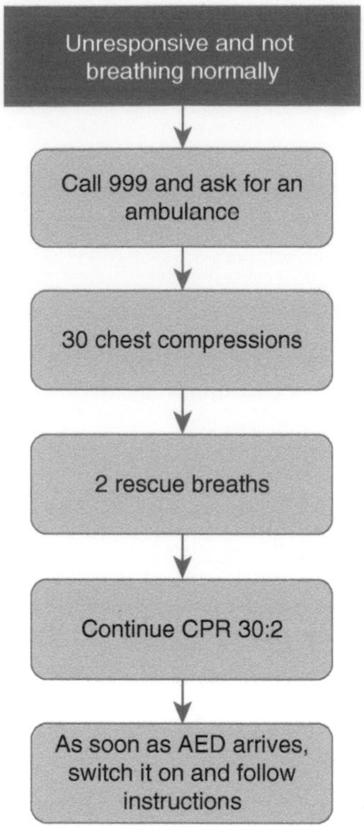

Figure 18.3 Flowchart for basic life support. *Source:* Resuscitation Council (2015). © 2015 Resuscitation Council.

Bleeding

Within an inpatient or community environment, you will come across patients with wounds from surgery or from injury within your nursing associate role. For a mental health setting, this could include self-injury wounds. Therefore, external signs of bleeding can stem from these wounds caused by an injury, an object or from surgery. Internal bleeding on the other hand can occur from surgery or an impact injury where bleeding enters the body cavity. If a patient is found, following your initial assessment, to be bleeding externally from a wound, you need to first call for help. Lie them down, raise the affected limb (if possible) to stem the blood flow and apply direct pressure, unless there is a foreign body or a bone protruding from the wound. Apply a dry non-adhesive dressing and bandage. When a foreign body or bone is located within the wound, apply the dressing around it. If bleeding from a surgical wound, for example, an abdominal wound, you should take care when applying pressure, with additional dressings, since this could cause the patient further pain. Monitor their vital signs, since they may be in shock. Avoid giving them food or fluids in case they need to return to theatre, which would necessitate a general anaesthetic. Continue observing for any changes in colour and sensation around the wound. If there is any internal bleeding, this will be evident through swelling, changes in conscious level and deterioration in the patient's vital signs. Remain with them whilst waiting for help and continue to monitor.

Shock

Anyone who experiences an unexpected injury, surgery, burns or a sudden allergic reaction is at risk of developing shock. It is a life-threatening condition where there is insufficient blood circulating within the body, triggering a reduction in oxygen and nutrients to sustain function to the vital organs. For all the different forms of shock (see Table 18.1), immediate medical help is required; however, fear can exacerbate this situation, so remember to remain calm and reassure the patient. Ask them to lie down if they are not already on the floor or bed. Raise their legs above the level of their heart to aid with circulation, loosen clothing and keep the patient warm. While waiting for help to arrive, monitor their vital signs. Avoid giving the patient fluids even if they complain of dryness and thirst in case surgery and a general anaesthetic is required. Monitor their airway and breathing at all times.

Burns

Burns can be classified in to three categories:

1. Superficial
2. Partial thickness
3. Full thickness

Table 18.1 Types of shock.

TYPES OF SHOCK	DESCRIPTION	GENERAL SIGNS AND SYMPTOMS
Hypovolemic	Severe blood or fluid loss resulting by insufficient circulating volume within the body. This can include internal and external blood loss.	• Tachycardia – a rapid, weak and thready pulse • Hypotension (low blood pressure) • Tachypnoea – rapid shallow breathing • Pale or cyanosed • Cool and clammy skin (warm in the case of distributive shock) • Reduced oxygen saturation levels • Nauseous and/or vomiting • Altered level of consciousness could be drowsy or unconscious • Urine output reduced
Cardiogenic	The heart is unable to pump due to damage, illness or trauma.	
Distributive (Septic)	Significant infection.	
Anaphylactic	Severe and life-threatening allergic reaction.	
Neurogenic	Disruption in autonomic nervous system, resulting from an illness, a drug or an injury blocking the impulses.	

Source: Jones (2018).

In the case of a superficial burn, only the outer layer (epidermis) is affected and will appear red, swollen and tender. Sunburn is a common cause for this type of burn and remedied by rehydrating the surface skin area. A partial-thickness burn is where the tissues below the surface of the skin have become damaged. These will be painful, blistered and red. A full-thickness burn can result in tissue, nerve, fat and muscle damage. Pain sensation is lost, and the skin will be charred requiring urgent medical attention. If someone in your care sustains a burn, you will need to act quickly as they may require specialist treatment. Burns include electrical, fire, chemical and scalds. If the burn is from an electrical source, ensure that the power is switched off before you approach the patient. Likewise, from a fire, ensure that it is safely extinguished. You will need to run cool water over the affected area for at least 10 minutes. Remove clothing and jewellery around the burn but only if possible; do not remove any stuck within it. Avoid bursting any blisters or applying anything to them. Once the area has been cooled, apply cling film around it to prevent infection and reduce pain. If none available, then apply a non-fibrous dressing. Avoid giving the patient anything to eat or drink in case they require a general anaesthetic later. Stay with the patient, reassure them and monitor their vital signs while waiting for help to arrive.

Blue Flag

While the person requiring assistance must be the priority of the nursing associate, if family members or relatives are also present at the scene, their needs may also need to be given consideration.

Supporting Evidence

It is very important to immediately cool the skin after a burn; this can help to stop the damage from the burning process. Putting butter or other greasy ointments on a burn could make things worse, as the grease will slow the release of heat from the skin. This causes more damage from the retained heat. The best way to release heat from the skin is with cool water. Using ice and ice water would be too harsh and can further aggravate already damaged skin. Cool water helps to gently remove heat from the area (Haveland 2019).

Fractures

A patient in your care can fall resulting in a fractured (broken) bone. This may be an open fracture where the broken bone protrudes breaking through the skin or closed where it does not break the skin. However, the limb may appear deformed and swollen. Once you have summoned help and performed a DR ABCDE assessment, reassure the patient and immobilise the affected limb. This will reduce the pain and risk of further damage to internal tissues, blood vessels and nerves. If an upper limb has been fractured, then immobilise it using a triangular bandage. If a leg has been fractured, then use the other leg as a splint and bandage them together. In the case of an open fracture, apply a padded non-fibrous dressing around the broken skin area, loosely wrapping a bandage to reduce the risk of infection, movement, pain and prevent further damage. Never press directly onto the protruding bone. Do not to allow the patient to eat or drink in case there is a need to have a general anaesthetic. Avoid moving the patient until help arrives, observing for any further deterioration in the affected limb, by assessing its colour, pulse and sensation.

Nosebleed

A nosebleed (epistaxis) is when the blood vessels within the nasal cavity rupture due to someone receiving an injury directly to their nose or head, for example, by falling. Alternatively, it could occur in a patient with an existing medical condition, for example, hypertension. First, you need to reassure the patient and remain calm; ask them to sit down and lean their head forward to allow the blood to drain away. Remember that you must always maintain a patent airway. Direct them to pinch their nose for 10 minutes, provide tissues and a bowl for the bleeding. Avoid telling them to put their head back, as this could result in blood being swallowed and cause vomiting which could compromise their airway. After 10 minutes, ask them to release their fingers to see if the bleeding has stopped. If not, apply pressure for another 10 minutes, then reassess again and repeat once more if necessary. If bleeding continues after 30 minutes, urgent medical help is required by contacting the medical staff or attending the nearest Emergency Department.

Seizures

Patients can have seizures due to medication, drug or alcohol withdrawal, head injury, photosensitivity or if they have epilepsy. Seizures can best be described as sudden uncontrolled electrical activity within the brain, which can cause psychomotor disturbances. This is where the patient's limbs jerk, otherwise known as a convulsion, together with a loss of consciousness. Sometimes, patients experience a warning of a seizure, known as an aura. This can include a specific smell or taste in their mouth or a strange sensation. If a patient has a seizure in your care, your priority is to maintain their safety while maintaining a clear airway. Keep calm, call for help and stay with the patient. It is important not to restrain them and avoid putting anything in their mouth since this could result in further injury to them or you. Once the seizure subsides, check the patient's airway, and if breathing, place them in the recovery position. Remain with them until they regain consciousness. Remember, it is vital that you time the length of the seizure. If the patient continues having reoccurring seizures without a period of consciousness or a seizure lasts longer than 5 minutes, this is known as convulsive status epilepticus (National Institute for Health and Care Excellence (NICE) 2018) that is an emergency requiring immediate medical attention.

Supporting Evidence

NICE is a body set up to provide national guidance and advice to improve health and social care within England. It develops pathways, guidance and standards for use in treatment and the provision of healthcare services. These are developed by a variety of healthcare professionals, invited for their expertise, through research. Visit its website: https://www.nice.org.uk

Touch Point

In any unexpected situation where you find a patient has sustained an injury or has suddenly fallen ill, you need to be fully aware of the emergency telephone numbers or call points in the area to be able to summon help promptly. Use a structured approach to undertake primary and secondary surveys using the DR ABCDE principles. Always remain as calm as possible, reassuring the patient at all times. Prevent any further deterioration and remain with them until help arrives. Observe their vital signs, conscious level and injury site. Report and record your observations once help has arrived.

This chapter has explored some of the common first aid situations that you, as a nursing associate, may encounter in your day-to-day practice or when off duty. The knowledge and skills have been identified alongside your role responsibilities. Now, visit companion website to take the test to see what you have learnt.

Touch Points Revisited

- Nursing associates are required to always act in the patients' best interest while adhering to the NMC code of conduct.
- There may be situations where the nursing associate is required to perform first aid, if they are the first person at the scene of an accident or to witness an injury.
- They must always remember to work with the boundaries of their role.
- If required, and if needed to summon help promptly, they must be fully aware of emergency telephone numbers or call points in the area to be able to request assistance.
- A structured approach is required so as to undertake primary and secondary surveys using the DR ABCDE principles.
- Remain as calm as possible and reassure the patient at all times.
- Their role is to prevent any further deterioration and remain with the person until help arrives.
- Observe vital signs, conscious level and injury site.
- Report and record observations once help has arrived.

References

Haveland, S. (2019) First aid, in Peate, I. (ed.) *Learning to care, the nursing associate*, Oxford: Wiley, Ch 19, 207–222.

Jones, N. (2018) Fluid and electrolyte imbalance and shock, in Peate, I. & Wild, K. (eds.) *Nursing practice knowledge and care*, Oxford: Wiley, Ch 25, 546–548.

National Institute for Health and Care Excellence (NICE). (2018) *Epilepsies: diagnosis and management, NICE.* [online] Available: https://www.nice.org.uk/guidance/cg137/chapter/Key-priorities-for-implementation. Accessed 30 April 2019.

Nursing Midwifery Council. (2018a) *The code of conduct*, London: NMC.

Nursing Midwifery Council. (2018b) *Standards of proficiency for nursing associates, NMC.* [online] Available: https://www.nmc.org.uk/globalassets/sitedocuments/education-standards/nursing-associates-proficiency-standards.pdf. Accessed 1 May 2019.

Resuscitation Council. (2015) *Adult basic life algorithm*. [online] Available: https://www.resus.org.uk. Accessed 25 April 2019.

St John Ambulance. (2014) *First aid manual* (10th edn), London: Dorling Kindersley Ltd.

Wilson, J. (2005) Nurses should learn basic first aid, *Nursing Standard*, 23(28): 31.

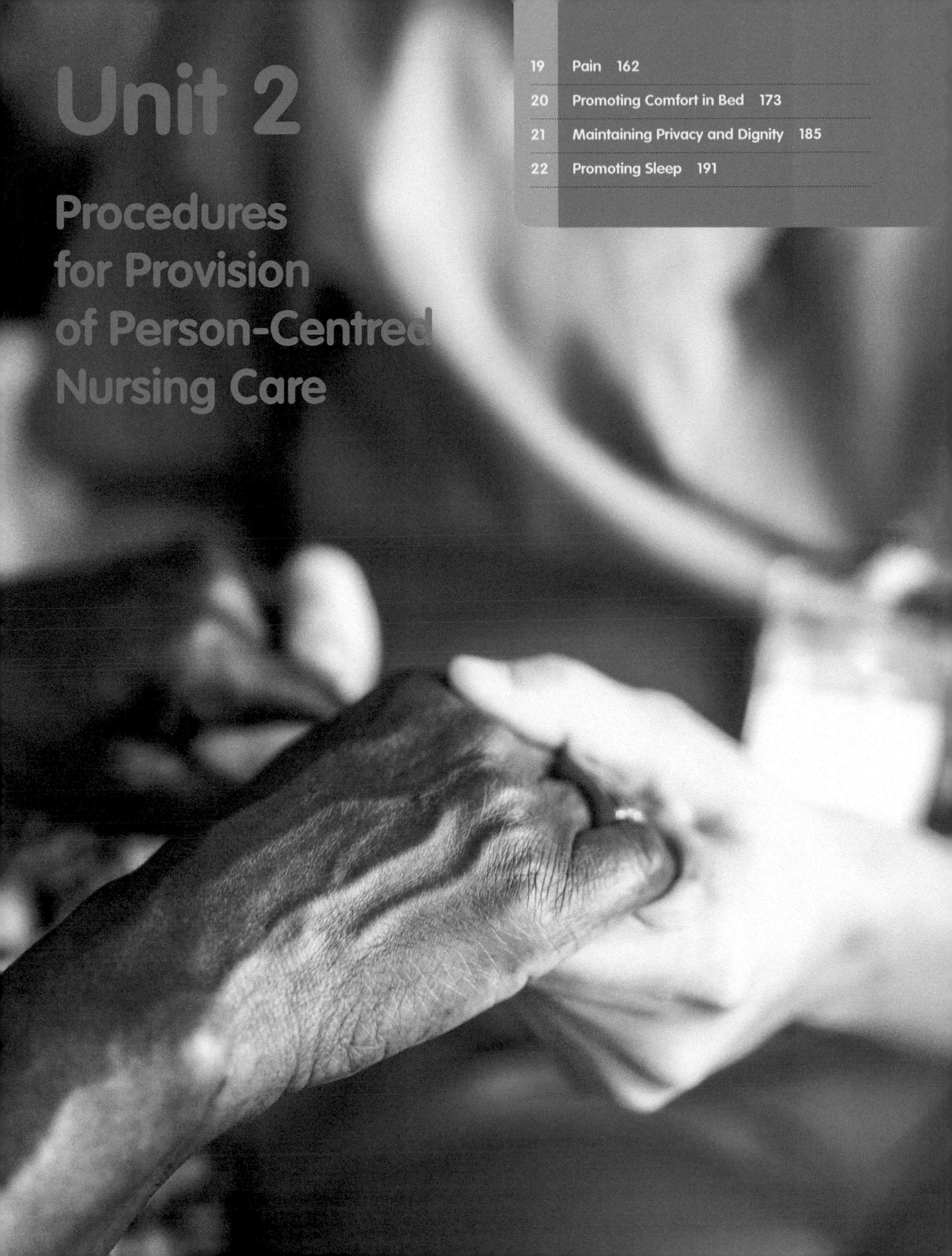

Unit 2

Procedures for Provision of Person-Centred Nursing Care

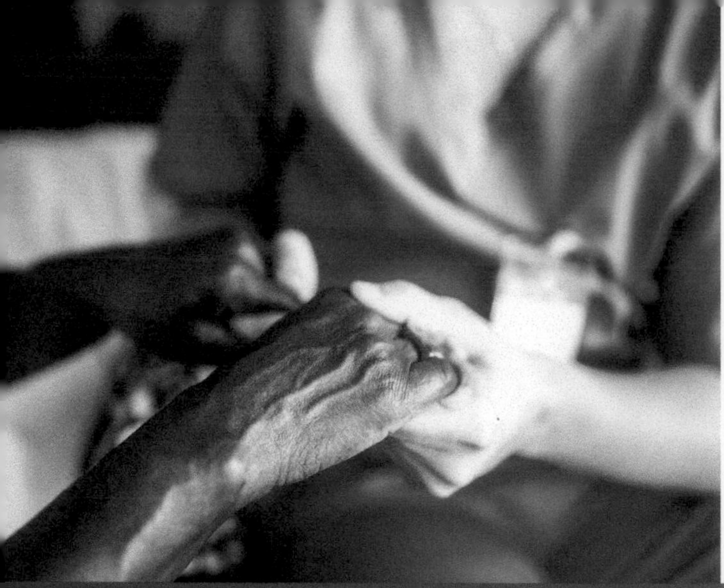

19

Pain

Anthony Wheeldon

University of Hertfordshire, UK

Chapter Aim

This chapter aims to provide the reader with an understanding of the skills, knowledge and attitude required to review and provide compassionate and holistic care to people in acute pain or people living with chronic pain.

Learning Outcomes

By the end of this chapter, the reader will be able to:

- **Gain insight into the difference between acute and chronic pain**
- **Effectively review the impact of acute and chronic pain on an individual's well-being**
- **Understand the care required by people in acute pain and people living with chronic pain**

Test Yourself Multiple Choice Questions

1. **What is pain?**
   A) **The sensation we feel when tissue is damaged**
   B) **A warning that something is wrong in your body**
   C) **Whatever the person in pain says it is**
   D) **An uncomfortable but short-lived feeling we experience when injured**
2. **Which of the following statement is true?**
   A) **Chronic pain is intense but short-lived**
   B) **Acute pain continues even after healing has occurred**
   C) **Pain that is an ever-present feature of a person's life would be described as chronic pain**
   D) **All of the above**

The Nursing Associate's Handbook of Clinical Skills, First Edition. Edited by Ian Peate.

Companion website: www.wiley.com/nursingassociate

3. **Unresolved pain will have a negative impact on which of the following?**
   A) **Breathing**
   B) **Healing**
   C) **Eating and nutrition**
   D) **All of the above**
4. **Which of the following best describes superficial pain?**
   A) **Pain that does not last too long**
   B) **Pain that emanates from structures close to the outer surface of the body**
   C) **Pain that is exaggerated by the patient**
   D) **Pain from an injury that is not life-threatening**
5. **Which of the following statements is true?**
   A) **Pain is an individual experience**
   B) **You can teach people to tolerate pain**
   C) **We all have different pain thresholds**
   D) **Analgesia should not be given until we know the cause of a patient's pain**

Introduction

This chapter explores the assessment (review) of pain and its impact on the individual. The initial section explores the nature of pain and reinforces the important concept of holistic pain management, which respects the fundamental nursing principle that pain is a personal experience and is whatever the individual in pain says it is. This is an important principle of care, which nursing associates, like all healthcare professionals, must adhere to. The fundamental aim of pain assessment is to ensure that individuals in acute pain or living with chronic pain are treated with dignity and compassion.

It is essential that nursing associates appreciate the complexities of pain assessment and how the range of available treatment options work. The second section, therefore, explores comprehensive pain assessment and pain management. Pain can be debilitating, and people living with long-term pain often experience difficulties with activities of living, such as eating, socialising and sleeping. Many experience depression and isolation as a result. Therefore, when assessing an individual in pain, nursing associates must ensure they are kind, considerate and attentive.

Platform 1 (Nursing and Midwifery Council (NMC) 2018a) requires the nursing associate to be an accountable professional. When nursing associates challenge popular assumptions and assess a patient objectively, this demonstrates they are able to be an accountable professional, establishing an understanding of and the ability to challenge discriminatory behaviour.

By being aware of the dangers of unresolved or badly managed pain, you will be demonstrating that you are able to respond to needs and plan care for patients in pain. Understanding pain requires you to exhibit and apply knowledge of body systems and homeostasis, human anatomy and physiology, biology, genomics, pharmacology and social and behavioural sciences when undertaking full and accurate person-centred nursing assessments and developing appropriate care plans (Nursing and Midwifery Council 2018a).

Listening to the patients and tailoring care to their needs enables you to show that you are proficient in providing and evaluating care for those living with chronic pain, accepting what is important to people and how to use this knowledge to ensure their needs for safety, dignity, privacy, comfort and sleep can be met, as well as acting as a role model for others as you provide evidence-based person-centred care.

Violet Flag

In some settings, for example, places of detention (secure environments), managing persistent pain presents clinicians with a number of challenges surrounding diagnosis, management and measuring meaningful outcomes of therapy. It is essential that every person in custody has access to evidence-based pain management strategies, and that these strategies ensure both effective pain control and the safety of analgesic medications.

What is Pain?

Pain is the most likely reason why people seek medical attention. It is also universal in that everyone experiences pain periodically throughout their life. While pain is an ever-present feature of life and healthcare, it is difficult to define. It can be described as an unpleasant and uncomfortable sensation, which occurs as a result of injury, inflammation or disease. However, pain can also be constant in people living with a long-term health condition, even when there is little evidence of tissue damage or healing is complete. *Pain* is also a term used to describe our emotional state. For example, we use the word *pain* to describe feelings of loss, bereavement, grief and unrequited love. The physiology of pain explains that pain is a unique and personal experience, and the way in which someone expresses and deals with their pain will depend on their culture, life experiences and personality. The intensity of pain sensation can also depend on what pain means to the individual. It is for these reasons that the following definition of *pain* is commonly cited by healthcare professionals:

> *'Pain is whatever the experiencing person says it is, existing when he says it does'.*
>
> McCaffery (1979, p. 11)

Pain Physiology

Pain is both physical and psychological. There are physiological changes that occur in response to tissue damage (as a result of injury, trauma, inflammation or infection, for example). However, there is also a psychological response to tissue damage, which entails the individual making sense of the pain and determining its severity.

In simple terms, the generation and sensation of pain follows three steps:

1. *Pain sensation* – where the nervous system detects injury, irritation or inflammation.
2. *Pain transmission* – where pain messages are transmitted from the site of injury, irritation and inflammation to the central nervous system.
3. *Pain interpretation* – where the brain receives the pain message and assesses the extent and significance of the injury, irritation or inflammation. It is at this point the individual feels pain (see Figure 19.1).

Pain Sensation

Pain is generated when the peripheral nervous system is stimulated by noxious substances generated by cells that are damaged as a result of trauma or injury, ulceration, infection, inflammation, extremes in temperature or even a lack of oxygen.

Pain Transmission

Messages of pain are transmitted to the brain via the ascending pain pathway. The ascending pain pathway consists of three linked neurons called *first-*, *second-* and *third-*order neurons (Figure 19.2). First-order neurons carry pain messages from the site of injury to the spine, second-order neurons carry pain messages up the spine towards the brain and third-order neurons carry pain messages through the brain.

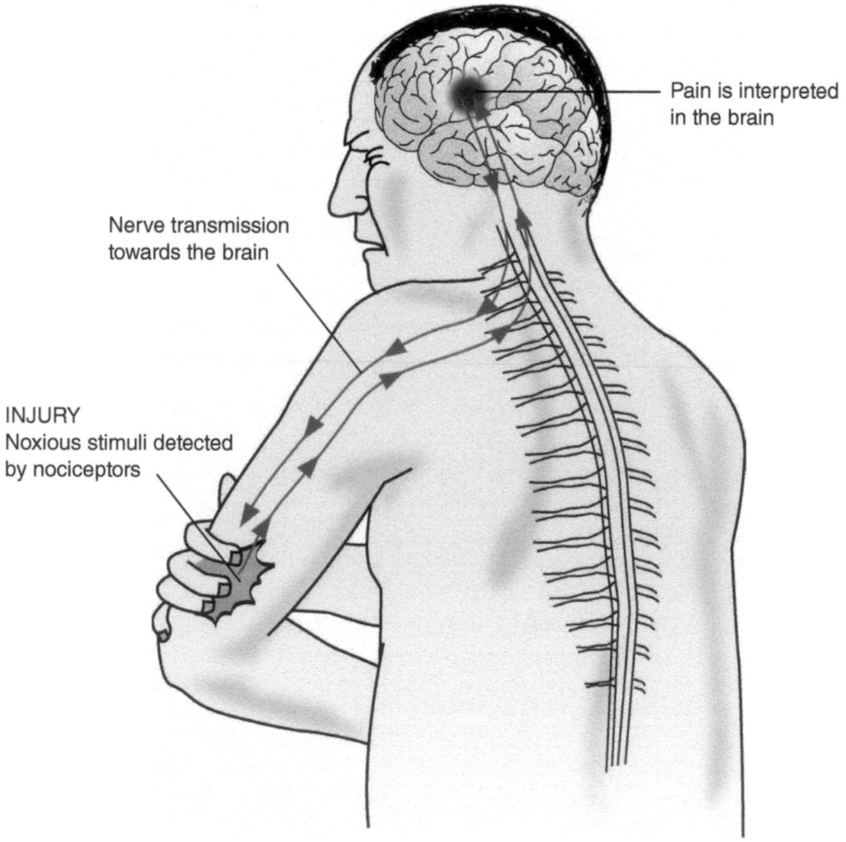

Figure 19.1 Pathway of pain transmission and interpretation. *Source:* Peate (2018), chapter 15, figure 15.1, p. 443. © 2018 John Wiley & Sons.

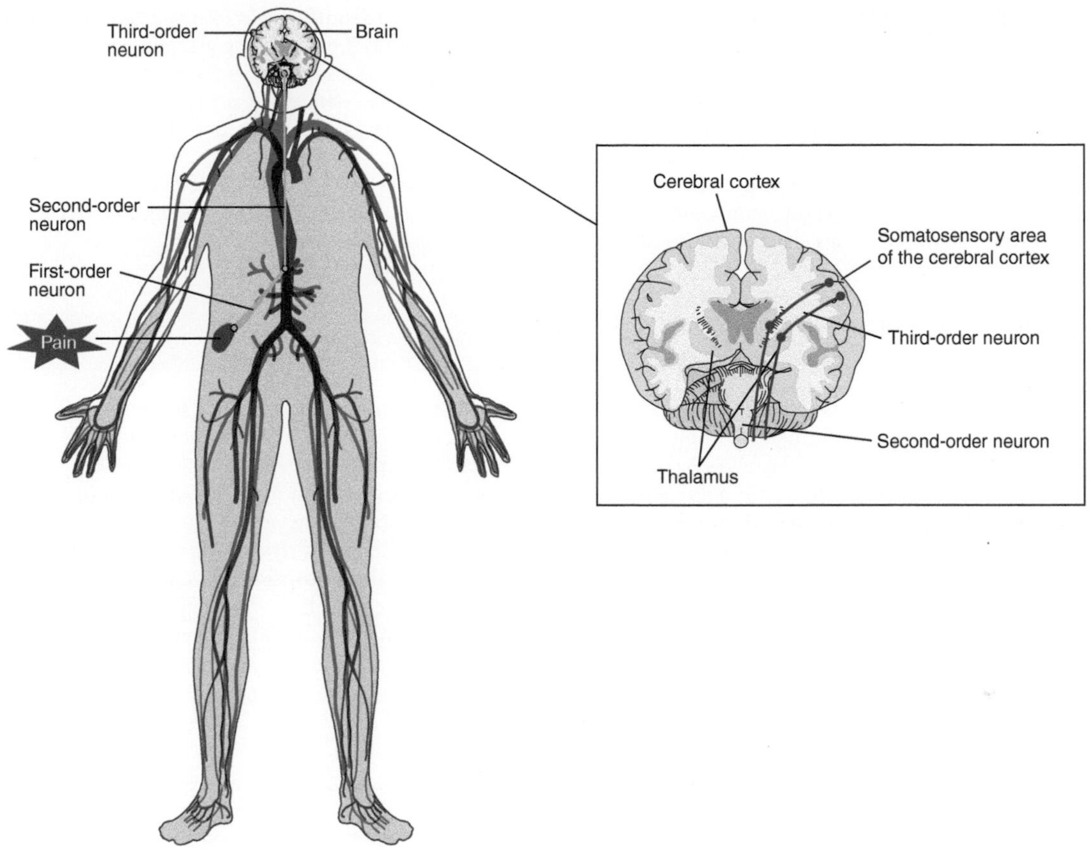

Figure 19.2 The ascending pain pathway. ***Source:*** **Peate (2018), chapter 15, figure 15.2, p. 444. © 2018 John Wiley & Sons.**

Pain is said to have two phases called *first pain* and *second pain*. First pain is the first pain sensation one senses and is often described as being sharp or pricking. Second pain soon follows and is a lengthier sensation, which is often described as being a dull, burning or aching feeling. The first-order neurons responsible for promoting first and second pain are the A-delta (Aδ) fibres and C fibres. Aδ fibres are thick and myelinated, which means they can transmit messages of pain much quicker than the thinner, non-myelinated C fibres. Aδ fibres are thought to promote the first pain sensation, whereas C fibres promote the lingering dull achy second pain.

The ascending pain pathway follows the same route as transmissions of sensations of heat and cold. The first-order neurons that transmit sensations of heat and cold are A-beta (Aβ) fibres. Aβ fibres are myelinated and thicker than Aδ fibres and as a result can transmit messages of heat and cold quicker than pain impulses. Heat and cold, therefore, may help minimise pain in certain circumstances. Examples of effective use of heat and cold include rubbing a mild injury, using a hot water bottle to alleviate menstrual pain or using cold compression to reduce muscle injury.

Pain Interpretation

Pain interpretation occurs in the brain. Indeed, pain sensation does not occur until pain signals sent through first-, second- and third-order neurons travel from the thalamus towards outer regions of the brain called the *cortex*. Pain interpretation involves locating the pain, describing the pain and discerning its severity. An area of the brain called the *limbic system* also produces an emotional response and ascribes meaning to the pain. The limbic system is influenced by our life experiences, personality and culture; therefore, an individual's response to pain is subjective and unique to them. An emotional response to pain, therefore, could range from mild irritation to anger and mild upset to distress; some individuals may even experience pleasure (Briggs 2010; Bell & Duffy 2009).

Yellow Flag **Pain and Culture**

We learn how to express our pain from the behaviour of those around us. The way in which a patient expresses their pain may be influenced by their culture, upbringing and experiences of close family members. In some cultures, it may be expected that individuals living with pain are stoical, and any betrayal of pain could be construed as weakness. In other cultures, the opposite may be true, and it is socially acceptable and expected to verbally express pain in public.

The meaning individuals ascribe to their pain will influence how they deal with their discomfort. For example, a patient having undergone surgery to remove a cancer may be able to tolerate their pain because for them their pain signifies healing and getting better, whereas an individual with abdominal pain may experience intense pain exacerbated by the anxiety of not knowing what the cause is and that it could potentially be something serious (Melzack & Wall 1988). Previous pain experiences could also determine pain intensity. For example, previous exposure to severe pain as a result of a medical procedure could lead to anxiety and greater pain levels as a result.

Pain interpretation leads to an attempt to inhibit the sensation of pain via the descending pain pathway, which involves the release of endogenous opiates, such as endorphins, encephalins and dynorphins, which have pain-reducing properties. Throughout the central nervous system, there are opiate receptors, which when stimulated by endogenous opiates can dampen the transmission of pain. Levels of endogenous opiates increase during periods of stress and excitement, which helps explain why humans can cope with pain in life-threatening situations.

Pain is an Individual Experience

Because pain interpretation is dependent on life experiences, personality and culture, as well as what we learn from others, we should conclude that pain is an individual experience that is unique to the individual we are looking after. It is also for this reason that McCaffrey states, *'Pain is whatever the experiencing person says it is, existing when he says it does'* McCaffery (1979, p. 11).

Despite being an individual experience, there are many assumptions made about people in pain or on the nature of pain. For example, it is often reported that different people have different thresholds to pain. However, pain threshold is the point at which we feel pain, and it is generally accepted that this tends to be the same in all humans. In other words, we will all sense pain and report pain at a similar time. Where humans differ is in the way they express their pain. Some may behave irrationally, and others may able to control their emotions, especially if they feel it is socially unacceptable to cry out or complain (Marieb & Hoehn 2007). The term *pain threshold*, therefore, may be unhelpful to nursing associates when they are trying to assess the impact of an individual's pain. There are many other popular misconceptions about the nature of pain, and it is essential that nursing associates are able to recognise them and ensure that their care decisions are based on reality. Table 19.1 lists some of the most common misconceptions on the nature of pain.

Take Note Pain Is What the Individual Says It Is

Poorly managed pain can have serious consequences for individuals, and therefore, an accurate assessment is paramount. However, there are many assumptions and misconceptions about the nature of pain, and the way we express pain is often influenced by culture. Whatever our upbringing, life experiences or culture, we must not project our perspective onto others or rely on popular assumptions to determine our assessment of an individual in pain. It is vital that we listen to our patients and allow them to express their pain, how it makes them feel and the impact it has on their life.

Deep or Superficial Pain

Pain can be *deep* or *superficial*. Superficial pain occurs in the structures close to or within skin, whereas deep pain occurs in within organs and structures deep within the body. An understanding of deep and superficial pain can help the nursing associate understand the individual's pain experience. The closer to the surface of the body the cause of pain is, the easier it is for the brain to locate it. The skin and nearby structures are

Table 19.1 Some common misconceptions about the nature of pain.

	COMMON MISCONCEPTIONS ABOUT THE NATURE OF PAIN
You can teach people to tolerate pain; the longer they have pain, the more used to it they become	This is not true. Tolerance to pain is an individual experience. In reality, people with prolonged pain tend to develop pain hypersensitivity.
Nurses and allied health professionals are the authority on pain and the nature of pain	This is not true. Only the patient experiencing the pain fully understands how it feels and its impact on their life.
Lying about the existence of pain or malingering is commonplace	In reality, very few people lie about the existence of pain, and fabrication of pain is very rare.
Visible symptoms of pain can used to verify its severity	Not always – a lack of pain expression does not equal lack of pain. People living with chronic pain may have the ability to carry on as normal.
Patients should not be given analgesia until a reason for their pain has been diagnosed	This would not ensure holistic or person-centred care. Pain should be treated even when there is no discernible cause. People seeking assistance for pain have the right to have their pain assessed, accepted and acted upon.

Source: Adapted from McGann (2007).

well served by nociceptors, the receptors that detect cell injury, and as a result, the brain can easily locate the source and location of injury. Structures and organs deep within the body, however, are served by fewer nociceptors. The brain, therefore, often has difficulties locating the source of deep pain, when the cause is deep within the body. Your patient may, therefore, find it difficult to explain to you or a doctor the precise location of their pain. Rather than pinpoint the source of the pain, you may observe individuals indicating a region that hurts or explain that their pain radiates from one place to another.

Take Note Acute Abdominal Pain

Abdominal pain is a common reason for admission to hospital. There are numerous organs in the abdomen (stomach, spleen, liver, pancreas, small and large intestine, kidneys, for example) and many potential causes of pain. However, because deep pain is hard to locate or pinpoint, it can be challenging for healthcare professionals to determine the precise cause. The anxiety associated with a lack of a quick diagnosis can exacerbate the intensity of the pain, further increasing the patient's distress. A calm and patient-focused approach to the care of the patient with acute abdominal pain is, therefore, paramount.

Acute and Chronic Pain

Pain is classified as being either *transient*, *acute* or *chronic*. Each of these classifications is distinct, and nursing associates need to be able to determine which classification of pain their patient has. This is to ensure that the patient is assessed appropriately and that they plan care appropriately. The duration of pain determines its classification, as follows:

- Transient pain – a short episode of pain, which occurs because of a minor injury. The pain can be intense and can cause upset. However, it will be short-lived and temporary. In most cases, the individual will consider the pain to be unimportant and will not seek medical attention.
- Acute pain – debilitating pain, which has a sudden onset and continues until healing begins. The pain experience will be prolonged and will continue until healing begins. Individuals in acute pain may describe it as intolerable and intense.
- Chronic pain – pain that continues even though healing is complete. The pain becomes an ever-present feature of an individual's life, which can have a lasting effect on their well-being.

Acute pain is associated with visible symptoms, which the nursing associate must look out for. Acute pain can cause a high pulse rate, high blood pressure, nausea, vomiting and excessive sweating. Individuals with acute pain often exhibit notable pain behaviours, such as facial grimace, guarding, irritability, anger and being upset. People in chronic pain, on the other hand, may not exhibit visible symptoms of pain or notable pain behaviours. However, their pain may be as intense as acute pain despite the lack of visible and physical symptoms. For this reason, chronic pain is often considered to be a syndrome or a medical condition.

Acute Pain

Acute pain is a symptom of an acute problem, which may result from burns, injury, trauma or abdominal pain. Patients can also experience acute pain after surgery. Acute pain is stressful, and many of the signs and symptoms are as a result of a 'fight or flight' nervous system response. Individuals in acute pain may also verbalise their pain and may visually project their suffering. When assessing acute pain, the nursing associate must look for the following signs and symptoms:

- Tachycardia – a heart rate faster than 100 beats per minute
- Hypertension – a diastolic blood pressure greater than 100 mmHg or a systolic blood pressure greater than 180 mmHg
- Excessive sweating
- Altered respiratory rate – people in pain may breathe fast, or they may breathe shallowly to reduce or minimise pain
- Increased muscle tension – people in acute pain may appear tense
- Cool and clammy skin, fingers and toes
- Nausea and vomiting
- Anxiety and fear – people in acute pain may appear frightened and distressed
- Altered facial expressions – people in acute pain may grimace
- Verbalisation of pain – this could include yelling, screaming or shouting
- Agitation, restlessness, anger and irritability
- Guarding

Red Flag Acute Pain

Acute pain is a medical emergency. Care priorities include a holistic assessment to aid diagnosis and swift treatment, the reduction of the sensation of pain and promotion of comfort.

Unresolved acute pain has a detrimental impact on all major body systems and has a significant impact on well-being. For example, acute pain can affect breathing, heart function, mobility and nutrition.

Acute Pain and Breathing

Pain in the thoracic region may result in shallow breathing as pain reduces muscle contraction in the chest and abdominal area. Clinicians often refer to this as 'muscle splinting', which means that muscles contract on either side of the injury in order to 'splint' the area and prevent movement. The glottis may also close, and the individual in acute pain can present with a 'grunting' breathing sound. This is a natural response to acute pain, which, along with muscle spasms, increases intra-abdominal and intra-thoracic pressure as the body braces against an impending injury or anticipated pain.

If left untreated, these changes in breathing will lead to reduced respiratory function. Splinting can also result in an inability to cough and clear chest secretions, increasing the likelihood of chest infections. Assessment of respiratory rate, depth, rhythm and symmetry are, therefore, integral elements of a pain assessment.

Acute Pain and the Heart

The stress response associated with the acute pain experience increases heart rate and blood pressure. The resultant escalation in effort the heart exerts increases the amount of oxygen it requires. Simultaneously, intensification of heart rate also reduces diastolic filling time, and oxygen delivery to heart muscle is reduced. In the patient with acute pain, there is a potential for a mismatch between oxygen demand and delivery of oxygen to heart muscle, which could lead to chest pain. This is particularly true for people living with pre-existing heart disease.

Acute Pain and Mobility

Acute muscular pain promotes muscle spasm and increased pain on movement. A lack of movement is associated with reduced muscle metabolism, muscle atrophy and a delayed return to normal muscle function.

Acute Pain and Nutrition

The stress response associated with acute pain slows down intestinal motility. Gastric stasis and paralytic ileus may occur also occur. Reduced intestinal motility may be detrimental to the patient's nutritional status as the process of digestion is prolonged.

The main care objectives for an individual in acute pain are to reduce discomfort and enhance breathing and movement. Care of the individual in acute pain should include:

- An accurate pain assessment
- Safe administration of prescribed analgesia
- Assess the impact of analgesic therapy
- Use of psychological interventions such as relaxation, distraction and imagery to complement pharmacological interventions
- Monitor patient for signs and symptoms of stress
- Regularly reassess pain intensity and evaluate success of pharmacological and psychological interventions

Orange Flag **Cognitive Behavioural Therapy (CBT)**

The psychological aspects of the pain experience are an integral element of the pain experience. Non-pharmacological methods of pain management can alleviate anxiety or stress helping the individual to cope with their pain. The most effective, evidence-based, psychological treatment for chronic pain is cognitive behavioural therapy or CBT (Ecclestone et al. 2009); this involves a series of structured, patient-focused sessions aiming to address the individual's psychological and emotional experience of their pain.

Take Note **Impact of Unresolved Pain on Well-being**

Pain has a major impact on the human body. Much of this impact is insidious, occurring over time but with serious effect. Nursing associates must be aware of the dangers of unresolved or badly managed pain and observe for their presence. Major examples include:

Infection – shallow breathing, suppressed cough and splinting can lead to retained secretions in the lungs, which can cause a chest infection. Reduced dietary intake and increased stress can lead to reduced immunity, which increases the risk of infection.

Embolism – reduced movement can lead to thrombus formation within deep vein circulation.

Chronic Pain

Chronic pain develops over time and is often classified as a psychological phenomenon or syndrome. There are many health conditions for which chronic pain is a feature, for instance, arthritis, neuropathy, chronic back pain and cancer. Unresolved acute pain can also lead to chronic pain, and it can also occur in the absence of any identifiable biological or physical cause. Fight or flight stress responses to pain are difficult to maintain over sustained periods of time; therefore, people living with chronic pain may not present with the symptoms associated with acute pain. Therefore, the assessment of chronic pain should explore the impact pain has on their day-to-day life. For instance, chronic pain can have an impact on their sleep, diet, libido, socialisation and their mood. Therefore, the care priorities for the individual living with chronic pain are to reduce the impact of pain on the quality of life. Care of the individual in chronic pain should include:

- An accurate pain assessment
- Safe administration of prescribed analgesia
- Monitor for evidence of the main side effects of opioid therapy
- Use of psychological interventions such as CBT relaxation, distraction and imagery
- Consider complimentary therapies
- Monitor the individual's quality of life
- Refer to chronic pain services

Touch Point **Listening to People Living with Chronic Pain**

Many people living with chronic pain may not present with the signs and symptoms of pain, such as tachycardia and hypertension. Furthermore, they may not present with the visible indicators of pain, such as grimacing, muscle tension or guarding. Nevertheless, the intensity of their pain may be the same as acute pain. It is vital that we listen to people living with chronic pain and believe their descriptions of their pain; pain is what the patient says it is.

Green Flag **Treat People as Individuals and Uphold Their Dignity**

Listening to people with chronic pain is essential for effective pain management and crucial if dignity is to be maintained. Always refer to the Code, which states you must avoid making assumptions and recognise diversity and individual choice.

Source: Nursing and Midwifery Council (2018b).

Supportive Evidence **The Royal College of Nursing (RCN)**

RCN – Subject guide – Pain. Accessible via https://www.rcn.org.uk/library/subject-guides/pain#tab3

The RCN library provides a comprehensive collection of resources, books, journal articles and reports to inform the care patients living with pain require.

Pain Assessment

Pain is a complex phenomenon, which is both a physical and psychological experience. Therefore, effective assessment is a challenge for all nursing associates. It is also important to remember that pain is a subjective experience, and therefore, healthcare professionals are also reliant on the individual's description of their pain. Some people may be unable to verbalise their pain, and, in such instances, the nursing associate must look for non-verbal indication of pain, such as facial expressions, irritability or guarding. The intensity of pain is often measured using structured pain assessments, which assign a number or description to the patient's pain.

Touch Point **The Importance of Non-verbal Cues**

Not everyone can verbalise their pain. It is vital, therefore, that nursing associates continually observe for non-verbal indications of pain. Questions nursing associates should ask include:

- Has the patient's facial expression changed? Are they grimacing?
- Are they sweating?
- Do they appear tense? Can you observe increased muscle tension?
- Are their fingers and toes cool? Is their skim clammy to touch?
- Have they been vomiting or complaining of nausea?
- Do they appear anxious, afraid, upset or distressed?
- Are they agitated, restless, angry or irritable?
- Is there any evidence of guarding?

Presence of any of the above could indicate that the patient is in pain.

Structured Pain Assessments

There are a wide variety of pain assessment tools at the nursing associate's disposal, ranging from simple single-dimension scales to comprehensive pain questionnaires. Three common single-dimension scales are:

1. Verbal rating scale
2. Visual analogue rating scale
3. Numerical rating

The verbal rating scale (see Figure 19.3) asks individuals to select an adjective, from a pre-determined list, which best describes their pain.

The numerical measure uses a numerical scale, normally 0–3 or 0–10, for example, from which the individual in pain selects the number which most accurately describes the intensity of their pain (see Figure 19.4).

The visual analogue simply consists of a rudimentary continuum that runs from no pain to the worst pain imaginable (see Figure 19.5).

Simple scales are easy to use and can be utilised swiftly to establish pain intensity while not overburdening the individual being assessed. However, it should be remembered that these scales only assess one aspect of pain, that is, its intensity, and there is an assumption that the patient will be literate (MacLellan 2006).

Supporting Evidence Pain Rating Scales

British Pain Society. (2019) *Outcome measures*. [Online] Available: https://www.britishpainsociety.org/static/uploads/resources/files/Outcome_Measures_January_2019.pdf

Outcome measures are a review of the evidence base for pain management, with a focus on the assessment of chronic pain. A wide range of assessment tools are reviewed, ranging from physical functioning to disability as well as anxiety and emotional functioning. It enables practitioners to make informed choices about how they can effectively assess an individual living with pain.

Assessing the Physiological Impact of Pain

Pain promotes a stress response. Assessing the presence of a physiological stress response can help the nursing associate to determine the impact of pain on an individual's homeostasis. The presence of a physiological impact could also help to determine pain in individuals who are unable to express their pain verbally.

The stress response is triggered by the autonomic nervous system, and its primary purpose is to prepare the human body for a perceived threat or challenge. Symptoms of a stress response include an increase in heart rate, increase in blood pressure, deeper and faster breathing and dilation of the pupils, a phenomenon referred to a 'fight or flight response'. Other associated symptoms include sweating, pallor, nausea and vomiting. As a minimum, a physiological assessment of pain must therefore include the following observations:

- Blood pressure – is the patient's blood pressure elevated above their normal?
- Pulse – is the patient's pulse fast, i.e. greater than 100 beats per minute?
- Respiratory rate – is the patient breathing faster than normal, i.e. greater than 20 respirations per minute?
- Are there any visible signs of stress, i.e. pallor, sweating or vomiting?
- Is the patient complaining of nausea?

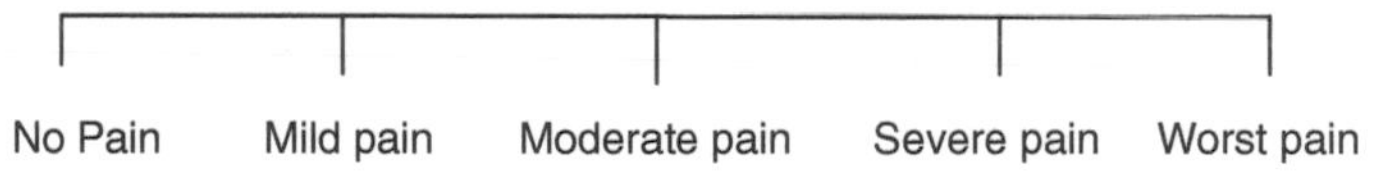

Figure 19.3 The verbal rating scale. ***Source:*** **Peate (2018), chapter 15, figure 15.15, p. 459. © 2018 John Wiley & Sons.**

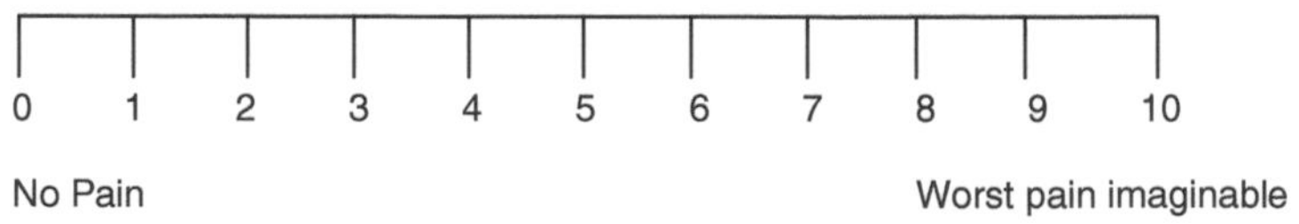

Figure 19.4 A numerical scale. ***Source:*** **Peate (2018), chapter 15, figure 15.14, p. 459. © 2018 John Wiley & Sons.**

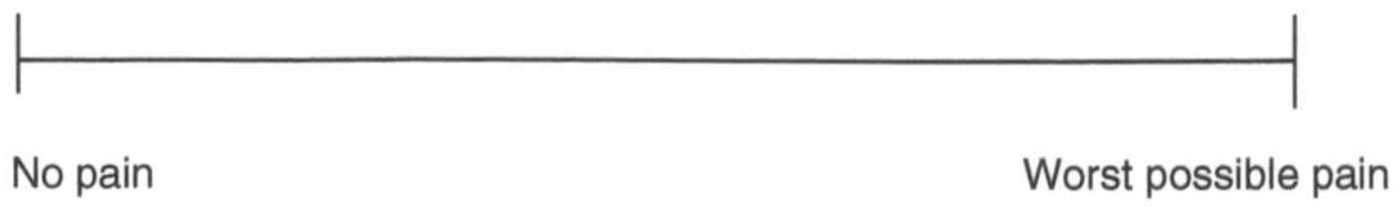

Figure 19.5 Visual analogue scale. ***Source:*** **Peate (2018), chapter 15, figure 15.14, p. 459. © 2018 John Wiley & Sons.**

Assessing the Impact of Pain on Well-Being

Both acute and chronic pain affect many body systems and can have a debilitating impact on well-being. In the longer term, chronic pain can be demanding and have a severe effect on the ability of the individual to live their life to the full. Structured pain assessments such as rating scales can be one dimensional and only provide insight into the intensity of the pain. Furthermore, chronic pain may not generate the common symptoms associated with a stress response. Therefore, in order to ensure a full, holistic pain assessment, a more comprehensive approach is required. A comprehensive pain assessment that fully assesses the impact of a patient's pain on the quality of life must include the following:

- The location of the pain
  - Where is the pain?
  - Can it be easily located?
  - Does it radiate anywhere?
- The duration of the pain
  - How long has the patient had the pain?
- Onset
  - When did the pain start?
    - What was the patient doing at the time?
- Frequency
  - How often does the pain occur?
- Intensity
  - How painful is it?
  - Does the level of pain change?
- Aggravating and relieving factors
  - What makes the pain worse?
  - What makes the pain feel better?
  - How does the individual cope with their pain?
- Other symptoms
  - Does the patient feel dizzy, nauseous or sweaty?
  - Do they feel short of breath?
  - Have they suffered a loss of appetite?
- Sleep
  - Is the patient's sleep disturbed by their pain?
- Expectations
  - What are the patient's expectations of any potential treatments?
  - What are the patient's treatment preferences?
- Concerns
  - What are the patient's concerns of the cause of their pain?
  - What are their fears and anxieties?
- Sexuality
  - Does the patient's pain have a negative impact on their libido or relationships?
- Socialisation
  - Is the patient able to maintain social activities or do they feel isolated?
- Mood and well-being
  - Does the patient express any feelings of anxiety, depression or despair?
- Spirituality
  - Does the individual have any personal or spiritual beliefs, which help them to cope with their pain?
- Acceptability
  - What does the individual consider to be an acceptable level of pain?
  - What level of pain would allow the individual to return to work or enjoy personal interests?

Blue Flag

Living with chronic pain can place a strain on all the important relationships in a person's life and it can have a ripple effect. Negative emotions, depression and anxiety that can accompany pain add to relationship problems.

Touch Point Holistic Approaches to Pain Assessment

Pain is an individual experience having a wide-ranging impact on someone's ability to live life to the full. Unresolved pain can disrupt many aspects of life, leading to people becoming withdrawn or depressed as they are no longer able to work, pursue interests or engage in social activities. When assessing the impact of pain, ask about all aspects of life, including sleep, relationships, socialisation, work as well as mood and anxieties.

Conclusion

Pain is a personal and individual experience. The way we express pain is dependent on our state of mind, personality, upbringing, culture, life experiences and the meaning we ascribe to the pain. Acute pain is often debilitating but is often short term; however, if left unresolved, it can become problematic and could potentially lead to the development of chronic pain. The accurate assessment of pain, therefore, is crucial if well-being is to be maintained. Nursing associates are ideally placed to assess the patient with pain, as long as they remember that pain is what the patient says it is.

References

Bell, L. and Duffy A. (2009) Pain assessment and management in surgical nursing: a literature review, *British Journal of Nursing*, 18(3): 153–156.

Briggs, E. (2010) Understanding the experience and physiology of pain, *Nursing Standard*, 25(3): 35–39.

British Pain Society. (2019) *Outcome measures*. [Online] Available: https://www.britishpainsociety.org/static/uploads/resources/files/Outcome_Measures_January_2019.pdf. Accessed 18 November 2019.

Eccleston, C., Williams, A. and Morley, S. (2009) *Psychological therapies for the management of chronic pain (excluding headache) in adults (review), Cochrane Database of Systematic Reviews,* (2). Doi: 10.1002/14651858.CD007407.pub2.

MacLellan, K. (2006) *Expanding nursing and health care practice: management of pain*, Cheltenham: Nelson Thornes.

Marieb, E. and Hoehn, K. (2007) *Human anatomy and physiology (7th edn)*, San Francisco: Pearson Benjamin Cummings.

McCaffery, M. (1979) *Nursing management of the patient with pain (2nd edn)*, New York: J.B. Lippincott Company.

McGann, K. (2007) *Fundamental aspects of pain assessment and management*, Gateshead: Quay Books.

Melzack, R. and Wall, P. (1988) *The challenge of pain* (2nd edn), London: Penguin.

Nursing and Midwifery Council. (2018a) *Future nurse: standards of proficiency for registered nurses*. [Online] Available: https://www.nmc.org.uk/globalassets/sitedocuments/education-standards/future-nurse-proficiencies.pdf. Accessed 18 November 2019.

Nursing and Midwifery Council. (2018b) *The code professional standards of practice and behaviour for nurses, midwives and nursing associates*. [Online] Available: https://www.nmc.org.uk/standards/code/. Accessed 18 November 2019.

Peate, I. (2018) *Fundamentals of pathophysiology (3rd edn)*, UK: Wiley Blackwell.

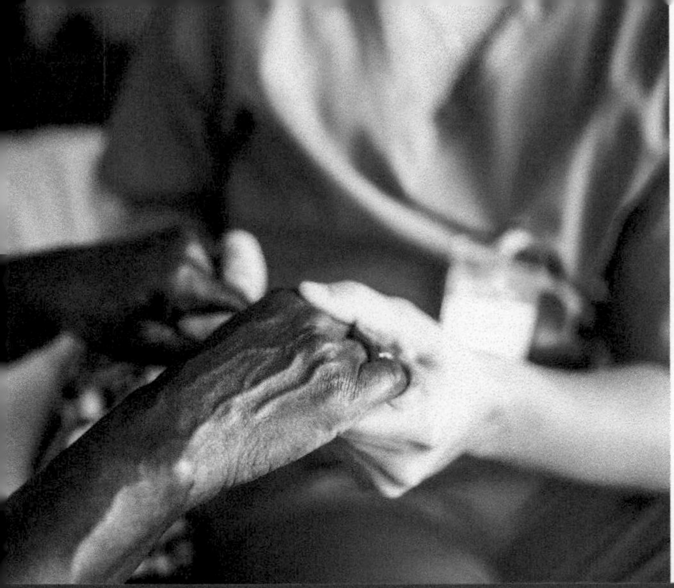

20

Promoting Comfort in Bed

Iain Mcgregor[1] and Ian Peate[2]

[1] Nottingham University Hospitals NHS Trust, UK
[2] School of Health Studies, Gibraltar

Chapter Aim

This chapter aims to provide the reader with knowledge and understanding to deliver care to patients who require assistance when in bed.

Learning Outcomes

By the end of this chapter, the reader will be able to:

- **List the commonly used patient positioning techniques for promoting comfort in bed**
- **Identify some of the common causes of pressure area damage**
- **Demonstrate an awareness of current best practice associated with patient positioning and comfort in bed**

Test Yourself Multiple Choice Questions

1. **Which of the options below are reasons why a patient's position should be changed regularly?**
   A) **Comfort of the patient**
   B) **Relieving pressure on affected areas**
   C) **Prevents contractures or deformities**
   D) **Improves cardiovascular function**
   E) **All of the above**
2. **Maintaining correct body alignment is a key principle for effective patient positioning.**
   A) **True**
   B) **False**

The Nursing Associate's Handbook of Clinical Skills, First Edition. Edited by Ian Peate.

Companion website: www.wiley.com/nursingassociate

3. **Every patient requires to be repositioned every 2 hours.**
   A) **True**
   B) **False**
4. **Bed and mattress choice should be considered for both the patient and staff members.**
   A) **True**
   B) **False**
5. **Lying patients on their front (prone position) for long periods of time is well used within clinical environments.**
   A) **True**
   B) **False**
   C) **Depending on the patient's condition and treatment plans**

Introduction

Nursing associates are responsible for ensuring the comfort of patients who are receiving nursing care in bed while maintaining their safety and well-being during a number of core care activities, such as eating, drinking and sleeping. National Institute for Health and Care Excellence (NICE) (2014) considers it as an essential component to nursing practice. There will also be times when other clinical risks and presentations will require you to position patients comfortably and safely, maximising care and recovery.

Supporting Evidence

NICE Guidance is available electronically within clinical practice for reference. It can be accessed at https://www.nice.org.uk/Guidance/CG179.

Healthcare Improvement Scotland have produced draft standards that can be accessed at: http://www.healthcareimprovementscotland.org/our_work/standards_and_guidelines/stnds/pressure_ulcer_standards.aspx.

This chapter addresses several of the key aspects of promoting comfort of individuals whilst in bed. It provides clinical scenarios of position choice for patients who are receiving nursing care; these can also be applied to any care area.

The Nursing and Midwifery Council (2018) requires all nursing associates to be accountable practitioners, to promote an individual's health and well-being, to provide and monitor care, to work in teams and to improve safety and quality of care It also requires meeting several of the skills in Annexes A and B of the standards of proficiency for nursing associates (Nursing and Midwifery Council 2018a).

Yellow Flag

Communication underpins everything that the nursing associate does. It is usually understood that the nursing associate and other clinicians have the knowledge and skills to communicate in a culturally sensitive way. To attest to culturally sensitive communication requires understanding and respect for individuals (Nursing and Midwifery Council 2018b).

Through verbal and non-verbal communication, the nursing associate attempts to identify individualised patient needs; however, effective culturally sensitive communication will also rely on nursing associates being able to critically reflect on their own values, beliefs, preferences and culture, including an understanding of traditions, perspectives and practices of culturally diverse individuals, families and their communities.

This chapter is specifically written for positioning patients in bed and can be applicable to a number of healthcare and social care settings. During practice and placements, you will be introduced to a range of specific care practices that are unique to that clinical area.

Violet Flag

Myfanwe Evans is a 77-year-old lady who had a stroke (cerebrovascular accident, CVA) 9 years ago. She lives at home with her husband, Michael, who is her main carer. She is normally mobile with a walking stick and keeps generally well but has become bedbound after a short illness. She now needs assistance to change position in bed, but this is difficult to manage as she shares a double bed with her husband. Social Care has become involved to offer support and equipment, but both Myfanwe and Michael have declined assistance or any new equipment. They feel that if they have to change the bedroom around and sleep in separate beds, then that will ruin their 55-year marriage. They do agree for the district nursing team to visit on a daily basis though to make sure that her condition is improving. The district nursing team working with Mr and Mrs Evans organise their sleeping arrangements to meet their individual needs.

The Importance of Patient Positioning

Being comfortable in bed is paramount for everyone; it allows us to feel rested and recharged. It is also a requirement of nursing care in certain settings where the patient is required to remain in bed for extended periods of time due to either their clinical presentation or personal abilities (Perry et al. 2014).

Remaining in any position for extended periods of time can become uncomfortable and then painful. People who are able to change their positions independently have the ability to recognise when it is time to change position and then do so.

A patient who is physically unable to change position may be able to voice when they are uncomfortable but due to their condition will require assistance to do so. Someone who has cognitive or sensory impairment may not be able to recognise this need.

There are four main reasons why a patient's position should be changed regularly:

1. Comfort of the patient
2. Relieving pressure on affected areas
3. Prevents contractures or deformities
4. Improving cardiovascular function

Red Flag

You are out shopping in a supermarket, and a man in front of you collapses. Initially, you are reluctant to help as you are not sure what you might find or become involved in, but you are the first person on the scene to help.

On the initial review, you find that he is unconscious but breathing; you are placing him in the recovery position while other help arrives. You are able to check again once in the recovery position that he is still breathing.

The emergency services are called and an ambulance requested, and they advise the caller that they are extremely busy and help will be with you as soon as possible. After 20 minutes, the ambulance still has not arrived. There is no change in his condition at present.

From your basic life support training, you recall that you have to change his position after a period of time to minimise the risk of pressure ulcers. As you are laying the gentleman on his back, you notice that he has stopped breathing and commence cardiopulmonary resuscitation. Emergency services are called again to update them on the condition change.

Key Principles of Patient Positioning

Along with the reasons to reposition a patient, there are also key principles for effective positioning.

1. Maintaining correct body alignment
2. Adequate support and positioning aids to help with alignment
3. Regular repositioning – based on risk assessments, clinical findings, patient's condition and choice

When reviewing patients and their position, it is important to observe them to determine if they are comfortable and to ask them how they feel. If something looks uncomfortable, that usually means it is.

Green Flag

The nursing associate needs to be aware that there are potential legal implications associated with the positioning of patients (from a variety of perspectives). It is important to undertake appropriate and relevant record-keeping concerning care interventions carried out, for example, risk assessments, skin examinations, care planning (including repositioning activities), the use of pressure- relieving devices and frequent skin reviews.

Principle 1 – Maintaining Correct Body Alignment

The aim of good body alignment is to position the patient so that the moveable parts of the body are aligned in such a way that there is no undue stress placed on the muscles or skeleton.

Good body alignment should be taken into consideration, maintaining correct lateral (side-to-side) as well as anterior–posterior (front-to-back) positioning.

Principle 2 – Adequate Support and Positioning Aids to Help with Alignment

Figure 20.1 demonstrates poor body alignment. There are a number of factors in play at this point that can potentially cause undue harm to the patient.

When a patient's body is poorly aligned from an anterior-to-posterior perspective:

- The patient's neck and chest is flexed, and chest expansion is limited. This can increase the risk of developing respiratory infections and prevent deep breathing and affect the ability to swallow.
- The arms across the chest can cause muscle strain on the shoulders and wrists.

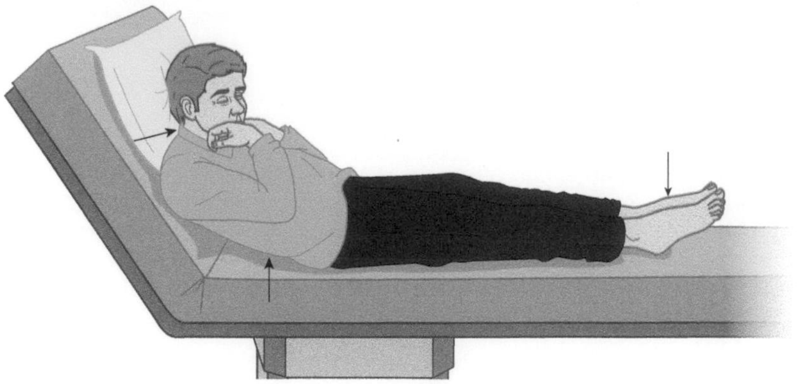

Figure 20.1 **Poor body alignment.**

- There is no support of the lower back which can cause hyperextension and strain on the abdominal and back muscles.
- Direct pressure on the sacrum can increase the risk of pressure damage.
- Knees are not flexed which can cause muscle strain.
- Foot drop can occur as the feet are hyperextended. This can cause problems with mobilising at a later time.

If a patient is poorly aligned from a lateral perspective:

- Circulation can be impaired in the arm under the patient.
- Not supporting the other arm can cause strain on the shoulder, elbow and wrist.
- Internal rotation of the hip joint can occur if the upper leg is not supported.

All of these can be addressed and increase the comfort of the patient, by flexing the elbows, hips and knees while the alignment of the body is maintained.

Take Note

Body alignment refers to the relationship of the moveable aspects of the body to one another. When good alignment is achieved, then there is no undue stress placed on the muscles, skeleton or underlying tissue.

A very common aspect of the nursing associate's practice is to change the patient's position. When left in any position, after a period of time, this will become uncomfortable, and then it becomes painful. Those who are unable to move their limbs freely in order to change their position or who are partially or totally dependent on the nursing associate and others due to injury or disease must be moved at regular intervals. Changing the dependant person's position is based on a review of a person's individual needs.

Positioning Aids

There are products in the market that can assist with positioning, although these are rarely seen within a formal care environment. The following are the main aids that are used: pillows, towels and face cloths (see Table 20.1).

Table 20.1 **The main aids: Pillows, towels and face cloths.**

POSITIONING AID	RATIONALE
Pillows	• Used to support various parts of the body • They are soft and can help reduce pressure • They are light, flexible and can be rolled and tucked under the body, maintaining a good position
Towels	• Used to support the patient's forearm and hand to prevent strain on the shoulder and wrist muscles • Towels can be folded for many purposes • They can be easily washed, maintaining good hygiene
Face cloths	• Used to make hand rolls and can be used for patients who are not able to move their hands. The hand roll should fit into the palm of the hand, with the thumb curved in a grasp position • Hand rolls are used to prevent the fingers of the hand from being in a tight fist which could cause contractures • Hand rolls can provide some extension to the fingers and helps in reducing skin breakdown

Principle 3 – Regular Repositioning – Based on Risk Assessments, Clinical Findings, Patient's Condition and Choice

It is essential that every patient be assessed individually with regards to repositioning, and advice should be sought from a registered nurse who is prescribing the care if any changes are noted.

How Pressure Ulcers Develop

Pressure ulcers develop when there is direct pressure or shear applied to the skin and the underlying tissues which cause damage to the capillary, venous or lymphatic networks. The cells around the area die, and if the pressure is not removed, the damage will spread.

The severity of the damage ranges from a small red area on the skin to large cavity wounds where damage has been caused to the muscles and potentially the bones. These are known as Category/Stage 1–4. There are two main risk factors for developing a pressure ulcer: intrinsic and extrinsic factors.

Intrinsic Factors

Intrinsic factors are considered to be internal to the patient and often difficult to manage without the patient's active involvement in their care and well-being.

Box 20.1 lists some potential risk factors.

Extrinsic Factors

Extrinsic factors are often caused by environmental changes or healthcare-related practices or equipment.

Box 20.2 identifies some potential risk factors.

Box 20.1 Some Intrinsic Risk Factors

- Reduced movement
- Cardiovascular disease
- Smoking
- Nutrition and hydration
- Medication
- Weight – both malnourished and obesity
- Reduced sensation
- Diabetes
- Neurological conditions
- Incontinence

Source: adapted from Peate & Stephens (2020)

Box 20.2 Some Extrinsic Factors

- Room temperature
- Room humidity
- Direct pressure from healthcare equipment, i.e. catheters, ventilators, nasogastric tubes
- Shear
- Friction
- Poor posture/alignment
- Number of staff available
- Staff education
- Type of mattress

Source: adapted from Peate & Stephens (2020)

Take Note

There are several factors that can cause a pressure ulcer to develop, and these are related to extrinsic and intrinsic factors. Being aware of the potential influencing factors can help the nursing associate take action prior any harm being incurred.

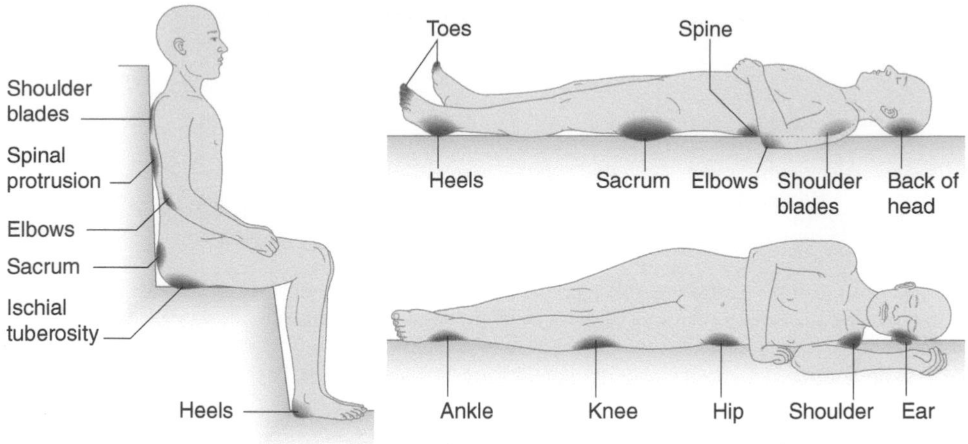

Figure 20.2 Areas of the body at risk. *Source:* Peate & Glencross (2019). © 2019 John Wiley & Sons.

Areas of the Body at Risk

Those areas of the body that are most at risk are detailed in Figure 20.2.

The structure of the skin along with assessment tools and equipment are being discussed in other chapters of this textbook, for example, Chapters 23 and 24; however, it is important to appreciate the importance of how these will affect pressure relief for patients and clinical decision-making during patient review.

Pressure Relief (Pressure Area Care)

The development of a pressure ulcer while receiving care and support is a key indicator of the quality and experience being delivered. Guest et al. (2017) suggest that up to 200,000 people were at risk of developing a new pressure ulcer in 2017–2018.

Patients who have sustained pressure damage are shown to have significant impact on their overall well-being and potentially leave permanent changes in their condition (Moore & Cowman 2009).

Within acute care settings, the development of a pressure ulcer can cause delays to further treatment and improvement to health. This will have an impact on the length of stay within a hospital environment and additional costs for treatment. It is suggested that, in 2012, the cost was £2.1 billion annually (Dealey et al. 2012).

The majority of pressure damage is preventable with appropriate care and repositioning; it is vital that regardless of how or when pressure ulcers are noticed, they are treated promptly with suitable review, treatment and reporting. A key part of this is to also have an open and honest conversation with the patients and their families regarding this. It would also be prudent to discuss with your mentor or line manager regarding Duty of Candour at this time, as it may be essential for this to be undertaken also.

Supporting Evidence

There are national programmes established which collate data and provide guidance on the prevention of pressure ulcers; further details can be found at: www.nhs.stopthepressure.co.uk.

Each incidence of pressure damage or development of a pressure ulcer should be reported also through the local reporting systems. These reports are not to apportion blame; they are used for monitoring purposes as well as for identifying trends.

If you are practising within a primary care environment that is inspected by one of the care regulators, i.e. Care Quality Commission or Care Inspectorate, pressure ulcers at Grade 3 or above also need to be reported to them.

Pressure-Relieving Equipment

There are significant amounts of pressure-relieving equipment available in the market, each of them slightly different but offering ultimately the same depending on the category they fall into. Choice must be based on individual review.

Your service will have specific equipment available, and the decisions to use these will have been based on several factors. Cost, reliability, availability and service/repair will all be considered. When nursing patients in bed, there will be several risk assessments that will guide you to making your choices on equipment (see Chapter 23 of this text).

Touch Point

The nursing associate must remember that the amount of support that is required for positioning will depend on the individual. When creating a care plan and positioning schedule for the person, employ an evidence-based approach and always consider the individual needs for the person.

Bed Choices

Many of the beds available in services are electric profiling beds, as these have been designed to reduce the risk of harm to the staff members when assisting patients to change position (see also Chapter 38). They enable the patients to alter their position independently using the controls, promoting independence as much as possible.

Some community services may still have manual profiling beds or divan-style beds; consideration needs to be made if this is suitable if a patient requires regular repositioning or has been identified as being at risk of developing a pressure ulcer. Divan-style beds and manual profiling beds are not always compatible with certain types of mattress, so this will need to be factored into decisions also.

When using electric profiling beds, thought has to be given to the potential risk of the patient rolling out of it, as there are usually two heights of beds available. There are low-profiling beds that offer the same abilities as a standard-height bed, although lower down, closer to the floor, reducing the risks again if the patient does roll out of bed.

Mattress Choice

There are many types of mattress available; however, the two main types used within a healthcare or social care setting are:

- Cut-foam mattress – The name of these mattresses is an accurate description of what it looks like inside. The mattress is usually the first-line choice in a secondary care setting, offering a supportive surface which will offload pressure over bony prominences. The brand and specific instructions regarding patient weight, recommended mattress time and use and cleaning instructions are provided by the manufacturer and your organisation (employer).
- Dynamic air mattress – There are two specific types – high risk and very high risk. Your organisation may have different brands available, and each will come with its own set of guidance and criteria for use. Both offer a pressure-relieving surface, oscillates gently moving the air through the mattress, relieving the pressure in key areas.

  Organisational protocols that outline care interventions are available, for example, for patients admitted with a fractured hip or pelvis.

Heel Protection/Offloading

There are a range of items that are potentially available for offloading heels when a patient is being nursed in bed. The most widely used are pillows, which should be positioned ideally from knee to ankle and allow the heel to float.

Heel boots and troughs may be available in your organisation – it is recommended that you discuss this with either your lead on tissue viability or the tissue viability specialist nurses. There are several exclusion criteria for using these with patients; therefore, local-level information is more applicable.

Take Note

Alignment and correct positioning will only be effective if the patient is comfortable and feels safe. Good body alignment should be maintained from lateral (side to side) and anterior–posterior (front to back).

Commonly Used Patient Positions

- **Fowler's** – The head of the patient's bed is placed at 45° or greater; Figure 20.3 shows Fowler's position.
- The patient's hips may or may not be flexed. This is a commonly used position to provide all aspects of patient care but can help with easing symptoms of respiratory or cardiac problems.

  In Fowler's position, gravity can move the diaphragm downwards allowing greater chest expansion.

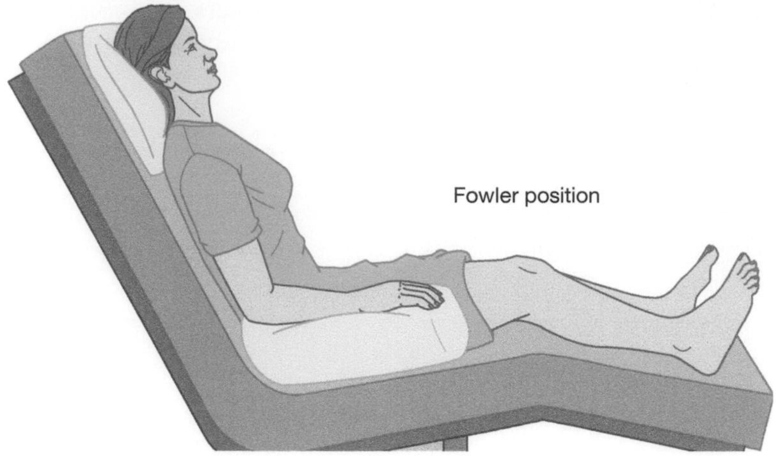

Figure 20.3 **Fowler's position.**

Patients should not be encouraged to remain in this position for a significant period of time due to the potential risks of shear, friction and pressure on the sacrum and coccyx.

Orange Flag

Being touched can make many people uncomfortable, people must give their consent to being touched. If the fear is intense and appears even when touched by family or friends and if it causes significant distress, this may be haphephobia.

Haphephobia is an anxiety disorder characterised by a fear of being touched. Haphephobia is different from a hypersensitivity to touch; this is known as allodynia. A person with allodynia may also avoid being touched, but they do so because it causes them to feel pain as opposed to fear.

Table 20.2 Steps to be taken along with the rationale for Fowler's position.

STEPS	RATIONALE	OTHER NOTES
1. Place one pillow under head and shoulders	Hyperextension of neck is prevented and alignment is maintained	*Patients may be suffering from kyphosis or lordosis and have limited neck extension. The pillow helps support the neck in good alignment*
2. Arms and wrists are supported on the bed parallel to the body or can be flexed and placed in a comfortable position on the patient's lap	Both positions prevent muscle strain on the shoulders	
3a. One pillow is placed under the thigh to flex the knee slightly 3b. Elevate the bed slightly at the feet or knee brace	This decreased knee and hip extension and relaxed the lower back Helps maintain a sitting position without sliding down the bed Relieves some of the pressure on the heels Avoids pressure on the lower back and prevents patient slipping down the bed which can cause shearing	*Shearing occurs when the skeleton and deep tissues slide downward while the skin and superficial tissues remain in the original position*
4. The heels are resting on the bed	This can be tolerated for short periods of time without causing pressure damage	*If the patient is identified as being high risk of pressure damage, a pillow may be placed under the lower leg to offload the heels*

Table 20.2 provides details concerning the steps to be taken along with the rationale for using Fowler's position.
In Table 20.2, steps 3a and 3b are listed separately as it may depend on what bed the patient is on and its capabilities.
The head of the bed should not be brought up to the full 90° position if the patient is not able to maintain their own balance.

- **Semi-Fowler's** – The head of the patient's bed is placed at a 30° angle or less. This position can be used to allow the patient to rest and relax or sleep. It is commonly used for patients who have a nasogastric tube.
  See Figure 20.4 for semi-Fowler's position.

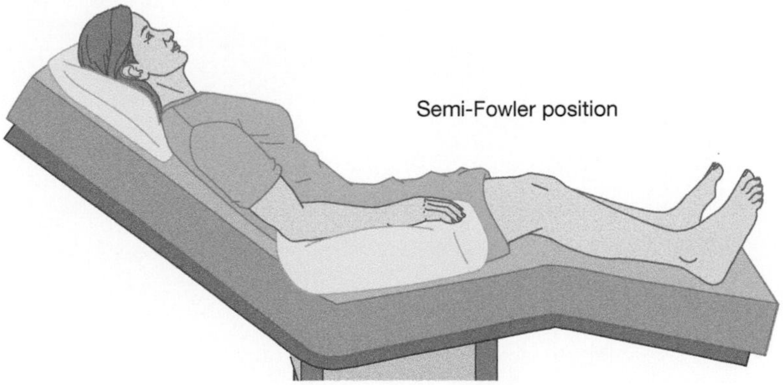

Figure 20.4 **Semi-Fowler's position.**

Table 20.3 **Details concerning the steps to be taken along with the rationale for semi-Fowler's position.**

STEPS	RATIONALE	OTHER NOTES
1. Place one pillow under head and shoulders	Hyperextension of the neck is prevented and alignment maintained	*Patients may be suffering from kyphosis or lordosis and have limited neck extension. The pillow helps support the neck in good alignment*
2. Arms and wrists are supported on the bed parallel to the body or can be flexed and placed in a comfortable position on the patient's lap	Both positions prevent muscle strain on the shoulders. The arms are also supported in good alignment	
3. Raise the foot of the bed slightly or flex the knee brace	This prevents the patient from sliding down the bed and causing shearing The slight flexion of the knees when the foot of the bed or knee brace is elevated promotes increased comfort and reduces the strain on the abdominal muscles and lower back	
4. The heels are resting on the bed	This can be tolerated for short periods of time without causing pressure damage	*Prolonged pressure on the heels is not recommended for periods over 30 minutes*

Table 20.3 provides details concerning the steps to be taken along with the rationale for semi-Fowler's position.

- **Lateral** – The formal description of the lateral position is where the patient lies on their side with the top leg over the bottom leg, and the uppermost arm and leg are supported on pillows. Within current practice, a variation of this is used to relieve pressure on the sacrum and back using a 30° tilt (see Figure 20.5).
  Table 20.4 provides details concerning the steps to be taken along with the rationale for the lateral position.
- **Tripod** – This is where the patient is sitting on the side of the chair or bed with head resting on an overbed table (or table) and supported by several pillows. Patients who are having difficulty breathing often will adopt this position as it allows them to breathe deeper (see Figure 20.6). There is a variation of this also, where the patient will remain in bed, but lean forward and be supported by pillows.
  Table 20.5 provides details concerning the steps to be taken along with the rationale for the tripod position.
  The tripod position can also be adopted by someone in a chair if required.

Less Commonly Used in Clinical Practice

Supine – This is where the patient is lying flat on their back (see Figure 20.7). There may be additional pressure-relieving devices in use if a patient is required to be cared for in this position for a protracted time period.

Prone – This is where a patient is positioned on their front, lying on their stomach with their head turned to one side (see Figure 20.8).

- **Trendelenburg** – This position involves the patient being in a supine position with the head lowered and feet raised, tilting the head into a downward position. Historically, it was used to treat patients with hypotension, although now more commonly seen in emergency situations or when a central line is being placed.
- **Recovery Position** – This position is widely recognised as one of the first-line measures taken when a patient or casualty is unconscious and breathing. There are many ways to describe the positioning of the arms including sleeping policeman or the 'how' position. The main aim of the recovery position though is to protect the patient's airway in a secure position allowing the first aider to monitor other aspects of the patient's condition.

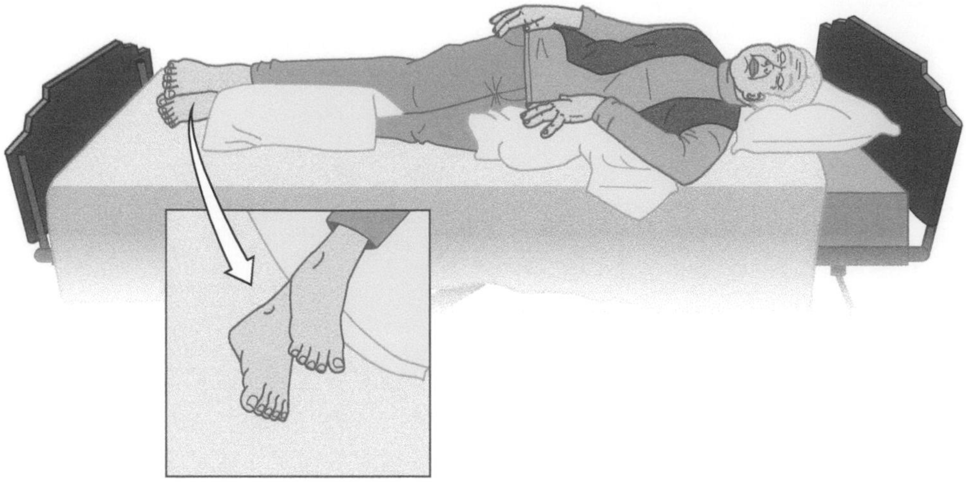

Figure 20.5 **Lateral position and 30° tilt.**

Table 20.4 **Details concerning the steps to be taken along with the rationale for the lateral position.**

STEPS	RATIONALE	OTHER NOTES
1. Place one pillow under the head and shoulders	Hyperextension of the neck is prevented and alignment is maintained	*If the head rests on the bed surface, pressure is placed on the lateral aspects of the face and ears*
2. One pillow is placed under the upper arm, slightly flexed with wrist supported and comfortable on the pillow at the back (or across the abdomen)	Prevents internal rotation of the shoulder	*Internal rotation of the shoulder and arm can cause pressure on the chest and restrict the expansion during breathing*
3. A second pillow is placed lengthwise and tucked in at the back. The patient is encouraged to lean back into the pillow	This supports alignment and maintains the position	
4. The patient's lower arm is supported, slightly flexed with wrist supported and comfortable on a pillow in the front	Give support and prevents internal rotation	*Make sure the patient is not lying on their arm* *If pillows are not available for this, then folded towels will be a suitable alternative*
5. The lower limbs are outstretched with knees slightly flexed, upper leg slightly forward of the lower leg The uppermost lower extremity is supported by a sufficient number of pillows to support the lower extremity in proper alignment with the trunk	Minimum extension of the legs minimises pressure on the trochanter to avoid excessive pull on the lower trunk This also prevents pressure on the knees and ankles	

Other Factors

Along with all of the other factors described in this chapter associated with patient positioning and preventing pressure ulcer formation, there are other core nursing aspects that should be included in all practice, included here as aide memoires.

Self-Care

It is impossible for any healthcare and social care practitioner to monitor an individual's skin 24 hours a day, and in busy clinical environments, it is important to prioritise care delivery to some patients; the principle of self-care and encouragement is useful to adopt in this situation.

Many organisations now have a patient or carer leaflet given on admission, explaining the importance of regular pressure area care and how, as an individual, they are able to assist in the prevention of this.

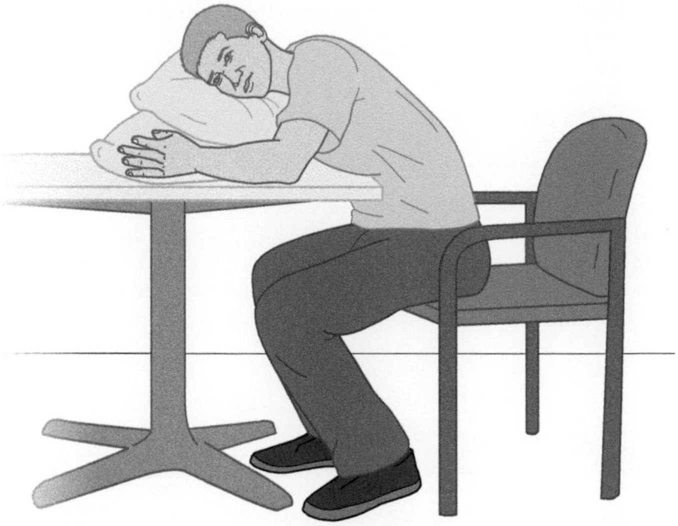

Figure 20.6 **Tripod position and lean forward position.**

Table 20.5 Detail concerning the steps to be taken along with the rationale for the tripod position.

STEPS	RATIONALE	OTHER NOTES
1. Assist the patient into a seated position on the edge of the chair	This allows patients to support themselves and expand their chest	
2. Place a table (or overbed table) in front of the patient	Allows patients to form the tripod position by leaning forward while maintaining stability	*Patients who have the ability to maintain their own sitting balance should only be considered for this position*
3. Place 1–2 pillows on the table (or overbed table) for the patient to lean forward	This position allows patients to relax their diaphragm and breathe deeper	Patients who have long-term respiratory problems will usually get themselves into this position if they are experiencing difficulty in breathing

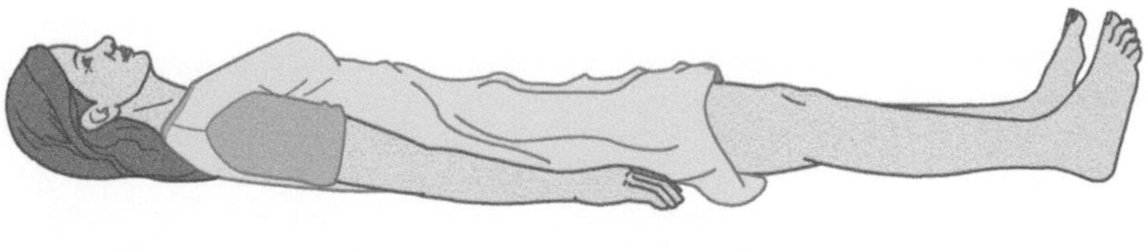

Figure 20.7 **Supine.**

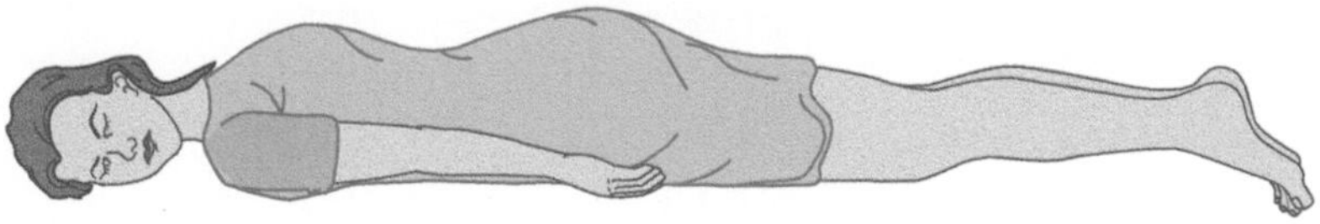

Figure 20.8 **Prone.**

Some patients may be at risk for a short period of time while recovering from an acute illness or surgery. Others will have an ongoing risk due to comorbidities or chronic reduction in mobility.

Hydration

When the nursing associate has any interaction with patients even if it is for the briefest of moments, it should be considered an opportunity to promote hydration of the patient. This can be done in the simplest of ways by topping up a water glass of a patient while chatting to them or asking them if they would like a drink prepared.

The opportunities during repositioning are immense for core nursing interventions and reviews, including promoting hydration; it is imperative that a drink should be left accessible once the repositioning has been completed so that the patient is able to continue with their hydration independently.

Nurse Call System

Once a patient has been assisted to reposition, it is paramount that we enable the patients to contact us if they need. Regardless of clinical environment and if the patient is visible by the nursing team, every patient should be able to contact or call for a member of the nursing team.

Patients who need assistance to reposition are more requiring of this than patients who are independent or mobile due to their current clinical condition. There may also be an element of fear if they are unable to contact someone, especially if they are positioned in such a way that they are not able to see people moving around the clinical area or if they are being cared for in a side room.

Blue Flag

The establishment of trust in the nursing associate–patient relationship has the real potential of promoting patient engagement, and it can also improve the likelihood that the patient will be an active member of the patient care team. Engaging the patient (and, if appropriate, their family) can result in care that is truly patient centred.

Conclusion

A nursing associate is required to possess and demonstrate skills in promoting comfort in bed; this includes positioning patients and utilising pressure-relieving techniques. This chapter has provided insight regarding the role and function of the nursing associate, highlighting the key responsibility they have in promoting comfort and ensuring that the patient is at the centre of all that is done.

References

Dealey, C., Posnett, J. and Walker, A. (2012) The cost of pressure ulcers in the United Kingdom, *Journal of Wound Care*, 21(6): 261–266.

Guest, J., Vowden, K. and Vowden P. (2017) The health economic burden that acute and chronic wounds impose on an average clinical commissioning group/health board in the UK, *Journal of Wound Care*, 26(6): 292.

Moore, Z.E.H. and Cowman, S. (2015) *Repositioning for treating pressure ulcers, Cochrane database of systematic reviews*, London: Wiley & Sons.

National Health Service Stop the Pressure. [*online] Available*: www.nhs.stopthepressure.co.uk/docs/Surface%20selection%20guide%20nov%2015%2c%20version%201%20author%20Lorraine%20Jones.pdf. Accessed September 2020.

National Institute for Health and Care Excellence (NICE). (2014) *Pressure ulcers: prevention and management. [online] Available*: https://www.nice.org.uk/guidance/cg179/resources/pressure-ulcers-prevention-and-management-pdf-35109760631749. Accessed December 2019.

Nursing and Midwifery Council. (2018a) *Standards of proficiency for nursing associates.* [online] Available: https://www.nmc.org.uk/standards/standards-for-nursing-associates/standards-of-proficiency-for-nursing-associates/. Accessed December 2019.

Nursing and Midwifery Council. (2018b) *The code, Professional standards of practice and behaviour for nurses, midwives and nursing associates.* [online] Available: https://www.nmc.org.uk/globalassets/sitedocuments/nmc-publications/nmc-code.pdf. Accessed December 2019.

Peate, I. and Glencross, W. (2019) *Wound care at a glance*, Oxford: Wiley.

Peate, I. and Stephens, M. (2020) *Wound care at a glance* (2nd edn), Oxford: Wiley.

Perry, A.G., Potter, P.A. and Ostendorf, W.R. (2014) *Clinical nursing skills and techniques*, St. Louis: Elsevier.

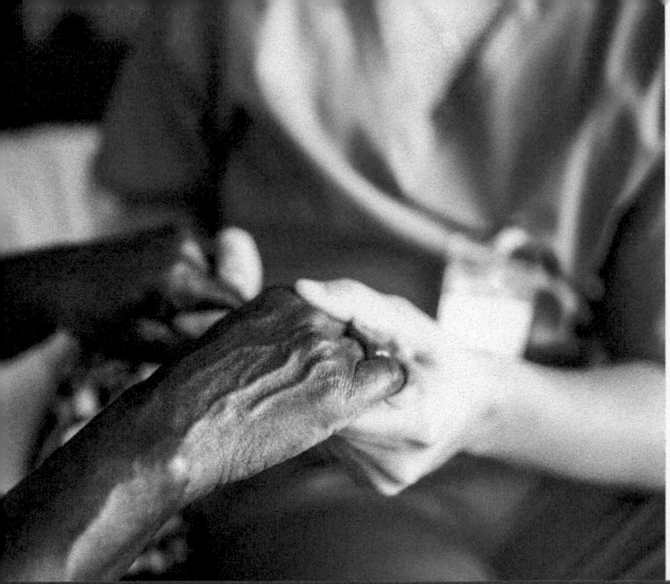

21

Maintaining Privacy and Dignity

Graham Patrick Jones

Teesside University, UK

Chapter Aim

- This chapter aims to appreciate and understand the importance of ensuring patient privacy and dignity.

Learning Outcomes

By the end of this chapter, the learner will be able to:

- Discuss what constitutes privacy
- Discuss what constitutes dignity
- Discuss the nursing associate's role in maintaining privacy and providing dignified care

Test Yourself Multiple Choice Questions

1. Subject to certain exceptions, who is the individual that confidential information can be disclosed to?
   A) The patient
   B) The family
   C) The police
   D) Social services
2. Who is a Caldicott Guardian?
   A) A senior person responsible for protecting the confidentiality of people's health and care information
   B) The patient's spouse who looks after their health and well-being
   C) A representative of the police, social services or armed forces
   D) A member of the patient advice and liaison service (PALS)

The Nursing Associate's Handbook of Clinical Skills, First Edition. Edited by Ian Peate.

Companion website: www.wiley.com/nursingassociate

3. **Which health services collect, store and share information?**
   A) Sexual health clinics
   B) Dental surgeries
   C) Doctors' surgeries
   D) All of the above
4. **What are beneficence and non-maleficence?**
   A) Tropical diseases
   B) Ethical principles
   C) Law within the United Kingdom
   D) Medication for anxiety
5. **What is the meaning of autonomy?**
   A) To have someone to help make decisions for you
   B) Safeguarding of a vulnerable individual
   C) Using patient's stored records to deliver care
   D) The ability to make your own decisions

Introduction

All patients have a right to be treated as individuals in a courteous dignified manner that demonstrates respect for autonomy and privacy. Nursing associates are at the front line of care delivery and as such must appreciate the multiple considerations associated with the delivery of care that maintains modesty, considers diverse cultural and religious needs and ensures that those in their charge are cared for in a compassionate non-discriminatory manner. To facilitate this, the nursing associate must possess multiple qualities, skills and attributes. The Nursing and Midwifery Code (2018a) details that nursing associates must 'respect a person's right to privacy in all aspects of their care, ensuring that patients are informed about how and why information is used and shared'. The Code also stresses that the nursing associate must only share necessary information with other healthcare professionals and agencies when it is in the best interests of the patient's safety and public protection. Platform 1 of the standards of proficiency for nursing associates (2018b) emphasises the importance of being an accountable professional.

Green Flag

The Nursing and Midwifery Code (2018a)
Standards of proficiency for nursing associates (2018b)
The Data Protection Act (2018)
The National Health Service Confidentiality Code of Practice (2010)
The Health and Social Care Act (2012)
The Equality Act (2010)

The terms privacy and dignity are often used synonymously; however, both terms are open to interpretation and are invariably seen to mean different things to different individuals. It is evident that both privacy and dignity are not simplistic notions but are entwined in the ethical complexities of autonomy, beneficence, justice and non-maleficence (Hawley 2007). The concepts encapsulate multidimensional considerations that involve duty of care, confidentiality and a professional, moral and legal commitment. A duty of care can simplistically be defined as doing the right thing in the right way. 'It denotes the obligations placed on individuals to act in a legal, ethical and professional way in accordance with the required standards of their profession'. The nursing associate is expected to deliver care that would be appropriate for any 'ordinarily competent practitioner', and their 'duty of care' is judged against the standards of whether it is 'reasonably foreseeable' that the 'practitioner might cause harm through their actions or omissions' (Duncan 2019). This chapter will discuss the important role the nursing associate plays in maintaining patient privacy and delivering care that ensures that all patients are cared for in a dignified manner.

Violet Flag

Regardless of where a person is, dignity is dynamic and can fluctuate; it is affected by interactions, events, the person's own feelings as well care environment factors. Patients' views about what is most important for their dignity might vary and differ, for example, a residential care setting. The nursing associate must acknowledge that these views may differ from our own views.

Privacy

As individuals, we all have a fundamental expectation that privacy is a basic human right. The concept of patient privacy in nursing practice is of monumental importance as it facilitates a secure environment in which the patient is to be cared for and reinforces confidence in 'health care and emphasises the importance of respect for patient autonomy' (Beauchamp & Childress 2009). The Nursing and Midwifery Council (2018a) identifies that nursing associates must 'respect a person's right to privacy in all aspects of their care'. Fundamentally, patient privacy can be separated into two basic categories: spatial privacy and informational privacy. Spatial privacy refers to personal space, secrecy, anonymity and choice, while informational privacy refers to data protection and the recording and storage of data.

Blue Flag

The Care Quality Commission asks providers a number of questions to ensure that they are helping people to develop and respect intimate personal relationships, and these include:

- Is there a relationship and sexuality policy?
- Does the organisation recognise people have different ways of experiencing and expressing sexuality?
- Are staff trained to support people with regards to personal relationship needs?
- Are there examples demonstrating positive support for relationships?
- Is there accessible information about, and links with, sexual health services?
- Is there a policy for allowing people to have guests staying overnight?
- How does the setting accommodate those in existing relationships?
- How are people encouraged and supported to develop relationships?
- Are people using the service given information and support about relationships and sexual health?
- Can people be signposted to a local organisation that provides this service?
- Are staff aware of what action to take if they have concerns that someone is at risk of harm or abuse?

Source: (Care Quality Commission 2018).

In relation to 'spatial privacy', the nursing associate must appreciate the importance of the patient's 'personal space'. Within the clinical setting, nurses will often move patient's belongings without asking permission. They may interact with a patient without introducing themselves; they may enter a room without knocking or fail to fully close bedside curtains. The nursing associate must consider the potential detrimental consequences of feeling that one's privacy has been compromised and actively strive to ensure that all possible considerations are explored to minimise breaches of patient privacy. There are multiple logistical considerations in relation to the maintenance of 'spatial privacy' (see Box 21.1).

In maintaining informational privacy, there is an inordinate amount of data that is immediately available through the medium of social media, and increasingly, technology is being used to gather and store data within the healthcare setting (Francis & Francis 2017). The utilisation of digital patient records and the increasing need for the sharing of data between different providers culminate in a need for better information security (Appari & Johnson 2010). The Data Protection Act (2018) makes provision in relation to the processing of personal data to ensure that stored details are kept private. There are multiple logistical considerations in relation to the maintenance of 'information privacy' (see Box 21.2).

Breach of Privacy/Confidentiality

The NHS Confidentiality Code of Practice (2010) requires all NHS staff to work within the parameters of the code and details very clear guidance on how confidential information should be recorded, stored and shared. Despite this, patient privacy may be compromised quite unintentionally; however, the consequences of such a breach can be extremely distressful. Inadvertent breaches are potentially commonplace on wards where medical notes may be left visible, confidential patient data such as handover documentation are not discarded appropriately or data

Box 21.1 Spatial Privacy

Follow trust policies in relation to patient information
Respect personal space
Knock on a patient's door before entering a room
Close the doors
Close the curtains and windows when delivering personal care
Lower your voice when discussing personal issues with patients, remembering curtains are not soundproof
Consider individual choice, sexuality, gender and transgender
Consider religious needs relation to privacy

Box 21.2 Information Privacy

Ensure that the nursing notes are stored securely
Log off from computers after accessing records
Change computer password regularly
Ensure information relayed to other healthcare professionals is on a 'need-to-know' basis only
Consider information offered over the telephone
Consider information offered to family members
Consider information offered to police/social services

encryption e-mail services are not used by both the sender and recipient. Fundamentally, breaches of privacy can occur when verbal, written or electronic date can identify a patient directly or indirectly (Blightman et al. 2014).

Take Note

There are occasions where breaches of privacy occur. When this happens, then mechanisms must be put in place to investigate the cause(s) and to take action to reduce the risk of reoccurrence.

The sharing of one's healthcare information without consent is a fundamental disregard for legality and ethical principles; however, there are exceptions. There are certain exemptions that may apply in law enforcement situations and in a court of law whereby the nursing associate may divulge patient information without consent. Data may be shared if the information is deemed to be in the public interest; however, there is a definitive difference in what is 'in the public interest and what the public are interested in'. Information may be disclosed if there is a perceived threat to public safety (Blightman et al. 2014).

The nursing associate may also share confidential information without consent if it is required by law or directed by a court. They can also divulge information to an appropriate person if they have legitimate concerns regarding a child or young person's safety weighing up the possible consequences of not sharing the information against the harm that sharing the information. It is also acceptable to breach confidentiality if information relayed has the potential to cause harm, for example, a patient may tell you that he is saving up all his daily medication and intends to take it all at the end of the week in an attempt to take his own life (National Health Service 2010).

Take Note

The nursing associate has a responsibility to ensure that any information given to them is protected and shared only with those need to know. There are exceptions to the duty of confidentiality; at all times, local policy and procedure and professional obligations apply.

Caldicott Guardians

A Caldicott Guardian is a senior person within a healthcare or social care organisation who ensures that data is processed in accordance with the seven Caldicott principles (see Box 21.3). The charge of the Caldicott Guardian is to ensure that information about individuals who use the service is used legally, ethically and appropriately and that privacy and confidentiality is maintained. 'All NHS organisations and local authorities which provide social services must have a registered Caldicott Guardian' (The UK Caldicott Guardian Council Report 2019).

Supporting Evidence

The UK Caldicott Guardian Council is the UK National Body for Caldicott Guardians. The aims of the Council are to:

- be a point of contact for all Caldicott Guardians and for health and care organisations seeking advice on the Caldicott principles,
- enable Caldicott Guardians to share information, views and experience,
- encourage consistent standards and training for Caldicott Guardians and
- help to develop guidance and policies relating to the Caldicott principles.

Its website (https://www.ukcgc.uk) has a number of useful resources that can help the nursing associate become Caldicott competent.

Dignity

It may be argued that dignity is itself not an easily definable phenomenon (Jacobson 2012); however, German philosopher Immanuel Kant postulated that dignity should be perceived as a moral imperative and an inherent human right (Szăwarsk 2019). Patients strive to maintain a level of normality during illness, maintaining self-determination, self-governance, self-care and self-management (Lindberg et al. 2014). By the

Box 21.3 Seven Caldicott Principles

To justify the purpose for using confidential information
To only use data when absolutely necessary
To use only the minimum amount of data required
To give access only on a strict need-to-know basis
To understand your responsibilities (Code of Confidentiality)
To understand and comply with the law
To understand that the duty to share information can be as important as the duty to protect patient confidentiality

Source: modified from Department of Health (2013)

very nature of illness, disease and hospitalisation, patients often feel a level of vulnerability, losing autonomy and control which in turn diminishes their perception of 'self-dignity'. Patient autonomy is defined as the ability to make informed decisions without pressure or bias about the care received (Entwistle et al. 2010).

Touch Point

Dignity should be seen as an inherent human right. Article 1 of the Universal Declaration of Human Rights proclaims that: 'All human beings are born free and equal in dignity and rights'.

To facilitate patient autonomy, nursing associates must first empower their patient to be confident and self-determined. *Empowerment* in healthcare is defined as a process through which people gain greater control over decisions and actions affecting their health (Risling et al. 2017). The empowerment of patients requires good communication and the transfer of knowledge to facilitate informed choices. Empowerment fosters the enablement of patients to be active participants in the decision-making process and requires a mutual and trustful relationship (Holmstrom & Röing 2010) between patients and the nursing associate.

Ostaszkiewicz (2019) highlights that one must portray empathy and understanding of the human experience to facilitate dignified care. Nursing associates must ensure the delivery of dignified patient care by demonstrating professional, moral and ethical values that can be viewed as prerequisites of the nursing profession. When delivering dignified care to patients, the nursing associate must consider a kaleidoscope of different issues, including compassion, awareness, engagement, communication, attentiveness, respect, identity, empowerment, autonomy involving the patient and seeing the patient as a unique individual (Sanakova & Cap 2019). In maintaining dignity, the nursing associate must be aware of the privileged position they find themselves in, developing a therapeutic relationship with their patients and acting as their advocate.

The Health and Social Care Act (2012) identifies the logistical complexities of delivering care that demonstrates dignity which recognises the need for careful consideration of the patient's individuality. What may be viewed as caring and compassionate to one patient may cause distress to another, for example, the use of therapeutic touch. Each patient should be spoken to in a respectful manner in the way they want to be addressed – for example, the use of Mr, Mrs, Ms or even a nickname. The nursing associate must ensure that the patient's dignity is maintained when they receive treatment, bathe or use the toilet. The relationship the patient has with their visitors, friends, family or relevant other persons should be respected, and privacy should be maintained. Patients using services must be cared for in a non-judgemental manner and not be discriminated against in any way in adherence with the Equality Act (2010).

Touch Point **Delivering dignified care**

Speak to the patient directly
Speak respectfully to and about the patient
People using the service should be addressed in the way they prefer
Create a respectful atmosphere
Always cover the patient up
Respect diversity
Assist the patient with personal hygiene needs
Assist the patient at meal times
Assist the patient with toileting needs
Communicate in a dignified manner
Promote self-esteem
Promote self-determination
Be conscious of the use of therapeutic touch
Ensure, where possible, that the patients are afforded the opportunity to wear their own clothing
Staff must respect people's personal preferences, lifestyle and care choices.

Yellow Flag

Therapeutic touch is a legitimate nursing intervention; however, there are some patients who may feel uncomfortable with it because of their personal beliefs. How touch is exchanged and planned is extremely important for the patient and the nursing associate, and if this is not done in appropriate manner, this has the potential to spoil relationships.

Conclusion

Platform 1, clause 1.11 of the Nursing and Midwifery Councils standards of proficiency for nursing associates (2018b), states that nursing associates must 'provide, promote, and where appropriate advocate for, non-discriminatory, person-centred and sensitive care at all times'. They must appreciate the diversity of their client group and ensure that the patient's values, beliefs, cultural characteristics, language requirements and preferences are at the forefront of all patient interaction to ensure that privacy is maintained and dignified care is delivered. It is apparent that the maintenance of privacy and the delivery of care that promote dignity are not, as many perceive, simplistic undertakings. What is extremely evident is the monumental importance of the two concepts in the delivery of optimum, patient-centred holistic care.

References

Appari, A. and Johnson, M.E. (2010) Information security and privacy in healthcare: current state of research, *International Journal of Internet and Enterprise Management*, 6(4): 279–314.

Beauchamp, T.L. and Childress, J.F. (2009) *Principles of biomedical ethics* (6th edn), Oxford: Oxford University Press.

Blightman, K., Griffiths, S.E. and Danbury, C. (2014) Patient confidentiality: patient confidentiality: when can a breach be justified? *Continuing Education in Anaesthesia, Critical Care & Pain*, 14(2): 52–56.

Care Quality Commission. (2018) Relationships and sexuality in adult social care services, *Guidance for CQC inspection staff and registered adult social care providers*. [online] Available: https://www.cqc.org.uk/sites/default/files/20190221-Relationships-and-sexuality-in-social-care-PUBLICATION.pdf. Accessed 10 December 2019.

Caldicott Guardian Council. (2019) *Caldicott guardian council Annual report 2018–19*. [online] Available: https://assets.publishing.service.gov.uk/government/uploads/system/uploads/attachment_data/file/826708/UKCGC_Annual_Report_2018_19_v1.3.pdf. Accessed 31 February 2020.

Department of Health. (2013) *Information: share or not to share government response to the Caldicott review*. [online] Available: https://assets.publishing.service.gov.uk/government/uploads/system/uploads/attachment_data/file/251750/9731-2901141-TSO-Caldicott-Government_Response_ACCESSIBLE.PDF. Accessed 10 December 2019.

Duncan, M. (2019) Employers' duty of care to district nursing team members: health and safety concerns with lone domiciliary visits, *British Journal of Community Nursing*, 24(8): 377–379.

Entwistle, V.A., Carter, S. M. Cribb, A. and McCaffery, K. (2010) Supporting patient autonomy: the importance of clinician-patient relationships, *Journal of General Internal Medicine*, 25(7): 741–745.

Equality Act. (2010) *Legislation.gov.uk*. [online] Available: http://www.legislation.gov.uk/ukpga/2010/15/contents. Accessed 10 October 2019.

Francis, L.P. and Francis, J.G. (2017) *Privacy: what everyone needs to know*, Oxford: Oxford University Press.

Hawley, G. (2007) *Ethics in clinical practice an interprofessional approach*, Harlow: Pearson Educational.

Health and Social Care Act. (2012) [online] Available: http://www.legislation.gov.uk/ukpga/2012/7/contents/enacted. Accessed 10 September 2019.

Holmstrom, I. and Röing, M. (2010) The relation between patient-centeredness and patient empowerment: a discussion of concepts, *Patient Education and Counselling*, 79(2): 167–172.

Jacobson, N. (2012) *Dignity and health, Nashville, TN: Vanderbilt* University Press.

Lindberg, C., Fagerstreom, C., Sivberg, B. and Willman, A. (2014) Concept analysis: patient autonomy in a caring context, *Journal of Advanced Nursing*, 70(10): 2208–2221.

National Health Service. (2010) *Confidentiality: NHS code of practice supplementary guidance: public interest disclosures*. [online] Available: https://assets.publishing.service.gov.uk/government/uploads/system/uploads/attachment_data/file/200147/Confidentiality_-_NHS_Code_of_Practice_Supplementary_Guidance_on_Public_Interest_Disclosures.pdf. Accessed 11 September 2019.

Nursing and Midwifery Council. (2018a) *The code: professional standards of practice and behaviour for nurses, midwives and nursing associates*, London: Nursing and Midwifery Council.

Nursing and Midwifery Council. (2018b) *Standards of proficiency for nursing associates*. [online] Available: www.nmc.org.uk. Accessed 10 November 2019.

Ostaszkiewicz, J. (2019) Defending patients' dignity: An under recognised and under resourced nursing role, *JARNA*, 22(2): 4–6.

Risling, T.R.N., Martinez, J., Young, J. and Thorp-Froslie, N. (2017) Evaluating patient empowerment in association with eHealth technology: scoping review, *Journal of Medical Internet Research*, 19(9): e329.

Sanakova, S. and Cap, J. (2019) Dignity from the nurses' and older patients' perspective: a qualitative literature review, *Nursing Ethics*, 26(5): 1292–1309.

Szawarsk, P. (2019) Classic cases revisited – Tony Nicklinson and the question of dignity, *Journal of the Intensive Care Society*, 21(2): 1–5.

The Data Protection Act. (2018) *Legislation.gov.uk. [online]* Available: http://www.legislation.gov.uk/. Accessed 1 September 2019.

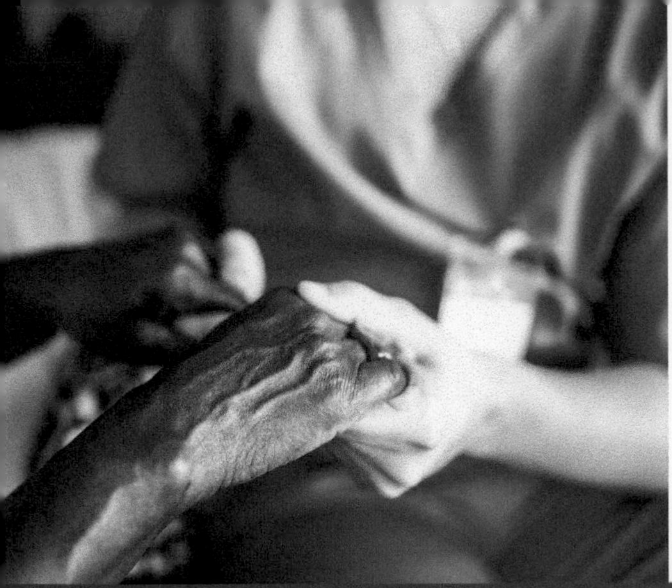

22

Promoting Sleep

Graham Patrick Jones

Teesside University, UK

Chapter Aim

- **This chapter aims to assist the reader in developing an understanding of the importance of sleep in maintaining holistic health and well-being.**

Learning Outcomes

By the end of this chapter, the learner will be able to:
- **Understand the fundamental physiology of sleep**
- **Discuss the stages of sleep**
- **Identify how much sleep is needed**
- **Explain sleep deprivation**
- **Explore the nursing associate's role in promoting sleep**

Test Yourself Multiple Choice Questions

1. **Which hormone do we associate with sleep?**
   A) **Melatonin**
   B) **Vasopressin**
   C) **Endothelin**
   D) **Insulin**
2. **What is the recommended daily sleep time for a newborn?**
   A) **22 to 23 hours**
   B) **14 to 17 hours**
   C) **12 to 14 hours**
   D) **8 to 12 hours**

The Nursing Associate's Handbook of Clinical Skills, First Edition. Edited by Ian Peate.

Companion website: www.wiley.com/nursingassociate

3. **What are the two fundamental types of sleep?**
   A) **Deep and NREM**
   B) **Coma and REM**
   C) **NREM and REM**
   D) **REM and EEG**

4. **What is Willis–Ekbom disease commonly known as?**
   A) **Insomnia**
   B) **Snoring**
   C) **Apnoea**
   D) **Restless Legs Syndrome**
5. **What does the term 'Sleep Hygiene' refer to?**
   A) **Showering before bedtime**
   B) **Ensuring bedsheets are clean**
   C) **Encouraging good sleep habits**
   D) **Providing the patient with wipes to clean hands**

Introduction

Each night, most of us depart from a level of waking consciousness and become submerged in an unconscious, unaware state that is characterised by periods of relaxation and reduced mobility. Approximately one-third of one's life is spent sleeping; it is an important part of our daily routine and is essential for physical, psychological and cognitive health and well-being, as emphasised by Roper et al. (1990) who identified sleep as one of the twelve activities of living (Williams 2015).

As a nursing associate, it is imperative that one possesses, demonstrates and maintains the standards of proficiency in relation to the delivery of high-quality, patient-centred holistic care that demonstrates awareness, identification and management of individuals whose sleep patterns may be compromised. This will require the nursing associate to be an accountable professional and to promote health and prevent ill health, provide and monitor care, work in teams and improve safety and quality of care while contributing to integrated care (Nursing and Midwifery Council 2018).

Fundamental Physiology of Sleep

Sleep is far from the simplistic process many take for granted; fundamentally, the sleep–wake cycle in humans is regulated by two significant physiological processes: homeostatic involvement and the endogenous circadian cycle. Homeostatic involvement encapsulates the maintenance of an internal state of equilibrium and stability within the body (Fisher et al. 2013). The circadian cycle is a complex process that involves, among other integrated process, the synthesis and release of melatonin by the pineal gland when exposed to darkness.

What are Circadian Rhythms?

The physical, mental and behavioural changes that follow a daily cycle such as being awake during the day and sleeping at night are known as *circadian rhythms*. Circadian rhythms can influence not only sleep–wake cycles but hormone release, eating habits and digestion, body temperature and other important bodily functions. Think of it as a 24-hour internal clock within the brain.

Controlling Circadian Rhythms

Within the brain, a group of neurons called the suprachiasmatic nucleus (SCN) forms part of the hypothalamus and controls the circadian rhythm. Often referred to as the 'master clock', this group of neurons interpret stimuli from the environment. The SCN receives information from the optic nerves in the eye (Ostrin 2019); as darkness falls, the SCN tells the pineal gland to release the hormone melatonin. Melatonin is synthesised and released by the pineal gland upon exposure to darkness, and it is suppressed by exposure to light. Melatonin is a neurohormone known to modulate a wide range of circadian functions, including sleep.

> Touch Point **Optic Nerves**
>
> **Controlling circadian rhythms**
>
> The synthesis and release of melatonin from the pineal gland is heavily influenced by light stimulation.

Suprachiasmatic Nucleus
Numbering some 10,000 neurons, the SCN is the 'master' circadian clock, directing the daily processes of behaviour and physiology.

Pineal Gland
The pineal gland is approximately 10 mm long, reddish brown in colour and surrounded by a capsule. The gland tends to atrophy after puberty and may become calcified in later life.

Melatonin
The hormone melatonin, secreted by the pineal gland, plays various functions within the human body, including influencing circadian rhythms. This neurohormone plays a key role in the co-ordination of the circadian system, otherwise referred to as the 'biological clock'.

Source: (Waugh & Grant 2018; Ostrin 2019; Hastings et al. 2018)

Stages of Sleep

Sleep can be seen to be a complex physiological process that can be divided into two fundamental types: non-rapid eye movement (non-REM) sleep and rapid eye movement (REM) sleep. Non-REM has three levels: Stage 1 represents the transition from wakefulness to sleep. In Stage 2, we enter a state of light sleep in which physiological changes occur, muscles relax and eye movement slows down, as does breathing, brain activity and heart rate. The transition into Stage 3 takes place, and one enters the most restorative stage of sleep; here, deep sleep occurs.

REM sleep is where we enter a dream state in which brain wave activity is seen to be similar to wakefulness. During REM sleep, rapid phasic eye movement is observed, and muscle tone is all but absent apart from constriction and expansion of the diaphragm (Gonfalone 2019).

Number of Sleep Hours

Individuals' need for sleep and their sleeping pattern alter as they progress through the life continuum, and the appropriate amount varies significantly across each individual of the same age. The National Sleep Foundation (2015) recommends appropriate sleep durations for specific age groups.

Take Note

Newborn (0 to 3 months)	14 to 17 hours
Infants (4 to 11 months)	12 to 15 hours
Toddlers (1 to 2 years)	11 to 14 hours
Preschool (3 to 5 years)	10 to 13 hours
School-age children (6 to 13 years)	9 to 11 hours
Teenagers (14 to 17 years)	8 to 10 hours
Adults (18 to 64 years)	7 to 9 hours
Older adults (over 65 years)	7 to 8 hours

Source: Modified from National Sleep Foundation (NSF) (2015).

Sleep Deprivation

What are the Causes of Sleep Deprivation?

Commentators discuss that there are multiple inter-related causes of sleep deprivation; some psychological, some physical and some social.

Red Flag

Emotional distress and anxiety	Apnoea
Relationship breakdown	Insomnia
Finance	Breathing problems
Work/school	Incontinence
Caffeine	Temperature
Discomfort/pain	Noise

Source: Modified from Hirotsu et al. (2015).

Consequences of Sleep Deprivation

Carter (2019) emphasises that individuals suffering from sleep deprivation can experience multiple pathologies which will impact upon their physical, psychological and social well-being. Troynikov et al. (2018) discuss that the consequences of poor-quality sleep are multifarious and involve reduced cognitive ability, mood, decision-making, stress, depression and limited task performance. Physiologically, poor-quality sleep may result in impaired immunity, cardiovascular and respiratory problems, hormonal changes and urological disease (Pierce & Chughtai 2019). The long-term consequences of sleep deprivation are identified by Munafo et al. (2018) who prescribes that 'individuals experiencing sleep deprivation are more likely to suffer from chronic diseases such as obesity, diabetes, hypertension, and depression, as well as cancer, increased mortality, and reduced quality of life and productivity'. A systematic review and meta-analysis conducted by Cappuccio et al. (2010) postulates that 'regularly sleeping less than 5 hours each night increases the chance of death, from all causes, by about 15%'.

Red Flag Sleep deprivation has been linked to multiple pathologies including

Low mood	Temperature regulation
Stress	Obesity
Anxiety	Diabetes
Cognitive impairment	Hypertension
Memory impairment	Appetite
Hallucinations	Decreased libido
Processing information	Muscle soreness and aching
Depression	Headaches
Suicide	Risk of heart attack and stroke

Source: Carter (2019); Larson (2018); Ludden (2018).

Chapter 20 provides further details concerning the promotion of comfort in bed. Also, the nursing associate can learn how to enhance comfort, aiding rest and enhancing sleep.

Sleep Disorders

Insomnia

Insomnia is defined as the inability to fall asleep, stay asleep throughout the night or waking up too early in the morning. The causes of insomnia are multiple and vary from one individual to another. Insomnia can be seen to have a detrimental effect upon quality of life and daily functioning contributing to the development of psychiatric disorders and chronic health conditions (Wright 2019).

Obstructive Sleep Apnoea

Obstructive sleep apnoea is defined as a sleep breathing disorder resulting from airway obstruction as a consequence of intermittent collapse of upper airway tissue during sleep. Obese individuals are at increased risk of airway obstruction 'because their anatomy often combines a large neck circumference with excess lateral pharyngeal adipose tissue resulting in a narrowed airway' (Willard et al. 2019).

Narcolepsy

Narcolepsy is a sleeping disorder that affects approximately 1 in 2,000 people with onset usually in the first three decades of life (Narcolepsy Network 2019). The condition, a neurological disorder, manifests as an uncontrollable inability to remain awake. Symptoms of the condition can vary from individual to individual with varying degrees of severity. Those who experience narcolepsy enter REM sleep almost immediately. Commentators suggest various causes of narcolepsy; however, many prescribe to the hypothesis that the condition is caused by the immune system mistakenly attacking sections of the brain that produce a neuropeptide called orexin; this chemical plays a part in regulating sleep patterns (Cohen et al. 2018).

Willis–Ekbom Disease

Many will not have heard of Willis–Ekbom disease; however, most people will know the condition by the more common term of 'Restless Legs Syndrome' (RLS). RLS symptoms often occur in the evening hours and can have an extremely detrimental impact upon an individual's ability to fall asleep. The condition manifests as an overwhelming propensity to mobilise the legs when at rest. The urge to move the legs is often accompanied by unpleasant sensations. RLS is categorised as early onset which is thought to have a genetic aetiology and late onset which occurs over the age of 45 years and is more severe and associated with chronic renal disease, anaemia and pregnancy (Chaiard & Weaver 2019).

Nursing Associate's Role in Promoting Sleep

In July 2019, the UK Government asked the National Health Service to explore what more could be done to ensure those in care settings were getting the amount of rest and sleep they needed. The government suggests an assessment of the current policies on sleep and the rollout of 'protected sleep time' in hospitals, where staff leave patients sleeping unless clinically necessary (Mitchell 2019). The role of the nursing associate is to deliver optimum, high-quality, patient-centred, individualised holistic care; this involves consideration of multiple factors including the sleep needs of those they are charged with caring for. It is apparent that sleep is not the simplistic event that many take for granted, but a complex process that encapsulates multiple variables and considerations.

We have learnt that sleep is a fundamental requirement of health and well-being; it is crucial for the maintenance of 'immune function, tissue healing, pain modulation, cardiovascular health, mental health, cognitive function, and learning and memory' (Ries 2018). Nursing associates will deliver care to patients in a variety of clinical environments: hospitals, hospice, nursing homes and many other settings; patients in these environments will present with varying degrees of illness and disability, often fragile with chronic illness or severe diseases. The nursing associate must deliver care based on the uniqueness of the patient and act as an advocate implementing appropriate strategies to facilitate optimum sleep.

A term often introduced in discussion pertaining to sleep is 'sleep hygiene'. Sleep hygiene is simply a term used to describe good sleep habits. The sleep hygiene agenda promotes a variety of different practices that are necessary to have a 'normal' quality night's sleep. These advocated 'habits' derive from cognitive behavioural therapy which is deemed to be an effective long-term treatment for individuals with chronic insomnia (see Box 22.1 for recommendations).

The hospital setting is not conducive to quality sleep with multiple disruptions that are hard to control, including environmental factors such as lights, noise and alarms; consequently, the nursing associate must at all times strive to implement innovative new ways of working that

Box 22.1 Recommendations for a Quality Night's Sleep

Reduce or avoid sleeping during the day
Limit or avoid caffeine, alcohol and nicotine before bedtime
Avoid going to bed hungry or too full
Try to have a relaxing bedtime routine
Keep the room quiet (this is challenging in the hospital setting)
Keep the room dark
Keep the room temperature comfortable
Do not force yourself to try to go to sleep
Get regular exposure to natural light (this is challenging in the hospital setting)
Ensure that clocks are not visible
A tidy room makes for a tidy mind and a restful night's sleep
No technology in the room (this can be challenging in the hospital setting)
No LED displays

Source: Modified from Sleep Council (2019).

promote sleep and minimise disruption. A review of relevant literature performed by Dubose & Hadi (2016) highlighted various initiatives that can be implemented to promote good-quality sleep, such as the more extensive use of complimentary interventions. These include the utilisation of interventions such as music, massage and aromatherapy which may prove effective in improving the quality of sleep and promote both the physical and psychological well-being of patients (Pagnucci et al. 2019).

Take Note Nursing associate interventions to promote sleep

Earplugs offer an easy and affordable solution for reducing noise
Eye masks improve sleep by blocking out light
Utilisation of techniques to induce relaxation such as music
Massage therapy
Aroma vaporisers
Aromatherapy
Do not sit and talk at the nurse's station
Wearing appropriate footwear.

Conclusion

During sleep, individuals have no conscious realisation of their environment; however, brain activity is constant, receiving sensory information, monitoring and processing stimuli. This subconscious awareness can, in appropriate circumstances, be beneficial; however, for those who are hospitalised and in need of rest, it can have a detrimental effect. Nursing associates must deploy innovative interventions to initiate a relaxing tranquil environment that facilitates optimum sleep.

References

Cappuccio, F.P., D'Elia, L., Strazzullo, P. and Miller, M.A. (2010) Sleep duration and all-cause mortality: a systematic review and meta-analysis of prospective studies, *Sleep*, 33(5): 585–592.

Carter, P. (2019) Remembering sleep: sleep deprivation and symptom management at home, *Cancer Nursing*, 42(5): 426–427.

Chaiard, J. and Weaver, T.E. (2019) Update on research and practices in major sleep disorders: part II—Insomnia, Willis-Ekbom disease (Restless Leg Syndrome), and narcolepsy, *Journal of Nursing Scholarship*, 51(6): 624–633.

Cohen, A., Jay Mandrekar, J., St. Louis, E.K., Michael, H., Silber, M.H. and Kotagal, S. (2018) Comorbidities in a community sample of narcolepsy, *Seep Medicine*, 43(2018): 14–18.

Dubose, J.R. and Hadi, K. (2016) Improving inpatient environments to support patient sleep, *International Journal for Quality in Health Care*, 28(5): 540–553.

Fisher, S.P., Foster, R.G. and Peirson, S.N. (2013) The circadian control of sleep, *Handbook of Experimental Pharmacology* (01 Jan 2013), (217): 157–183.

Gonfalone, A.A. (2019) Hypothetical role of gravity in rapid eye movements during sleep, *Medical Hypotheses*, 127: 63–65.

Hastings, M.H., Maywood, E.S. and Brancaccio, M. (2018) Generation of circadian rhythms in the suprachiasmatic nucleus, *Nature Reviews Neuroscience*, 19(8): 453–469.

Hirotsu, C., Tufik, S. and Andersen, M.L. (2015) Interactions between sleep, stress, and metabolism: From physiological to pathological conditions, *Sleep Science*, 8(3): 143–152.

Larson, E.B. (2018) Sleep disturbance and cognition in people with TBI, *Neuro Rehabilitation*, 43(3): 297–306.

Ludden, D. (2018) How lack of sleep strains relationships, *Psychology Today*, 51(2).

Mitchell, G. (2019) *Sleeping patient waking ban suggested in new green paper, Nursing Times, 23 July 2019. [online] Available*: https://www.nursingtimes.net/news/public-health/sleeping-patient-waking-ban-suggested-in-new-green-paper-23-07-2019/. Accessed 10 October 2019.

Munafo, D., Loewy, D., Reuben, K., Kavy, G. and Hevener, B. (2018) Sleep deprivation and the workplace: prevalence, impact and solutions, *American Journal of Health Promotion*, 32(7): 1644–1646.

Narcolepsy Network. (2019) [online] Available: https://narcolepsynetwork.org/about-narcolepsy/narcolepsy-fast-facts/. Accessed 10 December 2019.

National Sleep Foundation. (2019) [online] Available: https://www.sleepfoundation.org/. Accessed 10 September 2019.

Nursing & Midwifery Council. (2018) *Standards of proficiency for nursing associates.* [online] Available: www.nmc.org.uk [accessed 9 September 2019].

Pierce, H. and Chughtai, B. (2019) Impact of poor sleep quality on urologic disease, *Urology Times*, July 2019.

Pagnucci, N., Tolotti, A., Cadorin, L., Valcarenghi, D. and Forfori, F. (2019) Promoting nighttime sleep in the intensive care unit: alternative strategies in nursing, *Intensive & Critical Care Nursing*, 51(2019): 73–81.

Ostrin, L. (2019) Ocular and systemic melatonin and the influence of light exposure, *Optometry Australia: Clinical and Experimental Optometry*, 102(2): 99–108.

Ries, E. (2018) Promoting sleep not leap, *PTinMOTIONmag.org / October 2018.* [online] Available: https://www.apta.org/uploadedFiles/APTAorg/News_and_Publications/PT_in_Motion/2018/10/PTinMotionOct2018.pdf. Accessed 9 September 2019.

Roper, N., Logan, W.W. and Tierney, A. (1990) *The elements of nursing* (3rd edn), Churchill Livingstone: Edinburgh.

The Sleep Council. (2019) *Seven ways to a better night's sleep.* [online] Available: https://sleepcouncil.org.uk/seven-steps-to-a-better-nights-sleep/. Accessed 11 September 2019.

Troynikov, O., Watson, C.G. and Nawaz, N. (2018) Sleep environments and sleep physiology: a review, *Journal of Thermal Biology*, 78(2018): 192–203.

Waugh, A. and Grant, A. (2018) *Ross & Wilson anatomy and physiology in health & illness* (13th edn), Edinburgh: Elsevier.

Willard, C.E., Rice, A.N., Broome, M.E., Silva, S. and Muckler, V.C. (2019) Nasal ventilation mask for prevention of upper airway obstruction in patients with obesity or obstructive sleep apnoea, *AANA Journal*, 87(5): 395.

Williams, B. (2019) The Roper-Logan-Tierney model of nursing: a framework to complement the nursing process, *Nursing*, 45(3): 24–26.

Wright, W.L. (2019) Insomnia across the lifespan, *Continuing Education,* June 2019 Women's Healthcare.

Unit 3

Provide Care and Support with Hygiene and The Maintenance of Skin Integrity

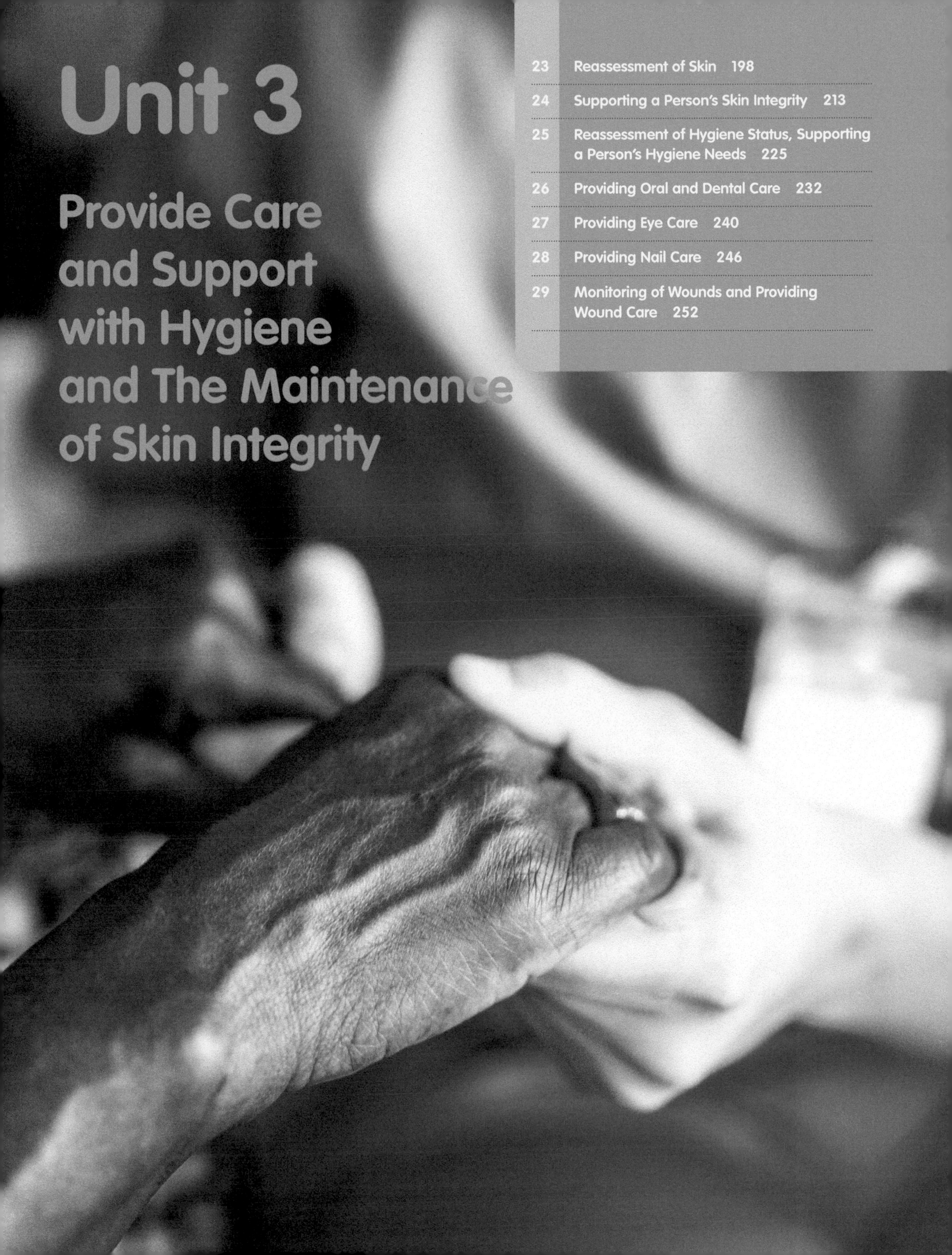

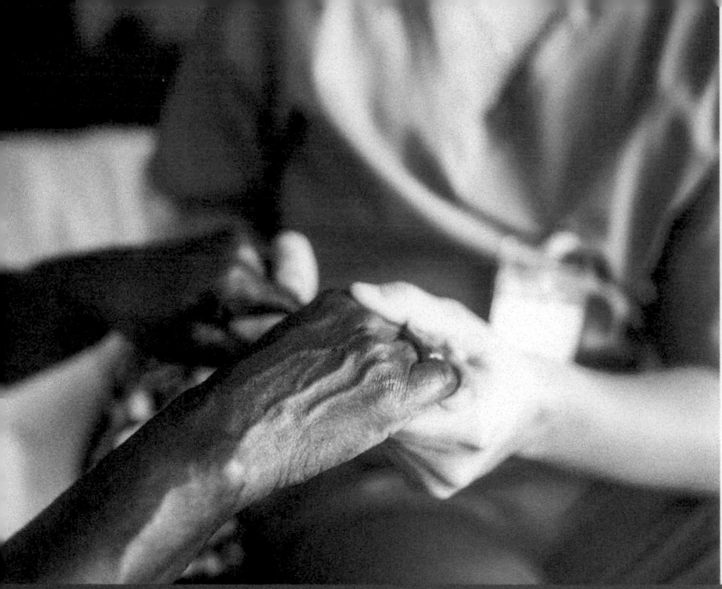

23

Reassessment of Skin

Nicole Blythe

University of Salford, UK

Chapter Aim

- **This chapter aims to provide the reader with the knowledge, skills and behaviours required to carry out an effective skin reassessment.**

Learning Outcomes

By the end of this chapter, the reader will be able to:
- **Identify factors affecting skin integrity**
- **Describe key concepts and the role of the nursing associate in skin reassessment**
- **Discuss a range of contemporary skin assessment tools and documentation**

Test Yourself Multiple Choice Questions

1. **Which is the largest organ in the human body?**
   A) **Heart**
   B) **Brain**
   C) **Skin**
   D) **Liver**
2. **SSKIN is a five-step model for:**
   A) **Psoriasis grading**
   B) **Pressure ulcer prevention**
   C) **Skin cancer detection**
   D) **Wound assessment**

The Nursing Associate's Handbook of Clinical Skills, First Edition. Edited by Ian Peate.

Companion website: www.wiley.com/nursingassociate

3. **Pressure ulcer risk assessment include a:**
   A) **Blood pressure check**
   B) **Skin assessment**
   C) **Review of resuscitation status**
   D) **Urinalysis**
4. **Extrinsic factors effecting skin integrity include (tick all that apply):**
   A) **Ultraviolet (UV) light**
   B) **Environmental pollutants**
   C) **Central heating**
   D) **Soaps and bubble baths**
5. **At the point of registration, a nursing associate is required to (tick all that apply):**
   A) **Identify and manage skin irritations and rashes**
   B) **Prevent and manage skin breakdown through appropriate use of products**
   C) **Observe and reassess skin and hygiene status using contemporary approaches**
   D) **Demonstrate an awareness of how requirements for procedures may vary across different health and care settings**

Introduction

In this chapter, the reassessment of skin is considered. While the initial holistic skin assessment may be carried out by the registered nurse, the same knowledge, skills and behaviours are required by the nursing associate for reassessment. Therefore, in this chapter, assessment is used interchangeably with reassessment.

The Nursing and Midwifery Council's (NMC's) (2018a) standards of proficiency for nursing associates require the nursing associate to be able to observe and reassess skin using contemporary approaches to determine the need for support and ongoing intervention at the point of registration.

Skin is the largest organ of the body, and there are many different skin conditions a nursing associate may come across that require a skilled, structured and appropriate assessment. With this in mind, the first section of this chapter explores a range of key considerations that can be applied generically across all skin conditions and associated assessments. The second section is dedicated to the skin reassessment of individuals at risk of developing pressure ulcers, and in the final section, documentation including a brief selection of assessment tools is discussed.

General Considerations

Skin Layers and Functions of the Skin

For nursing associates to perform a skin reassessment, they must understand not only the basic layers and functions of the skin but also the factors that underpin common skin problems as a whole. Skin has three main layers: the epidermis, dermis and the subcutaneous layer (sometimes also called the hypodermis). See Figure 23.1 for a representation of the skin and its associated structures.

The epidermis is the outermost layer of the skin. It is an elastic layer that is continuously regenerated. It comprises keratinocytes, corneocytes and melanocytes, and its main function is to provide waterproofing and serve as a barrier to infection. The dermis is the inner layer and includes sweats glands, sebaceous glands and hair follicles. All of these play a key role in temperature regulation. The subcutaneous layer lies under the dermis and is made up of connective tissue and fat. Fat, in particular, is a good insulator.

The following are the functions of the skin:

- Provides a protective barrier against mechanical, thermal and physical injury and hazardous substances
- Prevents loss of moisture
- Reduces harmful effects of ultraviolet (UV) radiation
- Acts as a sensory organ (touch, detects temperature)
- Helps regulate temperature
- Production of vitamin D
- Aesthetics and communication.

Factors underpinning skin problems can be categorised into two groups: internal (intrinsic) and external (extrinsic) factors; Table 23.1 shows some of these internal and external factors.

Take Note

The nursing associate will come across many different acute and chronic skin conditions that require a skilled, structured and appropriate assessment. Assessment tools are useful as an 'aide-memoire', but they do not replace clinical judgement, and the nursing associate should therefore not rely on them alone.

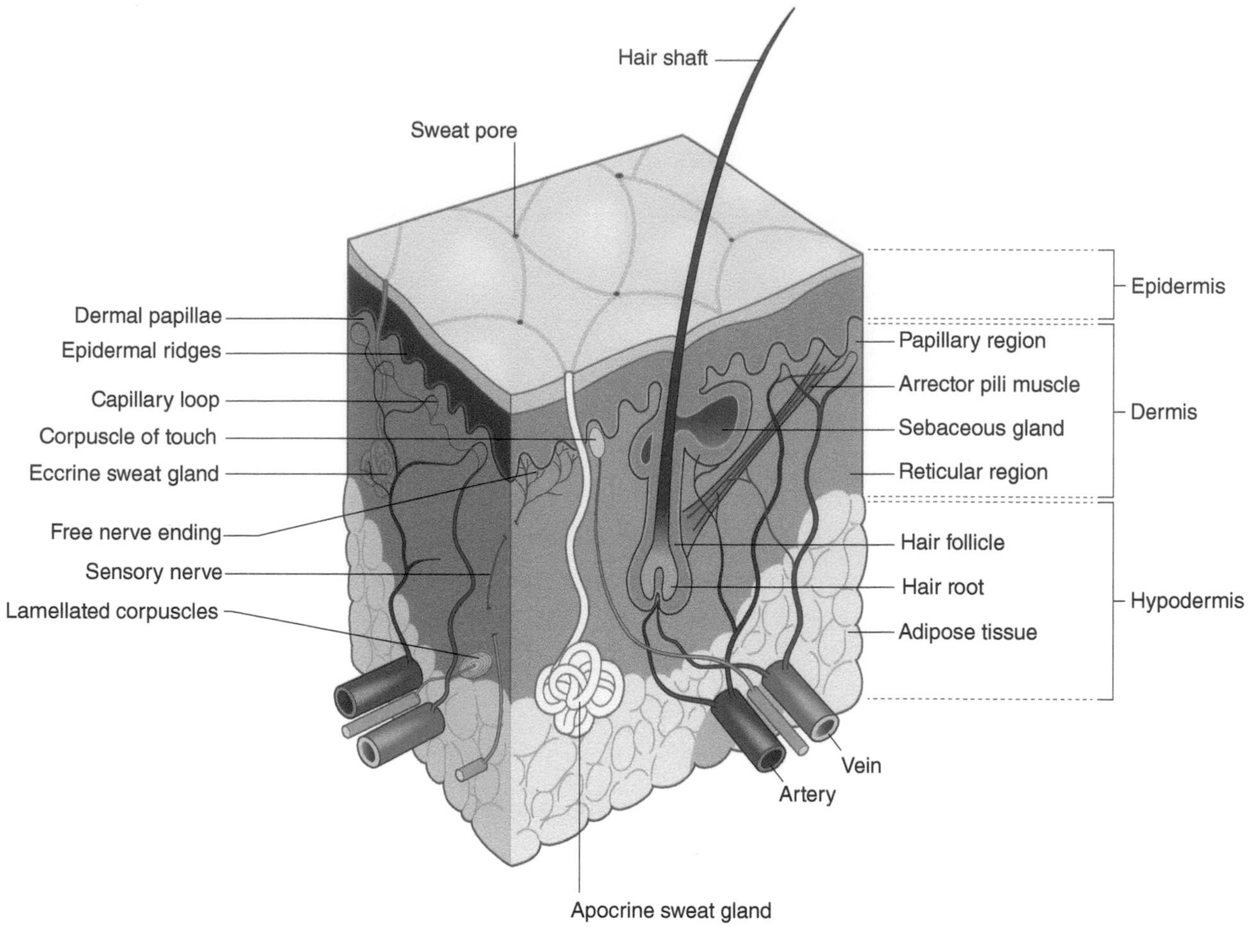

Figure 23.1 The three layers of the skin. *Source:* Peate and Nair (2015). © 2015 John Wiley & Sons, Ltd. Published 2015 by John Wiley & Sons, Ltd.

Table 23.1 Some internal and external factors underpinning skin problems.

INTERNAL FACTORS	EXTERNAL FACTORS
• Psychological, e.g. stress, anxiety and depression • Genetic, e.g. sickle cell disease, premature ageing disease and ichthyosis • Internal disease and comorbidities, e.g. diabetes mellitus, vascular impairment, cancer and hormone imbalance • Drugs, e.g. steroids, cytotoxic drugs, hormones, recreational drugs and alcohol • Infections, e.g. group A streptococcal infections and fungal infections • Inflammation, e.g. psoriasis and lupus	• Sunshine, e.g. exposure to UV light from the sun, sunburns and skin cancer • Heat and cold, e.g. injury to nerve and muscle tissues due to burns or chilblains • Allergens, e.g. plants, medication and food • Chemicals, e.g. acid, bleach and paint • Irritants, e.g. soaps, fragrances, creams and clothing • Infection, e.g. *Streptococcus pyogenes* and *Staphylococcus aureus* • Trauma, e.g. cuts, burns and lacerations • Friction, e.g. incorrect moving and handling and restraints • Pressure, e.g. medical devices, poor repositioning practices and inappropriate (prolonged) repositioning frequencies

Source: Arndt et al. (2015) Manual of dermatologic therapeutics, Wolters Kluwer Health.

Touch Point

Skin is the largest organ of the body. It comprises three main layers: the epidermis, dermis and subcutaneous layer. Its function includes the protection of the body, temperature regulation and sensation. Multiple factors can affect skin, and these are commonly categorised into two groups: internal (intrinsic) and external (extrinsic) factors.

Common Dermatological Conditions

There are many different skin conditions the nursing associate will come across when reassessing skin. Here is a short list of conditions the nursing associate should be familiar with:

- Atopic dermatitis and eczema (see Figures 23.2 and 23.3)
- Cold sores
- Hives (urticaria)
- Impetigo
- Itching
- Psoriasis
- Ringworm
- Scabies
- Skin cancer
- Vitiligo
- Warts and verrucas

For the assessment to be effective, nursing associates need to have the ability and underpinning knowledge to competently identify common skin irritations and rashes. Consideration should be given to skin appearance (e.g. dry, scaly, redness, pus-filled, raised or swollen), parts of the body that are affected (e.g. localised to one area or generalised all over the skin), symptoms that the patient is experiencing (e.g. pain, itch, tension or pressure), whether the condition is contagious and spread of the disease (e.g. skin-to-skin contact, contaminated objects or surfaces). Head-to-toe inspection of the skin is essential, including the back of the head, feet and mucous membranes.

Touch Points Revisited

Holistic and effective skin reassessment carried out by the nursing associate includes the following:

- Skin appearance (e.g. dry, scaly, redness, pus-filled, raised or swollen)
- Part of the body affected (e.g. localised in one area or generalised all over the skin)
- Symptoms (e.g. pain, itch, tension or pressure)
- Spread of the disease (contagious: yes/no).

Atopic dermatitis (eczema)

- Erythema, wet 'weeping' areas, dry scaly, thickened skin
- Intensely itchy
- Risk of secondary bacterial (staphylococcal) and viral (herpes zoster) infection
- Often linked with other atopic problems, e.g. asthma and hay fever
- Some cases linked with food and environmental allergens
- Breast-feeding may reduce risk of eczema
- Treat with moisturising creams to prevent skin drying
- Cream (water based) to wet areas
- Ointment (oil based) to dry areas
- Wet wraps to prevent drying and reduce scratching
- Topical steroids to persistent inflamed areas
- Topical (tacrolimus) and oral (ciclosporin) immunomodulators if severe
- Family support and follow-up important for chronic condition

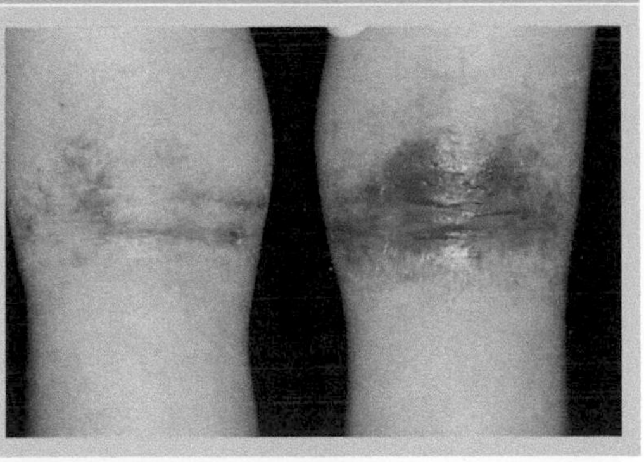

Figure 23.2 Atopic dermatitis. *Source:* Peate & Wild (2018).

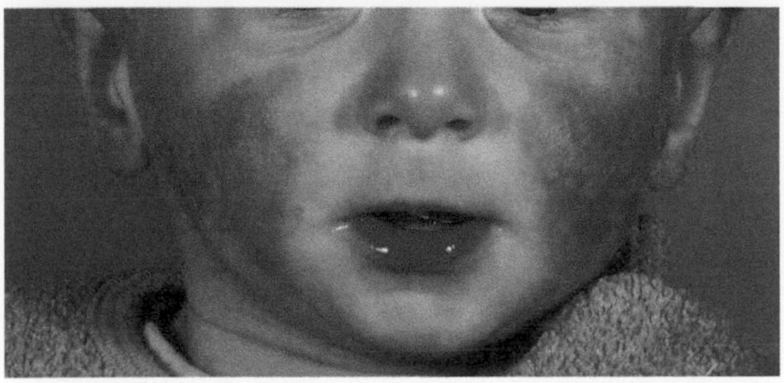

Figure 23.3 Eczema. Buxton & Morris-Jones (2013). Reproduced with permission of John Wiley & Sons Ltd.

Red Flag

Anaphylaxis is a severe and potentially life-threatening reaction to a trigger such as an allergy (allergen). It is also known as an *anaphylactic shock*. The nursing associate should look out for:

- Skin rashes, itching and hives
- Swelling of the lips, tongue or throat
- Shortness of breath, trouble breathing and wheezing (whistling sound during breathing)
- Dizziness and/or fainting
- Stomach pain, vomiting or diarrhoea
- Feeling like something awful is about to happen

Blue Flag

Smith (National Institute for Health and Care Excellence [NICE 2012]) states: 'Psoriasis is much more than a skin irritation. The condition can have profound functional, psychological and social effects on a person's life'. Nursing associates need to appreciate the impact of body image on a person's physical and mental health and well-being and how the impact of altered body image can affect an individual's personal and intimate relationships. Consideration of how body image may affect a person should form an integral part of any holistic skin reassessment. The nursing associate should consider that:

- Psoriasis may alter individuals' perception of their body image and impact on their thoughts, their self-esteem and confidence, thus leading to decreased body image and sexual function.
- A person in their care may experience feelings of guilt or shame.

Negative body image may interfere with sexual response, experience and sexual behaviour, which may affect not only the individuals but also their relationship with intimate/sexual partners (see Figure 23.4 for an example of psoriasis).

Yellow Flag

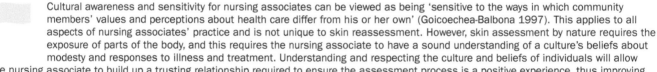

Cultural awareness and sensitivity for nursing associates can be viewed as being 'sensitive to the ways in which community members' values and perceptions about health care differ from his or her own' (Goicoechea-Balbona 1997). This applies to all aspects of nursing associates' practice and is not unique to skin reassessment. However, skin assessment by nature requires the exposure of parts of the body, and this requires the nursing associate to have a sound understanding of a culture's beliefs about modesty and responses to illness and treatment. Understanding and respecting the culture and beliefs of individuals will allow the nursing associate to build up a trusting relationship required to ensure the assessment process is a positive experience, thus improving continuity of care and patient satisfaction.

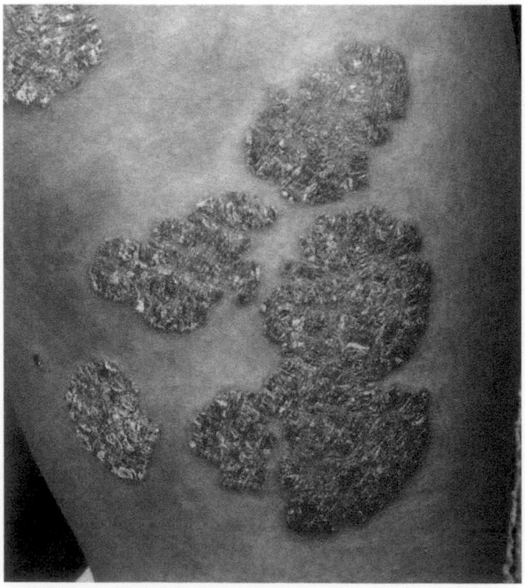

Figure 23.4 Psoriasis. ***Source:*** **Buxton & Morris-Jones (2013). Reproduced with permission of John Wiley & Sons Ltd.**

Supporting Evidence

Rashes in babies and children are common. This National Health Service (NHS) website offers simple information about a range of common rashes and what to do about it:
www.nhs.uk/conditions/rashes-babies-and-children/

Consent

Informed consent must be sought by the nursing associate prior to performing any skin reassessment. To ensure the consent is valid, the nursing associate needs to consider the following:

- The individual has the capacity to give consent
- There was no pressure or coercion on the individual to give consent
- The individual was fully and appropriately informed about the nature and purpose of the skin reassessment as well as implications of giving or refusing consent

Nursing associates must pay particular attention when seeking consent of 'vulnerable' individuals, such as those with learning disabilities or mental impairment or children. They should assume that individuals have the capacity to make their own decisions unless it is proven otherwise. If capacity is impaired or of concern, then the principles outlined in the Mental Capacity Act 2005 will provide the nursing associate with guidance and direction. If there are concerns, the nursing associate should seek advice from a more senior member of staff.

Privacy and Dignity

A full skin inspection requires the patient to undress; therefore, a sensitive approach is essential to help avoid patients feeling uncomfortable or vulnerable. Fundamental principles such as treating the patient with respect, care and compassion need to be upheld at all times. During the assessment, as little skin as possible should be exposed at any given time. The nursing associate needs to ensure that curtains, blinds or doors are closed, and the assessment is not interrupted. Every effort should be made to consider the individual's personal preferences such as requesting staff of a specific gender. The use of a chaperone should always be considered and offered to the patient.

Supporting Self-Care

A nursing associate needs to possess sound communication and interpersonal skills to establish a meaningful relationship with the patient, striving to create a compassionate, warm and positive patient experience that will not only allow the person to carry out the task more easily but will engage them in their care. Once readiness and ability to self-care has been determined, patients should be supported and taught to check their own skin for signs of improvement or deterioration. In supporting the patient, the nursing associate can:

- Work with the patient to develop a daily skin monitoring routine
- Include significant others such as carers (where appropriate)
- Assist in developing knowledge of areas most at risk of skin breakdown
- Aid in the acquisition of knowledge allowing for identification and detection of early signs of skin changes
- Encourage the reporting of skin changes to appropriate professionals
- Assist in the use of aids such as mirrors to allow for self-monitoring

Pain Assessment

During any skin reassessment, 'history taking' should be conducted, and patients need to be asked if they are experiencing any pain or discomfort. The nursing associate needs to consider the following verbal and non-verbal signs of pain:

- Type of pain (e.g. stabbing and throbbing)
- Duration (e.g. new onset)
- Location (e.g. localised to one area of the body)
- Frequency (e.g. intermittent or continuous)
- Intensity (e.g. 10/10 with 10 being the worst pain)
- Radiation (e.g. into joints or surrounding skin)
- Analgesia (have they taken analgesia, and if so, what was it and when)
- Patient's ability to answer the question (cognitive impairment, dementia, children and language)
- Facial expressions indicative of pain (e.g. grimacing, frowning, looking sad or withdrawn)
- Sounds indicative of pain (moaning, groaning, whimpering, crying or screaming)
- Other considerations (agitation, moving more frequently or not wanting to move, guarding the area of pain)
- Changes to physiological observations (e.g. tachycardia, hypertension or hyperpnea)

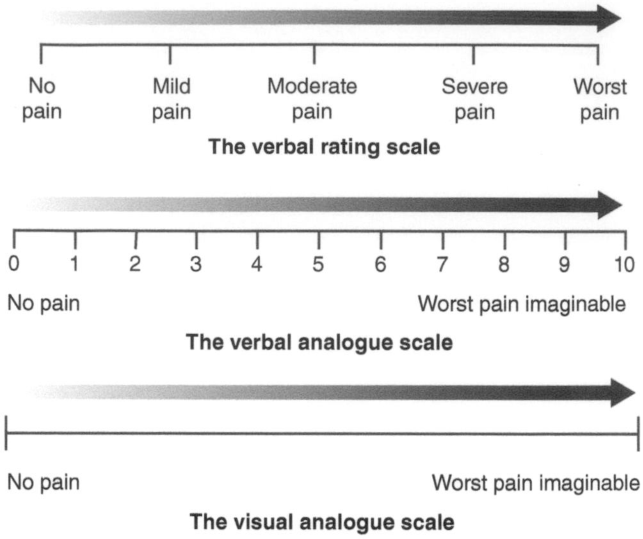

Figure 23.5 A type of pain assessment. Visual analogue scale. *Source:* Peate & Wild (2018).

The nursing associate should use a pain assessment tool appropriate for the patient to ensure that the assessment is both comprehensive and systematic. See Figure 23.5 for an example of a pain assessment tool. Please see Chapter 19 for the management of pain and discomfort.

Escalation of Skin Changes

Platform 1 of the NMC's standards of proficiencies for nursing associates sets out that the nursing associate must recognise and work within the limits of their competencies. In the context of skin reassessment, this means that any changes identified during the skin assessment need to be reported to an appropriate professional of the nursing and/or multidisciplinary team, for example, the named nurse, tissue viability specialist nurse, leg ulcer specialist nurse, dermatologist, pain team or pharmacist. This will allow for expert help and advice as well as prompt and appropriate amendment of the patient's care plan. It will also ensure the implementation of more appropriate treatment options. Any acute changes such as anaphylaxis need to be escalated following an emergency protocol. It is therefore of paramount importance that the nursing associate is familiar with local and national emergency phone numbers for the hospital as well as community setting.

Nursing associates take personal responsibility to ensure that any concerning skin changes are documented clearly and in line with local and national organisational frameworks, legislation and regulations. Relevant information needs to be shared according to local policy, and appropriate immediate action is to be taken by nursing associates to provide adequate safeguarding of all patients in their care. Risks identified need to be reported and unambiguously documented. Any actions required as a result of the escalation need to be implemented by the nursing associate as instructed by the expert professional.

Violet Flag

Poor housing, overcrowding, poor sanitary facilities and poverty may all have a directed impact on the skin health of individuals. During the assessment process, the nursing associate should take note of the socio-economic and socio-demographic circumstances of the individual such as low income, level of education, immigration status and living conditions, all of which can be linked to one or multiple skin problems.

Common skin conditions related to poor household infrastructure are:

- Bacterial skin infections such as Group A Streptococcal infection (e.g. impetigo)
- Pyoderma (any skin disease that has pus) attributed to Group A Streptococcus and exacerbated by overcrowding, humidity and poor hygiene
- Chickenpox, mumps and measles associated with missed vaccinations
- Scabies, blisters, scaling and rashes (particularly if larger numbers of young children live in the same household, access to household or personal cleaning products is limited and carpeted flooring is contaminated)
- Inflammatory skin conditions (e.g. acne and folliculitis)
- Pigmentary disorders associated with malnutrition

(see Figure 23.6. for common types of bacterial skin infections).

BACTERIAL INFECTION OF THE SKIN	COMMONEST CAUSATIVE BACTERIA	SIGNS, SYMPTOMS AND COMPLICATIONS	SITE
Folliculitis: bacterial infection of the hair follicle 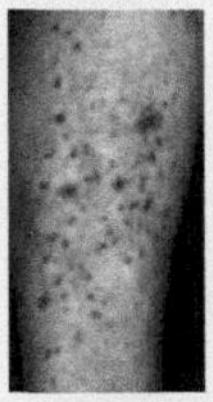	*Staphylococcus aureus* and *Pseudomonas aeruginosa*	Inflammation, pustules and lesions seen at the hair follicle. Discomfort ranging from slight burning to intense itching. Complication of abscess formation	Scalp, face of bearded men (sycosis barbae), eye (stye) and extremities on the legs of women who shave
Furuncles (boils): inflammation of the hair follicle 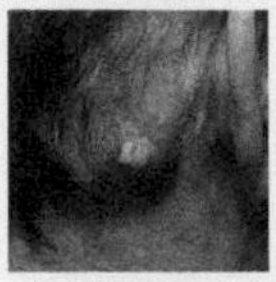	*Staphylococcus aureus*	Deep, firm, red, painful nodule 1–5 cm in diameter. After few days the nodule changes to large painful cystic nodule draining infected, purulent pus	Any part of the body that has hair, particularly neck, face, flexures and buttocks
Carbuncles: group of infected hair follicles	*Staphylococcus aureus*	Firm mass located in the subcutaneous tissue and lower dermis. Mass becomes painful and swollen and has multiple openings to the skin surface. Patient may experience chills, fever and malaise	Neck, back and lateral thighs
Cellulitis: localised infection of the dermis and subcutaneous tissue	*Streptococcus pyogenes*	Red, swollen and painful area. Vesicles may form over the cellulitic area, accompanied by chills, fever, malaise, headache and swollen lymph glands	Anywhere on the body. Common areas are lower legs in adults and eye and perianal area in children
Erysipelas: infection of the skin	*Streptococcus pyogenes*	Chills, fever and malaise (4–20 hours) precede a skin lesion appearing. Lesion(s) appear as firm red spots enlarging to form a circumscribed, bright red, raised, hot lesion. Petechiae, necrosis and blistering can occur if not treated early	Face, ears and lower legs

Figure 23.6 Common types of bacterial skin infections. ***Source:*** **Peate & Wild (2018).**

Yellow Flag **Psychosocial Impact of Skin Conditions**

Patients with visible dermatological conditions are more likely to have a poorer quality of life, suffer from depression, anxiety, low self-esteem, social isolation and suicidal thoughts compared to those who do not have such a condition. Treating the psychological impact is therefore as important as treating physical symptoms. Nursing associates can support patients in a variety of ways by showing compassion, empathy and excellent communication skills and by working alongside specialist practitioners (e.g. dermatology nurse consultants, specialist nurses and counsellors) to help with:

- Acceptance of the condition
- Managing treatment expectations of patient (and family)
- Finding coping strategies to deal with sometimes debilitating discomfort
- Finding the right words to explain their visible symptoms to others
- Regaining life satisfaction and improving self-esteem
- Engaging with the treatment process

Pressure Ulcers

By definition, a pressure ulcer is 'a localized damage to the skin and underlying soft tissue usually over a bony prominence or related to a medical or other device'. The injury can present as intact skin or an open ulcer and may be painful (National Pressure Ulcer Advisory Panel 2016). They can develop at any age, and it is simply a myth that they are only a problem in the elderly. See Figure 23.9 for a diagram on how pressure ulcers develop.

To carry out an accurate skin assessment, the nursing associate needs to understand and appreciate this definition. Without this, the patient may come to harm as a result of missed opportunity for implementation of preventative measures, leading to conflict with the values and principles set out in the 2018 NMC Code (Nursing and Midwifery Council 2018b). In the context of pressure ulcers and skin reassessment, the NMC Code (Nursing and Midwifery Council 2018b) alerts the nursing associate directly and indirectly at various points of the importance of skin assessment. For example:

- 1.2 make sure you deliver the fundamentals of care effectively
- 6.2 maintain the knowledge and skills you need for safe and effective practice
- 13.1 accurately identify, observe and assess signs of normal or worsening physical and mental health in the person receiving care
- 13.5 complete the necessary training before carrying out a new role
- 17.1 take all reasonable steps to protect people who are vulnerable or at risk from harm, neglect or abuse

Skin Assessment

According to the European Pressure Ulcer Advisory Panel (2016), ongoing assessment of the skin is necessary in order to detect early signs of pressure damage, especially over bony prominences. Following a structured risk assessment using an appropriate risk assessment tool (RAT), an individual identified to be 'at risk' of developing a pressure ulcer should be offered a full skin assessment. For nursing associates to carry out this assessment, they must have received adequate education and training about completing the assessment, how to identify a pressure ulcer and when and how to escalate for senior support. Furthermore, the nursing associate should have sufficient understanding that allows for a meaningful discussion with patients and carers about pressure ulcer prevention.

- Current guidelines by National Institute for Health and Care Excellence (2019) recommend that a skin assessment considers skin integrity in areas of pressure (commonly over bony prominences such as sacrum, ischial tuberosities, greater trochanters, shoulders and heels), variations in temperature condition and moisture, pain and discomfort reported by the patient as well as colour changes or discoloration. Figure 23.7 outlines the common sites for pressure ulcers.

Here are some examples indicative of (or associated with) pressure ulcer development the nursing associate should be alert to:

Skin Integrity in Areas of Pressure

Are there any signs of trauma (cuts, incisions or lacerations), bleeding, bruising, infection, benign or malignant lesions, scarring and evidence of healed pressure ulcers?

Variations

Temperature: does the high-risk area feel warmer or cooler to touch compared to adjacent skin?

Tissue consistency: does the area feel firm, soft, swollen, mushy or boggy? Is it dry, scaly or inflamed? Are there signs of induration (hardening of the skin)?

Moisture: has the at-risk area been exposed to high levels of moisture or humidity, for example, urine, faeces, wound exudate or sweat?

Pain and Discomfort

Does the patient report or display signs of pain, discomfort or tenderness during the carrying out of clinical procedures and at rest?

Colour Changes or Discoloration

One of the earliest signs of a pressure ulcer is a non-blanchable erythema (redness) that may present as a colour change or discolouration, particularly in darker skin tones. To determine if skin is blanching or not (non-blanching), the nursing associate should carry out a simple,

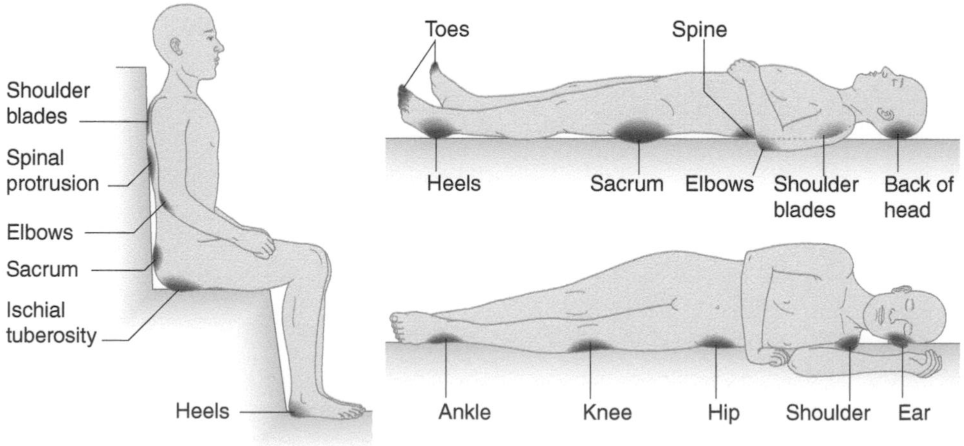

Figure 23.7 Common site for pressure ulcers. *Source:* Peate & Glencross (2015), figure 34.2, p. 74. © 2015 John Wiley & Sons, Ltd. Published 2015 by John Wiley & Sons, Ltd.

non-invasive test using gentle finger palpation or diascopy (using a disc of plastic or glass). This will determine whether the erythema or discolouration identified during the skin assessment is blanchable. If skin is non-blanchable, further assessment of the tissue is required to determine the extent of the pressure ulcer.

The pressure ulcer should be classified according to the level of tissue loss (European Pressure Ulcer Advisory Panel/National Pressure Ulcer Advisory Panel 2016). A consistent and accurate approach to definitions is essential to identify, treat and report pressure ulcers and also raise the profile of 'hidden' categories such as deep tissue injuries and medical devise damage (NHS Improvement 2018). Nursing associates therefore need to understand and follow the current categorisation (or staging) system recommended in international guidelines.

Pressure Ulcer Categories

Category 1: Non-Blanchable Erythema of Intact Skin

This stage is characterised by an intact skin with non-blanchable redness of a localised area usually over a bony prominence. This may be difficult to detect in darkly pigmented skin, but the colour may nevertheless still differ from the surrounding skin. It is important that nursing associates recognise, clearly document and report this redness as a category 1 pressure ulcer and not simply as 'redness'. Please note that colour changes at this stage do not include purple or maroon discoloration. These may indicate much deeper damage as a 'deep tissue injury'.

Category 2: Partial-Thickness Skin Loss with Exposed Epidermis

A category 2 pressure ulcer is one where there is partial-thickness skin loss presenting as a shallow, open ulcer with a red pink wound bed, without slough. This pressure ulcer may also present as an intact or open/ruptured serum-filled blister. Please note that blood-filled blisters do not fall into this section. The nursing associate must not use this category to describe skin abnormalities such as skin tears, burns, bruises or excoriation. See Figure 23.8 for an example of a category 2 pressure ulcer.

Category 3: Full-Thickness Skin Loss

In this stage, subcutaneous tissue may be visible, but bone, muscle or tendons are not exposed. Slough may be present but does not obscure the depth of the tissue loss. This stage may include undermining and tunnelling. Here, the nursing associate must be aware that the depth of the tissue damage varies by anatomical location. For example, a category 3 pressure ulcer at the bridge of the nose will be shallow due to the lack of subcutaneous tissue. In contrast, a Stage III pressure ulcer in an area with significant adipose (fat) tissue such as buttocks can develop deep wounds. In any event, underlying structures such as muscle, bones or tendons will not be visible or palpable.

Category 4: Full-Thickness Skin and Tissue Loss

This stage exhibits full-thickness skin and tissue loss where bone, tendon or muscle is exposed, and slough or eschar may be present on some parts of the wound bed. This category often included tunnelling or undermining (damage that also extends under the skin, beneath the wound opening). Like a category 3 pressure ulcer, the depth of the category 4 pressure ulcer varies by anatomical location. The nursing associate needs to be aware that these pressure ulcers can extend into the muscle and supporting structures such as fascia or joint capsules, making osteomyelitis (infection of the bone) possible. If slough or eschar obscures the extent of tissue loss, this is an 'unstageable pressure ulcer'.

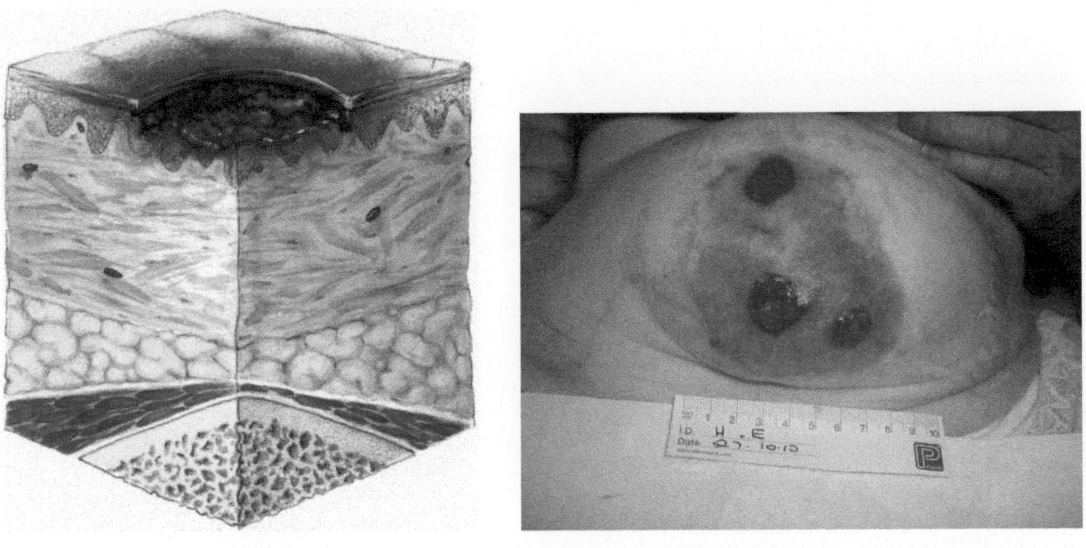

Figure 23.8 Stage II pressure ulcer. *Source:* Flanagan (2013). Reproduced with permission of John Wiley & sons Ltd.

Unstageable/Depth Unknown: Obscured Full-Thickness Skin and Tissue Loss

An unstageable pressure ulcer is a full-thickness skin loss in which the base of the ulcer is covered by slough and/or eschar in the wound bed. Slough can appear yellow, tan, brown, green or grey. Eschar will be brown, black or tan. For skin assessment, the nursing associate needs to appreciate that until the full depth of the wound bed is exposed through the removal of slough and/or eschar, the true stage of the pressure ulcer cannot be determined. The nursing associate should not attempt to categorise this type of pressure ulcer; instead, it must be recorded as 'unstageable/depth unknown'.

Suspected Deep Tissue Injury: Persistent Non-Blanchable Deep Red, Maroon or Purple Discoloration

The localised area will be purple or maroon coloured and present as intact skin or a blood-filled blister due to damage of underlying tissue. Pain and temperature change often precede skin colour changes. It is therefore important that the nursing associate assesses if the area feels firm or mushy, warmer or cooler compared to surrounding tissue and asks the patients if they experience any pain in the damaged area. This will help in the assessment process, particularly in individuals with dark skin tones in whom it may be difficult to detect deep tissue injuries.

Medical Device–Related Pressure Ulcer

Pressure ulcers related to medical device use are not a new category of pressure ulcer and should be classified according to level of tissue loss using the International National Pressure Ulcer Advisory Panel (NPUAP)/European Pressure Ulcer Advisory Panel (EPUAP) Pressure Ulcer Classification System. Commonly used equipment associated with this category are nasal cannulas, catheters, pulse oximeters and oxygen face masks.

Timing and Frequency of Reassessment in Accordance with Nice Guidance

Guidance about the timing of skin assessment has been available for many years, yet confusion, disparity and ritualistic practices remain a common problem in many healthcare settings. This, however, provides the nursing associate with an ideal opportunity to lead by example, educate and make a real difference to individuals at risk of developing a pressure ulcer (and to those with an existing pressure ulcer).

The initial skin assessment forms part of the initial pressure ulcer risk assessment and is carried out as soon as possible but no later than the first 6 hours of admission (or the first visit in community settings). Subsequent reassessments should be carried out effectively and appropriately timed. It is imperative that this is done in accordance with NICE guidelines. The nursing associate should conduct a comprehensive skin reassessment:

- As part of every pressure ulcer risk assessment.
- Ongoing assessment based on the clinical setting and the individual's degree of risk.
- In response to changes in an individual's condition (deterioration or improvement). If this occurs, the frequency of the reassessment needs to be increased appropriately.
- At least twice daily under and around medical devices (e.g. oxygen masks or indwelling urinary catheters).
- Prior to the individual's discharge.

Ideal opportunities for the nursing associate to carry out brief ad hoc skin reassessment include:

- Each time the patient is repositioned
- When hygiene needs are attended to (e.g. washing, bathing or showering a patient)
- When assisting a patient with their bowel or bladder needs

How to Carry Out an Effective Skin Assessment

- The principles of consent, dignity and privacy and duty of candour apply to skin assessment in the same way as they would for all other assessments. The standards outlined in the NMC Code (2018b) must be upheld by the nursing associate throughout.
- A skin assessment is an intimate and personal procedure that requires a sensitive, compassionate and caring approach from the nursing associate. Effective communication skills are of paramount importance here. This is to ensure that the individual assessed feels comfortable, at ease, protected and, most of all, safe.
- Remember to close doors, curtains or blinds; fully explain the assessment purpose and procedure to the patient; avoid interruption; expose only as much of the body as needed; and ensure that the room is warm enough to avoid the patient from feeling or getting cold and that lighting is adequate to allow for detection of changes in the skin colour.
- Remove footwear, socks and compression stockings prior to heel inspection.
- Remove bandages and dressings if safe to do so.
- Conduct a head-to-toe assessment with particular focus on skin overlying bony prominences including the sacrum, shoulders and ischial tuberosities, as well as areas a medical device could contribute to pressure ulcer development (e.g. catheter or oxygen masks).
- Assess skin temperature, changes in tissue consistency in relation to surrounding tissue and evidence of oedema during each reassessment.
- Apply the technique of either gentle finger palpation or diascopy (disk method) for identifying blanching response, localised heat, oedema and induration and differentiate whether the skin redness is blanchable or non-blanchable.
  - Finger palpation method: a finger is pressed gently on the redness for 3 seconds, and blanching is assessed following removal of the finger.
  - Diascopy (transparent disk method): a transparent disk is used to apply gentle pressure equally over an area of redness, and blanching can be observed underneath the disk.

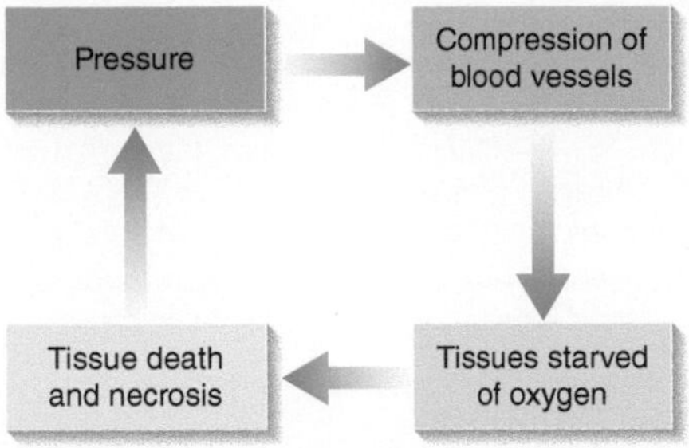

Figure 23.9 Pressure ulcer development. *Source:* Peate & Glencross (2015), figure 34.1, p. 74. © 2015 John Wiley & Sons, Ltd. Published 2015 by John Wiley & Sons, Ltd.

- Darkly pigmented skin: The nursing associate needs to be aware that Stage I pressure ulcers are underdetected in individuals with darkly pigmented skin because areas of redness are not easily identified. The nursing associate must therefore ask the patient about localised pain, discomfort or tenderness and palpate (touch) the skin to feel its temperature, consistency and moisture level and be observant to other variations indicative of pressure ulcer development.
- Ask all individuals who are able to respond reliably to report areas of localised pain, discomfort or tenderness. The use of a pain scale should be considered. For patients who are unable to respond and those unable to articulate their symptoms accurately, the nursing associate needs to apply other assessments appropriate to their needs. Assessments should also be carried out with cultural sensitivity in mind. For example, pain or emotions may be expressed differently in different cultures, and this can have a profound impact on the assessment and patient outcome. The nursing associate may need to modify questions and communication accordingly.

Green Flag

Pressure ulcers may occur as a result of neglect in both adults and children. Where concerns are raised regarding skin damage as a result of pressure, there is a requirement to raise it as a safeguarding concern within the organisation.

An adult at risk of developing a pressure ulcer as a result of neglect may be a person who:

- is elderly and frail due to ill health, physical disability or cognitive impairment,
- has a learning disability,
- has a physical disability and/or a sensory impairment,
- has mental health needs including dementia or a personality disorder,
- has a long-term illness/condition,
- misuses substances or alcohol and
- is unable to demonstrate the capacity to make a decision and is need of care and support.

(Department of Health and Social Care 2016)

Supporting Evidence

Richard developed an avoidable pressure ulcer during respite at a nursing home. The experience has inspired him and his carer wife Doreen to help inform and educate.

This is his story: www.nhs.stopthepressure.co.uk/patient-stories.html

Touch Point

Pressure ulcers are classified/staged according to the level of tissue loss using the current system recommended in the 'international guidelines' (European Pressure Ulcer Advisory Panel, National Pressure Ulcer Advisory Panel and Pan Pacific Pressure Injury Alliance 2014).

Category1/Stage I: Non-blanchable erythema
Category/Stage II: Partial-thickness skin loss
Category/Stage III: Full-thickness skin loss
Category/Stage IV: Full-thickness tissue loss
Unstageable: Depth unknown
Suspected deep tissue injury: Depth unknown
Medical device–related pressure ulcer

Take Note

Recognising early signs of pressure ulcer development is pivotal in the prevention of deeper and long-lasting skin damage. One of the earliest signs of a pressure ulcer is non-blanching erythema. It is important that nursing associates recognise, clearly document and report this redness as a Stage I pressure ulcer and not simply as 'redness'. By doing so, appropriate and patient-centred preventative measures can be implemented without unnecessary delay.

Documentation

Findings of all skin assessments must be documented clearly, legibly and unambiguously by the nursing associate. Both comprehensive and ad hoc reassessments need to be documented. Assessment tools and generic documentation and the manner in which they are recorded may, however, differ depending on the healthcare provider. In any event, nursing associates need to ensure that they have received adequate preparation to complete documentation accurately. Mistakes made at this stage are likely to lead to errors in subsequent care planning as well as care delivery, thus jeopardising the health and well-being of the individual.

There are many assessment and documentation tools available, and it is not possible to explore them all. For this reason, only a small selection of widely used tools will be discussed in the next section of this chapter.

Pressure Ulcer Risk Assessment

Before exploring a selection of pressure ulcer RATs, it is important to draw the attention of the nursing associate to the fact that there is no single universally used assessment tool. An abundance of RATs using a validated scale are available, all of varying levels of detail and complexity. What the nursing associate must remember is that RATs are merely 'aide-memoires', and clinical judgement is as much part of the assessment process as the use of the scale. Crucially, it is the action that follows that makes the difference to the individual. The action (e.g. repositioning, pressure relieving equipment, nutrition and hydration) must never be forgotten.

1. PURPOSE T: Pressure Ulcer Risk Primary or Secondary Evaluation Tool: Developed in 2015, it aims to identify adults at risk of pressure ulcer development in a hospital or community setting and make a distinction between primary prevention (applicable to 'at risk' patients) and secondary prevention (applicable to individuals who already have a pressure ulcer) (Nixon et al. 2015).
2. Norton: It was developed in the 1960s to identify 'at risk' adult patients. The scale contains five subscales ranging from 5 to 20. The lower the score, the higher the risk of developing pressure ulcers (Norton et al. 1962).
3. Waterlow: Developed in the mid-1980s and revised in 2005, it aims to assess pressure ulcer risk. The higher the score, the higher the risk (Waterlow 1985).
4. Braden: It was developed in the late 1980s to identify 'at risk' adult patients. The scale consists of six subscales, and the total scores range from 6 to 23. Generally, the lower the score, the higher the risk of developing pressure ulcers (Bergstrom et al. 1987a, 1987b).
5. Braden Q: It is an adaptation of the Braden scale for use in paediatric patients (Bergstrom et al. 1987a, 1987b).

Psoriasis Assessment

Psoriasis Area and Severity Index (PASI): The PASI assessment tool (Fredriksson & Pettersson 1978) combines the assessment of the area of body involved, including the head and neck, upper extremities, trunk and lower extremities. The following are the three signs of psoriasis used when scoring in PASI:

- The erythema (redness of the plaques)
- The amount of scaling
- The thickness of the plaques (induration)

Impact of Skin Disease Assessment

Dermatology Life Quality Index (DLQI): The DLQI (Finlay & Khan 1994) is a simple but reliable 10-question patient self-report questionnaire that assesses the impact of skin disease on a person's overall quality of life over the last week. It asks, for example, about the impact of the skin disease on activities such as shopping or gardening, a person's choice of clothing, as well as the impact on relationships with partners, friends or family. The questionnaire should be completed unaided unless there is confusion about its content.

Occupational Skin Disease Questionnaire

In Europe, skin diseases such as work-related contact dermatitis, contact urticaria and infections are the second most common occupational diseases after musculoskeletal conditions (Health and Safety Executive 2018). A variety of tools are available to question factors such environmental exposure, type of work, demographics, occupational history, atopic symptoms, self-reported hand or forearm eczema, exacerbating factors, consequences and impact of the condition on quality of life.

Body Maps

The purpose of 'body mapping' is to complement the recording of findings ascertained during the skin assessment. A body map is a valuable tool that can be used in addition to other forms of written documentation or visual recording (photography). In its simplest form, it will contain two outlines of the body, labelled 'front' and 'back' (see Figure 23.10). The nursing associate will document a minimum of two patient identifiers such as the patient's name and date of birth (World Health Organisation 2007) before proceeding to record information such as general appearance, location, type, colour, smell and number or size of skin changes by:

- Drawing on the map
- Providing a brief description of each of the findings (e.g. what you see and what it feels like)

If visual recording (photography) is used alongside written documentation, the nursing associate needs to respect and follow ethical principles of consent and confidentiality as outlined in the NMC Code (Nursing and Midwifery Council 2018b). Specific consent may be required especially if a patient does not have capacity. Obtaining this type of consent may fall outside the limitations of the nursing associate's role and may need to be gained by a doctor or specialist nurse. For this, the nursing associate needs to be familiar with and follow relevant local and national guidelines. In any event, photographs taken as part of patients' care are part of their medical record and must be treated in the same way as any other medical records (General Medical Council 2013).

Touch Point

Every pressure ulcer risk assessment needs to include a head-to-toe assessment of the skin, and findings need to be accurately recorded. However, there is no universally approved documentation tool, and tools are merely an 'aide-memoire' to be used in conjunction with sound clinical judgement.

Take Note

Skin assessment forms part of every pressure ulcer risk assessment, but crucially, it is the action that follows that makes the difference to the individual.

Touch Points Revisited

Nursing associates play an integral part in holistic skin reassessment of patients in a variety of settings.

Skin reassessment is undertaken in a skilled, confident and compassionate manner, requiring underpinning knowledge and understanding of key considerations such as factors affecting the skin, common skin conditions or the identification and escalation of early signs of pressure ulcer.

Working competently and effectively within the multidisciplinary team, nursing associates are making a valid contribution to the physiological and psychological management of patients at risk of skin damage and to those with existing skin problems.

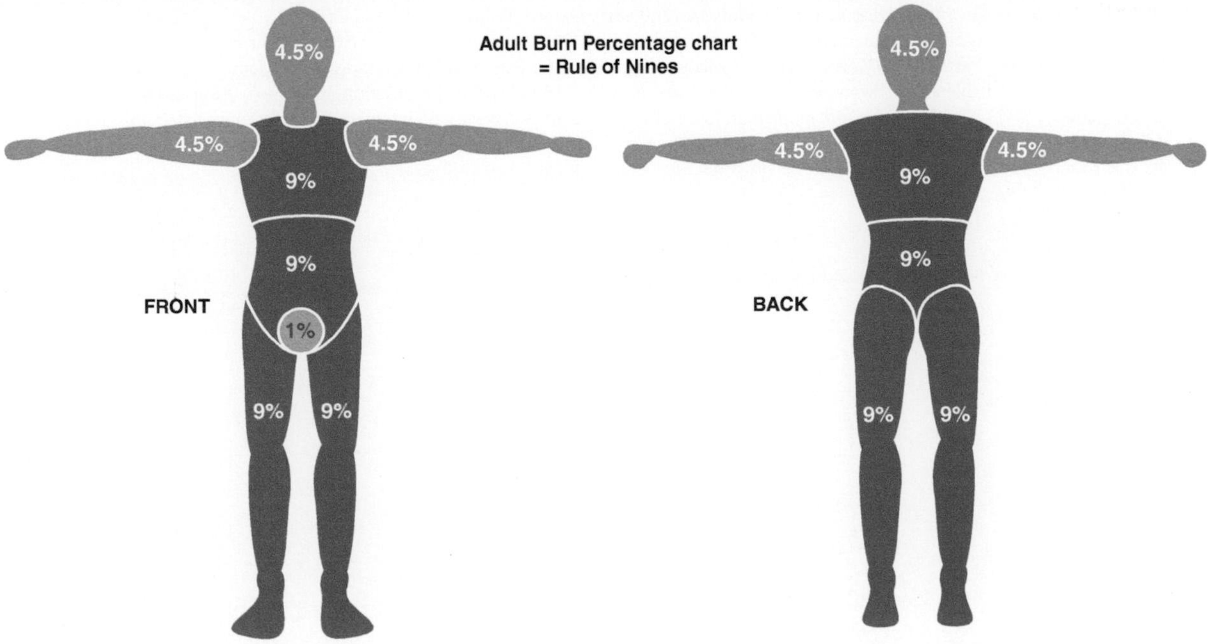

Figure 23.10 An example of a body map. *Source:* adapted from Burns & Scalds, in Peate & Glencross (2015), figure 45.2, p. 97.

References

Arndt, K.A., Hsu, J.T.S., Alam, M., Bhatia, A.C. and Chilukuri, S. (2015) *Manual of dermatologic therapeutics, Wolters Kluwer Health*, 2014. ProQuest Ebook Central. [online] Available: https://ebookcentral-proquest-com.salford.idm.oclc.org/lib/salford/detail.action?docID=2031621. Accessed 1 October 2019.

Bergstrom, N., Braden, B.J., Laguzza, A. and Holman, V. (1987a) The Braden scale for predicting pressure sore risk, *Nursing Research*, 36(4): 205–210.

Bergstrom, N., Demuth, P.J. and Braden, B.J. (1987b) A clinical trial of the Braden scale for predicting pressure sore risk, *Nursing Clinics of North America*, 22(2): 417–429.

Buxton, P.K. & Morris-Jones, R. (2013) *ABC Dermatology*, 5th edn. John Wiley & Sons Ltd, Chichester.

Department of Health and Social Care. (2016) Safeguarding adults' protocol, *Pressure ulcers and the interface with a safeguarding enquiry*, London: Department of Health and Social Care. Crown (2016) Published to gov.uk. [online] Available: https://assets.publishing.service.gov.uk/government/uploads/system/uploads/attachment_data/file/756243/safeguarding-adults-protocol-pressure-ulcers.pdf. Accessed 6 October 2019.

European Pressure Ulcer Advisory Panel. (2016) Prevention and treatment of pressure ulcers, *Quick reference guide*. [online] Available: http://www.epuap.org/wp-content/uploads/2016/10/quick-reference-guide-digital-npuap-epuap-pppia-jan2016.pdf. Accessed 3 October 2019.

European Pressure Ulcer Advisory Panel, National Pressure Ulcer Advisory Panel and Pan Pacific Pressure Injury Alliance. (2014) *Prevention and treatment of pressure ulcers: clinical practice guideline*, Osborne Park, Western Australia: Cambridge Media.

Finlay, A.Y. and Khan, G.K. (1994) Dermatology life quality index (DLQI): a simple practical measure for routine clinical use, *Clinical and Experimental Dermatology*, 19(3): 210–216.

Flanagan, M. (2013) *Wound Healing and Skin Integrity. Principles and Practice*. John Wiley & Sons, Chichester.

Fredriksson, T. and Pettersson, U. (1978) Severe psoriasis--oral therapy with a new retinoid, *Dermatologica*, 157(4): 238–244.

General Medical Council. (2013) *Making and using visual and audio recordings of patients*. [online] Available: https://www.gmc-uk.org/-/media/documents/making-and-using-visual-and-audio-recordings-of-patients_pdf-58838365.pdf?la=en. Accessed 6 October 2019.

Goicoechea-Balbona, A. (1997) Culturally specific health care model for ensuring health care use by rural, ethnically diverse families affected by HIV/AIDS, *Health and Social Work*, 1997(22): 172–180.

Health and Safety Executive. (2018) *Work-related skin disease in Great Britain, crown (2018) health and safety executive V1 10/18*. [online] Available: http://www.hse.gov.uk/statistics/causdis/dermatitis/skin.pdf. Accessed 6 October 2019.

National Institute for Health and Care Excellence. (2012) *Psoriasis, the assessment and management of psoriasis*. [online] Available: https://www.nice.org.uk/guidance/cg153. Accessed 15 September 2019.

National Pressure Ulcer Advisory Panel. (2016) *NPUAP pressure injury stages*. [online] Available: https://npuap.org/page/PressureInjuryStages. Accessed 6 October 2019.

NHS Improvement. (2018) *Pressure ulcers: revised definition and measurement. Summary and recommendations, London: NHS Improvement. [online]* Available: https://improvement.nhs.uk/documents/2932/NSTPP_summary__recommendations_2.pdf. Accessed 6 October 2019.

Nixon, J., Nelson, E.A., Rutherford, C., Coleman, S., Muir, D., Keen, J., McCabe, C., Dealey, C., Briggs, M., Brown, S., Collinson, M., Hulme, C.T., Meads, D.M., McGinnis, E., Patterson, M., Czoski-Murray, C., Pinkney, L., Smith, I.L., Stevenson, R., Stubbs, N., Wilson, L. and Brown, J.M. (2015) *Pressure ulcer programme of research (PURPOSE): using mixed methods (systematic reviews, prospective cohort, case study, consensus and psychometrics) to identify patient and organisational risk, develop a risk assessment tool and patient-reported outcome Quality of Life and Health Utility measures*, Southampton (UK): NIHR Journals Library; 2015 Sep. [online] Available: https://www.ncbi.nlm.nih.gov/books/NBK321049/. Accessed 3 October 2019.

Norton, D., McLaren, R. and Exon Smith, A. (1962) *An investigation of geriatric nursing problems in hospital* (1st edn), London: Churchill Livingstone.

Nursing and Midwifery Council. (2018) *Standards of proficiencies for nursing associates*. [online] Available: https://www.nmc.org.uk/globalassets/sitedocuments/education-standards/nursing-associates-proficiency-standards.pdf. Accessed 3 October 2019.

Nursing and Midwifery Council. (2018b) *The code - professional standards of practice and behaviour for nurses, midwives and nursing associates*. [online] Available: https://www.nmc.org.uk/globalassets/sitedocuments/nmc-publications/nmc-code.pdf. Accessed 3 October 2019.

Peate, I. and Glencross, W. (2015) *Wound care at a glance*, Oxford: Wiley.

Peate, I. and Nair, M. (2015) *Anatomy and physiology for nurses at a glance* (1st edn), Oxford: Wiley.

Peate, I. and Wild, K. (eds) (2018) *Nursing practice: knowledge and care* (2nd edn), Oxford: Wiley.

The Mental Capacity Act. (2005) [online] Available: www.legistation.gov.uk/ukpga/2005/9/contents. Accessed 6 September 2020.

World Health Organisation. (2007) *Patient identification,* WHO Collaborating Centre for Patient Safety Solutions Aide Memoire, Patient Safety Solutions (2007) PS-Solution2.pdf. [online] Available: https://www.who.int/patientsafety/solutions/patientsafety/PS-Solution2.pdf?ua=1. Accessed 6 October 2019.

World Health Organisation. (2018) *Housing and health guidelines*. [online] Available: https://www.who.int/sustainable-development/publications/housing-health-guidelines/en/. Accessed 6 September 2020.

Waterlow, J. (1985) A risk assessment card, *Nursing Times*, 81(48): 49–55.

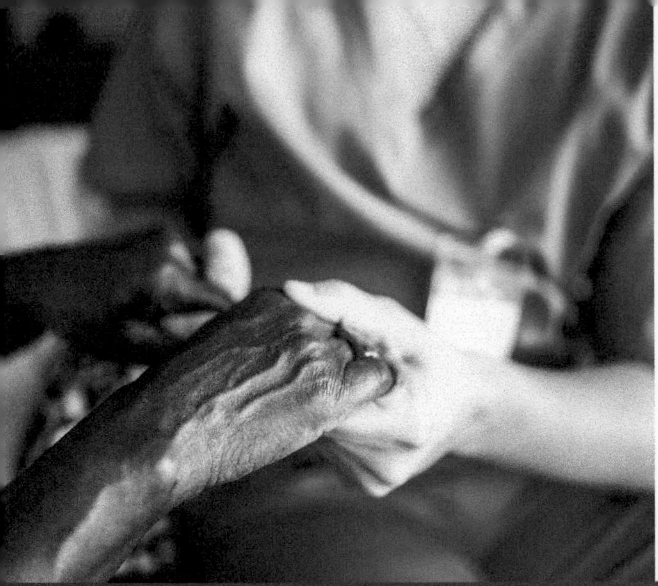

24

Supporting a Person's Skin Integrity

Nicole Blythe

University of Salford, UK

Chapter Aim

- This chapter aims to provide the reader with the knowledge, skills and behaviours required to implement approaches needed to support a person's skin integrity.

Learning Outcomes

By the end of this chapter, the reader will be able to:

- Consider factors affecting skin integrity
- Describe key considerations and the role of the nursing associate in supporting skin integrity
- Discuss a range of contemporary approaches to support and manage skin integrity through the appropriate use of products

Test Yourself Multiple Choice Questions

1. Moisture can affect a person's skin integrity.
   A) True
   B) False
2. Supporting skin integrity may require the nursing associate to support a patient referral to:
   A) Continence Advise Services
   B) Tissue viability specialist nurse
   C) Dermatology nurse consultant
   D) Job centre
3. Holistic skin assessment should include a:
   A) Radial pulse check
   B) Visual inspection of bony prominences
   C) Moving and handling risk assessment
   D) Blood test

The Nursing Associate's Handbook of Clinical Skills, First Edition. Edited by Ian Peate.

Companion website: www.wiley.com/nursingassociate

4. **Intrinsic factors affecting skin integrity include (tick all that apply):**
   A) **Malnutrition**
   B) **Endocrine comorbidities**
   C) **Pressure**
   D) **Sunshine**
5. **At the point of registration, a nursing associate is required to (tick all that apply):**
   A) **Observe and reassess skin and hygiene status using contemporary approaches to determine the need for support and ongoing intervention**
   B) **Prevent and manage skin breakdown through appropriate use of products**
   C) **Observe and reassess skin and hygiene status using contemporary approaches**
   D) **Use appropriate positioning and pressure relieving techniques**

Introduction

In this chapter, holistic care and support to maintain a person's skin integrity is considered. It will discuss how skin integrity can be managed through the delivery of conservative nursing actions as well as the appropriate use of products.

The Nursing and Midwifery Council (2018a) Standards of Proficiency require the nursing associate to be able to provide care to support the maintenance of skin integrity at the point of registration.

Skin is the largest organ of the body. It is made up of three main layers: epidermis, dermis and subcutaneous tissue. Every square inch of skin contains millions of cells and hundreds of sweat glands, sebaceous (oil) glands, blood vessels and nerve endings (Thibodeau & Patterson 2008). Figure 24.1 shows the three layers of the skin and glands.

Skin provides a protective barrier against mechanical, thermal and physical injury, infections and hazardous substances. It prevents loss of moisture, reduces harmful effects of ultraviolet radiation and acts as a sensory organ. It also helps to regulate temperature, synthesises vitamin D and acts as a medium for communication and aesthetics.

There are many different factors affecting skin integrity such as physical, environmental, emotional, psychological, social and economic. Factors are often interlinked, and if not rectified, resolved or reduced, skin integrity may not be maintained, improved or restored. Table 24.1 highlights factors affecting skin integrity, and Figure 24.2 shows a visual illustration of how factors can affect each other.

Take Note

Skin is not only the largest organ in the body, it is also a major sensory organ. Skin expresses emotions detectable by others through pallor, coldness, 'goose bumps', redness, warmth or sweating. It is visible and can be touched by self and others. Today and throughout history, people with visible skin disorders have often been stigmatised or even treated as outcasts bringing carried a much higher psychological or emotional burden. To support a person's skin integrity, factors affecting skin integrity need to be understood. However, whilst science has a good understanding of how, for example, mechanical or environmental factors affect skin, little is still known about how the mind can influence the skin and skin disorders.

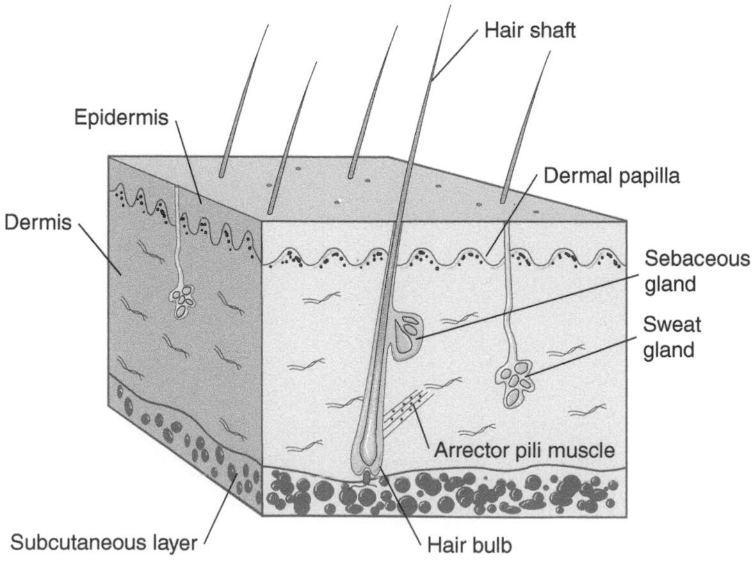

Figure 24.1 **Three layers of the skin sweat and sebaceous glands.** *Source:* Peate & Nair (2017). John Wiley & Sons, Incorporated, 2nd edition.

Table 24.1 Some factors underpinning skin integrity.

FACTOR	EXAMPLE
Economical	Finances (low income) impacting on food choices, footwear, bedding, personal and household cleaning products
Emotional	Worries and fears, bereavement, pain, loneliness, unmet religious or spiritual needs
Environmental	Pressure, friction, moisture, pollution, chemicals, allergens, irritants such as fragrances
Physical	Age, gender, weight, internal disease and comorbidities, infections, genetics, medication, trauma
Psychological	Stress, anxiety, neurological conditions, mental health issues, impaired mental capacity
Social	Poor housing/living conditions, overcrowding, loneliness, social isolation, lifestyle

Source: Based on Arndt et al. (2015).

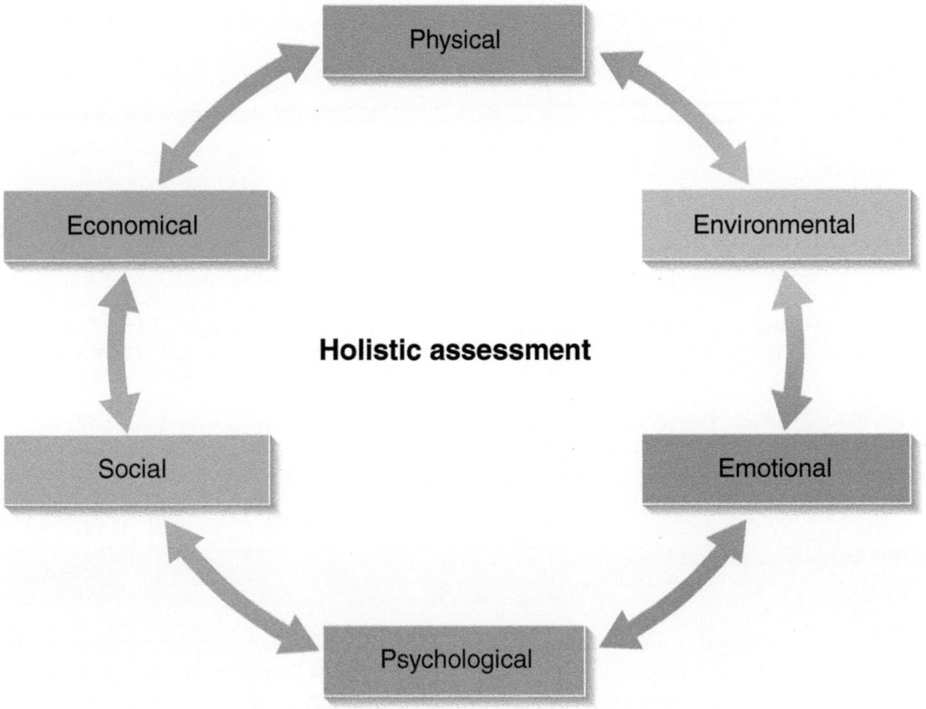

Figure 24.2 Factors affecting skin integrity. ***Source:*** **Peate & Glencross (2015), figure 10.1, p. 22. Wiley & Sons 2015.**

Supporting Evidence

Skin stories: The stories shared by individuals affected by skin disease can be found in the following websites:
https://www.britishskinfoundation.org.uk/blogs/case-studies
https://www.melanomauk.org.uk/pages/category/patient-stories
https://www.skinhealthinfo.org.uk/getting-treated/patient-journeys/

Touch Point

Supporting a person's skin integrity requires the nursing associate to understand the impact of factors that can affect the skin. For skin integrity to be maintained, improved or restored, affecting factors need to be identified and eliminated. If this is not possible, then as minimum, they should be reduced.

The nursing associate is required to care for people in various care settings. These care settings can include caring for people in their own homes, residential care settings, outpatient departments, general practice, places of detention and those without homes (the homeless).

Violet Flag 'Sleeping Rough' and Skin Health

Homelessness is a growing problem in much of the world including the United Kingdom. Death rates amongst people sleeping rough is high and so is the rate of co-occurring health problems such as drug and alcohol addiction, mental health problems, heart and lung disease and skin disorders (Office for National Statistics 2019). Skin health is often significantly compromised due to poor physical health including malnutrition and vitamin deficiencies as a result of poor diet, dehydration, high levels of stress and difficulty maintaining personal hygiene. Precursors for good health including the access to adequate sanitation infrastructure, showers and handwashing facilities are limited or not available at all. Poor mental health and substance misuse can either impact on skin integrity, which may become worse under stress, or on a person's motivation or ability to maintain their own skin health. Additional physical or mental disabilities and/or cognitive or visual impairment often exacerbate the problem.

An understanding of the needs of the rough sleeping person is essential as is respect for the complexity of the task. The nursing associate can support healthy skin in this highly vulnerable group of people by participating in the provision of practical advice about:

- Skin assessment: check own skin (and feet) for changes such as infections; bacterial, viral or fungal infestation; irritations or rashes; injuries and trauma; vascular problems or maceration
- Keeping skin clean and dry (dry clothes, socks and shoes) and how to apply topical treatment
- Nutrition (high calorie, high protein, staying hydrated, local emergency hot/cold food supplies)
- Accessing local services: emergency accommodations (hostels, night shelters), public wash and toilet facilities, food banks, homeless support services
- Accessing primary care and allied health services (general practitioner (GP), dietician, podiatrist, pharmacist, dentist, smoking cessation, sexual health, mental health in-reach and out-reach teams).

Source: (Public Health England 2019).

Supporting Evidence

Supporting homeless people to access health care:

- National Health Service (NHS) England has produced a leaflet that people who are homeless can use when they need to register with a GP.
- Read this case study on a new approach to engaging the rough sleeping and homeless community to attend tuberculosis screening session: https://www.gov.uk/government/case-studies/new-approach-to-engaging-rough-sleeping-and-homeless-community

Real-life homeless stories:

- https://www.crisis.org.uk/get-involved/everybody-in/real-life-homeless-stories/?sb=date
- https://centrepoint.org.uk/youth-homelessness/real-stories/
- https://blog.shelter.org.uk/2014/12/the-christmas-story-of-homeless-children/

Key Considerations

The skin, a multifunctional organ, is affected by many different factors. Before the nursing associate implements any actions to support skin integrity, the effects of potential factors impacting on the person's skin integrity must be reviewed. Simply identifying a skin abnormality or making a subjective judgement about how 'at risk' a person may develop skin breakdown will not allow for the implementation of appropriate and individualised supporting actions; this may indeed cause the individual unnecessary harm and suffering, for example, developing a pressure ulcer. It is crucial that this review is carried out in a logical and concise manner prior to planning and implementing supporting measures (Brown & Flanagan 2013).

Prevention of Skin Breakdown

1. Identify causes responsible for skin breakdown
   a. For example, pressure, shear, friction, increased skin moisture, poor nutrition, poor oxygenation and perfusion
2. Review and act on skin status
   a. Consider skin turgor, elasticity, hydration status (dehydration/oedema), fragility and vulnerability (newborn skin to aging skin)
   b. Identify skin irritations, rashes, acute and/or chronic skin disease, blistering
3. Review the hygiene status of the individual and implement supporting actions
4. Review continence status and implement supporting interventions
   a. Urinary incontinence
   b. Faecal incontinence
   c. A combination of urinary and faecal incontinence
5. Review and act on activity/mobility status
   a. Use appropriate positioning and pressure-relieving techniques
   b. Determine an individualised repositioning frequency considering tissue tolerance, level of activity and mobility, general medical condition, overall treatment objectives, skin condition and comfort

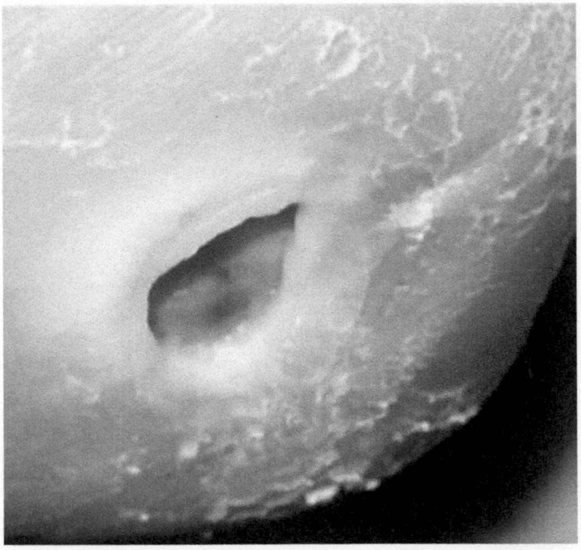

Figure 24.3 **Pressure ulcer to the plantar aspect of the heel. *Source:* Karen Ousey & Caroline McIntosh (2009). Reproduced with permission of John Wiley & Sons Ltd.**

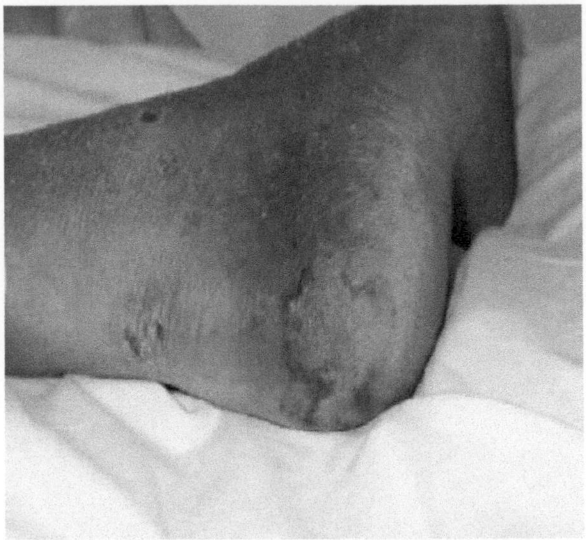

Figure 24.4 **Pressure ulcer to the heel. *Source:* Karen Ousey & Caroline McIntosh (2009). Reproduced with permission of John Wiley & Sons Ltd.**

   c. Apply correct moving and handling techniques
   d. Consider the impact of mobility limitations on pressure ulcer risk and avoid positioning the individual on an area of redness (erythema) whenever possible
   e. Consider the appropriateness of support surface (mattress) or seating equipment (e.g. chair, stool, seat cover or cushion)
6. Use only appropriate products to prevent and manage skin integrity
7. Provide adequate nutrient and hydration
   a. Complete nutritional assessment and screening using a valid and reliable screening tool such as the Malnutrition Universal Screening Tool (MUST) (British Association for Parenteral and Enteral Nutrition 2003) and take into consideration factors affecting unintended weight changes such as stress or medication (e.g. steroids)
   b. Consider the person's ability to eat and drink independently and assist if they cannot do so on their own
   c. Ensure the person is adequately nourished and hydrated (e.g. calories, protein, vitamins and minerals, fluid requirements)
   d. Develop and follow an individualised nutritional care plan
8. Review skin of individuals 'at risk' or with an existing pressure ulcer
   Skin assessment in relation to pressure ulcers has already been discussed in Chapter 23. Here is a brief summary of key points:
   - Skin assessment is necessary in order to detect early signs of pressure damage, especially over bony prominences.
   - Moisture from incontinence can cause the skin to become macerated or excoriated. Once this occurs, skin is much more vulnerable to the effects of pressure and/or shear. The person is, therefore, at greater and faster risk of pressure ulcer development.
   - For a nursing associate to carry out this assessment, they must have received adequate education and training about completing the assessment, how to identify a pressure ulcer and when and how to escalate for senior support.
   - Skin assessment should consider skin integrity in areas of pressure (commonly over bony prominences such as sacrum, ischial tuberosities, greater trochanters, shoulders and heels), variations in temperature, condition and moisture, pain and discomfort reported by the patient as well as colour changes or discoloration (European Pressure Ulcer Advisory Panel 2016).
   - Nursing associates should have sufficient understanding that allows for a meaningful discussion with patients and carers about skin assessment and pressure ulcer prevention.

Figures 24.3 and 24.4 are reminders of what pressure ulcers can look like, and Figures 24.5 and 24.6 demonstrate category 4 pressure ulcers that originated poorly managed moisture lesions.

Moisture Lesions

Excessive moisture combined with the acidic nature of bodily fluids easily disrupts the barrier properties of the stratum corneum (in the epidermis). This can cause maceration or excoriation, leaving the skin vulnerable to injury and infection (Beeckman et al. 2015). It is important to note that skin damage from moisture is not a pressure ulcer, but the presence of skin damage from moisture can increase the risk of pressure ulceration. Skin, therefore, needs to be protected with the use of a barrier product and/or moisturised using a skin moisturiser to hydrate dry skin in order to reduce risk of skin damage.

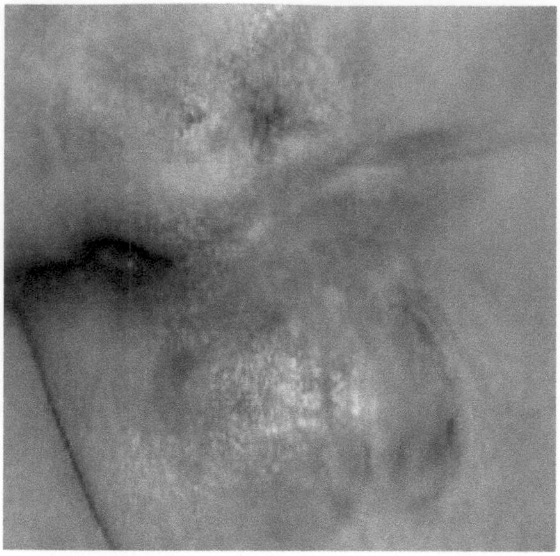

Figure 24.5 Incontinence-associated dermatitis. *Source:* Ian Peate & Wyn Glencross (2015). Reproduced with permission of John Wiley & Sons Ltd.

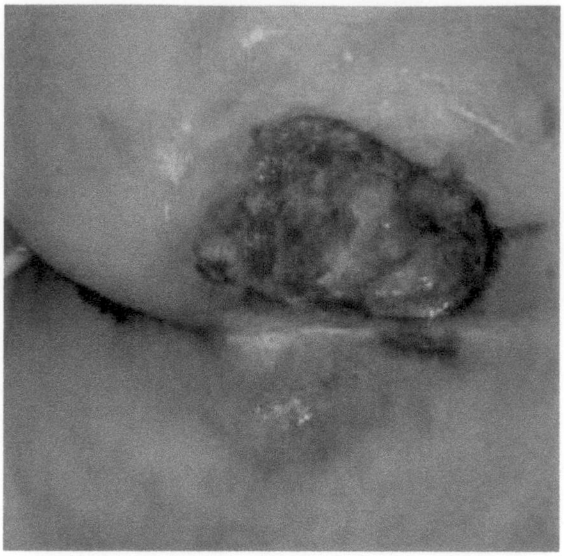

Figure 24.6 Pressure ulcer exacerbated by moisture lesion. *Source:* Ian Peate & Wyn Glencross (2015). Reproduced with permission of John Wiley & Sons Ltd.

Red Flag Incontinence-Associated Dermatitis

Incontinence-associated dermatitis (IAD), a painful and distressing condition, is largely preventable. It presents as inflammation and/or disruption of skin integrity due to urinary or faecal incontinence, or combination of both. Excessive moisture combined with the acidic bodily fluids easily disrupts the barrier properties of the stratum corneum (in the epidermis). This can cause maceration or excoriation, leaving the skin vulnerable to injury and infection (Beeckman et al. 2015). IAD is a form of moisture lesion, but the two should not be confused. A *moisture lesion* is a general term used for all damage caused by any excessive moisture including damage caused by wound exudate, perspiration, vomit, urine or a combination, whilst *IAD* is a specific term used only to describe damage associated with urine or stool (Ousey et al. 2012). Figure 24.5 shows the red, wet skin of IAD.

IAD and category 2 pressure ulcers are two very different skin conditions, yet due to the similarity in appearance, the two are frequently mistaken or misdiagnosed. This can then lead to inappropriate treatment and management of the damaged skin, which can cause unnecessary suffering and have a negative impact on the individual's quality of life. It is crucial that the nursing associate understands the differences between the two conditions, their causes, preventative measures as well as treatment choices. This can ensure that the person receives the most appropriate treatment intervention (Mahoney 2019).

Using Appropriate Products to Prevent and Manage Skin Breakdown

Cleansing Vulnerable Skin

See Table 24.2 that demonstrates an example of a good skin cleansing regimen.

Emollients

Emollients are grease-based products and are generally indicated for all skin conditions that cause dry or scaling skin (e.g. psoriasis, eczema, pruritus). They can help to repair, hydrate or soothe the skin. It is believed that emollients work in two ways:

1. By either preventing water loss from the skin and
2. By penetrating deep into the skin (stratum corneum) and mimicking its natural barrier effect.

To prevent and manage skin breakdown, an emollient can be used during washing as a soap substitute to maintain the normal pH level of the skin, or immediately after washing to moisturise skin. They should be applied in the direction of hair growth to reduce the risk of folliculitis. If the emollient is kept in a tub, a clean spoon or spatula must be used to remove the preparation to avoid bacterial contamination (Joint Formulary Committee 2019). The choice of an appropriate emollient depends on:

- The severity of the condition
- Site of application
- Patient preference
- Cosmetic acceptability or tolerability.

Table 24.3 shows the most common emollient types.

Table 24.2 An example of a good skin cleansing regimen.

Cleanse	• Use a pH neutral cleanser/soap substitute after each episode of incontinence • Avoid aggressive rubbing of the area during drying
Protect	• Select an appropriate barrier product according to severity of incontinence and skin damage • Ensure that the skin regimen is reviewed at regular intervals to evaluate effectiveness of interventions
Restore	• Replenish lipid barrier function of the skin by using emollients, adding barrier product if required

Source: Mahoney (2019).

Table 24.3 Emollient types and descriptions.

EMOLLIENT TYPES	DEFINITION
Bath additives	Added to water (bath or basin) and are not rinsed off
Soap substitutes	Have cleansing properties and are rinsed off the skin
Lotions	Topical application: Contain the least amount of grease and oil and are the lightest and most easily absorbed
Creams	Topical application: Higher oil content than lotion, which is absorbed by the skin
Ointments	Topical application: High grease and oil content. Is the most obvious when applied, tends to sit on top of the skin longer before absorption and can stain clothing Ointments are effective for very dry skin

Source: Dingwall (2010).

The following are the side effects and risks associated with emollients:

- Increased temperature due to interference with the body's natural ability to sweat and cool down,
- Increased risk of slipping in the bath or shower,
- Contact dermatitis,
- Folliculitis (inflammation of the hair follicle) and
- Allergic reaction caused by the preservatives (usually in creams).

The nursing associate should note that there is a risk of severe and fatal burns with paraffin-containing and paraffin-free emollients. There is a fire risk with all paraffin-containing emollients, regardless of paraffin concentration, and it cannot be excluded with paraffin-free emollients.

Nursing associates should advise patients not to smoke or go near naked flames as clothing, bedding, dressings and or other fabrics that have been in contact with an emollient or emollient-treated skin can rapidly ignite (Medicines and Healthcare Products Regulatory Agency 2018).

Barrier Products

Barrier products can be used on intact skin to prevent skin breakdown. They are commonly used on the skin around wounds, stomas and areas at risk of pressure ulcer development (usually over bony prominences). Barrier products can help prevent skin breakdown caused by moisture (urine, faeces, sweat, etc.) by providing a water-repellent barrier. They are NOT a substitute for adequate nursing care (Joint Formulary Committee 2019).

The most common types of barrier products are creams, films and sprays. Figure 24.7 demonstrates a range of barrier products.

Skin Cleansers

There is an abundance of skin cleansers available, ranging from the humble bar of soap to prescription-only products. Much will depend on the person's skin condition, underlying skin disease as well as personal preference and acceptability of a specific product. Before selecting a specific product, the nursing associate should consider what they are trying to achieve and why the use of a skin cleanser is indicated: Is it to treat a skin condition? Is its use preventative? Or is it simply to meet the fundamental hygiene needs of a person who is unable to do this independently but has otherwise healthy skin not with risk of breaking down.

There is evidence that harsh surfactants such as sodium lauryl sulphate (SLS) used in skin cleansers, shampoos or moisturisers are damaging to the skin barrier causing burning, stinging, itching or redness (British Association of Dermatologists 2019). It is recommended that people with compromised skin (e.g. atopic dermatitis) use mild, unperfumed, pH-neutral wash products with some emollient ingredients. An emollient cream (not containing SLS) can be used as a soap substitute, or as an alternative, an emollient bath oil or shower product may be preferred. Aqueous cream may still be used as a wash-off soap substitute, but its use as a leave-on moisturiser is no longer advised because it contains SLS (National Institute for Health and Care Excellence 2017). Table 24.4 outlines considerations for cleaning the compromised skin.

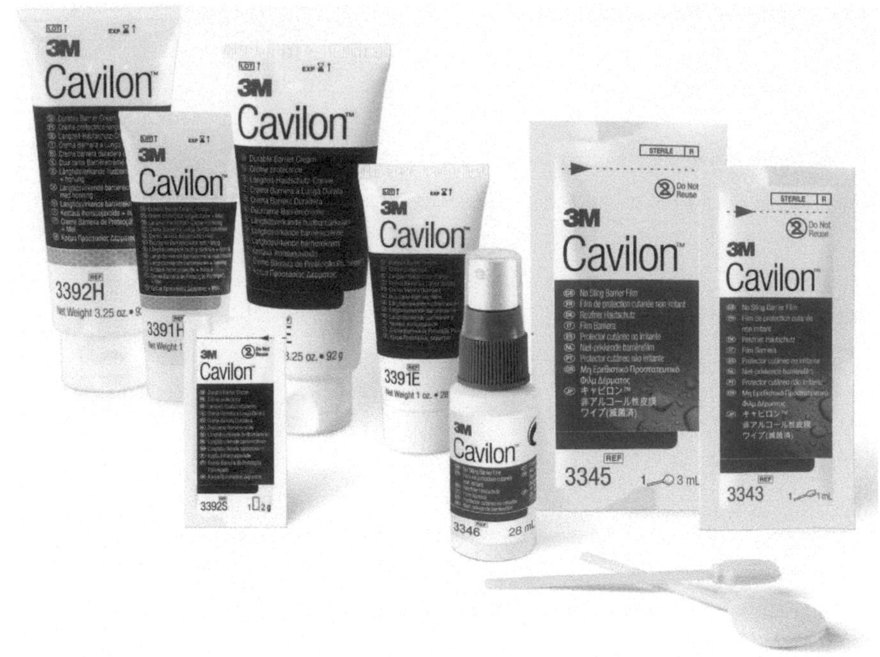

Figure 24.7 The Cavilon range of products, which act to protect the skin from excessive moisture, e.g. from body fluids. *Source:* Ian Peate & Wyn Glencross (2015). Reproduced with permission of John Wiley & Sons Ltd.

Table 24.4 Cleaning the compromised skin.

- Offer the individual a choice of unperfumed emollients to use every day for washing, bathing and moisturising
- Encourage the use of emollients and/or emollient wash products instead of soaps and detergent-based wash products
- Consider the use of emollients and/or emollient wash products instead of shampoo, and avoid washing hair in bath water
- Consider and offer alternative products if a particular one causes skin irritations such as stinging, burning, itching or redness
- On discharge from hospital or in the community, encourage the person to ensure availability and accessibility of the chosen skin care product in workplace, school, nursery, leisure or sports facilities or when on holiday
- To avoid wasting resources, it is reasonable to use low-cost, SLS-free products although some patients may need more complex and expensive products due to allergies, infections or irritations
- Offer educational support for self-care and self-use of skin cleanser
- If a person with compromised skin has a physical disability, or cognitive or visual impairment, offer advice and practical support about skin cleaning taking into account the person's individual needs.

Source: Modified from British Association of Dermatologists (2019).

Green Flag

Nursing associates support and manage the skin integrity of people of all ages, from different background, cultures and beliefs. To do this effectively, they must follow the four themes of The Code:

1. Prioritise people
2. Practice effectively
3. Preserve safety
4. Promote professionalism and trust.

They must also be able to carry out procedure outlined in Annexe B: *Procedures to be undertaken by the nursing associate*. Here are some of the skills the nursing associate needs to be proficient in when supporting a person's skin integrity:

1.6 Recognise and escalate signs of all forms of abuse

2.3 Use appropriate positioning and pressure-relieving techniques

2.4 Take appropriate action to ensure privacy and dignity at all times

3.1 Observe and reassess skin and hygiene status using contemporary approaches to determine the need for support and ongoing intervention

3.4 Prevent and manage skin breakdown through appropriate use of products

3.5 Identify and manage skin irritations and rashes

3.6 Monitor wounds and undertake wound care using appropriate evidence-based techniques

5.1 Observe and monitor the level of urinary and bowel continence to determine the need for ongoing support and intervention, the level of independence and self-management of care that an individual can manage

5.2 Assist with toileting, maintaining dignity

10.3 Exercise professional accountability in ensuring the safe administration of medicines to those receiving care

Table 24.5 Medications to support skin integrity.

Topical therapies	• emollients • topical steroids • antihistamines • antiseptics • topical antibiotics
Oral therapies	• antihistamines for symptomatic relief • antibiotics (e.g. flucloxacillin) for bacterial infections • antifungals (e.g. fluconazole) • antivirals (e.g. aciclovir) for secondary herpes infection • immunosuppressants (e.g. oral prednisolone, azathioprine, ciclosporin)

Source: Modified from British Association of Dermatologists (2019).

Medications to Support Skin Integrity

The nursing associate must meet and adhere to all procedural competencies required by the NMC when administering medicines and exercise professional accountability in ensuring safe administration to those receiving care (Nursing and Midwifery Council 2018a).

When supporting a person's skin integrity, the nursing associate is likely to administer medication via the topical or oral route. It is crucial that they understand all medicines need to be prescribed including emollients and barrier products. Manufacturer's instructions on how to apply products must always be followed and local policy and procedure adhered to. Medications used to support skin integrity are highlighted in Table 24.5.

Consent

Valid consent must be gained by the nursing associate prior to delivering any type of nursing care to support a person's skin integrity; consider the following:

- The individual has the capacity to give consent.
- There was no pressure or coercion on the individual to give consent.
- The individual was fully and appropriately informed about the nature and purpose of the intervention as well as implications of giving or refusing consent.

Nursing associates must pay particular attention when seeking consent of 'vulnerable' individuals such as those with learning disabilities, mental impairment or children. They should assume that a person has the capacity to make their own decisions unless proven otherwise. If capacity is impaired or of concern, the principles outlined in the Mental Capacity Act (2005) provide the nursing associate with guidance and direction. If there are concerns, the nursing associate should seek advice from a more senior member of staff.

Privacy and Dignity

When skin care is delivered by the nursing associate (e.g. the application of topical treatment, repositioning or a skin reassessment), the nursing associate must interact sensitively with the person and apply fundamental principles such as treating the patient with respect, care and compassion without exception. The nursing associate needs to ensure that as little skin as possible is exposed at any given time; curtains, blinds or doors are closed and unnecessary interruption by others is avoided. Cultural awareness, sensitivity and a sound understanding of a person's cultural beliefs about modesty and responses to illness and treatment (Goicoechea-Balbona 1997) is a prerequisite. The use of a chaperone must always be considered and offered to the patient. Every effort should be made to consider the individual's preferences such as requesting staff of a specific gender to perform the review.

Yellow Flag **Spiritual and Religious Aspects of Skin**

'The skin projects to self and others both physical health or illness and emotional reactions and responses. Skin, hair and nails at times may reflect inner issues of the body, emotions, psychological states and spiritual being and meaning' (Dethlefsen & Dahlke 1990). Skin and skin disorders have had spiritual and religious aspects since ancient times (Scheinfeld 2007). Tattoos, for example, are as old as human history, the ancient Egyptians mastered the art of bandaging and mummification and the ancient Greeks already managed localised pain by applying opioids as a 'skin patch' (Adrian et al. 2012). Today, spiritual and religious significances continue to be revealed in many different ways. It is important that the nursing associate understands, respects and demonstrates sensitivity to spiritual and religious aspects when implementing measures to support a person's skin integrity. They need to appreciate that spirit, mind, emotions and body are one holistic unit. They need to recognise that maintaining or healing the skin of an individual can be hindered until the spiritual aspect affecting its integrity is sufficiently addressed. Here are a number of spiritual/religious significances the nursing associate should be aware of:

- What and how much skin is exposed (e.g. type of clothing, covering up or nude/none)
- Length of scalp hair (short, long, styled, accessorised)
- Skin appearance (e.g. colour, condition, temperature, intentional scarring)
- How and why skin is painted or decorated (e.g. piercings, tattoos, makeup, body paint, wigs and hair pieces)
- Individual beliefs (e.g. attitude toward life, making sense of life, relating to others and seeking unity with the transcendent)
- Religious and cultural beliefs, norms, values and taboos (e.g. reactions and acceptance of skin disorders, stigmatisation, acceptance of treatment choices).

Source: Shenefelt & Shenefelt (2014).

Supporting Self-Care and Patient Education

The nursing associate needs to employ effective communication and interpersonal skills and have the ability to establish a meaningful relationship with the patient when delivering not only skin care but any type of care. They need to strive to create a compassionate, warm and positive patient experience that promotes independence and engages patients in their care.

The ability to manage skin problems independently varies from patient to patient and is influenced by factors such as cognitive ability, physical ability and the extent of the skin problem itself (Dingwall 2010). Once readiness, ability and appropriateness to self-care have been determined, patients should be supported and taught to check their own skin for signs of improvement or deterioration and how to administer treatments to support the skin integrity of their skin. In supporting the patient, the nursing associate can:

- Participate in the education of the individual about their care and/or treatment
- Work with the patient to develop a daily skin care routine
- Include significant others such as carers (where appropriate)
- Assist in developing knowledge of areas most at risk of skin breakdown
- Aid in the acquisition of knowledge allowing for identification and detection of early signs of skin changes for example cancer, pressure ulcers and allergic reactions
- Teach individuals to do 'pressure-relief lifts' or other pressure-relieving manoeuvres as appropriate
- Encourage the reporting of skin changes to appropriate professionals
- Assist in the use of aids to allow self-administration of treatment and self-monitoring of skin integrity.

Documentation and Reporting Concerns

Nursing associates take personal responsibility to ensure that care delivered is documented clearly and in line with local and national organisational frameworks, legislation and regulations (Nursing and Midwifery Council 2018a). Relevant information needs to be shared according to local policy. If a patient is identified to be 'at risk' of harm (or further harm), then appropriate immediate action is to be taken by the nursing associate to provide adequate safeguarding of the individual. Risks identified need to be reported and unambiguously documented. Any actions required as a result of the reporting need to be implemented by the nursing associate as instructed by the expert professional.

Take Note

Maintaining skin integrity requires a multifaceted approach and can at times be challenging and complex. For the nursing associate's practice to be safe and effective, they must always ensure that the care they deliver and any products they have chosen to use to support skin integrity are based on a holistic assessment, are prescribed and are always in accordance with manufacturer recommendations.

Blue Flag The Impact of Skin Disease and Wounds on Body Image and Relationships

Skin conditions and wounds can have extensive and detrimental effects on all aspects of a person's life. It can affect their relationships, schooling, work, social interactions, sexuality and ultimately their mental health. We are living in a society in which considerable importance is attached to the appearance of a person. People may make judgement about another person based on their skin appearance, affecting how that person may feel about themselves, their body image, self-esteem and confidence (Dingwall 2010). Figure 24.8 illustrates the impact of altered body image on a person.

Skin disease may provoke psychosocial comorbidities such as anxiety, depression or behavioural problems, and psychosocial stresses may in turn provoke skin disease; a perfect spiral of cause and effect. Multidisciplinary teams, which may include nursing professionals, dermatologists and psychiatrists, have been associated with better clinical outcomes.

Orange Flag Psychological and Social Implications of Aging Skin with Skin Disease

Older adults with skin disease have a substantial burden of psychosocial suffering as a result of intentional and unconscious stigmatisation. This is often intensified if skin disease is superimposed on the already aging skin, particularly if highly visibly areas such as the face, head or hands are affected. To holistically and effectively support an older adult with additional skin disease with the maintenance of their skin integrity, the nursing associate needs to be aware of how the combination of age and disease may impact the individual. They should consider that:

- The awareness of one's compromised appearance makes interpersonal relationships uncomfortable and promotes social withdrawal.
- Having a rough, itchy, aged skin is associated with a significant level of both physical and psychological discomfort.
- Skin that does not look or feel good is emotionally burdensome.
- Skin disease can erode self-esteem of the individual, causing anxiety, depression and social withdrawal.
- Skin disorders in the elderly are often the bane of their existence, the source of a significant amount of discomfort and distress, having an adverse effect on almost every area of life.
- People whose body image and self-esteem are less stable have been observed to exhibit dysmorphic tendencies, an obsession with personal appearance and depression as a reaction to skin disease (Farage et al. 2017).

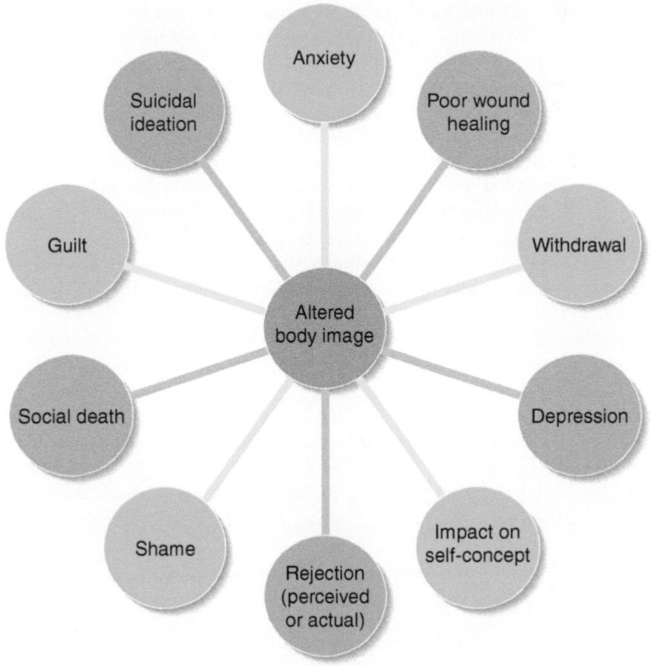

Figure 24.8 The impact of a wound on a person's self-esteem and body image. *Source:* Peate & Glencross (2015), figure 4.1, p. 8. © Wiley & Sons 2015.

Touch Points Revisited

- Maintaining skin integrity requires a multifaceted approach and can at times be challenging and complex.
- Supporting a person's skin integrity requires a holistic and patient-centred approach by the nursing associate.
- The nursing associate is required to provide fundamental nursing care such as washing, bathing and adequately nourishing a patient as well as an understanding of deeper and more complex issues such as respecting a person's spiritual and religious beliefs, understanding the psychological effects of skin diseases and wounds and an awareness of the challenges the most vulnerable people of society face when trying to maintain their skin integrity.
- The nursing associate is required to demonstrate competence and confidence when implementing the various approaches required to support a person's skin integrity.

References

Adrian, P.H., Steen, H.H. and Else, M.B. (2012) Transdermal opioid patches for pain treatment in ancient Greece, *Pain Practice*, 12(8): 620–625.

Arndt, K.A., Hsu, J.T.S., Alam, M., Bhatia, A.C. and Chilukuri, S. (2015) *Manual of dermatologic therapeutics*, Wolters Kluwer Health, 2014. ProQuest Ebook Central. [online] Available: https://ebookcentral-proquest-com.salford.idm.oclc.org/lib/salford/detail.action?docID=2031621. .

British Association for Parenteral and Enteral Nutrition (BAPEN). (2003) *Malnutrition universal screening tool*. [online] Available: www.bapen.org.uk [accessed 13 October 2019].

Beeckman, D., Campbell, J., Campbell, K., Chimentão, D., Coyer, F., Domansky, R., Gray, M., Hevia, H., Junkin, J., Karadag, A., Kottner, J., Arnold Long, M., McNichol, L., Meaume, S. Nix, D., Sabasse, M., Sanada, H., Yu, P., Voegeli, D. and Wang, L. (2015) *Incontinence associated dermatitis: moving prevention forward, Addressing evidence gaps for best practice, Wounds International*. [online] Available: www.woundsinternational.com [accessed 9 October 2019].

British Association of Dermatologists (BAD). (2014) *Dermatology: a handbook for medical students and junior doctors* (2nd edn). [online] Available: http://www.bad.org.uk/shared/get-file.ashx?itemtype=document&id=3632. Accessed 13 October 2019.

British Association of Dermatologists (BAD). (2019) Position statement on the place of bath emollients in the treatment of atopic dermatitis (AD). [online] Available: http://www.bad.org.uk/healthcare-professionals/clinical-standards. Accessed 13 October 19.

Brown, A. and Flanagan, M. (2013) Assessing skin integrity, in Flanagan, M. (ed.) *Wound healing and skin integrity: principles and practices*, Wiley & Sons, Chapter 4, 52–64.

Dingwall, L. (2010) *Personal hygiene care*, Hoboken, NJ: John Wiley and Sons, Incorporated.

Dethlefsen, T. and Dahlke, R. (1990) *The healing power of illness: the meaning of symptoms and how to interpret them*, Shaftesbury, UK: Element Books Ltd.

European Pressure Ulcer Advisory Panel (EPUAP). (2016) Prevention and treatment of pressure ulcers, Quick reference guide. [online] Available: http://www.epuap.org/wp-content/uploads/2016/10/quick-reference-guide-digital-npuap-epuap-pppia-jan2016.pdf. Accessed 3 October 2019.

Farage, M.A., Miller, K.W., Berardesca, E. and Maibach, H.I. (2017) Psychological and social implications of aging skin: normal aging and the effects of cutaneous disease, in Farage, M., Miller, K. & Maibach, H. (eds.) *Textbook of aging skin*, Berlin, Heidelberg: Springer.

Goicoechea-Balbona, A. (1997) Culturally specific health care model for ensuring health care use by rural, ethnically diverse families affected by HIV/AIDS, *Health and Social Work*, (22): 172–180.

Joint Formulary Committee. (2019) *Emollient and barrier preparations. British National Formulary (online)*, London: BMJ Group and Pharmaceutical Press. [online] Available: http://www.medicinescomplete.com. Accessed 16 October 2019.

Mahoney, K. (2019) Incontinence-associated dermatitis: diagnosis and treatment. *Journal of Community Nursing*, 33(3): 20–26,28.
Medicines and Healthcare Products Regulatory Agency (MHRA). (2018) *Emollient cream build-up in fabric can lead to fire deaths.* [online] Available: www.gov.uk [accessed 12 October 2019].
Nursing and Midwifery Council. (2018a) *Standards of proficiencies for nursing associates.* [online] Available: https://www.nmc.org.uk/globalassets/sitedocuments/education-standards/nursing-associates-proficiency-standards.pdf. Accessed 3 October 2019.
Nursing and Midwifery Council. (2018b) *The code - professional standards of practice and behaviour for nurses, midwives and nursing associates.* [online] Available: https://www.nmc.org.uk/globalassets/sitedocuments/nmc-publications/nmc-code.pdf. Accessed 3 October 2019.
Office for National Statistics (ONA). (2019) *Death of homeless people in England and Wales.* [online] Available: www.ons.gov.uk/peoplepopulationandcommunity/birthsdeathsandmarriages/deaths/bulletins/deathsofhomelesspeopleinenglandandwales/2018 [accessed 13 October 2019].
Ousey, K. and McIntosh, C. (2008) *Lower Extremity Wounds: A Problem-Based Approach, 1e.* Oxford: Wiley.
Ousey, K., Bianchi, J., Beldon, P. and Young, T. (2012) Identification and treatment of moisture lesions, *Wounds UK*, 8(2): S1–S20. [online] Available: https://www.wounds-uk.com/journals/issue/30/article-details/supplement-82-the-identification-and-management-of-moisture-lesions. Accessed 9 October 2019.
Peate, I. and Glencross, W. (2015) *Wound care at a glance*, Oxford: Wiley.
Peate, I. & Nair, M. (2017). *Fundamentals of anatomy and physiology: for nursing and healthcare students* (2nd edn). Oxford: Wiley.
Public Health England. (2019) *Guidance – health matters: sleeping rough.* [online] Available: www.gov.uk/government/publications/health-matters-rough-sleeping [accessed 13 October 2019].
Scheinfeld, N. (2007) Tattoos and religion, *Clinics in Dermatology*, 25(4): 362–366.
Shenefelt, P.D. and Shenefelt, D.A. (2014) Spiritual and religious aspects of skin and skin disorders, *Psychology Research and Behavior Management*, 7: 201–212. https://dx.doi.org/10.2147%2FPRBM.S65578
The Mental Capacity Act (2005) [online] Available: www.legistation.gov.uk/ukpga/2005/9/contents. Accessed 6 September 2020.
Thibodeau, G.A. and Patton, K.T. (2008) *Structure & function of the body* (13th edn), St Louise: Mosby/Elsevier.

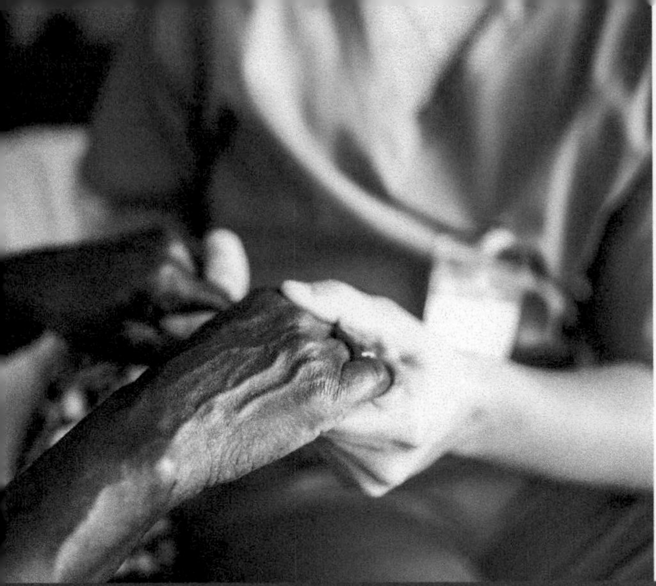

25

Reassessment of Hygiene Status Supporting a Person's Hygiene Needs

Abby Hughes

University of Salford, UK

Chapter Aim

- This chapter aims to provide the reader with the knowledge and skills required to support a person's personal hygiene.

Learning Outcomes

By the end of this chapter, the trainee nursing associate will be able to:

- Describe how a patient's personal hygiene can be reassessed
- Discuss the core principles which need to be applied when supporting a patient's personal hygiene

Test Yourself Multiple Choice Questions

1. What might be the impact of not maintaining personal hygiene?
   A) Skin infection
   B) Reduced mental well-being
   C) Body odour
   D) All of the above

The Nursing Associate's Handbook of Clinical Skills, First Edition. Edited by Ian Peate.

Companion website: www.wiley.com/nursingassociate

2. **Why might a patient not be able to maintain their own personal hygiene?**
   A) **Age**
   B) **Illness**
   C) **Immobility**
   D) **All of the above**

3. **Which nursing staff should be involved in assisting with patient's personal hygiene?**
   A) **Registered nurses**
   B) **Nursing associates**
   C) **Healthcare assistants**
   D) **All of the above**
4. **Which is not an important principle that needs to be considered when assisting a patient with their personal hygiene?**
   A) **Privacy and dignity**
   B) **Infection control**
   C) **Promoting independence**
   D) **Antibiotic stewardship**
5. **What patient preferences should be taken into account when reassessing and providing personal hygiene care?**
   A) **Timing**
   B) **Products used**
   C) **Frequency**
   D) **All of the above**

Introduction

This chapter will consider the nursing associate's role in providing and reassessing a patient's personal hygiene. Personal care is described by the Care Quality Commission (CQC) (2013) as the provision of care to persons who, for a variety of reasons, cannot provide it to themselves. Providing this type of care is a fundamental nursing activity, and as such, it is contained within the Standards of Proficiency for Nursing Associates (2018a). The reassessment of personal hygiene, as well as supporting a person with their personal care, is an important skill the nursing associate must possess.

The standards of personal care provided in healthcare are very important to patients and their families. Failure to adequately provide personal care has been a prominent feature of recent care shortcomings and investigations such as The Francis Report into the deficiencies at the Mid Staffordshire Hospital (2013). The importance that the patients and their families still place on this fundamental aspect of nursing today is demonstrated by personal care remaining the third most common reason for complaints about the National Health Service (NHS) treatment in 2017–2018 (NHS Digital 2018).

Supporting Evidence

The Francis Report into the Mid Staffordshire Hospital including the concerns and recommendations from the enquiry can be found here: https://webarchive.nationalarchives.gov.uk/20150407084231/http://www.midstaffspublicinquiry.com/report

The Nursing and Midwifery Council (NMC) Standards of Proficiency (2018a) require the nursing associate to provide care and support to people with their hygiene needs and the maintenance of skin integrity. The nursing associate has to observe and reassess skin and hygiene status using contemporary approaches to determine needs for support and ongoing intervention.

The maintenance of personal hygiene is important for all individuals throughout their life course in order to maintain physical and mental well-being and encompasses activities such as washing, grooming and oral hygiene. Failing to maintain personal hygiene may lead to physical issues such as body odour, halitosis or skin infections and psychological issues such as diminished self-belief related to personal appearance.

Orange Flag

Failing to maintain personal hygiene can lead to physical and mental health and well-being issues such as skin infections and diminished self-belief.

Reassessment of Personal Hygiene Needs

Throughout their careers, nursing associates are required to provide and monitor care (NMC 2018a). In order to provide care for a patient's personal hygiene, the nursing associate will be required to continually review the person's ability to provide their own personal hygiene and the level of care required.

Green Flag

Nursing associates are required in their standards of proficiency and skills annex (NMC 2018a) to care for patient's personal hygiene:
3. Provide care and support with hygiene and the maintenance of skin integrity:
3.1 observe and reassess skin and hygiene status using contemporary approaches to determine the need for support and ongoing intervention

In order to achieve this, they will also need to apply the NMC Code of Conduct (2018b) and the themes within it of:

1. Prioritise people
2. Practice effectively
3. Preserve safety
4. Promote professionalism and trust.

In order to review personal hygiene needs, a variety of data and information sources should be used. Directly questioning the patient can be a useful source of information; however, the nursing associate should employ all of their communication skills when doing this, as personal hygiene can be a sensitive topic to talk about and may cause embarrassment for some patients (see Chapter 1 of this text regarding theories and models of communication). If a patient is unable to answer questions, for example, due to age or illness, family members or carers could be used as a source of information with the patient's consent. Although potentially subjective data, questions can be a useful way of gathering information. For example, the nursing associate can ask the patient their preferences such as frequency of bathing, timing of bathing, which method of bathing they prefer, preference of bathing product, patient's equipment needs such as bath seats, raised shower chairs and patient's usual personal hygiene routine.

Yellow Flag

It is important to follow patient's personal beliefs and values when assisting with personal hygiene. For example, some patients who follow a vegan lifestyle may require only vegan bathing products to be used such as vegan soaps and shampoo.

Further data can be obtained from observation of the patient and their environment. For example, the nursing associate can observe a patient's physical ability to provide their own personal hygiene, and personal preferences may be ascertained from observation of the patient's belongings and their environment.

Assessment Across the Life Course

Many factors affect a person's ability to maintain their own personal hygiene. Age is a key factor that needs to be considered when reviewing a patient's ability to provide their own personal care. Parents and carers provide personal hygiene to babies and children until they are physically and cognitively able to do this for themselves. Safety must always be maintained when assisting with personal hygiene for children or patients with cognitive impairments. For example, a child or a patient with a learning disability or dementia may not understand the risk from scalding water or be able to protect themselves from the risk of drowning in bath water.

Some older patients may no longer be physically able to provide their own personal hygiene due to fragility. Acute illness, such as sepsis, or acute injuries, such as fractures, may suddenly affect a patient's ability to care for their own personal hygiene due to pain, medical interventions or medical devices. Acute cognitive impairment, such as delirium, or chronic cognitive impairment, such as dementia or learning disability, may also affect the person's ability to provide their own personal care. Patients with cognitive impairment may need additional assistance with their personal hygiene. The use of usual routines may be helpful when assisting patients with cognitive impairment with their personal hygiene.

All patients need to be assessed on an individual basis and, as stated by the NMC (2018a), constantly reassessed by the nursing associate for any improvement or deterioration in their ability to care for their own personal hygiene. Any changes should be responded to, clearly documented in the patient's notes and escalated to the registered nurse for investigation if needed.

Promotion of Independence with Personal Hygiene

The nursing associate should always promote the patient's independence whilst maintaining patient safety (NMC 2018a). This is in keeping with the Code of Conduct (2018b), which requires nursing associates to respect the contribution that patients can make to their own health and well-being. When the nursing associate fails to promote a patient's independence, this can negatively impact the patient both physically and psychologically. Therefore, the level of personal care assistance provided should be based on the nursing associate's review of the patient's need for assistance, whilst promoting their independence and ensuring patient safety. The needs of the patient can quickly change. For example, a patient in acute pain may not be able to provide themselves with their usual level of personal hygiene if the pain is reducing their mobility. Or a patient who has an acute urinary tract infection may suffer with incontinence not usually experienced due to the infection or associated delirium, and therefore, need additional assistance from the nursing associate. Due to the possibility that patient's needs may rapidly change during illness, the nursing associate should be constantly reassessing and evaluating the patient's personal care needs and level of assistance required.

Promoting patient's independence to aid recovery, encourage mobilisation and normalisation of care received has been the focus of a recent NHS England campaign (2018) to end PJ paralysis in hospitals. Nursing associates can participate in this campaign during personal care by promoting their patient's independence. For example, when completing personal hygiene care, the nursing associate should ensure that patients are given the opportunity to self-care, hence not losing their functional ability during illness. In practice, this would vary depending on the individual ability of patients, but it could mean promoting a patient to walk to the bathroom if safe and able to do so, or just promoting the patient to wash their own face.

Supporting Evidence

Find out more about the national #endPJparalysis campaign including the background to the programme, videos and resources associated with the programme here: https://endpjparalysis.org

In order to maximise independence, a variety of equipment is available to assist patients to maintain their own personal hygiene. These include:

- shower seats
- grab rails
- walk in baths.

If the nursing associate feels that equipment to assist with personal hygiene care is required, appropriate referrals to the physiotherapist or occupational therapist, according to local policy, should be made.

Take Note

When caring for patients, independence should be maintained as much as possible to avoid them losing the functional ability to care for their own personal hygiene needs.

Communication

Some key nursing principles should be remembered when assisting patients with their personal hygiene needs. First, the nursing associate should use their communication skills to enable the development of a strong therapeutic relationship with the patient. This will be particularly needed when there is a requirement for the nursing associate to assist the patient with personal hygiene activities, which are usually done privately and may cause embarrassment. The nursing associate should ensure that care is delivered in a person-centred way, and choices and wishes are upheld. Therefore, in the reassessment of care, effective communication skills are required to explore what these preferences are.

Green Flag **Legislation/ Professional Issues**

A chaperone may be considered to protect the patient and the nursing associate if the care required is of an intimate nature. The NMC Code (2018b) and local chaperone policies should be used to guide the trainee nursing associate (TNA) in this situation.

Take Note

The nursing associate needs to quickly develop a therapeutic relationship with the patient when caring for their personal hygiene, as assistance with personal care may cause embarrassment for the patient.

As detailed in the NMC Code of Conduct (2018b), valid consent must be obtained from the patient by the nursing associate before any assistance with personal hygiene can be provided (Department of Health 2009; NMC 2018b). Some patients may prefer to be assisted with their personal hygiene by a particular gender of staff, and this preference should be facilitated. Some patients may prefer any assistance they require to be provided by family members. With the consent of the family member, this should be accommodated, and any education and support for the family members should be provided by the nursing associate. These details should be documented in the patient's care notes.

Privacy and Dignity

Privacy and dignity are two other key principles which need to be maintained whilst assisting patients with their personal hygiene needs. The Royal College of Nursing (RCN) (2019) includes privacy and dignity as a core principle of nursing practice which can be expected of all nursing professionals. Privacy and dignity must be maintained during any communication with the patient about their personal hygiene care as well as during any aspect of care delivery. Any communication with the patient must be confidential (DH 2003) including that about personal hygiene. Privacy and dignity can be maintained by considering the environment in which the care is occurring. Where possible, a closed environment such as a lockable bathroom should be provided for patients to allow both privacy and sound barriers. However, emergency access into the bathroom should be available in case it is needed. The nursing associate should review whether by using equipment, the patient's personal hygiene can be facilitated in a bathroom rather than at the bedside. Where it is not possible to provide the patient access to a lockable bathroom, curtains or screens should be used, and care should be taken to prevent other people including other healthcare professionals from coming behind the curtains or screen during care episodes. The nursing associate should ensure that any environment in which personal care is being provided is warm and draft free. This is both for patient comfort and to avoid vulnerable patients such as babies and the elderly being exposed to extremes of temperature.

Privacy and dignity can also be maintained during the care episode by not exposing areas of the patient's body unnecessarily. For example, if assistance is being given to wash the patient's chest, the lower half of their body should remain covered. This can easily be achieved with the use of clean towels to cover the patient to maintain their dignity.

Touch Point

Consider ways in which you can ensure that privacy and dignity is maintained when assisting a patient with their personal hygiene in your workplace.

Infection Control/Risk Management

The Standards of Proficiency for Nursing Associates (2018a) and the NMC Code of Conduct (2018b) explain how infection control must be maintained at all times. This includes when reassessing and caring for a patient's personal hygiene. National and local infection control policies and processes should always be followed. As the nursing associate is likely to come into contact with body fluids whilst assisting with personal hygiene and to prevent cross-contamination, personal protective equipment (PPE) should be used such as gloves (see Chapter 45 of this text for more discussion on PPE). Aprons should also be used during personal care to protect the nursing associate's uniform and prevent cross-contamination within the healthcare environment. All equipment used for assisting patients with their personal hygiene should be single-patient use or cleaned following local policy between patients. For example, bath chairs should be cleaned following local policy between use, towels should be laundered and bathing products should be single-patient use. Single-patient products include items such as soap or shampoo, where the patient may use this item repeatedly, but this item must not be used by more than one patient to avoid cross-contamination. Although not an exhaustive list, other safety aspects that need to be considered when caring for a patient's personal hygiene include:

- Falls risk assessments
- Water temperature
- Level of supervision required.

The nursing associate should be constantly reassessing the risk during personal hygiene care, for example, a patient may be a higher falls risk due to a postural blood pressure drop following a hot bath or shower, or they may be a higher falls risk due to removing their non-slip footwear in the bathroom.

Patient Preferences

Person-centred care is contained in the first platform in the Standards of Proficiency for Nursing Associates (2018) and therefore should be practiced at all times. This requires the nursing associate to put the needs of the patient first (RCN 2016) and compels flexibility in the way in which personal hygiene care is delivered. Patients must be viewed as equal partners in their care (Keogh 2013), and therefore, patient preferences should be taken into account when reassessing and providing personal hygiene care. For example, some patients may prefer baths, some showers. Some patients may bathe every day, others may bathe every other day. Some patients may prefer to bathe in the morning, others in the evening. Some patients may have religious or cultural preferences, which relate to their personal hygiene care, which needs to be upheld. Common options available to maintain a patient's personal hygiene include bathing, showering, bed bathing or washing at the bedside; patient's preference for how they wish to cleanse should be taken into account.

Violet Flag

Patients who are homeless, living in substandard housing or living in poverty may not be able to bathe and maintain their personal hygiene as frequently as they would wish to. This may be due to inadequate washing and bathing facilities or the cost of warm water.

Patient's preference for cleansing agent is another issue the nursing associate needs to consider. For some patients such as babies, soap products may not be appropriate due to the impact of the pH on the babies' skin. Soap may not be appropriate for an older patient's skin, due to the risk of skin dehydration caused by the alkaline soap. Other alternatives to soap include dry cleansing foam and antimicrobial washes. Some hospitals ask patients to cleanse in antimicrobial washes prior to, or after admission. If this is required, the nursing associate should confirm that the patient has no allergies, which would prevent its use and then ensure that the product is used correctly to maximise its antimicrobial effect.

Some patients may prefer additional products to be used as part of their personal hygiene such as deodorant, perfumes and moisturisers. This should be facilitated where possible to uphold patient preference and maintain their psychological well-being. Equipment is available to facilitate personal preferences in personal hygiene care. Examples include bath hoists, which can allow bedbound patients to maintain their personal hygiene in a bath rather than having to rely on bed baths. The nursing associate should refer to occupational therapists and physiotherapists for equipment and assessments according to local policies. The manufacturer's instructions must be followed at all times (Chapters 37 and 38 provides further information on provision and support with mobility and safety).

Touch Point

Consider what is important to you when caring for your own personal hygiene and consider the impact on your health and well-being if these preferences were not followed.

Skin

As discussed in other chapters in this text (for example, Chapters 23 and 24), the health of the skin should be considered when assisting patients with their personal hygiene. When patients with fragile skin liable to pressure damage are assisted with their personal hygiene, care must be taken to avoid damaging their skin. Skin cleansing agents should be chosen carefully to avoid disturbing the skin's pH. Rubbing skin dry after personal hygiene should be avoided, as this friction can damage the vulnerable skin. However, on all patients, the nursing associate should ensure all areas of the body are dry after personal hygiene to avoid moisture damage. If any discrepancies are noted, this should be reported and documented, so appropriate action can be taken.

Red Flag

When assisting with personal hygiene needs, the care provided should ensure that the patient's skin integrity is not compromised.

Female Personal Hygiene

Special consideration should be given to the personal hygiene requirements of women during menstruation. The nursing associate should ensure that the woman has access to appropriate feminine hygiene products such as sanitary towels or tampons when required. The nursing associate should ensure that the woman is given privacy and dignity to avoid the patient feeling any embarrassment or shame. Patient preferences should be maintained during menstruation such as the type of feminine hygiene product used or changes in a patient preference in their bathing habits.

Violet Flag

Some women are not able to access appropriate feminine hygiene products due to their cost. This has led to global campaigns to end period poverty. You can find out more about this here: https://www.actionaid.org.uk/about-us/what-we-do/womens-economic-empowerment/period-poverty. Not being able to access appropriate feminine hygiene products can negatively impact a woman's physical and psychological health.

Conclusion

This chapter has discussed the knowledge and skills the nursing associate requires when supporting a person's personal hygiene. It has described why personal care is a part of the nursing associate's role and why it is important for patients and their families. It has described some of the key professional and legal aspects, which must be taken into account when supporting a patient with their personal hygiene such as maintaining safety, person-centred care, respecting patient preferences and privacy and dignity. Special considerations such as promoting independence and supporting patient during menstruation have also been discussed.

References

CQC. (2013) *Personal care.* [online] Available: https://www.cqc.org.uk/sites/default/files/documents/ra_1_personal_care.pdf [accessed 24 November 2019].

Department of Health. (2003) *Confidentiality: NHS code of practice.* [online] Available: https://www.gov.uk/government/publications/confidentiality-nhs-code-of-practice [accessed 24 November 2019].

Department of Health. (2009) *Reference guide to consent for examination or treatment* (2nd edn). [online] Available: https://assets.publishing.service.gov.uk/government/uploads/system/uploads/attachment_data/file/138296/dh_103653__1_.pdf [accessed 24 November 2019].

Francis, R. (2013) *Report of the mid Staffordshire NHS foundation trust public inquiry*, London: The Stationery Office.

Keogh, B. (2013) *Review into the quality of care and treatment provided by 14 hospital trusts in England: overview report.* [online] Available: https://www.nhs.uk/nhsengland/bruce-keogh-review/documents/outcomes/keogh-review-final-report.pdf [accessed 24 November 2019].

NHS Digital. (2018) *Data on written complaints in the NHS 2017-2018.* [online] Available: https://digital.nhs.uk/data-and-information/publications/statistical/data-on-written-complaints-in-the-nhs/2017-18 [accessed 24 November 2019].

NHS England. (2018) *End PJ paralysis campaign.* [online] Available: https://endpjparalysis.org/ [accessed 24 November 2019].

Nursing and Midwifery Council (NMC). (2018) *Standards of proficiency for nursing associates.* [online] Available: https://www.nmc.org.uk/standards/standards-for-nursing-associates/standards-of-proficiency-for-nursing-associates/ [accessed 24 November 2019].

Nursing and Midwifery Council (NMC). (2018) *The code: professional standards of practice and behaviour for nurses, midwives and nursing associates*, London: Nursing and Midwifery Council.

Royal College of Nursing (RCN). (2016) *What person-centred care means.* [online] Available: https://rcni.com/hosted-content/rcn/first-steps/what-person-centred-care-means [accessed 24 November 2019].

Royal College of Nursing (RCN). (2019) *Principles of nursing practice.* [online] Available: https://www.rcn.org.uk/professional-development/principles-of-nursing-practice [accessed 24 November 2019].

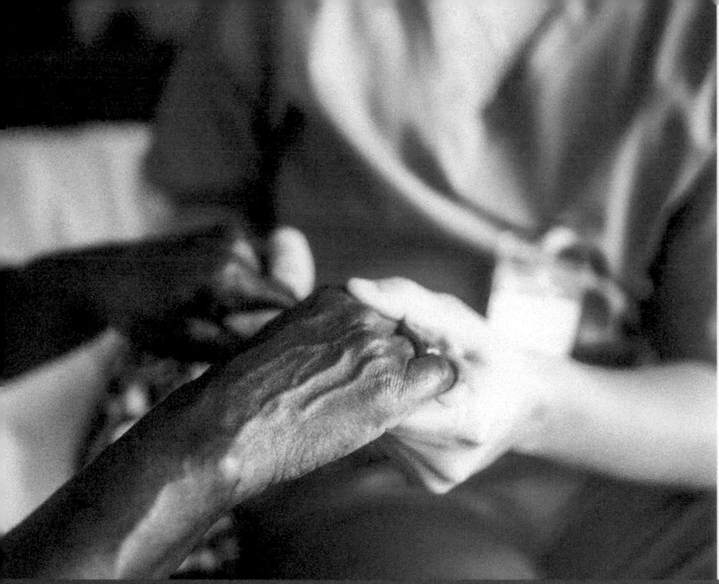

26

Providing Oral and Dental Care

Phill Hoddinott[1] *and Angela Chick*[2]

[1] Buckinghamshire New University, London, UK
[2] Chelsea and Westminster Hospital NHS Foundation Trust, London, UK

Chapter Aim

- **This chapter provides the reader with an overview of oral and dental healthcare, emphasising the importance of oral and dental review.**

Learning Outcomes

By the end of this chapter, the reader will be able to:
- **Describe and understand the structures of the mouth**
- **Explain how to complete an oral healthcare review and understand the interventions required in order to maintain oral/dental health**
- **Understand the professional requirement and when an onward referral is needed in order to maintain oral/dental health**

Test Yourself Multiple Choice Questions

1. **What are the symptoms of poor oral/dental health?**
   A) **Pain**
   B) **Dribbling saliva**
   C) **Not smiling**
2. **Which of the following people may need a greater assistance with maintaining their oral and dental health?**
   A) **People who are independent**
   B) **People who have not got a toothbrush**
   C) **People who have symptoms of poor oral/dental health**

The Nursing Associate's Handbook of Clinical Skills, First Edition. Edited by Ian Peate.

Companion website: www.wiley.com/nursingassociate

3. **What protective equipment do you need when preforming mouth/dental care?**
   A) **Sterile gloves**
   B) **Apron**
   C) **Waterproof jacket**
4. **What should dentures be cleaned with?**
   A) **A soft tufted toothbrush**
   B) **A cloth**
   C) **Just soak them in hot water**
5. **Saliva is important for which of the following?**
   A) **Movement of the lips**
   B) **Swallowing food**
   C) **A natural way to clean teeth**

Introduction

This chapter relates to the Nursing and Midwifery Council's (NMC's) (2018a) standards of proficiency for nursing associates. The nursing associate is required to demonstrate the knowledge, skills and ability to act as required to meet people's needs concerning oral care and to provide and monitor care. Also, the nursing associate is required to identify the need for and provide appropriate oral care and inform others when an onward referral is needed.

All nursing associates must adhere to the tenets within the NMC's Code of Conduct (Nursing and Midwifery Council 2018b); the Code is structured around four themes:

1. Prioritise people
2. Practise effectively
3. Preserve safety
4. Promote professionalism and trust

The nursing associate must ensure that the patient is at the centre of all that is done.

Oral and dental health is an important aspect of a person's identity and is an indicator of an individual's overall general wellness. Through publishing its toolkit, Public Health England (2019) has demonstrated that good oral and dental health has a direct correlation with a person's well-being. It has also been recognised that there are inequalities with oral and dental health across the United Kingdom and within healthcare provision in both primary and secondary care.

There are many definitions of what good oral and dental health is. Morely & Lotto (2019) recognise that it is broadly centred on the absence of pain, discomfort and disease. Delivering quality-assured, evidence-based oral and dental care is a fundamental aspect of nursing. Nursing associates should understand how to plan, implement and evaluate evidence-based care to ensure that quality-assured oral and dental care can be delivered at the point of care and, where required, expert onward referral can be sought. Delivering quality-assured, evidence-based oral and dental care is a fundamental aspect of nursing which all nursing associates should have a full understanding of in order to ensure that the best oral and dental care can be delivered.

Red Flag

Evidence from The National Institute for Health and Care Excellence (NICE) (2016) demonstrates the impact of good oral and dental care and has shown that complications such as aspiration pneumonia and other hospital-associated infections can be significantly reduced when intensified oral and dental hygiene procedures take place within the acute care setting. This considerably increases patient experience and outcome, as well as reduces the length of stay in acute care settings, leading to fewer complications and a cost reduction in both primary and secondary care.

Anatomy and Physiology of the Oral Cavity

The oral cavity has a number of structures with important functions which must be healthy in order for these to function effectively. The structures of the oral cavity can be seen in Figure 26.1.

Some of the key features of the oral cavity that the nursing associate must know include:

- The oral mucosa is all around the mouth, lips and gums and provides a first line of support against oral and respiratory infections
- The teeth are covered in enamel and are important for the mastication and grinding of food
- The tongue is where taste buds are housed and has a function in swallowing food and in the articulation of speech
- The hard and soft palate is involved in the mastication and swallowing of food as well as in speech production
- Saliva is important in the mastication and swallowing of food as well as in speech production and has an antibacterial action
- The mouth also plays a role in pleasure and sexual activities such as kissing and showing sexual affection

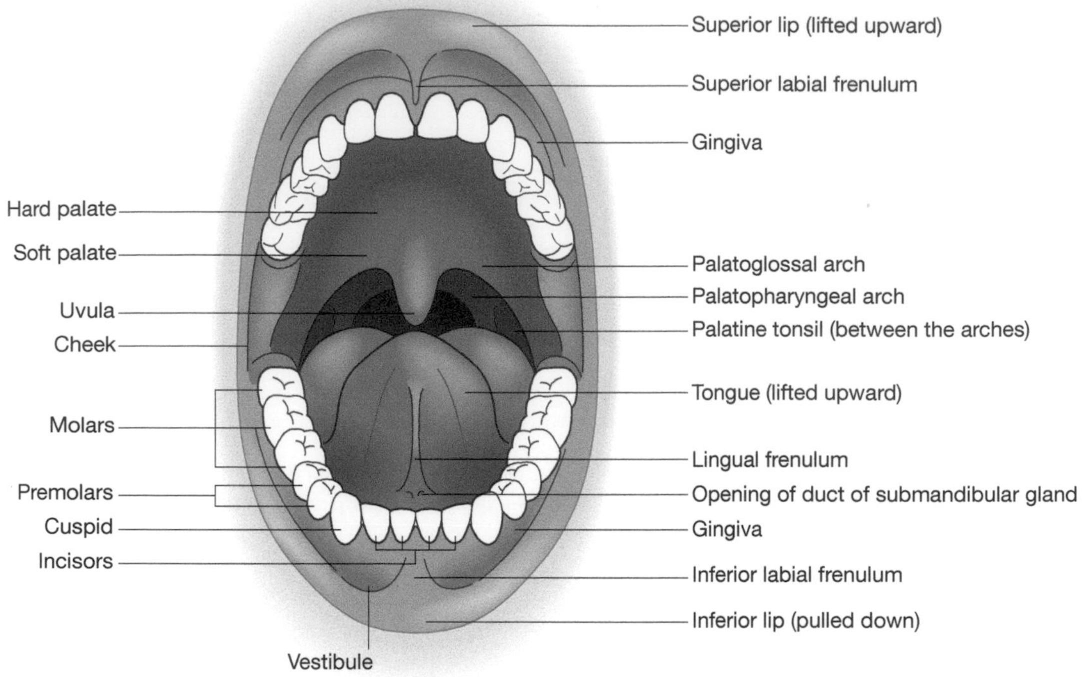

Figure 26.1 Structures of the mouth. *Source:* **Peate & Wild (2018), chapter 29, figure 293, p. 63. © John Wiley & Sons 2018**

Some Causes of Poor Oral and Dental Health

Inadequate oral and dental care can lead to decay and infection. There are many reasons why a person may have poor oral and dental health, which may be associated with social or health-related problems. A person's underlying health issues, their ability to source and use dental and oral hygiene products and their lifestyle choices around the use of alcohol, tobacco or diet may all impact oral and dental health. Some of the key causes of poor oral and dental health that the nursing associate should know include:

- Lifestyle issues such as poor diet, smoking and an increased alcohol intake can lead to ongoing mouth and dental issues such as tooth decay.
- People who have existing poor oral and dental health may not have had access to a dentist, appropriate equipment or the support and individualised care required to maintain their own oral and dental health effectively.
- Factors such as age and physical or cognitive function could prevent a person from meeting their oral and dental care requirements. Neurological conditions and injuries such as dementia, stroke and Parkinson's disease can also impact upon a person's ability to independently maintain their own oral and dental health.
- People who have a reduced oral intake or who are unable to eat and drink including those who are temporally nil by mouth. This could include people who are unable to feed themselves and those who are being fed via other routes such as nasogastric tube or percutaneous endoscopic gastrostomy. It may also include those awaiting surgery or procedures and those who are receiving end-of-life care.
- The person who is taking medications such as steroids, chemotherapy or other medicines that may have an impact on the immune system (immunosuppressants) resulting in people being more prone to infections such as candidiasis (thrush). The treatment of certain illnesses such as those associated with endocrine and oncological conditions often involve the use of these medicines which require specialist care including special attention to oral and dental care.
- Short-term therapies and treatments such as oxygen therapy can cause the oral mucosa to rapidly dry out.

Touch Point

The nursing associate should find opportunities to provide health promotion on oral and dental care whenever possible and offer advice to help the person independently maintain their own oral and dental health.

Consequences of Poor Oral and Dental Health

Poor oral and dental health can affect a person's self-esteem, quality of life and general well-being. It can reduce the person's sense of taste and, therefore, affect their desire to eat and communicate effectively, impacting on their day-to-day life. This may also impact upon a person's recovery from illness by limiting their independence or preventing them from being able to swallow medications.

Table 26.1 Consequences of poor oral and dental health and descriptions.

CONDITION/CONSEQUENCE	DESCRIPTION
Xerostomia (dry mouth)	Maybe due to a person being nil by mouth or a reduced food and fluid intake. Can also be a side effect of certain medications that reduce the flow of saliva to the mouth, such as some medicines used to treat Parkinson's disease.
Gingivitis (inflammation of the gums)	A common symptom of gum disease and can be a consequence of poor brushing technique that does not remove dental plaque or bacteria. Can be painful and may lead to further inflammation of the gums and supporting structures of the teeth known as periodontitis, a leading cause of tooth loss.
Oral infections	These include oral candida. Can be caused by a person's own natural defence mechanisms breaking down. Oral candida appears as creamy white patches (lesions) on the tongue, inner cheeks and palate of the mouth. People receiving chemotherapy or radiotherapy as well as those requiring prolonged, high dose or broad-spectrum antibiotic therapy are at greater risk.
Mouth ulcers	These may be caused by trauma or viral infections, are common and can affect anyone. They can be found on the cheeks, lips and tongue; are white, red, yellow or grey in appearance and are often swollen and painful.
Tooth decay	A leading cause of poor oral and dental hygiene. A build-up of plaque due to sugar, bacteria and other debris can damage the enamel of the teeth causing pain, infection and further decay. This could result in the loss of the tooth and damage to the gums and other structures of the oral cavity.
Poorly fitting dentures	These may cause irritation to the gums and oral mucosa resulting in pain and open sores in the mouth which could lead to infection of the oral cavity.

Source: Modified from Dougherty et al. (2015).

Some of the general implications of poor oral and dental health such as pain, difficulties communicating, eating and maintaining dignity have been discussed. The key consequences linked to some of the above causes of poor oral and dental health that the nursing associate should be aware of are detailed in Table 26.1.

Red Flag

Mouth ulcers can be a sign of a more serious condition such as an underlying disease, for example, an infection or cancer. If a mouth ulcer is worsening or has been present for more than 2 weeks, refer to a medical physician/dentist.

Take Note

Any adverse findings such as those listed in Table 26.1 must be documented and escalated to an appropriate person. Referral to a specialist/medical physician/dentist should be considered (see referral section).

Assessment of The Oral Cavity

Green Flag

The NMC Code (2018b) states that the nursing associate should always recognise and work within the limits of their competence and should accurately identify, observe and assess signs of normal or worsening physical and mental health in the person receiving care.

The nursing associate must always follow their organisation's local policy when assessing and delivering oral and dental care.

The use of comprehensive, evidence-based oral and dental care assessment must be used as per the nursing associate's local policy. The oral and dental care assessment must take into account the person's level of capacity; nutritional intake; the appearance of the lips, tongue, teeth/dentures and saliva as well as other factors discussed. A numerical score is sometimes used to help the healthcare professional plan the care around the findings of the assessment (see Table 26.2).

Table 26.2 Oral hygiene assessment tool.

LEVEL OF ALERTNESS/CAPACITY		NUTRITIONAL INTAKE		LIPS	
Alert and compliant	1	Normal	1	Smooth, pink, moist	1
Reduced insight and reduced independence	2	Modified	3	Dry/cracked	2
Sedated	8	NBM/oral trials/Enteral or parental feeding	11	Bleeding	3
Uncooperative/Delirium	10			Ulceration	4
GCS <8					
TONGUE		TEETH/DENTURES		SALIVA/SECRETIONS	
Clean, pink, moist	1	Clean, no debris	1	Normal	1
White/yellow coating, Shiny, red oedema	2	Debris/plaque, ill-fitting dentures	2	Thick stringy or dry mouth	2
Blistered, cracked, dry	3			Dried or pooling of secretions	3
				Absent	4
OTHER FACTORS					
None	0				
Steroid therapy/diabetes	1				
Oxygen Therapy	3				
Mouth Breathing	4				

Source: From Chelsea and Westminster NHS Foundation Trust (2018).

Appendix C

SCORE	PROTOCOL
6–7	A
8–15	B
16–40	C

A (score 6–7)

- Staff to assist as appropriate
- Brush teeth **twice** daily using a toothbrush, fluoride toothpaste.
- Dentures should be removed, cleaned with appropriate denture product twice a day and rinsed well before refitting. Dentures should be removed and soaked overnight. Use denture cleaner as directed by manufacturer.
- Mouth moisturiser to be applied regularly and accessible to patient. Encourage adequate fluid intake

B (score 8–15)

Care delivered as above and including. . .

- Use **thickened fluids** if recommended by the SALT. Use suction equipment as required.
- Ensure patient is in an upright position during mouth care.
- Encourage fluid intake and consider use of oral gels for dry mouth.
- Provide mouth care after each meal, clearing all debris using oral gel and standard sponge foam sticks or toothbrush.
- Refer to medical team if infection/pain/bleeding is present. Treat as prescribed. Ensure medication is effective and given at regular intervals.

C (score 16–40)

Care delivery as above and including. . .

- Provide mouth care using **SAGE Q4 Oral Care Kit** every 4 hours following procedures outlined during training. If oral cavity particularly coated, provide mouth care in between SAGE disposable applicator system using standard sponge foam sticks.
- Refer to medical team if infection/pain/bleeding is present. Treat as prescribed. Ensure medication is effective and given at regular intervals.
- Dentures to be removed and cleaned with an appropriate denture product twice a day. For patients with reduced level of alertness, dentures should be removed, cleaned and then stored in clean, dry container.

Box 26.1 Key Points Regarding Mouth and Dental Care Assessment

- A thorough oral and dental care assessment should be completed within 24 hours of admission/implementation of care to establish the condition of the mouth and teeth. This allows the appropriate individualised care to be implemented.
- Following completion of the assessment, appropriate actions should be taken ensuring that the person's mouth and dental care needs are effectively met. All people who you offer care to must be reassessed if their clinical condition changes. Daily documentation of care must be recorded on an appropriate form according to local policy and protocol.
- People requiring a high level of mouth and dental care such as those who are nil by mouth, those with difficulty swallowing and those who require a high level of assistance with maintaining their own personal care should have this provided at a minimum of 4 hourly intervals.

Source: Modified from Dougherty et al. (2015).

Some of the key points concerning mouth and dental care assessment can be found in Box 26.1.

Take Note

All people who you offer care to must have their oral and dental health assessed as part of their admission/initial assessment.
Assessment is not a one-off practice and should be repeated daily in order to check for oral and dental health maintenance, improvement or deterioration.

Interventions to Maintain Oral and Dental Health

Oral and dental care

Where possible, the nursing associate should encourage the person to maintain their own oral and dental health and, where required, offer evidence-based advice and guidance. Opportunities can be taken to offer health promotional advice around diet, smoking cessation, alcohol/ drug use and visiting a dentist every 6 months. Health promotion is a key role of the nursing associate (Nursing and Midwifery Council 2018a, 2018b), and advice on how to maintain good oral and dental health can help to reduce poor health.

For people who are not able to maintain their own oral and dental health, the nursing associate should follow the local policy which could include the below examples of evidence-based practice listed in Box 26.2. It is essential that nursing associates work within their scope of professional practice and within the limits of The Code (Nursing and Midwifery Council 2018b).

Take Note

It is vital that the effectiveness of all interventions is fully evaluated and documented. Reassessment must take place using the assessment tools in order to deliver effective and person-centred care.

Denture Care

Dentures should be cleaned and maintained in the same way a person would care for their own teeth (as described in Box 26.2). Some of the key points concerning denture care include:

- Use the person's own denture brush or soft tufted toothbrush to clean dentures to remove plaque and food debris. Dentures should be cleaned over a bowl or sink using a denture cleaning paste or liquid soap. Toothpaste should not be used; this can damage the dentures.
- Dentures should be removed overnight and left in a designated storage container, ensuring the person's name is on it. Dentures can be soaked in cold water or a denture cleaning solution; hot water should be avoided. This can alter the shape of the denture resulting in fitting complications.
- If a person has oral candida, dentures should be removed as often as possible until the infection has resolved. Dentures may be soaked in a 0.2% Chlorhexidine solution. However, some denture manufacturers indicate that soaking of dentures should be avoided. The manufacturer or dental practitioner guidance should always be referred to.

Take Note

Lost or damaged dentures can significantly impact a person's well-being. It can be highly distressing for a person and affects their dignity and ability to eat and drink. Always ensure that great care is taken not to lose or damage a person's dentures while they are in your care.

Box 26.2 Oral and Dental Care

- Consider personal protective equipment (PPE) in order to keep yourself and the person receiving care safe at all times (Chapter 45 considers PPE in more detail), for example, disposable gloves, aprons and eye protection (goggles or a visor).
- Gain informed consent and explain what you are going to do and the rationale for the procedure.
- Gather the required equipment, for example, water, a fluoride-based mouthwash, toothpaste containing at least 1,350 parts per million (ppm) (which is a way of expressing very dilute concentrations) of fluoride and a small soft tufted toothbrush.
- Some mouthwash solutions contain alcohol; it is important that considerations are made and alternatives found for people who do not wish to use alcohol; this could be due a personal or cultural perspective.
- The use of wall-mounted or portable suction should be considered where possible in order to prevent any risk of aspiration, particularly in those who have difficulty swallowing (dysphagia).
- Gently brush teeth and the oral cavity (including gums and tongue) with the toothbrush to reduce the build-up of plaque and to prevent avoidable infections. A bite block can be used to prevent biting down on the toothbrush if clinically indicated while cleaning the teeth and oral cavity. People who are unable to expectorate independently will benefit from the use of suction during this procedure to avoid potentially swallowing any bacteria.
- Brushing of the teeth with a soft tufted toothbrush should be done in a horizontal motion against the teeth for approximately 2 minutes. All surfaces of the mouth and teeth should be covered. The nursing associate, and the person receiving care, should also be advised to ensure that the mouth is not rinsed straight away with water or a mouthwash; this is because such a method causes concentrated fluoride in the toothpaste that has remained in the mouth to be rinsed away. It is also recommended not to eat or drink for approximately 30 minutes after cleaning teeth.
- Toothbrushes should be changed regularly or when required at least every 1 to 3 months.
- Additional water-based mouth care moisturiser can be applied if available, in line with the manufacturer's guidelines. There are now many non-flammable medical products that can be used to coat both the inside and outside of the mouth cavity and is particularly important for people requiring longer-term oxygen therapy, for example.
- The use of foam swabs is controversial, and there is evidence to suggest that these should not be used for oral and dental care. The Medicines and Healthcare Products Regulatory Agency (MHRA) published an alert in 2012 that foam heads of oral swabs may detach from the stick during use. This may present a choking hazard. Nursing associates should follow local policy and be aware of the MHRA actions around this alert. If a patient's mouth is particularly coated then mouth care using a standard foam sponge stick could be utilised alongside a toothbrush. All swabs should only be moistened prior to use and never left to soak in solution, as this has been linked to the foam head coming off. Reconsider their use in people who are at risk of biting them and the potential for using a bite block if available.
- A mouthwash solution may be considered for short-term use as a mouth rinse in addition to usual plaque control with tooth brushing. A 0.2% Chlorhexidine solution should be used in this case which should be prescribed and used alongside a care plan. 0.2% Chlorhexidine solution may also be used to treat mouth/dental infection such as gingivitis.

Source: Public Health England (2019); The Medicines and Healthcare Products Regulatory Agency (2012)

Referral

Regular dental check-ups are essential in order to maintain oral and dental health. Public Health England (2019) found that only 61% of adults in England reported they attended the dentist for a regular check-up. Everyone should see a dentist every 6 months, and those who have symptoms (such as pain) should see a dentist as soon as possible in order to prevent further deterioration in oral and dental health and commence any required treatment as early as possible.

Violet Flag

It is vital that dental care is made available to all; the nursing associate has an important role in ensuring that those who are accessing services outside of acute inpatient care (such as community, residential nursing and custodial care) can also access a dentist every 6 months.

Green Flag

The NMC Code (2018b) states that the nursing associate should preserve safety.

13 Recognise and work within the limits of your competence

13.2 make a timely referral to another practitioner when any action, care or treatment is required

Nursing associates must always follow their employer's/organisation's local policy when onward referral is required.

A multidisciplinary team approach should be taken in order to help a person maintain oral and dental health. Specialist nurses and practitioners, physicians, dentists and pharmacists can advise and support you in planning a person's care.

Touch Point

By conducting an early mouth and dental care assessment, using evidence-based interventions and monitoring effectiveness, any improvements or deterioration can be quickly identified. Escalation to others in the multidisciplinary team and rapid onward expert referral are required in order to maintain oral and dental health.

Supporting Evidence

Health Education England (2019) Mouth Care Matters: https://mouthcarematters.hee.nhs.uk

A website associated with the 'Mouth Care Matters' programme by Health Education England which aims to create a healthcare team that is more responsive and personalised for patients and delivers better clinical outcomes.

The Medicines and Healthcare products Regulatory Agency (2012) *Medical Device Alert – Oral swabs with a foam head*: https://assets.publishing.service.gov.uk/media/5485ac0440f0b60241000271/con149702.pdf

Full details of the MHRA alert regarding the use of oral swabs with a foam head can be found in the aforementioned website.

The National Institute for Health and Care Excellence (2016) Healthcare-associated infections: https://www.nice.org.uk/guidance/qs113/resources/healthcareassociated-infections-pdf-75545296430533

A web page around the quality standard for organisational factors in preventing and controlling healthcare-associated infections in secondary care settings.

Conclusion

The nursing associate should now better understand the importance of oral and dental health and the impact that poor oral and dental health has on an individual. A timely and comprehensive assessment can quickly identify issues, and evidence-based interventions are essential in order to improve oral and dental health for people who are cared for. Opportunities can be taken to provide health promotion, and, where required, the nursing associate should initiate referral to a professional with additional expertise in order to uphold good oral and dental health and manage symptoms.

References

Chelsea and Westminster NHS Foundation Trust. (2018) *Oral hygiene protocol for nursing and allied health professions*, London, UK: Chelsea and Westminster NHS Foundation Trust.

Dougherty, L., Lister, S. and West-Oram, A. (2015) *The royal Marsden manual of clinical nursing procedures* (9th edn), West Sussex: Wiley Blackwell.

Morely, P. and Lotto, R. (2019) An exploration of student nurses' views of oral health care in the hospitalised child: a qualitative study, *Nurse Education in Practice*, 38: 79-83.

Nursing and Midwifery Council (NMC). (2018a) *Standards of proficiency for nursing associates*, London, UK: NMC.

Nursing and Midwifery Council (NMC). (2018b) *The code*, London, UK: NMC.

Peate, I. and Wild, K. (2018) *Nursing practice: knowledge and care* (2nd edn), United States: John Wiley and Sons.

Public Health England. (2019) *Delivering better oral health: an evidence-based toolkit for prevention.* [online] Available https://www.gov.uk/government/publications/delivering-better-oral-health-an-evidence-based-toolkit-for-prevention. Accessed December 2019.

The Medicines and Healthcare Products Regulatory Agency (MRHA). (2012) *Medical device alert oral swabs with a foam head*, London, UK: MRHA.

The National Institute for Health and Care Excellence (NICE). (2016) *Healthcare-associated infections Healthcare-associated infections*, United Kingdom: NICE.

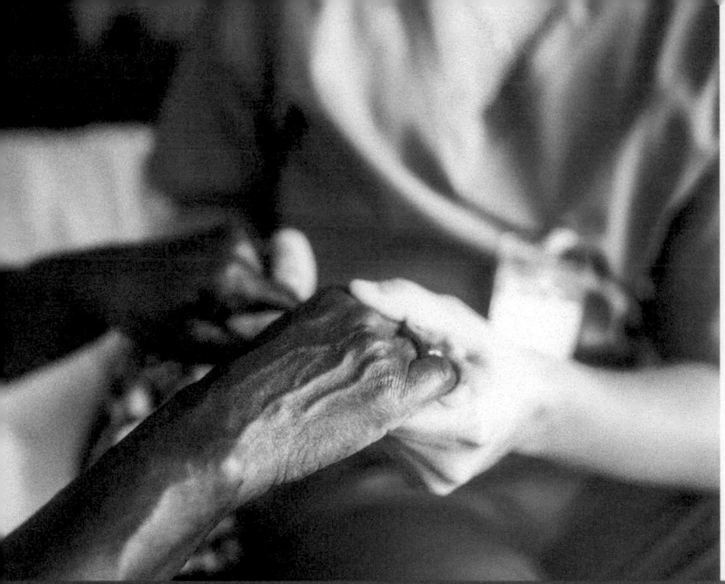

27

Providing Eye Care

Ally Sanderson

Teesside University, UK

Chapter Aim

- **This chapter aims to help the reader understand the importance of eye (ocular) care and recognition of visual changes in order to promote the health and well-being of patients.**

Learning Outcomes

By the end of this chapter, the reader will be able to:

- **Facilitate and maintain ocular health**
- **Recognise any deterioration in vision and ocular health, leading to appropriate care provision**

Test Yourself Multiple Choice Questions

1. **What is the primary function of the eyelids?**
   A) **Protection**
   B) **Lubrication**
   C) **Production of ocular lubricants**
   D) **Reduce photophobia**
2. **What is a cataract?**
   A) **Skin over the eye**
   B) **Opacity of the retina**
   C) **Opacity of the cornea**
   D) **Opacity of the lens**

The Nursing Associate's Handbook of Clinical Skills, First Edition. Edited by Ian Peate.

Companion website: www.wiley.com/nursingassociate

3. **What are two of the main causes of sight loss?**
   A) **Trauma and age-related changes**
   B) **Dry eyes and corneal abrasion**
   C) **Cataracts and age-related macular degeneration**
   D) **Ingrown eyelashes and retinal detachment**
4. **In the process of vision, what is the order that light passes through the eye?**
   A) **Lens, pupil, vitreous humour, retina, macula**
   B) **Cornea, pupil, lens, vitreous humour, fovea**
   C) **Tear film, lens, fovea, vitreous humour**
   D) **Pupil, lens, cornea, macula**
5. **You have a patient who has severe sight impairment, and they request to have a shower. What do you do?**
   A) **Help them with everything as they cannot see, hence will not be able to manage**
   B) **Offer them a bowl by their bed, as this is safer and easier**
   C) **Take them to the shower and stay with them to help**
   D) **Ask them what their needs are and how much help they require**

Introduction

The eyes and associated structures are complex sensory organs, which enable the process of vision. If there is no visual problem, then the light rays are bent (refracted) as they pass through the various layers of the tear film, cornea, pupil, lens, vitreous humour and finally arriving at the macula on the retina. Here, the light is changed into nerve impulses, which travel via the optic nerve to the occipital lobe in the brain for processing and recognition of images (Peate 2020). Many problems with systemic health can be detected through eye examination, and the role of a nursing associate is fundamental in the early recognition of changes and the promotion of health and the prevention of ill health, in relation to ocular care.

The terms *sight impairment* (SI), severe sight impairment (SSI) and *sight-impaired person* (SIP) will be used throughout this chapter.

Orange Flag

People who are newly diagnosed or living with sight loss, also known as SI or SSI, are at risk of low mood and potentially depression. Hence, support is required, and the nursing associate should liaise with other healthcare professionals to contribute to integrated care. The person may be anxious and frightened as they learn to adapt to this change.

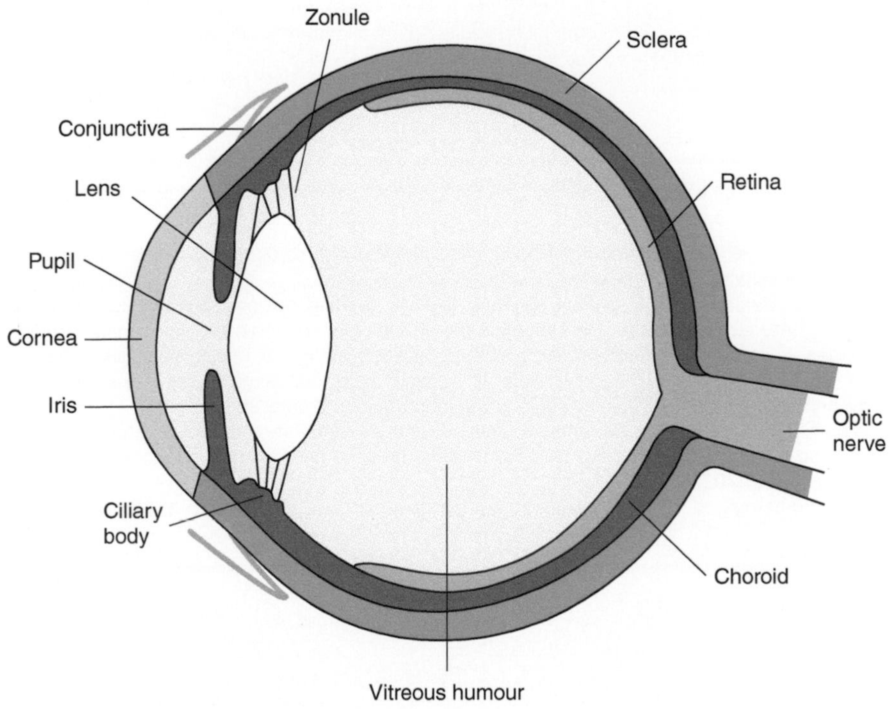

Figure 27.1 Cross-section of the eye. ***Source:*** **Peate (2017), figure 19.4, p. 568. © John Wiley & Sons.**

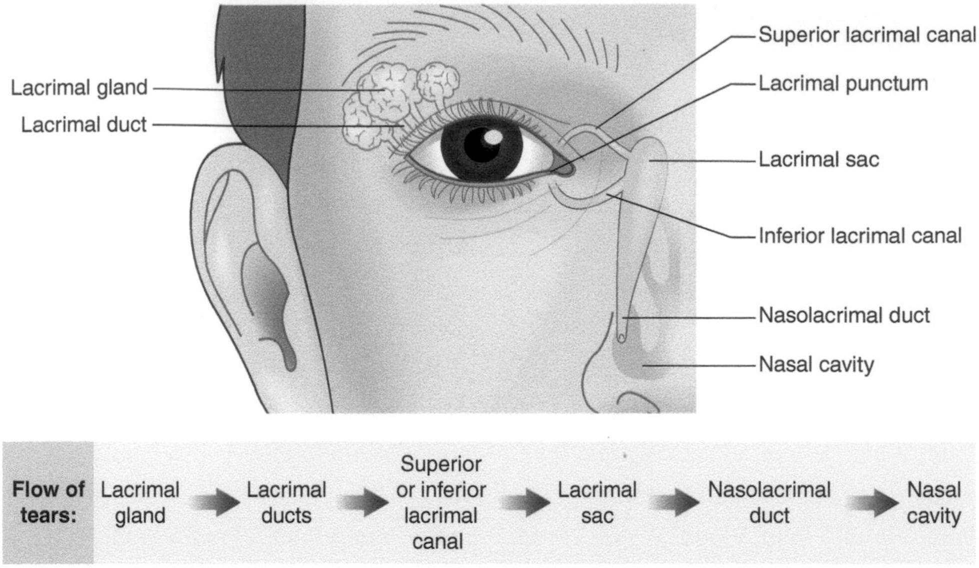

Figure 27.2 Eyelids and nasolacrimal system. *Source:* Peate & Wild (2018), figure 36.12, p. 865. © John Wiley & Sons.

There are a number of proficiencies identified in the Nursing and Midwifery Council's (NMC's) (2018) standards of proficiency for nursing associates that relate to this chapter, and they include:

- Being an accountable practitioner
- Promoting health and preventing ill health
- Improving safety and quality of care
- Providing and monitoring care
- Contributing to integrated care
- Working in teams

Touch Point

Maintaining a safe environment is vital, as SIPs are at increased risk of falls. Hence, an environment which is well lit; free from clutter, rugs and any trip hazards; and has secure flooring is paramount in improving safety and quality care (Newton & Sanderson 2013).

It is essential to fully orientate the SIPs to their current environment.

Red Flag

The nursing associate should be alert to any issues that could denote significant changes in ocular pathology. Any concerns must be escalated to a senior practitioner and then referred to appropriate ocular healthcare professional.

- Sudden loss of vision can be linked to numerous causes, including trauma, cardiovascular disease, hypertension or diabetes mellitus.
- Trauma to the eye(s) resulting from penetration, chemicals or blunt injuries.
- Gradual loss of central vision, when the patient has difficultly with reading, seeing faces and colour perceptions, can be linked to age-related macular degeneration (AMD). The incidence of AMD is increased in people who smoke (Rennie et al. 2012) and have cardiovascular disease, so health promotion, part of the nursing associate role, is also appropriate here.
- Ocular pain: Review the nature of the pain, using an appropriate pain assessment tool. Acute pain with sudden onset can be indicative of raised intraocular pressure and a duller ache can be linked to ocular inflammation (Peate 2020).
- Ocular infections, such as a hypopyon (pus inside the anterior chamber of the eye) will require urgent referral. More minor conditions such as conjunctivitis are contagious, so the spread of infection must be avoided through handwashing and using separate towels (National Institute for Health and Care Excellence (NICE) 2018).
- A red eye(s) can be related to numerous conditions, ranging from minor to sight threatening, so always escalate any concerns and changes to a senior practitioner.

Supporting Evidence

People with visual changes are at an increase in frequency of falling (Newton & Sanderson 2013), so a falls risk assessment should be completed as well as reviewed by an optometrist. Visit the Royal National Institute for the blind at https://www.rnib.org.uk/ for more information.

Table 27.1 Effect of health conditions on the eye and associated structures

CONDITION	EFFECT ON THE EYE AND ASSOCIATED STRUCTURES
Eczema or psoriasis	Blepharitis, inflammation of the eyelids, causing itching, redness and irritations.
Hypertension	Subconjunctival, retinal and vitreous haemorrhages.
Diabetes mellitus	Retinal or vitreous haemorrhages. Diabetic retinopathy and maculopathy can develop if this condition is not effectively managed.
Thyroid imbalance	Dry eyes, blurred vision and exophthalmos (bulging eye).
Multiple sclerosis	Ocular pain, squint, ptosis and irregular pupil size.
Migraines	Visual auras of lights and shapes, pain.
Inflammatory disorders such as irritable bowel syndrome and arthritis	Iritis (uveitis), the inflammation of the iris, ciliary body and choroid.
Asthma/chronic obstructive pulmonary disorder	Early cataracts if frequent use of oral steroidal medications.
Cerebrovascular accident (stroke)	Sudden sight loss due to central retinal artery occlusion Hemianopia (loss of half of visual field in each eye)
Hyperlipidaemia	Corneal arcus and xanthelasma

In Table 27.1, a number of systemic conditions that can affect the eyes and associated structures have been outlined.

Touch Point

Early recognition and detection of eye problems and changes to sight can help improve outcomes for the person. As a nursing associate, accountable professional, observational and communication skills are key to achieve early recognition. Involving family, carers and other healthcare professionals in the care planning will help the facilitation of working in teams. However, it is important to note that this is dependent upon the actual eye problem, as some eye conditions are progressive.

Eye Care

This is an important aspect of holistic and person-centred care. Remember to promote independence by encouraging the patients to be involved in their care decisions and interventions, as they are able. Some of the main care interventions and skills that you require as a nursing associate in the remit of providing and monitoring care include:

a. Eye bathing

This should be performed as a clean technique, using normal saline in a clinical environment or cooled boiled water in a community location (for example, the person's home).

Soak a cotton wool ball or gauze, then gently wipe, once, from the medial (inner) to lateral (outer) canthal region. This should be repeated until any discharge is removed. Wash hands thoroughly before and after; gloves can be worn as per local infection prevention and control policies.

Blue Flag

Social interactions and relationships can be affected if the person is struggling to cope with their sight loss and social isolation is a risk. It is important to recognise these changes and signpost to appropriate support networks.

b. Instillation of eye drops and eye ointment

Any use of medications should follow local policies, with expiry dates and guidance adhered to at all times, as showed in Box 27.1.

In addition, avoid dropping the solution onto the sensitive cornea, as this causes discomfort and will trigger a reflexive squeezing shut of the eye, and it is essential that all eye drop regimens are fully completed.

Box 27.1 outlines the procedure for instillation of eye drops/ointment and information for patients.

Box 27.1 Instilling Eye Drops (Information for Patients)

1. Read the instructions carefully before using eye drops.
2. Store eye drops at room temperature and away from heat, moisture and direct light (or as directed).
3. Do not use the drops if they change colour or are out of date.
4. Do not use the drops if they have debris (bits) floating in them.
5. Wait for 10–15 minutes before using a different kind of eye drop.
6. Wash hands before and after instilling eye drops.
7. Gently shake the bottle.
8. Do not touch the tip of the bottle to the eye.
9. Tilt the head back and pull down the lower eyelid with the index finger.
10. Gently squeeze the bottle to drop the correct number of drops into the eye.
11. Wait for 1 minute between each drop.
12. Replace the cap on the bottle.
13. Close the eyes. Press the index finger against the inside corner of the eye next to the nose for 1 minute, to reduce systemic absorption (punctal occlusion).
14. Gently wipe away any extra liquid with a tissue.
15. Wash hands.
16. Do not rub the eyes.

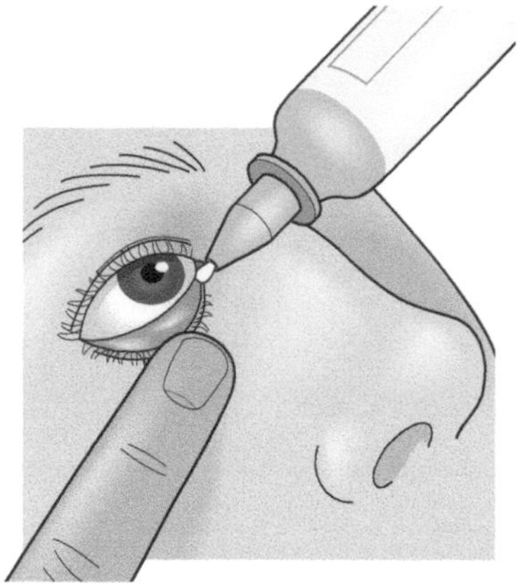

Source: Peate & Wild (2018), pp. 872–873. © John Wiley & Sons.

Green Flag

As a nursing associate, the emphasis is on safe and person-centred care. Changes in sight and potential impairments can be recognised through observation of the person's behaviour, noting any changes in their appearance or general mood and asking their family or significant other if they are aware of any changes.

c. Care of contact lens and glasses

Glasses should be stored safely in a case to minimise the risk of damage, when not worn. The lens should be carefully cleaned with soap and water and then dried with a non-fluffy cloth. Ensure that glasses are damage free and well fitting, as poor position will hinder vision.

If a person wears contact lens, they should be advised to follow the manufacturer's guidance with usage. If a person has a red eye, then contact lens should not be worn until this is resolved.

Touch Point

Ensuring regular eye checks by an optometrist is part of every person's care. Annual checks are advised if the person has a sight problem or associated family history such as glaucoma. Otherwise, every 2 years is sufficient for health screening.

Many optometrists offer a domiciliary service, so check local services; if people are housebound, then this may be suitable for them.

(NICE guidelines NG81 2017)

d. Care of an artificial eye and the eye socket

An artificial eye (AE) should be cleaned daily with warm water and normal soap and then rinsed thoroughly to ensure that no deposits of chemicals or debris remain before reinsertion into eye socket. The nursing associate should check this to avoid inflammation or infection in the socket. Also, if there is any damage to the AE, then this should be sent to the National Artificial Eye Service for repair.

If the eye socket appears infected, this should be irrigated using normal saline and treated with a topical antibiotic ointment, ensuring a safe aseptic technique. The artificial eye should not be inserted until the infection and redness has been resolved (National Artificial Eye Service 2019).

Yellow Flag

As a nursing associate, it is essential to understand that everyone living with an SI will have different needs and abilities. Many SIPs lead an independent life.

SSI can be due to corneal injury or disease, and, in certain circumstances, the only solution is a corneal graft from a donor eye. An awareness of organ donation and new legislation of opting out, introduced in Spring 2020 is important. Further information can be found at https://www.nhsbt.nhs.uk/.

e. How to safely guide SIPs.

As their sighted guide, you should offer them their preferred elbow, which they should hold as though gripping a glass. This naturally puts the guide one step ahead, so they can safely lead. As their sighted guide, you need to explain the journey and highlight any changes such as steps, narrower spaces and going through doors. Do not give too much advanced warning and make the conversation natural.

Violet Flag

Effective and safe discharge planning for all persons is key. In order to promote and maintain independent living, the SIPs may require adaptations to their home environment. A referral to social services should be made for possible financial support, and, if their sight is deteriorating, the option of being registered as an SSI or SI should be discussed. The latter is normally done, after a consultation with ophthalmologist, and it is the person's choice.

Touch Points Revisited

- Ensure regular eye checks with an optometrist or attendance eye clinic appointments in order to maintain eye health, detect any sight problems and changes.
- Early recognition and detection of eye problems and changes to sight can help with improved outcomes for the person, in some cases.
- Maintaining a safe environment for SIPs, as they are at increased risk of falls. The environment should be well lit; free from clutter, rugs and any trip hazards; and should have secure flooring in order to achieve improved safety and quality care.
- It is essential to fully orientate the SIPs to their current environment.

References

National Artificial Eye Service. (2019) [online] Available: https://www.naes.nhs.uk/. Accessed 16 October 2019.

National Institute for Health and Care Excellence (NICE). (2017) *Glaucoma: diagnosis and management NG81. [online] Available*: https://www.nice.org.uk/guidance/ng81. Accessed 16 October 2019.

National Institute for Health and Care Excellence (NICE). (2018) *National institute for health and care excellence (NICE) clinical guidelines for the red eye.* [online] Available: https;//cks.nice.org.uk/red-eye. Accessed 18 October 2019.

NHS Blood and Transplant. (2019) [online] Available: https://www.nhsbt.nhs.uk/. Accessed 16 October 2019.

Newton, M. and Sanderson, A. (2013) The effect of visual impairment on patients falls risks, *Nursing Older People*, 25(8): 16–21.

Nursing and Midwifery Council. (2018) *Standards of proficiency for nursing associates.* [online] Available: https://www.nmc.org.uk/standards/standards-for-nursing-associates/standards-of-proficiency-for-nursing-associates/. Accessed September 2019.

Peate, I. (2017) *Fundamentals of applied pathophysiology: an essential guide for nursing and healthcare students* (3rd edn), Oxford: Wiley.

Peate, I. (2020) *Alexander's nursing practice Hospital and Home*, 5th edition. Elsevier.

Peate, I. and Wild, K. (Eds) (2018) *Nursing practice: knowledge and care* (2nd edn), Oxford: Wiley.

Rennie, C.A., Stinge, A., King, E.A., Sothirachagan, S., Osmond, C. and Lotery, A.J. (2012) Can genetic risk information for age-related macular degeneration influence motivation to stop smoking? A pilot study, *Eye*, 26: 109–118.

Royal National Institute for the Blind (RNIB). (2019) [online] Available: https://www.rnib.org.uk/. Accessed 16 October 2019.

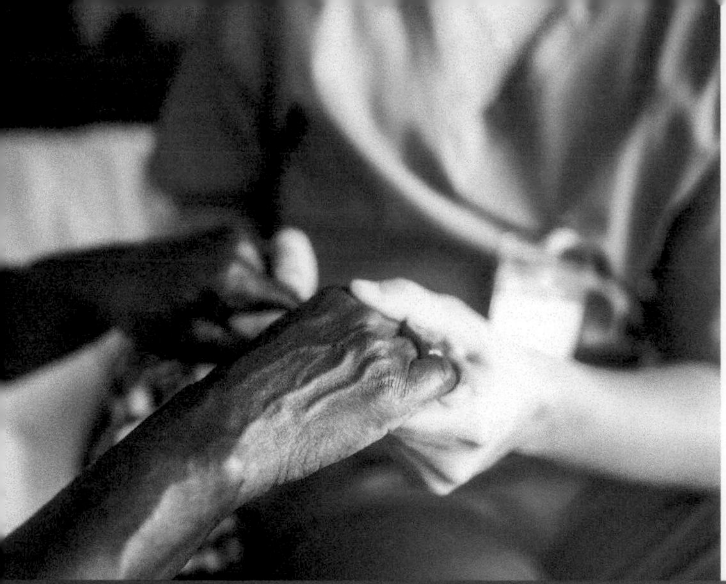

28

Providing Nail Care

Ally Sanderson

Teesside University, UK

Chapter Aim

- This chapter aims to help the reader understand the importance of care of the nails in the health and well-being of patients.

Learning Objectives

By the end of this chapter, the reader will be able to:
- Provide safe and effective person-centred care in order to promote the maintenance of healthy nails
- Recognise the significance of abnormalities of nails and how this is linked to illness and disease

Test Yourself Multiple Choice Questions

1. What are the two main functions of nails?
   A) Appearance and protection
   B) Protection and sensory function
   C) Dexterity and protection
   D) Dexterity and appearance
2. What are the nail structures called?
   A) Nail dish, nail base, cuticle, nail turns, luna and matrix
   B) Nail plate, nail bed, cuticle, nail folds, lunula and matrix
   C) Nail bowl, nail bed, cuticle, nail folds, luna and matrin
   D) Nail bowl, nail base, cubicle, nail turns, lunula and matrix
3. Which system do the nails belong too?
   A) Immune
   B) Endocrine
   C) Integumentary
   D) Cardiovascular

The Nursing Associate's Handbook of Clinical Skills, First Edition. Edited by Ian Peate.

Companion website: www.wiley.com/nursingassociate

4. **Which grows quicker?**
   A) **Fingernails**
   B) **Toenails**
   C) **Grow at same rate**
   D) **Depends on the individual person**
5. **Which illnesses or diseases can be detected from abnormalities of the nails?**
   A) **Leukaemia, cardiac disease, pneumonia and psoriasis**
   B) **Fungal infections, malnutrition, iron deficiency and pseudomonas**
   C) **Both A and B**
   D) **No diseases or illnesses are detectable by looking at the nails**

Introduction

The nails provide a protective covering for the ends of the fingers and toes. Nails are tightly packed, dead hard keratinised epidermal cells forming a clean, solid covering over digits (see Figure 28.1).

Nails are not essential for life. Fingernails and toenails help us to pick up objects and grasp them more firmly. They also allow people to pick, itch, peel, grab, climb, dig, tear and a number of other tasks; we are able to manipulate things with fingernails allowing us to do much more with them than without them.

The physical appearance of a person's fingernails and toenails can be indicative of systemic illnesses and disease; the nursing associate, as an accountable practitioner, should recognise any abnormalities and plan care accordingly (Nursing and Midwifery Council (NMC) 2018a). Nails are a window of health.

Orange Flag

Onychophagia – nail biting. A habit that can be associated with anxiety and stress in patients; the nursing associate should determine if there is an underlying cause and offer support to the person as needed.

Nursing associate has to be able to demonstrate proficiency in a number of areas related to nail care; this chapter considers these areas, for example, the nursing associate has to practise in an accountable manner, promote health and prevent ill health, improve safety and quality of care, provide and monitor care delivered, make a contribution to integrated care and work in teams (Nursing and Midwifery Council 2018b).

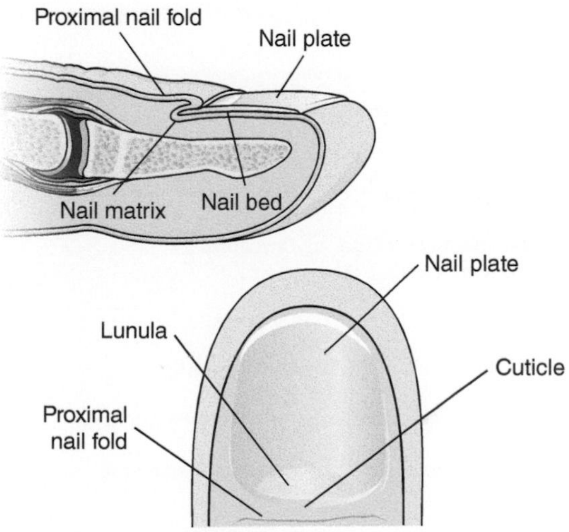

Figure 28.1 The nail. ***Source:*** **Peate & Nair (2017), figure 17.6, p. 562. © John Wiley & Sons**

Red Flag

The nursing associate should be alert to issues that denote serious pathology. If the nursing associate has any concerns, then these should be escalated to a senior practitioner, and the issues should be documented as per local policy and procedure.

- Beau lines – a groove crossing the nail horizontally. This happens when the nail stops growing for a period of time due to serious illness, such as cancer or pneumonia.
- Clubbing – the nail will curve over the fingertip; this can be linked to congenital cardiac conditions and chronic respiratory conditions.
- Paronychia – nails will have tiny vertical haemorrhages (splinter); this is associated with bacterial endocarditis.
- Onycholysis –the nail separates from the nail bed and can fall out. This can occur when patients have had chemotherapy treatment.
- Pseudomonas nail infection – the nail will lift from the nail bed and a green, odorous discharge will form between.
- Onychomycosis – fungal infection of the nail. This common problem results in thickening of the nail, causing cutting to be difficult and can result in onycholysis. Regular cutting and monitoring are needed to avoid ingrown nails.
- Ingrown nails – usually affects toenails. Can lead to inflammation and localised infection of the skin. Foot care should be part of routine screening, in the prevention of ulcers and infections; they are complex to manage if not diagnosed early, especially in patients with Diabetes Mellitus.
- Onychogryphosis – also known as *Ram's horn*. The nail will be thick, discoloured and growing away from the nail bed. Can cause problems with footwear, balance and increase the risk of falls, so a multi-disciplinary approach is needed and referral to chiropody.
- Psoriatic nails – linked to people who have arthritic conditions and dermatological conditions, such as eczema or psoriasis. The nail will be discoloured, and thickening of toenails is a common presentation.
- Koilonychias – nails will appear concave, like a spoon; this is due to iron deficiency.
- Trauma – can result from crush, penetration or avulsion injuries. The patient should be referred for review and appropriate management.

Supporting Evidence

The risk of foot problems in those with diabetes is increased, principally as a result of either diabetic neuropathy (nerve damage or degeneration) or peripheral arterial disease (poor blood supply due to diseased large- and medium-sized blood vessels in the legs), or both.

Foot complications are common in people with diabetes with an estimated 10% of people with diabetes experiencing a diabetic foot ulcer at some point in their lives. A foot ulcer can be defined as a localised injury to the skin and/or underlying tissue, below the ankle, in a person with diabetes.

Source: National Institute for Health and Care Excellence (2015)

In Table 28.1, a number of conditions that can affect the nail and the nail bed have been outlined.

Table 28.1 Common conditions and the effect on the nail bed.

CONDITION	EFFECT ON NAIL BED
Anxiety, depression or compulsive disorders	Nail biting, paronychia and periungual warts
Median nail dystrophy usually caused by an underlying psychological condition	Longitudinal depression along the nail bed with an enlarged lunula
Psoriasis	Pitting of the nail plate, onycholysis (separation of the free edge of the nail plate which whitens) and dystrophy (thickened, opaque and discoloured nail)
Alopecia areata, eczema, Reiter's syndrome and pemphigus	Pitting of the nail bed
Eczema, lichen planus, periungual warts, fungal infections of the nail, iron-deficiency anaemia, thyrotoxicosis and sarcoidosis	Onycholysis
Psoriasis acrodermatitis continua of Hallopeau	Dystrophy
Eczema	Nail shedding
Trauma, rheumatoid arthritis and bacterial endocarditis	Splinter haemorrhages
Systemic lupus erythematosus, dermatomyositis, sarcoidosis and human immunodeficiency virus (HIV)	Periungual erythema
Terry's half and half-nail (proximal part whitens)	Renal failure, liver cirrhosis, congestive cardiac failure and type 2 diabetes

Source: Stephens (2018).

Touch Point

Using the skills of observation and communication, the nursing associate can identify any potential health and well-being issues.

Nail Care

Nail care is an important aspect of holistic care, and as such, this is an essential component of total patient care. Foot care, for example, is essential for mobility, independent functioning and comfort. Every attempt should be made to ensure nails are clean in order to prevent spread of infection and also to promote the person's health and well-being. Person-centred care should be promoted by asking about preferences with length and how the person wishes their nails to look, if they are unable to maintain them independently.

Blue Flag

Artificial, gel, shellac or painted nails – this is a choice linked to how patients wish to express themselves. If they have limited independence, it is important for nursing associates to address this important aspect of their personal care. It is important to note that if a patient is due to have a surgical procedure, a pulse oximeter to monitor oxygen saturations will be used and gel/shellac nails make this inaccurate, so nails should be natural.

The majority of patients are able to perform nail care for themselves, and they usually do this as a part of their daily hygiene routine. The nursing associate may need to provide nail care for those patients who are unable to perform this activity themselves, for example, an unconscious person, a person with severe sight impairment, those with dexterity problems, a person who may be confused, a patient who has a tremor, those who are in casts or traction and those with learning disabilities. Individual assessment of needs is a requirement.

Touch Point

Most people are able to care for their own nails. The nursing associate may be required to assist with this essential aspect of nursing care. Nail care brings with it immediate and tangible benefits to patients; it can boost self-esteem and enhance a sense of well-being.

Nail care includes regular trimming, gentle cleaning under the nails and cuticle care (Williams 2018). Ensure that the nails are kept clean and trimmed according to patient preference (their cultural preferences, values and beliefs) and that you always adhere to local policy and procedure.

Yellow Flag

- Loss of nails – Any deformities or loss of nails may cause concerns for the person about their appearance.
- Personal values – Each individual will have a preference to how they like their nails to look, the length, how often they are cut and whether they use scissors or clippers. Ensure person-centred care, undertake a review of their preferences and provide safe and quality care.
- Cultural beliefs – Certain cultures will have beliefs and preferences. Some people from Haiti, USA, for example, have short and polished nails for hygiene purposes, and in the Hindu religion, nails should not be cut on a Saturday as this brings bad luck (Colin & Paperwall 2003).

Each healthcare provider is likely to have a policy and procedure associated with nail cutting, for example, cutting the toenails of a patient with diabetes or circulatory disease of the lower extremities may only be undertaken by a chiropodist. Policy and procedure must be checked to determine if it is acceptable for the nursing associate to trim the fingernails of people with diabetes. The nursing associate has to have been deemed competent and confident to undertake nail care; they will have received training from a competent person prior to undertaking any nail care procedure.

- Gather equipment (this will depend on individual needs and local policy and procedure).
- Wash hands and wear disposable gloves and apron.
- Explain the procedure to the patient and gain verbal consent.
- Ensure that the patient is in a comfortable position and the nails are easily accessible.
- If possible, soak the nails in warm soapy water for 5 to 10 minutes.
- Assess the nails to ensure that there are no complications that might require a referral to another healthcare professional.
- Gently, using an orangewood stick, clean under the nails (a metal nail file can make the nails rough and trap dirt).

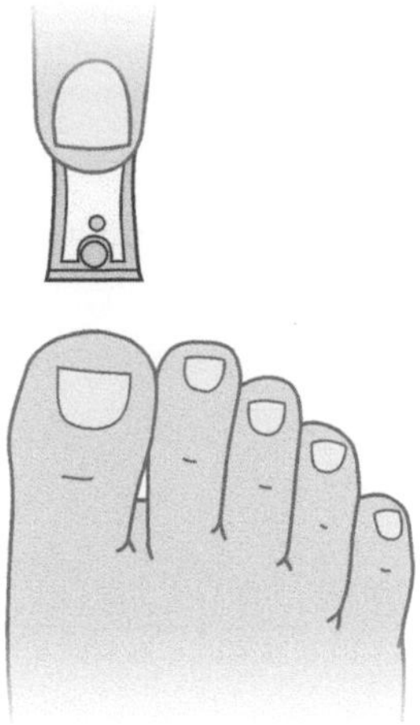

Figure 28.2 **Cut the toenail straight across and then smooth the corners.**

- Gently push cuticles back with the stick to prevent hangnails (these are pieces of skin that are partially detached at the base of the fingernail); they can be painful and a possible source of infection.
- Using nail clippers, cut the nails straight across; this prevents them from growing into the skin along the sides which can result in pain or infection and may lead to ingrown toenails. Often ingrown toenails require a surgical procedure to correct (see Figure 28.2).
- After clipping, dispose of the nail trimmings in the paper towel and dispose of in clinical waste bin.
- If needed, assist the patient to replace any socks, shoes or slippers and maintain a comfortable position.
- Remove gloves and apron.
- Wash hands.
- Document procedure recording which instruments (i.e. clippers) have been used.

Source: (Malkin & Berridge 2009)

Green Flag

General appearance: If the person is unkempt, with dirty nails and appears to have a neglected appearance with their clothing and personal hygiene standards, these may be personal choices. This can also be signs of abuse or neglect for the older person. The nursing associate must bear in mind that abuse and neglect can occur anywhere, and raise their concerns to a senior practitioner.

In order to prevent cross-infection, all patients should have their own equipment just as they would have their own toothbrush. The equipment should be cleaned with detergent and dried after use.

Violet Flag

Mees lines: These thin white lines which cross the nail horizontally is a sign of carbon monoxide poisoning. Urgent review of the individual and any other family members is priority, as well as a review of the home environment by social agencies and possible fire service for fitting of carbon monoxide monitor.

Touch Points Revisited

The physical appearance of a person's nails can be indicative of systemic illnesses and disease; the nursing associate should recognise this and plan care accordingly.

Person-centred care should be promoted by asking about preferences with length and how the person wishes their nails to look, if they are unable to maintain them independently.

References

Colin, J.M. and Paperwall, G. (2003) People of Haitian heritage, in Purnell, L.D. & Paulanka, B.J. (eds.) *Transcultural health care: a culturally competent approach* (2nd edn), Philadelphia: F.A. Davis, 517–543. https://www.in.gov/isdh/files/Haiti_Cultural_and_Clinical_Care_Presentation_Read-Only.pdf. Accessed 18 October 2019.

Malkin, B. and Berridge, P. (2009) Guidance on maintaining person hygiene in nail care, *Nursing Standard*, 23(41): 35–38. doi: 10.7748/ns2009.06.23.41.35.c7048.

National Institute for Health and Care Excellence. (2015) Guideline NG19, *Diabetic foot problems: prevention and management.* [online] Available: https://www.nice.org.uk/guidance/ng19. Accessed 4 October 2019.

Nursing and Midwifery Council (NMC). (2018a) *Standards of proficiency for nursing associates.* [online] Available: https://www.nmc.org.uk/standards/standards-for-nursing-associates/standards-of-proficiency-for-nursing-associates/. Accessed September 2019.

Nursing and Midwifery Council (NMC). (2018b) *The code: professional standards of practice and behaviour for nurses, midwives and nursing associates.* [online] Available: http://www.nmc.org.uk/globalassets/sitedocuments/nmc-publications/revised-new-nmc-code.pdf. Accessed September 2019.

Peate, I. & Nair, M. (2017). *Fundamentals of anatomy and physiology: for nursing and healthcare students* (2nd edn). Oxford: Wiley.

Stephens, M. (2018) The person with a skin disorder, in Peate, I. & Wild, K. (eds.) *Nursing practice, knowledge and care* (2nd edn), Oxford: Wiley, Ch 38, 909–930.

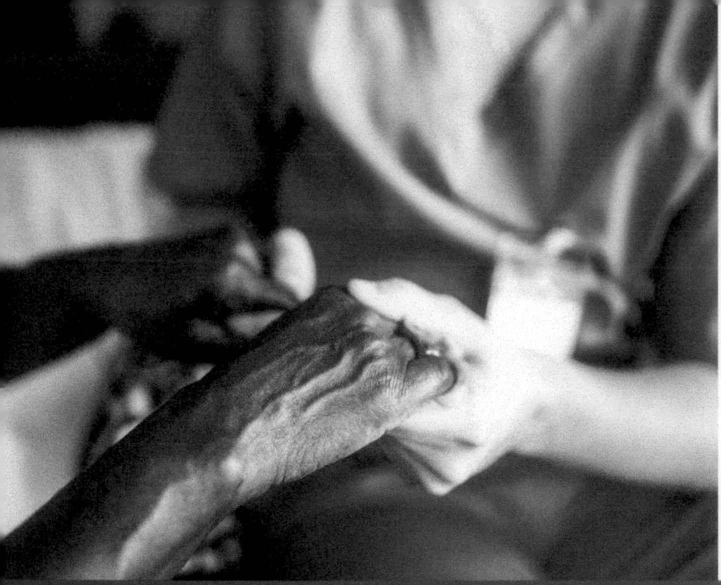

29

Monitoring of Wounds and Providing Wound Care

Ian Peate

School of Health Studies, Gibraltar

Chapter Aim

- **This chapter provides the reader with an outline of the principles associated with caring for people with wounds.**

Learning Outcomes

By the end of this chapter, the reader will be able to:

- **Define a wound**
- **Identify the causes of wounds**
- **Identify factors associated with healing and the monitoring of wounds**
- **Describe the principles of effective wound care**

Test Yourself Multiple Choice Questions

1. **The two layers of the skin are known as:**
   A) **The dermis and prodermis**
   B) **The dermis and epidermis**
   C) **The antedermis and dermis**
   D) **The dermal node and epidermal node**
2. **From birth until death:**
   A) **The skin and subcutaneous tissue grow, mature and age; the skin changes with age**
   B) **The skin hypotrophies and retracts**
   C) **The skin and subcutaneous tissue stop growing and cease to mature**
   D) **The skin and subcutaneous tissue stop growing**

The Nursing Associate's Handbook of Clinical Skills, First Edition. Edited by Ian Peate.

Companion website: www.wiley.com/nursingassociate

3. **A *wound* is defined as:**
   A) **An infected lesion**
   B) **A defect or breach in the continuity of the skin**
   C) **A defect or breach in tissue causing a visible scar**
   D) **Macerated tissue and high temperature**
4. **Each step of the wound-healing process is dependent on:**
   A) **Sunshine, nutrients, circulating amino acids, lipids and carbohydrates**
   B) **Sunshine, nutrients, circulating amino acids, lipids, carbohydrates and normal blood pressure**
   C) **Nutrients, circulating amino acids, lipids and carbohydrates**
   D) **Sunshine, nutrients, circulating amino acids, lipids, carbohydrates and glucose**
5. **The term angiogenesis means:**
   A) **Pain on pressure**
   B) **Swelling of the lips**
   C) **High temperature accompanied with high blood pressure**
   D) **The formation of new blood vessels**

Introduction

This chapter discusses the principles of wound care with a focus on defining what a wound is. This chapter will also help identify factors that may influence the healing process and aid the healing process.

It is essential that the nursing associate uses a structured, evidence-based approach in order to select the most appropriate wound dressing. If best patient outcomes are to be realised, then the application of evidence-based wound management knowledge and skills is key. The type of wound and the wound aetiology (cause) are factors that must be given much thought. At all times, there has to be a holistic focus with the patient at the centre of all that is done.

Blue Flag

The nursing associate needs to consider the effect of the wound on the patients' life and their family, reviewing their preferences and values. Actions and procedures have to be explained; the pros and cons of treatment options must be offered in clear terms that are free of jargon. Patients have the right to know about the benefits, risks and side effects of their wound care treatment and to be a part in the development of a treatment plan with the multidisciplinary team. It is important for the patient to be part of the informed decision-making process; this has the potential to help develop trust and rapport.

The standards of proficiency for nursing associates (Nursing and Midwifery Council (NMC) 2018a) require that, upon registration, the nursing associate must demonstrate they have the appropriate level of knowledge, the skills and the ability to meet the needs of people related to wound care and, as such, skin integrity. They are required to be proficient in monitoring wounds and undertaking wound care using appropriate evidence-based techniques.

Green Flag

The NMC Code (Nursing and Midwifery Council 2018b) makes clear that you:

- Put the interests of people using or needing nursing services first
- Assess needs and deliver or advise on treatment or give help (including preventative or rehabilitative care) without too much delay, to the best of your abilities, on the basis of best available evidence
- Make sure that patient and public safety are not affected
- Uphold the reputation of your profession at all times

These four overarching themes apply to the care of people with wounds.

The Skin

The skin is the largest organ of the body consisting of accessory organs: glands, hair and nails (the appendages). It is a multifunctional organ performing the following functions:

- Acts as a barrier against the external environment protecting against biological invasion, physical/mechanical damage and ultraviolet radiation
- The nerve endings provide sensation, temperature, pain and an alert for potential damage
- Controls heat through sweating and the regulation of blood flow

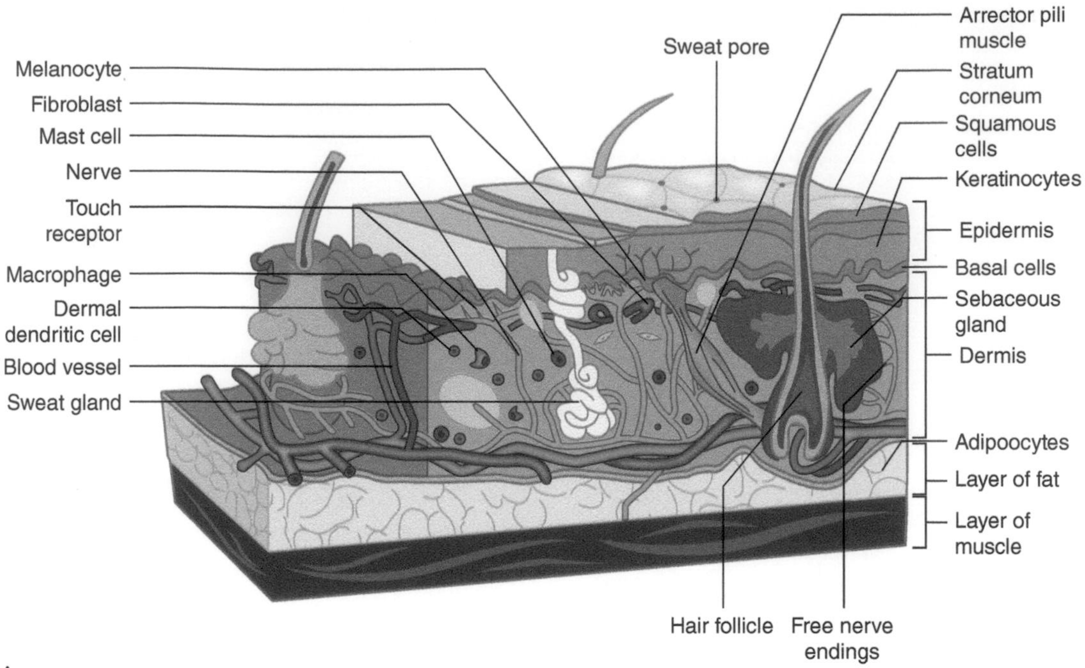

Figure 29.1 The skin.

- As an endocrine organ, it synthesises vitamin D, steroids and thyroid hormone
- Sweat excretes salts and small amounts of waste
- Aesthetics and communication.

The skin has two layers (see Figure 29.1 for a diagrammatic representation of the skin). Skin health has a great impact on the overall health of the individual and is of profound psychological importance.

The health of skin is influenced by a number of internal and external factors; these factors influence wound healing. To support the health of skin and the healing of wounds, nursing associates need to understand and recognise the complex nature of skin and what lies beneath.

Orange Flag

The skin is a window between the mind and body and the external environment. The physical presence of the skin as the largest organ of the body is significant concerning psychological and social perspectives. The skin has psychological and social components; it can lead to discrimination and has the ability to reveal how we are from a health and well-being perspective. When the nursing associate understands this complex relationship, they will be able to offer assistance with regards to the various coping mechanisms that can be used by people to help them live with wounds – healed or healing.

Table 29.1 considers some of the underlying structures that are required for movement, support, protection and production of blood components and the implications and effects on wounds.

Touch Point

For nursing associates, knowledge of the anatomy and physiology of skin and the healing process is key to prevent, review, treat and manage acute and chronic wounds effectively.

Skin Changes and Age

The changes in skin quality over a lifetime can be due to internal and external influences to cellular and molecular structure. A baby's skin, for example, is generally smoother and more supple than an adult's skin. From birth until death, the skin and subcutaneous tissue grow, mature and age; the skin changes with age.

Infant Skin

There are many ways in which infant skin differs from adult skin. The thickness of infant skin is 40% to 60% that of adult skin (Thappa 2016). Weak rete ridges offer limited surface attachment to the dermis which is immature. The infant's body surface area-to-weight ratio is up to five

Table 29.1 Some underlying structures required for movement, support, protection and production of blood components and wounds.

STRUCTURE	FUNCTION	EFFECT ON WOUNDS
Epidermis	Provides protection against trauma and harmful environment and organisms	If the epidermis is damaged, abrasion occurs.
Dermis	Provides skin flexibility and strength	Bleeding occurs, and the body's first line of defence is breached.
Arterial blood	Delivers oxygen to the body	Poor arterial flow leads to ischaemia and impaired healing.
Venous blood	Removes metabolic waste products from the body	Venous hypertension leads to oedema and hinders healing.
Lymph fluid	Removes waste and supports immune response	Lymphoedema often accompanies venous oedema and may hinder healing.
Subcutaneous tissue	Offers protection, cushioning, insulation and energy storage	Poorly vascularised tissue will result in slow healing.
Fascia	Gives structure, protection, support	Entry into fascia leads to infection.
Muscles	Perform movement	Muscles are highly vascularised and tear easily.
Tendons	Attaches muscle to bone	Exposed tendons should be kept moist. They are poorly vascularised and slow to heal. Loss of tendon results in loss of function.
Ligaments	Attach bones to bones, forming a joint	Exposed ligaments should be kept moist. They are poorly vascularised, slow to heal. Loss of ligament means loss of function.
Bones	Provide protection, strength and support	Exposed bone can lead to osteomyelitis. Bone should not be allowed to dry out.
Joints	Enable movement and mechanical support	Joint involvement in wounds can lead to osteomyelitis.

Source: Modified from Jarvis (2015).

times to that of an adult. These factors place the infant at greater risk for skin damage. Usually, baby skin contains slightly higher water content. While an infant is estimated to be roughly 75% water, adults are closer to 65% water, and the elderly are closer to 55% water.

Adolescent Skin

Adolescence is seen as the transitional stage of physical maturation and psychosocial development, usually occurring from puberty to adulthood. Adolescence brings about the maturation of the hair follicles, sebaceous glands and sweat glands in the skin. Stimulation of the sebaceous glands is caused by an increase in the sex hormones – oestrogen, androgen and progesterone; this results in an increased production of oil or sebum.

The Older Adult's Skin

As people age, their skin goes through a number of changes as a result of genetics, the environment, their lifestyle and existing chronic diseases. Despite these individual differences, the normal ageing process of all skin causes several predictable changes.

As age increases, there is a decrease in the turnover of the epidermal layer, and the pH of the skin becomes more neutral and more susceptible to bacterial growth and infections. The outer epidermal layer thins and can cause a decrease in collagen per year leading to wrinkling. Blood supply is reduced, and the dermis becomes increasingly avascular as the body ages. Changes occur in collagen and elastin, the connective tissues underlying the skin, which give the skin its firmness and elasticity.

Kottner (2015) states that ageing is a normal biological process that affects every organ and biological system. However, compared to the skin of youth, aged skin is compromised in many ways. Preventive skin care strategies are therefore of the utmost importance in maintaining skin integrity in our increasing elderly population.

Types of Wound

Wounds can be described in many ways, for example, by its aetiology, by its anatomical location, by whether it is acute or chronic, by the method of closure, by its presenting symptoms or by the appearance of the predominant tissue types in the wound bed. All definitions have an important role to play in the assessment and appropriate management of the wound through to symptom resolution or, if feasible, healing.

A wound is defined by Fletcher & Anderson (2019) as a defect or breach in the continuity of the skin. A wound results in a breakdown in the protective function of the skin with a loss of continuity of epithelium, with or without loss of underlying connective tissue (i.e. muscle, bone, nerves). Wounds can occur following injury to the skin or underlying tissues/organs caused by surgery, a blow (trauma), a cut, chemicals, heat/cold, friction/shear force, pressure or as a result of disease, for example, leg ulcers or cancer.

Classification of Wounds

There are two main categories of wounds: acute and chronic; along with this, there are two subcategories that identify the phases of the wound-healing process and the tissue type(s) on the wound bed. The classification of wounds enables the nursing associate to accurately review patient care for any given wound from a holistic perspective. In some cases, an acute wound will undoubtedly become chronic due to underlying comorbidities.

Acute Wounds

An acute wound is caused by trauma or surgery. An acute wound heals by primary intention any traumatic or surgical wound heals by secondary intention; these wounds are expected to progress through the phases of normal healing, resulting in the closure of the wound. There are many different causes of trauma:

Incision – This wound is usually induced by a sharp object (e.g. scalpel, knife, shard of glass or a metal sheet) causing a 'slice' to the skin. Usually, there is very little tissue loss, and the edges are often very clearly defined. The depth can vary from superficial to deep.

Laceration/skin tear – This is frequently caused by a blow against a blunt object causing the skin to 'split'. Often, there is swelling with some tissue loss with the creation of a skin flap that can be very thick or very thin in depth. A *skin tear* is usually caused by the tearing of the skin by a sharp object, for example, a nail, a fingernail, or by clothing/belts or rough handling; the older person's skin is often subject to this type of trauma. The depth is usually superficial and confined to the skin; however, it can affect deeper tissues.

Burn – This is caused by heat (fire), cold (frostbite), chemicals and electricity. It is essential to identify the cause of the burn in order to treat it appropriately. These wounds can vary in depth from superficial to deep.

Scald – This type of injury can be caused by hot liquids and steam and must be quickly cooled; damage can vary in depth from superficial to deep.

Puncture – This is a penetrating wound that can be of varying depth caused by pointed objects such as nails, wooden stakes, pins, needles or teeth (i.e. cat bites). These can appear insignificant due to the small opening on the skin; however, underlying structural damage and risk of infection are associated with this type of wound.

Contusion – This is a bruise caused by the rupture of superficial blood vessels due to the trauma, with no break to the skin itself. Bruising disperses in around 14 days via venous and lymphatic drainage. The darker the discolouration, the deeper the damage.

Friction – It is the erosion of superficial (and sometimes deeper) tissues caused by the sudden or constant rubbing of the skin against a rougher surface.

Pressure – This is tissue death creating a wound, caused by unrelieved and prolonged pressure applied against the skin.

Shearing – It is a closed wound where tissues attached to bone are torn away from the bone due to opposing forces of two tissue types. The affects are deep seated and can be painful due to inflammation of the bursa tissues at the site of trauma (bursitis). This type of injury is not usually visible to the eye but will make the patient more vulnerable to rapid onset of pressure damage.

Chronic Wounds

A chronic wound is defined as a being induced by a variety of causes and does not progress through the phases of wound healing leading to a prolonged or static wound as a result of underlying causes, usually of a duration longer than 4 to 6 weeks. The following wound types may become chronic, but any wound from any cause can become chronic due to underlying factors affecting the healing rates:

- Leg ulcers (venous or arterial ulceration)
- Diabetic foot ulceration
- Pressure ulcer
- Some skin conditions (such as eczema, psoriasis, blistering)

With chronic wounds, wound healing is delayed by the presence of intrinsic and extrinsic factors; these include medications, poor nutrition, comorbidities or inappropriate dressing selection.

Supporting Evidence European Wound Management Association

Atypical wounds

https://ewma.org/it/what-we-do/ewma-projects/atypical-wounds/

This document provides an overview of recent knowledge and evidence about atypical wounds. These are defined as those wounds that cannot be placed in the primary categories of non-healing wounds.

The document offers an overview about wounds considered atypical and present the diagnostic criteria, comorbidities and diagnostic tools for these types of wounds. It presents the best available documented treatment options and the various treatment options of these wounds.

Wound Healing

When the skin is damaged or wounded, it makes efforts to regenerate itself so that it can continue to offer protection. Wounds heal by primary intention or secondary intention depending upon whether the wound is closed with sutures or left to repair; damaged tissue is restored by the formation of connective tissue and the re-growth of epithelium.

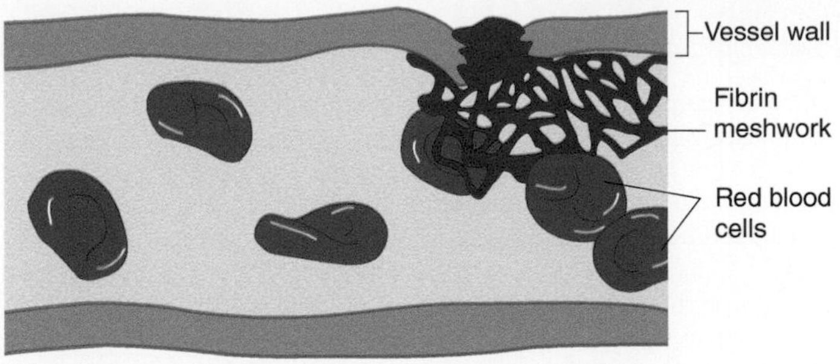

Figure 29.2 Fibrin meshwork and formation is a clot. *Source:* Peate & Glencross (2015), chapter 6, figure 6.2, p. 24. © John Wiley & Sons.

Wound healing is a complex and dynamic process that varies according to the location and type of wound; it is an organised process that follows in stepwise manner and involves the stages of haemostasis, inflammation and repair. Generally, from injury to resolution, wounds go through the following four phases:

1. Haemostasis
2. Inflammation
3. Proliferation
4. Remodelling

When wounds heal, fibrin formation occurs, and a protective wound scab is formed (see Figure 29.2). Scab formation provides a surface beneath which cell migration and movement of the wound edges can occur. As the inflammatory process develops, nutrients are brought to the area of the wound, debris and bacteria are removed and makes available chemical stimuli for wound repair to begin to occur. Repair begins immediately after wounding and proceeds quickly through the processes of epithelialisation, fibroplasia and capillary proliferation into the healing area. Different tissues have their own normal rates of growth as the healing process occurs. The ideal rate of healing happens when there are factors present that are advantageous to healing and factors that have the ability to disturb or hinder the healing processes that are controlled or absent.

Red Flag

Nutrition plays an important role in wound healing. Each step of the wound-healing process is dependent on nutrients, circulating amino acids, lipids and carbohydrates. Iron, zinc and vitamins A and C are seen as the most important micronutrients associated with wound healing. When there are deficiencies in the intake of proteins and vitamins (particularly common in the older population), wound healing can be delayed. Wounds that are infected often require that patients increase their nutritional intake.

The nursing associate is required to pay attention to nutritional requirements. There is no doubt that a healthy, balanced diet is invaluable in keeping the body functioning well. Issues can arise in those who are unable to fulfil the recommended daily intake for the required nutrients, and this is when wounds in older adults can fail to heal as a result of nutrient deficiency.

Monitoring Wounds

The overall aim of wound management is to prevent the build-up of unwanted tissue types on the wound bed and at the same time encouraging the growth of granulation and epithelial tissue in order to repair the wound. Tissue types are commonly documented in the following colours that can be used as part of documentation (Peate & Stephens 2020). The types of tissue commonly found on a wound bed are:

Necrotic tissue – (black) wet or dry tissue adhered to the wound bed consisting of red blood cells, skin cells, bacteria, varying levels of wound exudate (if moist or wet) and any other debris that may be on the wound, for example, dressing fibres or foreign bodies. Necrotic tissue can also consist of gangrene (tissue death), and it is important for the nursing associate to identify what type of necrotic tissue is on the wound. This is unwanted tissue. If the nursing associate has any concerns, this must be escalated or referred to a more senior clinician.

Slough – (yellow) wet or dry tissue consisting of congealed wound exudate, debris, skin cells, bacteria and blood cells. The colour of slough varies depending on the ingredients within it. A grey slough, for example, will have red blood cells, while a yellow slough contains many white blood cells. A green slough will have a bacterium known as pseudomonas within it; however, it must be noted that infection is not identified by the colour of slough. Slough is unwanted tissue.

Granulation tissue – (red) this is wanted tissue, consisting of angiogenesis used in tissue repair. The aim is to maintain a 'red' granulating wound while preventing the build-up of unwanted tissue types.

Epithelial tissue – (pink) this tissue type demonstrates the covering of skin over the granulation tissue as the wound fills with new tissues. Once the wound is entirely covered with epithelial tissue, the wound is regarded as closed (healed).

Wound Care

Successful treatment of wounds requires assessment of the entire patient and not just the wound. Often, systemic problems will hinder wound healing; conversely, wounds that are non-healing may be a sign of systemic pathology. There are several reasons why wounds may not heal in a straightforward manner; these reasons can be classified as intrinsic (something internal to the individual) or extrinsic (something external to the individual). On some occasions, factors may be both intrinsic and extrinsic. Individual review is paramount so that influencing factors of delayed healing rates can be identified and addressed as far as possible; following this, the wound itself can be reviewed.

The nursing associate should consider the negative effects of endocrine diseases – for example, diabetes mellitus and hypothyroidism; haematological conditions, including anaemia, polycythaemia and myeloproliferative disorders; cardiopulmonary problems, such as chronic obstructive pulmonary disease and congestive heart failure; gastrointestinal problems that result in malnutrition and vitamin deficiencies; obesity; and peripheral vascular pathology including atherosclerotic disease, chronic venous insufficiency and lymphoedema (Peate & Stephens 2020).

The lack of adequate wound care skills and techniques among healthcare professionals is a common reason for delayed wound healing. This can include the use of inappropriate dressings, causing trauma on removal of the dressing, which results in the wound reverting back to the beginning of the healing process; leaving a dressing in situ for too long, causing saturation and subsequent maceration/excoriation of the wound and peri-wound tissues. The guidelines/principles of wound management are detailed in Box 29.1.

Review and Assessment

The nursing associate is required to document clearly and comprehensively all aspects of wound care (Nursing and Midwifery Council 2018b); this includes any reviews, treatment and management plans, implementation and review. There are professional and legal reasons why high-quality documentation standards must be produced at all times and the implications for failure to adhere to these high standards bring with it consequences; effective documentation is a non-negotiable skill that all nursing associates must possess.

Reviewing and assessing a wound involves taking note of the wound's anatomical site, dimensions, depth (if a pressure ulcer, this will be by grade), tissue type on the wound, levels and type of wound exudate, condition of the surrounding skin (observing for maceration, excoriation, heat on touch and erythema, blistering or any other lesions), pain levels and aggravating or relieving factors of pain and whether or not there is malodour from the wound (see Box 29.2).

Box 29.1 Principles Underpinning Wound Care

- Adopt a multidisciplinary approach to care provision.
- Initial patient and wound review is essential and also whenever there is a change in condition.
- Consider the psychological implications of a wound, understanding pain that is associated with the wound and dressing changes.
- If appropriate, with the patient, ascertain the goal of care and anticipated outcomes.
- Respect the fragile wound environment.
- Maintain bacterial balance and use aseptic technique when undertaking wound procedures.
- Maintain a moist wound environment.
- Maintain a stable wound temperature. Avoid using cold solutions or wound exposure.
- Maintain an acidic or neutral pH.
- A heavily draining wound should be permitted to drain freely.
- Eliminate dead space but never pack a wound tightly.
- Select the most appropriate dressing and techniques based on assessment and best available evidence.
- Instigate appropriate adjunctive wound therapies, for example, the use of compression, splinting and pressure redistribution equipment, off-loading orthotics.
- Follow the principles for managing acute and chronic wounds.

Source: Benbow (2011); Carville (2017)

Box 29.2 Considerations to be Taken into Account when Conducting Initial and Ongoing Wound Reviews

- Type of wound – acute or chronic
- Aetiology – surgical, laceration, ulcer, burn, abrasion, traumatic, pressure injury, cancer
- Location and surrounding skin
- Tissue loss
- Clinical appearance of the wound bed and stage of healing
- Measurement and dimensions
- Wound edge
- Exudate
- Presence of infection
- Pain
- Previous wound management interventions.

Source: Peate & Stephens (2020)

This information can be recorded on a wound assessment chart, by photography or by tracing the wound on an acetate. Each care area will have their own form of documentation, and the nursing associate must adhere to local policy and procedure. Figure 29.3 provides an example of a wound assessment chart.

When the review is completed, the nursing associate, with the patient if appropriate, establishes the goals to be achieved in order to promote healing. A care plan is devised for each wound identified, providing instruction for others on the management of each wound. The plan must include as a minimum, identification of the site of the wound, the aim of the care plan, the type of dressing(s) to be applied to the wound, the frequency of dressing changes and a date when the wound has to be reviewed. The plan must be clear and concise, allowing others to deliver the care that has been planned.

Blue Flag

The value of a good rapport with patients is sometimes underestimated. Relationships with the nursing associate and other service providers are often valued more than treatment options or therapies provided; it is important to attend to this basic human need first. The therapeutic relationship is one that offers the other respect, trust and care.

When carrying out wound care, an aseptic technique must be used, using sterile dressings. Once the care has been delivered, this must be documented on the evaluation chart, the content of which should reflect the directions on the care plan.

The dressing must be observed at least once on every shift for signs of wound exudate strikethrough (i.e. the staining on the outer dressing). Whether or not there is any strikethrough must then be recorded on the care plan review document. Once the dressing shows evidence of strikethrough, the dressing requires changing so as to avoid saturation and increased risk of a wound infection. On removal of the dressing, the nursing associate must check the wound in order to establish whether or not the wound shows clinical changes and that the care plan remains appropriate if the findings are unchanged.

Adaptations to the care plan may be required. This may include increasing the frequency of dressing changes, or a different dressing choice to manage the exudate levels more appropriately. The rationale for any adaptations to the care plan must be documented in the care plan review.

In the event that the clinical findings are noted to have changed when re-dressing the wound (e.g. increased exudate levels, signs of infection, increased pain and deterioration in the wound), the nursing associate must review the wound once again and seek advice from a more senior clinician. All findings must be recorded and reported on the review and the care plan amended or re-written accordingly so as to reflect the changing requirements and goals. If there are no clinical changes noted, then a review must be completed at intervals established by either clinical judgement or by weekly/fortnightly/monthly time frames.

Violet Flag

Services can adopt an outreach approach; for those who are classed as 'hard to reach', this is an effective strategy in reaching and targeting these populations providing a service that is accessible and flexible in approach. While outreach is important and valuable, it is just as important to ensure that centre-based services are designed in such a way that they can accommodate the 'hard to reach'. Those providing wound services, for the homeless, for example, should commit themselves to establishing imaginative and innovative responses to meet the needs of this vulnerable group.

Measuring a Wound

Wound measurement is an essential aspect of wound assessment. It must be recorded and reported on initial presentation and at regularly defined intervals as part of review. Monitoring changes in dimensions is a key indicator and may also predict healing. There are a number of different methods available to enable wound measurement, and the same method must be used each time, with the patient in the same position. There are several sophisticated methods for measuring wounds; these include cameras that provide 3D images of the wound bed. These are likely to provide the most accurate measurement; however, they are not always available.

Continuous monitoring of changes in wound size is an important way of evaluating response to treatment. Measuring wounds:

- Provides a baseline measure
- Monitors healing progress
- Monitors rate of healing
- Can predict which wounds are unlikely to heal with conventional treatment
- Can help set wound care goals
- Monitors effectiveness of treatment
- Identifies delayed healing/static wounds and prompt review of the patient
- Provides positive feedback to the patient, helping with motivation and concordance.

Wound Assessment Chart
(Use a separate chart for every wound)

Patient ID________________ **Wound Type**________________ **Wound Site**________________

	Initial assessment date	Evaluation date	Evaluation date	Evaluation date	Evaluation date	Evaluation date	Evaluation date
Wound presentation % N – Necrotic (black) G – Granulation (bright red) S – Sloughy (yellow) E – Epithelialisation (pink)							
Exudate colour 1 – Straw colour 2 – Blood-stained 3 – Purulent *							
Level of exudate 4 – None 5 – Minimal (contained within primary dressing) 6 – Moderate (extends to secondary dressing) 7 – High (secondary dressing saturated)							
Other clinical signs of infection 1 – Non-healing / deterioration 5 – Bleeding 2 – Increased exudate 6 – Malodour 3 – Increased pain 7 – Pus 4 – Increased erythema							
Wound traced? Yes or No (please circle)	Y / N	Y / N	Y / N	Y / N	Y / N	Y / N	Y / N
Wound photographed? Yes or No (please circle)	Y / N	Y / N	Y / N	Y / N	Y / N	Y / N	Y / N
Consent for photography obtained? (please circle)	Y / N	Y / N	Y / N	Y / N	Y / N	Y / N	Y / N
Wound dimensions – width, depth, length (cms) **EPUAP Grade of Pressure Ulcer** 1 – Increasing * 2 – Decreasing 3 – Static * (review treatment)							
Doppler Ultrasound assessment carried out? (for leg ulcers) Yes or No	Y / N	Y / N	Y / N	Y / N	Y / N	Y / N	Y / N
Wound odour (a) none (b) malodorous *							
Wound infection - are there 2 or more clinical signs? Yes or No (circle)	Y / N	Y / N	Y / N	Y / N	Y / N	Y / N	Y / N
Wound swab taken? Yes or No (please circle)	Y / N	Y / N	Y / N	Y / N	Y / N	Y / N	Y / N
Antibiotics prescribed? Yes or No (please circle) (refer to path report)	Y / N	Y / N	Y / N	Y / N	Y / N	Y / N	Y / N
Condition of wound margins e.g. flat, raised, irregular, undermined							
Condition of surrounding skin 1 – Healthy 4 – Oedematous * 7 – Dermatitis / Eczema 2 – Inflamed * 5 – Blistered 3 – Macerated 6 – Ischaemic							
Pain assessment score (see pain assessment documentation)							
Onset of pain caused by? (e.g. walking, dressing change. Please state)							
Pain is relieved by? (e.g. analgesia, elevation. Please state)							
Signature & Designation							

Patient's own description of the pain: ....

....

....

....

Additional Information: ....

....

....

....

Figure 29.3 An example of a wound assessment chart. *Source:* Peate & Glencross (2015), chapter 10, figure 20.1, p. 44. © John Wiley & Sons.

Touch Point

Measuring wounds is an essential part of review and provides important information regarding the progress of the wound over time and the prediction of time to healing. There are a number of methods available to measure wounds; while there are limitations with all options, these can be reduced by using the same method at each review, with the patient in the same position. All measurements, tracings and photographs must be documented and stored securely (aligned to local policy and procedure) in the patient's care records and be accessible to all healthcare practitioners providing wound care to the patient.

Wounds should be measured when they are discovered and then at subsequent intervals, based on local policy and procedure.

Ruler/Linear Measurement

The easiest and quickest measurement method is linear. This is also known as the 'clock' method. This involves measuring the greatest length, width and depth of the wound, imagining the body as the face of a clock, with the head being 12 o'clock and the feet 6 o'clock.

Establish the wound's length (direct line from 12 o'clock to 6 o'clock) and width (9 o'clock to 3 o'clock) using a disposable, single-use-only paper ruler. Readings will never be absolutely accurate because of the variety and irregularity of wound shapes; they can only give an indication of changes.

The measurements should be documented at least weekly in centimetres; if the measurements are taken in exactly the same position each time, the wound progress will be evident. The depth can be assessed using a sterile cotton-tipped bud, which is then placed against the ruler to give the greatest depth measurement.

Photography

Photography is becoming an increasingly popular method of recording wound assessment and monitoring progress. When using photography to chart the progress of a wound, at least two photographs should be taken at each assessment. One should be taken about 10 cm from the wound and one that shows the position of the wound on the body.

Photographs must always have a ruler in them as this provides an objective view of size and should preferably be taken at the same distance from the wound each time, with the patient in the same position. Photography is a useful method of recording wound assessment but must not be used in isolation. Measurements are still required otherwise the photograph becomes meaningless.

Grids

By tracing wounds onto an acetate grid and counting the squares, the nursing associate can quickly calculate an accurate surface area. Tracing a wound is an easy and inexpensive method and has advantages over length times and width measurements. It provides more information about the shape of the wound.

Different regions of necrosis, granulation and slough can be marked on the acetate and can provide a comparison tool. When the acetate is placed on the wound, it will 'fog' up, and the wound margins may be difficult to define, but this can be overcome by wiping the acetate with alcohol prior to application. Care must be taken to ensure that the alcohol surface does not touch the wound, as this can cause pain for the patient.

In this method, the nursing associate uses a clear film layer; this is applied over the wound, and an acetate layer is placed on top. A fine-tipped permanent marker is used to draw around the wound outline, and then the wound contact layer is disposed of in the clinical waste, and the acetate sheet is stored in the patient's record after being clearly dated and labelled.

Wound Depth

Establishing the depth of a wound is an important aspect of the assessment process and to ascertain whether there is any sinus or undermining present. The recommended method for measuring depth is to use a sterile cotton tip swab, gently insert it into the area of undermining and then grasping it at the wound edge measure against a ruler (Morgan 2012). Plastic probes are also available that are pre-marked with centimetre markings. The cavity should be gently explored to establish any areas of pocketing or undermining and then the depth recorded at the deepest part of the wound.

Record also the amount of dressing required to fill the cavity; a reduction in the volume of packing required will also indicate healing progress. If there is tracking or undermining present, then the direction and depth must be recorded. It is also important to note which position the patient is lying in and to make sure that the same position is used at each review. If there is necrotic or sloughy tissue on the wound bed, then the depth will not be visible until the wound has been debrided.

Take Note

When reviewing the effectiveness of a treatment regimen, the nursing associate should be able to clearly state the wound type and what the treatment aims were. Failing to determine these factors means that the goal and any products selected are random and will not be based on best practice recommendations.

Conclusion

Accurate and continuous measurement of wounds along with consistent and clear documentation are essential to ensure good outcomes for patients. Wounds are more likely to heal if their progress is monitored and the nursing associate treats them appropriately. Documentation of wound care is a professional and legal requirement; failure to complete documentation can lead to legal proceedings if a patient sustains harm and there is no documentation to demonstrate that appropriate, evidence-based care was provided.

References

Benbow, M. (2011) Wound care: ensuring a holistic and collaborative assessment, *British Journal of Community Nursing*, 16(9): S6–16.

Carville, K. (2017) *Wound care manual* (7th edn), Osborne Park, Western Australia: Silver Chain Foundation.

Fletcher, J. and Anderson, I. (2019) Tissue viability and manging chronic wounds, in Peate, I. (ed.) *Alexander's nursing practice hospital and home* (5th edn), Edinburgh: Elsevier, Ch 22, 561–583.

Jarvis, C. (2015) *Physical examination and health assessment* (7th edn), St Louis: Elsevier.

Kottner, J. (2015) Of youth and age-what are the differences regarding skin structure and function? *European Wound Management Association Journal*, 15(2): 11–13.

Morgan, N. (2012) *Measuring wounds*. [online] Available: https://woundcareadvisor.com/measuring-wounds/. Accessed January 2020.

Nursing and Midwifery Council (NMC). (2018a) *Standards of proficiency for nursing associates*. [online] Available: https://www.nmc.org.uk/standards/standards-for-nursing-associates/standards-of-proficiency-for-nursing-associates/. Accessed January 2020.

Nursing and Midwifery Council (NMC). (2018b) The code, *Professional standards of practice and behaviour for nurses, midwives and nursing associates*. [online] Available: https://www.nmc.org.uk/globalassets/sitedocuments/nmc-publications/nmc-code.pdf. Accessed January 2020.

Peate, I. and Glencross, W. (2015) *Wound care at a glance*, Oxford: Wiley.

Peate, I. and Stephens, M. (2020) *Wound care at a glance* (2nd edn), Oxford: Wiley.

Thappa, D.M. (2016) *Clinical pediatric dermatology* (2nd edn), St Louis: Elsevier.

Unit 4

Provide Support with Nutrition and Hydration

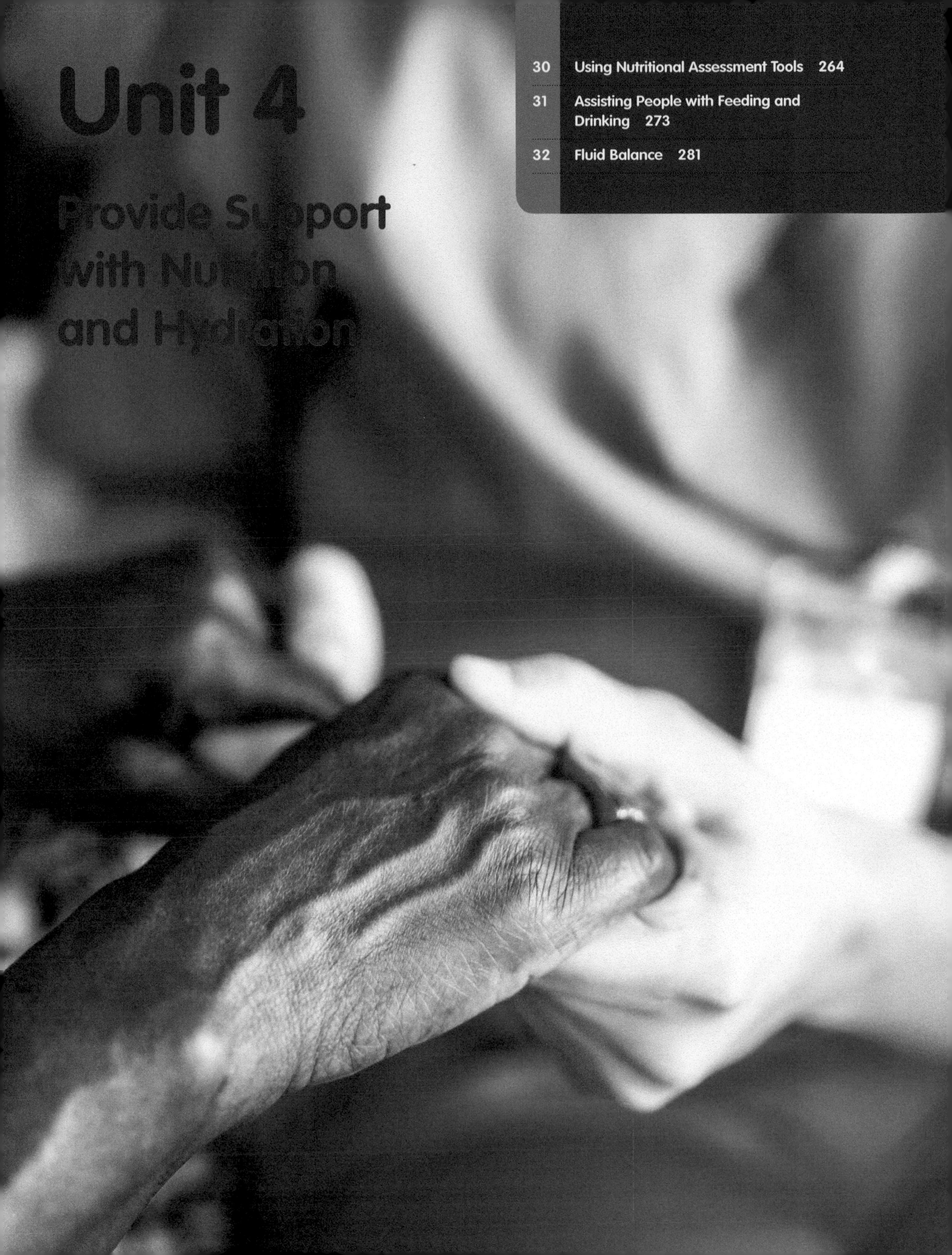

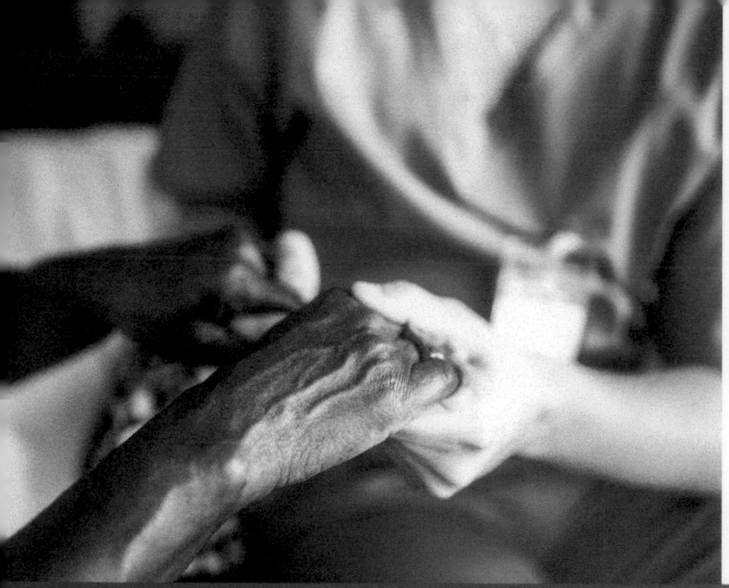

30

Using Nutritional Assessment Tools

Louise McErlean

Department of Nursing, School of Health and Social Work, Ulster University, Northern Ireland, UK

Chapter Aim

- **This chapter aims to explain the importance of nutrition for a range of people in a variety of care settings.**

Learning Outcomes

By the end of this chapter, the reader will be able to:

- **Understand the importance of nutrition for people of all ages**
- **Understand how the nutritional needs of people are different depending on their individual circumstances**
- **Understand how to effectively use nutritional assessment tools to improve nutrition**

Test Yourself Multiple Choice Questions

1. **What is malnutrition?**
   A) **Overnutrition**
   B) **Undernutrition**
   C) **Obesity**
   D) **All of the above**
2. **Which of the following is a sign of malnutrition in children?**
   A) **Failure to thrive**
   B) **High energy levels**
   C) **Weight gain**
   D) **Increasing height**

The Nursing Associate's Handbook of Clinical Skills, First Edition. Edited by Ian Peate.

Companion website: www.wiley.com/nursingassociate

3. **What does MUST stand for?**
   A) **Malnutrition Universal Scoring Test**
   B) **Mass Undernutrition Score Total**
   C) **Malnutrition Universal Screening Tool**
   D) **Maternal Universal Significance Test**
4. **How many days of little or no nutrition due to physiological or psychological ill health would be a red flag for the nutritional assessment?**
   A) **2 days**
   B) **3 days**
   C) **4 days**
   D) **5 days**
5. **Which of the following methods of nutritional support pertains to nutrition administered out with the digestive system?**
   A) **Parenteral nutrition**
   B) **Enteral nutrition**
   C) **Nutrition via percutaneous endoscopic gastrostomy**
   D) **Nutrition via a nasojejunal tube**

Introduction

Nutrition is important for maintaining health, for tissue repair and healing, and the act of eating and drinking contributes to our psychological well-being. Within healthcare, nursing associates have a duty to assist patients with their nutritional needs (Nursing and Midwifery Council (NMC) 2018a, 2018b). Failure to monitor and manage nutritional needs can lead to malnutrition, delayed healing and longer stays in hospital.

Promoting Health and Preventing Ill Health

The British Association for Parenteral and Enteral Nutrition (BAPEN) (2018) defines malnutrition as:

> 'a state of nutrition in which a deficiency or excess (or imbalance) of energy, protein and other nutrients causes measurable adverse effects on tissue/body form (body shape, size and composition) and function and clinical outcome'.

It is important to remember that malnutrition includes undernutrition and overnutrition. Overnutrition is more commonly referred to as obesity. The term malnutrition often refers more specifically to undernutrition.

Age UK (2016) reports the statistics associated with malnutrition in the United Kingdom. It notes that there are three million people in the United Kingdom who are malnourished. One-third of this group are aged 65 years and older. It reports that 93% of those who are malnourished live in community settings (Age UK 2016).

Orange Flag

Emerging research suggests that poor nutrition may have an impact on mood and conditions such as depression (Owens et al. 2020). Depression can lead to a lack of interest in food and further exacerbate the lack of micronutrients thought to be required to improve mood (Harbottle 2019). As depression and anxiety illnesses increase in society more research is required into the role of nutrition, nutritional supplements and the promotion of a healthy diet and how they can contribute to the prevention and/or treatment of depression. Nursing associates concerned about a patient who appears depressed should escalate this concern to the team caring for the patient.

Many people are affected by malnutrition. People who have mental health conditions or long term conditions are at increased risk of malnutrition. The risk is also high for people who require major surgery and people at the end of their lives. (Royal College of Nursing (RCN) 2019). There are physical, social and psychological reasons that can contribute to the development of malnutrition.

Physical Health Factors

In children, the most common causes of malnutrition are linked to the presence of long-term conditions such as congenital heart disease, cystic fibrosis, cerebral palsy or inflammatory bowel disorders. In adults, there are many conditions that can have malnutrition as a symptom, and these include the following:

- Inflammatory bowel diseases such as Crohn's disease or ulcerative colitis which can lead to the inability to absorb nutrients
- Dementia leading to an inability to communicate needs or ability to feed oneself
- Cancer leading to pain and nausea and lack of appetite
- Liver disease leading to pain and nausea
- Depression or schizophrenia leading to an inability to care for oneself

- Dysphagia – difficulty in swallowing for any reason but often secondary to stroke
- Vomiting and/or diarrhoea
- Eating disorders such as anorexia nervosa
- Conditions where there is an increased demand for energy, for example, chronic obstructive pulmonary disease, Parkinson's disease, following trauma or burns

There are barriers to healthy eating that can lead to a state of malnutrition. People, because of their individual circumstances, may find it difficult to get to the shops or use internet shopping; they might find it physically difficult to cook due to a medical condition, for example if they are recovering from illness. The loss of the sense of smell or taste can lead to a loss of appetite as can poorly fitting dentures, toothache or pain in the oral cavity.

Social Factors

Social circumstances can lead to malnutrition, for example, people living alone often skip meals. Recently, widowed people may struggle if they have lost a partner who did all of the cooking. People with alcohol or drug dependency will often not eat in order to buy alcohol and drugs or not have any great appetite for food. Low income and poverty are increasingly becoming problems in society with many people reliant on food banks. The Trussell Trust reported that food bank use in the United Kingdom had increased by 73% in the last 5 years (Trussell Trust 2019).

Violet Flag

In the United Kingdom, it is rare for malnutrition to occur due to poverty. However, the 2017 report, Poverty and Children's Health: Views from the Frontline, suggests that increasing poverty is affecting the nutrition of children. It reports an increased reliance on food banks, an inability to afford healthy choices leading to an increase in obesity levels and increasing anxiety in children (Royal College of Paediatrics and Child Health 2017). Therefore, in the United Kingdom, children are at risk of neglect, living in poverty or abuse. They may present with symptoms of malnutrition. It is the duty of the nursing associate to report concerns about child welfare to their employer's social services team.

Psychological Factors

Psychological or behavioural issues can lead to malnutrition. Eating disorders affect 1.6 billion people in the United Kingdom (Anorexia and Bulimia Care 2019). Eating disorders typically begin at the age of 14 years. Grief, depression and anxiety can lead to loss of appetite.

Malnutrition is complex and a combination of physical health factors, social factors and psychological factors can contribute to its development.

Touch Point

Holistic patient assessment is essential to recognise and understand why malnutrition has occurred. Holistic assessment should include consideration for the physical, psychological and social circumstances of the patient with regard nutritional status.

Provide and Monitor Care – Nutritional Assessment

Nutritional assessment begins with an understanding of the patient's history. The patient and their family (if appropriate) will be able to discuss any concerns and recent changes that have been identified. A nutritional assessment requires the nursing associate to be aware of the signs and symptoms associated with malnutrition (see Box 30.1).

Promoting Health and Preventing Ill Health

Within the United Kingdom, children have health and development reviews undertaken by a health visitor until they are 2 years old. This is recorded in the Personal Child Health Record (PCHR), known more commonly as the red book. The National Child Measurement Programme (healthy weight) is an optional programme looking at the height and the weight of children in reception and in year 6. The measurements are undertaken by a school nurse and shared with the family. The data provides a national picture of height and weight trends within the country. When children are admitted into hospital or being seen by a medical professional, they should be asked to bring their red book with them.

Box 30.1 Signs and Symptoms of Malnutrition

The signs and symptoms of malnutrition in children include:
- Tiring easily and having poor energy levels
- Behavioural changes
- Increasing irritability
- Increasing anxiety levels
- Acting more sluggishly compared to others
- Changes in skin or hair
- Failure to thrive

The signs and symptoms of malnutrition in adults include:
- Unplanned and/or unexplained weight loss
- Loss of appetite
- Feeling tired and lethargic
- Feeling cold
- Inability to concentrate
- Poor mood, feeling depressed
- Lack of libido
- Increased risk of developing infections and/or illnesses
- Increased recovery time from illness and /or infections
- Body mass index (BMI) less than 18.5
- Increased risk of developing pressure ulcers
- Poor wound healing

Supporting Evidence

National Institute for Health and Care and Excellence (NICE) (2006) Clinical Guideline [CG32]: Nutrition support for adults: oral nutrition support, enteral tube feeding and parenteral nutrition.

This guidance was written in 2006 but has been updated in 2017. The guidance contains a section on the risk of malnutrition and the screening required in the community and in the hospital setting. There is information on nutritional supplements, and enteral feeding. The evidence based recommendations within the clinical guidance are a useful source of information for the nursing associate.

https://www.nice.org.uk/guidance/cg32/chapter/1-Guidance#screening-for-malnutrition-and-the-risk-of-malnutrition-in-hospital-and-the-community

Providing and Monitoring Care – Nutritional Assessment

All patients admitted to hospitals or to outpatient departments should have a nutritional screening undertaken (National Institute for Health and Care and Excellence 2016). Screening should be repeated weekly for those who are inpatients, and it should be repeated for those who are outpatients if there is a clinical concern.

Care homes should undertake nutritional screening on admission and where a clinical concern is identified.

Green Flag

The Health and Social Care Act 2008 (Regulated Activities) Regulations 2014: Regulation 14 requires people who use social care services have adequate nutrition and hydration to sustain life and good health and to reduce the risks of malnutrition and dehydration while they are receiving care and treatment. In order to meet this regulation, where it is part of their role, care home providers have to make sure that people have enough to eat and drink so as to meet their nutrition and hydration needs and to receive the support they need to do so. People must have their nutritional needs assessed, and food must be provided to meet those needs. This includes where people are prescribed nutritional supplements and/or parenteral nutrition. People's preferences, religious and cultural backgrounds have to be taken into account when providing food and drink.

General practitioner (GP) surgeries should undertake nutritional assessment when a person joins the practice, during routine appointments for other reasons (for example, vaccinations and routine investigations) or where a clinical need has been identified. The nursing associate should make every contact count.

Nutrition Assesment Tools

There are a variety of nutritional assessment tools available. The assessment tool selected is often based on the age range or setting that it is being used in. The, including the Malnutrition Universal Screening Tool (MUST) (British Association for Parenteral and Enteral Nutrition 2018) is used for adult patients in acute hospital environments. The Mini Nutritional Assessment is often used in social care environments for older adults. The Paediatric Yorkhill Malnutrition Score (PYMS) (NHS Scotland 2019) and the Screening Tool for the Assessment of Malnutrition in Paediatrics (STAMP) (McCarthy *et al.* 2012) are seen in settings where children are cared for.

The assessment tool selected will be determined by local policy and be appropriate to the patient group it is being used to assess. Whichever assessment tool is selected, there are several features that are common to all.

Height and Weight

Nutritional assessment begins with a measure of height and weight. This is straightforward for adults. As children are still developing and growing centile growth charts are used to determine where the child's height and weight is compared to 100 of their peers. All measures used in the PCHR fall within the normal range for children. (Scientific Advisory Committee on Nutrition and Royal College of Paediatrics and Child Health 2007).

Measuring Height and Weight

Height and weight measurements should occur in an environment with a comfortable temperature and where the patient's privacy and dignity can be maintained. Table 30.1 shows how to measure weight.

Table 30.2 outlines the steps to measure height.

Body Mass Index

The BMI is a starting point in identifying those people who are at risk of malnutrition and who may require a nutritional care plan. The patient's weight in kilogram is divided by the height in m^2.

$$\text{BMI} = \frac{\text{Weight}(\text{kg})}{\text{Height}(\text{m}^2)}$$

The calculated score is then categorised in Table 30.3.

Table 30.1 How to measure weight.

1	The weighing scales should be class III scales and must be calibrated (Evans 2014)
2	If the using a chair scale, ensure the brakes are on
3	Ensure the scale has been zeroed
4	Ask the patient to remove their shoes and outdoor clothing For children under 2 years old, all clothing and nappies should be removed
5	Ask the patient to stand on the scale or sit on the chair scale
6	The weighing scales for babies and toddlers contain a tray that the baby or toddler is placed in, You must ensure the safety of the toddler at all times when using this scale
7	Check that the patient is not supporting themselves, which will affect the measure
8	Record the weight (in kilograms) on the documentation
9	Share the recording with the patient or parent/carer (with consent)
10	Scales should be cleaned according to the manufacturer's instruction and aligned to local policy and procedure

Table 30.2 How to measure height.

1	Use a wall-mounted stadiometer (see Figure 30.1)
2	Ensure the patient has taken their shoes off
3	Ask the patient to keep their heels together and stand as straight as possible, facing forward, under the stadiometer
4	The bar should be pulled down until it touches the top of the head
5	Record the height in metres on the documentation
6	Share the recording with the patient or parent/carer (with consent)
7	Be aware that a height measurement for babies and toddlers can be very difficult to accurately achieve

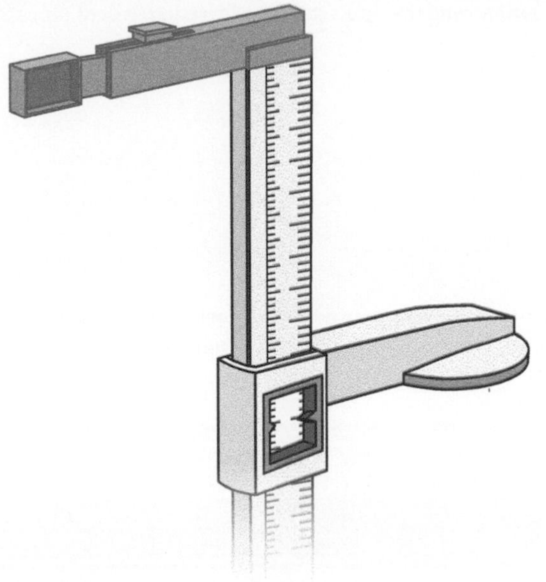

Figure 30.1 **Stadiometer.**

Table 30.3 **BMI score and categories.**

CATEGORY	BMI SCORE
Underweight	less than 18.5
Healthy weight	18.5–24.9
Overweight	25–29.9
Obesity I	30–34.9
Obesity II	35–39.9
Obesity III	40+

The BMI should not be used to assess pregnant women. It does not directly measure fat; muscle is denser than fat which can lead to a false categorisation of an athlete, for example. A normal BMI will not assess the amount of muscle that has wasted during an acute or chronic illness (Dougherty *et al.* 2015).

For some patients, assessment can be more difficult, for example, wheelchair users who cannot stand. If height cannot be measured, then ulna or knee length can be used to provide an estimated height measure (British Association for Parenteral and Enteral Nutrition 2011). Mid Upper Arm Circumference (MUAC) measures can be used to provide an estimated range of what the BMI may be in the absence of a height and weight measure (British Association for Parenteral and Enteral Nutrition 2011).

Orange Flag

Cerebral palsy described as a brain injury (static encephalopathy) which occurs as a result of a lack of oxygen to the brain before, during or immediately after birth. Cerebral palsy can be mild or severe, and as such, some people will have a learning disability associated with cerebral palsy and others will not.

Cerebral palsy, in some cases, can lead to motor dysfunction and permanent physical disability. Spinal deformity can make it difficult to accurately measure height due to the inability of the person to stand upright. A better indicator of height and BMI might be achieved using forearm or knee length to estimate height or MUAC to estimate BMI.

Weight Loss History

Nutritional assessment must consider any recent weight loss. This is calculated as a percentage of their usual weight.

$$\frac{\text{Original weight}\left(\text{before loss}\right)\text{in kg} - \text{current weight in kg} \times 100 = \%\text{weight loss}}{\text{Orginal weight}\left(\text{before loss}\right)\text{in kg}}$$

Nutritional assessment needs to consider unintentional weight loss. A person losing 5–10% or more of their body weight over a time period of 3–6 months unintentionally would be identified as a red flag, and this would require further intervention.

History of Illness

Acute illness will affect nutritional status. Loss of appetite during acute ill health will affect nutritional intake. The nature of the illness is a factor. If the illness affects the gastrointestinal tract or the persons ability to eat (for example dysphagia) then the risk to nutritional status increases. Nutritional requirements can increase during ill health due to an increased metabolic rate as seen in burns, trauma or sepsis. During periods of acute illness, daily weights may be required as part of ongoing nutritional assessment. No nutritional intake over a period of 5 days or more would be a trigger for nutritional intervention.

The nursing associate must consider a holistic approach to assessment and monitoring that takes into consideration, recent illness, lifestyle factors, ethnicity and age which can all have an impact on the nutritional assessment.

Supporting Evidence

BAPEN, a charity working to improve nutritional care, is responsible for the development of the MUST tool, and its website contains lots of useful information on nutrition: https://www.bapen.org.uk/

Take Note

Nutritional assessment requires the use of a validated nutritional assessment tool, consideration of the patient's previous and recent medical history, weight and height as well as their percentage unintentional weight loss.

Nutritional Intervention

Nutritional support is recommended in the presence of malnourishment as defined by National Institute for Health and Care and Excellence (2006):

- Low BMI of less than 18.5
- Unintentional weight loss of more than 10% in the preceding 3–6 months
- BMI of 20 and unintentional weight loss of more than 5% in the preceding 3–6 months
- Little or no intake for more than 5 days, and it is anticipated that this will continue for the following 5 days and beyond
- Poor absorption of nutrients from the gastrointestinal tract
- Increased nutritional requirements from catabolism, for example, burns/trauma
- Swallowing difficulties (for example, post stroke)
- A combination of factors

Types of Nutritional Intervention

Oral Nutritional Intervention

A food chart can be commenced to monitor oral intake and the requirement for further intervention. The dietician will calculate the calories required to meet the patient's metabolic needs. Oral nutritional supplements may be prescribed. Oral nutritional supplements are not intended to replace normal diet but to supplement it during the period of ill health. There are a variety of oral nutritional supplements available; they can contain proteins and carbohydrates as well as macro and micronutrients. The flavour of the supplements can be sweet or savoury and the texture can be liquid or thickened as a milkshake or soup. The oral nutritional supplements should be recorded on the food intake chart to allow the multidisciplinary team to review the patient's nutritional requirements. Consideration should be given to food preferences, oral hygiene and the taste and smell of the food. Stimulating the person's appetite is important. An example of a food chart is depicted in Table 30.4.

Table 30.4 An example of a daily food intake chart.

MEAL	FOOD TYPE	QUANTITY OF PORTION					INITIALS
		NONE	¼	½	¾	FULL PORTION	
Breakfast							
Mid-morning							
Lunch							
Mid-afternoon							
Evening meal							
Supper							
Snacks or overnight							

Enteral Tube Nutrition

If the patient is malnourished and oral intake is insufficient, an alternative source of nutrition is required. If the gastrointestinal tract is not compromised, then enteral tube feeding should be given considered. The need for enteral feeding should be assessed on a daily basis and can be stopped as soon as it is no longer required (National Institute for Health and Care and Excellence 2006).

Nasogastric tube feeding is the most commonly used route. It is suitable to be used for a period of 2–4 weeks (Dougherty *et al.* 2015). Fine-bore feeding tubes are placed via the patient's nose and into the stomach (nasogastric) or into the jejunum (nasojejunal). Nasogastric tubes are inserted by competed registered nurses. The nurse is responsible for ensuring the position of the feeding tube and the requirement for x-ray to confirm the position and prevent aspiration of enteral feed into the lungs.

Complications of Nasogastric Feeding

Despite initial checks of the position off the eneteral feeding tube, there is always a risk that the tube position can have altered and therefore there is a risk of aspiration. If there is any indication that the position has changed; the feed should be stopped, the registered nurse should be asked to assess the tube position. Aspiration of the stomach contents via the tube to check for an acidic pH is an essential additional check to ensure the position of the tube. NHS England (2016) continues to report the risks of misplaced tubes and reiterates the need to use approved CE pH paper for checking the pH of the aspirate and the use of radio-opaque fine-bore feeding tubes. The position of the tube should be checked after insertion, daily, if there is a change in respiratory observations, following vomiting and if there is a suspicion that the tube may have moved, for example the patient is coughing more or regurgitating feed.

Gastrostomy and jejunostomy tubes are placed directly into the stomach (gastrostomy) or jejunum (jejunostomy) via the abdominal wall. These tubes are selected when there is a requirement for more long-term feeding (more than 4 weeks). The jejunal routes are selected, for example, when the stomach is not suitable due to surgery or if delayed gastric emptying has been identified.

Gastrostomy and jejunostomy may be more comfortable than the nasal tubes. Gastrostomy tubes are inserted either under X-ray (Radiologically Inserted Gastrostomy) or during endoscopy (Percutaneous Endoscopic Gastrostomy).

Complications of Gastrostomy Feeding Tubes

Infection and tube dislodgement can be a complication associated with gastrostomy tubes. The nursing associate should pay attention to any of the following complications:

- Pain on feeding
- Prolonged or severe abdominal pain
- Leaking of gastric contents
- Bleeding

These complications could be indicative of peritonitis which could have serious consequences for the patient. The feed should be stopped immediately. The gastrostomy should be reviewed as a matter of urgency by the doctor and further investigations undertaken. Any issues or concerns with the gastrostomy feeding should be reported to a more senior clinical colleague. Document your findings and the actions taken.

Parenteral Nutrition

For people who are identified as malnourished but for whom the gastrointestinal route is not functioning, cannot be accessed or is perforated, then parenteral nutrition may be required (National Institute for Health and Care and Excellence 2006). Parenteral nutrition is nutrition delivered intravenously. As with enteral feeding, parenteral feeding should be reduced and withdrawn as oral intake improves. The risks associated with parenteral nutrition include infection and thrombosis.

Working in Teams – Nutritional Intervention

Nutritional assessment and the management required as a result of nutritional assessment are essential to providing holistic, person-centred care. There are many professionals in the multidisciplinary team who are involved in nutritional management. They include the nursing team, the dietician, the doctor and the Speech and Language Therapist. Radiographers and the theatre team will assist with feeding tube placement, and nursing associates. Nutrtional assessment and care takes place in a variety of settings including the patients home and across the lifespan. Assisting people with eating and drinking will be discussed in Chapter 31.

Conclusion

Nutritional assessment is complex and requires the nursing associate to consider many aspects of the patient's life. Nutritional assessment includes a comprehensive patient history, an assessment of current nutritional status and a team effort to improve nutritional care for people.

References

Age UK. (2016) *Policy Position Paper, Nutrition and hydration (England).* [online] Available: https://www.ageuk.org.uk/globalassets/age-uk/documents/policy-positions/health-and-wellbeing/ppp_nutrition_and_hydration_england.pdf. Accessed 23 October 2019.

Anorexia and Bulimia Care. (2019) *Statistics.* [online] Available: http://www.anorexiabulimiacare.org.uk/about/statistics. Accessed December 2019.

Dougherty, L., Lister, S. and West-Oram, A. (2015) *The royal Marsden manual of clinical nursing procedures* (9th edn), Chichester: Wiley Blackwell.

BAPEN. (2011) *The 'MUST' explanatory booklet, A guide to the 'malnutrition universal screening tool' ('MUST') for adults.* [online] Available: https://www.bapen.org.uk/pdfs/must/must_explan.pdf. Accessed 23 October 2019.

Evans, L. (2014) Accurate assessment of patient weight, *Nursing Times*, 110(12): 12–14.

Harbottle, L. (2019) The effect of nutrition older people's mental health, *British Journal of Community Nursing*, 24(Suo7): S12–S16.

McCarthy, H., Dixon, M., Crabtree, I., Eaton-Evans, M.J. and McNulty, H. (2012) The development and evaluation of the screening tool for the assessment of malnutrition in paediatrics (STAMP©) for use by healthcare staff, *Journal of Human Nutrition & Diet*, 25: 311–318.

NHS England. (2015) *10 key characteristics of 'good nutrition and hydration care'.*[online] Available: https://www.england.nhs.uk/commissioning/nut-hyd/10-key-characteristics/. Accessed 7 September 2020.

NHS England. (2016) *Nasogastric tube misplacement: continuing risk of death and severe harm.* [online] Available: https://www.england.nhs.uk/2016/07/nasogastric-tube-misplacement-continuing-risk-of-death-severe-harm/. Accessed 30 October 2019.

NHS Scotland. (2009) Paediatric Yorkhill malnutrition score, *Information and user's guide.* [online] Available: http://www.knowledge.scot.nhs.uk/media/2592959/pyms%20user%20and%20info%20guide.pdf. Accessed 23 October 2019.

NICE. (2017). *Nutrition Support for adults: oral nutrition support, enteral tube feeding and parenteral nutrition, CG32.* [online] Available: https://www.nice.org.uk/guidance/cg32/chapter/1-Guidance#screening-for-malnutrition-and-the-risk-of-malnutrition-in-hospital-and-the-community. Accessed 23 October 2019.

Nursing and Midwifery Council (NMC). (2018a) *Standards for pre-registration nursing associate programmes.* [online] Available: https://www.nmc.org.uk/standards/standards-for-nursing-associates/standards-for-pre-registration-nursing-associate-programmes/. Accessed 16 December 2019.

Nursing and Midwifery Council (NMC). (2018b) The code, *Professional standards of practice and behaviour for nurses, midwives and nursing associates.* [online] Available: https://www.nmc.org.uk/globalassets/sitedocuments/nmc-publications/nmc-code.pdf. Accessed 16 December 2019.

Owens, M., Watkins, E., Bot, M., Brouwer, I.A., Roca, M., Kohls, E., Penninx, B.W.J.H., van Grootheest, G., Hergerl, U. and Gili, M. (2020). Nutrition and depression: summary of findings from the EU funded MoodFOOD depression prevention randomised controlled trial and a clinical review of the literature. *Nutrition Bulletin.* 1–12. [online] Available: https://onlinelibrary.wiley.com/doi/full/10.1111/nbu.12447. Accessed 7 September 2020.

Royal College of Nursing. (2019) *Nutrition essentials.* [online] Available: https://www.rcn.org.uk/clinical-topics/nutrition-and-hydration/nutrition-essentials. Accessed 23 October 2019.

Royal College of Paediatrics and Child Health. (2017) *Poverty and children's health: views from the front line*, London: RCPCH.

Scientific Advisory Committee on Nutrition, Royal College of Paediatrics and Child Health. (2007) *Application of the WHO growth standards in the UK*, Norwich: Stationary Office.

Trussell Trust. (2019) *End of year stats.* [online] Available: https://www.trusselltrust.org/news-and-blog/latest-stats/end-year-stats/. Accessed 23 October 2019.

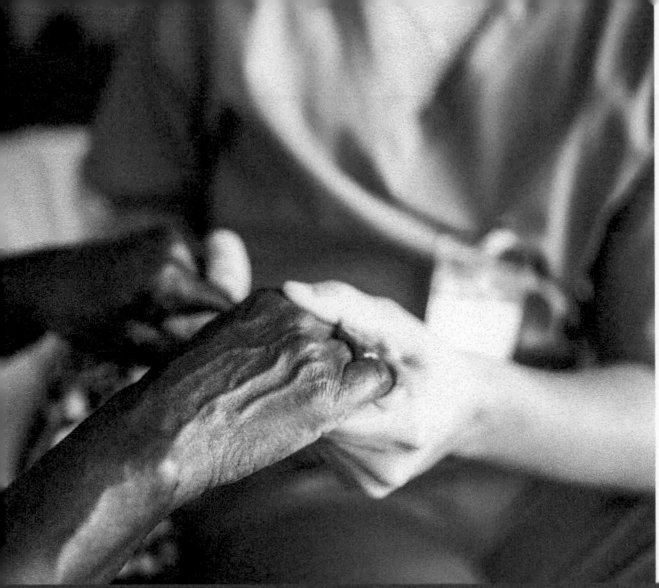

31

Assisting People with Feeding and Drinking

Louise McErlean

Department of Nursing, School of Health and Social Work, Ulster University, Northern Ireland, UK

Chapter Aim

- **This chapter aims to provide the reader with an understanding of a person-centred approach to assisting people with eating and drinking.**

Learning Outcomes

By the end of this chapter, the reader will be able to:

- **Understand the importance of providing nutrition to people who may struggle with this**
- **Understand the difficulties associated with dysphagia**
- **Understand how to assist patients with eating and drinking**

Test Yourself Multiple Choice Questions

1. **The correct medical term for *difficulty in swallowing* is:**
   A) Aphasia
   B) Dysphagia
   C) Ataxia
   D) Dysuria
2. **Which of these conditions has difficulty in swallowing as a symptom?**
   A) Multiple sclerosis
   B) Cholecystitis
   C) Chronic renal disease
   D) All of the above

The Nursing Associate's Handbook of Clinical Skills, First Edition. Edited by Ian Peate.

Companion website: www.wiley.com/nursingassociate

3. **Which of these is a symptom of aspiration pneumonia?**
   A) Coughing
   B) Pyrexia
   C) Hypoxia
   D) All of the above
4. **Which healthcare professional undertakes the swallow assessment?**
   A) Nursing associate
   B) Dietician
   C) Social worker
   D) Speech and language therapist
5. **Which of these investigations would be useful in diagnosing dysphagia?**
   A) Chest X-ray
   B) Head and neck CT
   C) Barium enema
   D) Videofluoroscopy

Introduction

Good nutritional care and hydration is essential to well-being and health. Malnutrition and dehydration have an undesirable effect on the body and contribute to poor wound healing, breakdown of the skin, an increased risk of developing sepsis and hospital-acquired infections, for example, chest and urinary tract infections. It is important that people have access to fluids and a balanced diet. Assistance with eating and drinking may be required by people at different times in their lifespan. The provision of high-quality, holistic patient care means that adequate nutrition and hydration are given high priority.

The Nursing and Midwifery Council (NMC) (2018a) requires the nursing associate to provide support with nutrition and hydration to people who need it. A key aspect of the nursing associate's role is to assist people with feeding and drinking and make use of appropriate feeding and drinking aids.

Green Flag

The NMC Code (Nursing and Midwifery Council 2018b), when discussing the fundamentals of care, includes nutrition and hydration. The Code makes it clear that it is essential to ensure that those receiving care have adequate access to nutrition and hydration and for the nursing associate to make sure that they provide help to those people who require assistance with eating and drinking.

Reasons Why People Require Assistance

Some medical conditions result in people having difficulty with eating and drinking. Stroke can result in difficulty in swallowing (dysphagia). Dysphagia increases the risk of the person aspirating on their oral intake and therefore support is required. A further complication of stroke is hemiparesis. Hemiparesis is paralysis affecting one half of the body. Hemiparesis makes it physically difficult to cut up and eat food. Conditions such as motor neurone disease (MND), multiple sclerosis (MS), myasthenia gravis, Huntington's disease and traumatic brain injury are less commonly occurring conditions but will also hinder the person's ability to manage eating and drinking independently. These conditions affect the physical ability of the person to manage oral intake.

Traumatic brain injury, major surgery and cancer can lead to loss of appetite and weight loss. Dementia can affect people's ability to remember to eat and drink. There is also loss of appetite, an inability to communicate needs, likes and dislikes, lack of concentration to focus on eating and drinking, poor coordination and difficulty with buying or cooking food. Childhood cerebral palsy can result in impairment of the facial muscles making it difficult to suck, chew and swallow food. Down syndrome is associated with several issues that can affect nutritional intake. Poor muscle tone and enlarged tongue (macroglossia) coupled with a small oral cavity leads to difficulty in chewing and swallowing and increases the risk of aspiration.

Supporting Evidence

The Scottish Intercollegiate Guidelines Network (2010). Management of patients with stroke: identification and management of dysphagia. A national clinical guideline: https://www.sign.ac.uk/assets/sign119.pdf

The guidance provides information on assessing the risk of aspiration and the importance of the swallow test and other useful investigations.

Red Flag

Dysphagia means difficulty in swallowing. It is a symptom of many diseases. A failure to swallow properly has two potentially serious consequences for people:

1. Choking
2. Aspiration pneumonia

Nursing associates, as part of basic life support training, should know how to manage a choking patient. It is important that the nursing associate recognises the risks, signs and symptoms of aspiration and escalates concerns appropriately.

Being an Accountable Professional

The NMC (2018) includes nutrition and hydration as part of the fundamentals of care. The Code (2018) discusses the importance of not only ensuring that people have access to food and drink but that people are assisted to eat and drink when this is required. A failure to recognise and assist people with eating and drinking is therefore a breach of the NMC Code.

Some people with learning disabilities, for example, are at greater risk of having difficulties with eating and drinking (Wright et al. 2018). When offering care to people with a learning disability, it is important to assess their ability to eat or drink independently by asking them and, if appropriate, their carer about eating and drinking, undertaking an assessment when they are eating or drinking or referring them to speech and language therapy (SALT) for a more formal assessment.

The Association of UK Dieticians has produced a professional consensus statement on the nutritional care of adults with a learning disability in care settings. This statement sets the standard of nutritional care that should be achieved for adults with a learning disability in care settings. The document considers all aspects of care specific to those with a learning disability and nutrition. This includes assessment, care planning, menu design, food preparation and presentation. There are recommendations for education and training of the care teams. Communication strategies are included as additional requirements, for example, pictures may be required to allow informed choices to be made (British Dietetic Association 2017).

All patients should have their risk of malnutrition assessed using assessment tools such as the Malnutrition Universal Screening Tool (adult) or the Paediatric Yorkhill Malnutrition Score (children) on admission. Chapter 30 provides details concerning the use of nutritional assessment tools.

The nursing associate should ascertain the normal eating habits of those in their care as part of the admission process. If the patient is unable to provide the information, a relative or carer may be asked. It is important to find out about the following:

- Usual ability to manage independently
- Amount of assistance required
- Food allergies
- Dietary preferences
- Special diets to meet medical or cultural requirements
- Oral health
- Physical difficulties that may affect ability to eat and drink

This information must be documented within the patient's nutritional care plan. The nursing associate should observe for signs that may indicate that there could be dysphagia. The signs of dysphagia include:

- Coughing during a meal
- Regurgitating food
- Food and secretions leaking from the mouth during eating
- Complaining of food sticking and not going down into the stomach
- A wet voice
- Excessive saliva

The risk associated with dysphagia is aspiration of the food and/or drink into the lungs which can lead to aspiration pneumonia. Aspiration pneumonia may present as recurrent infections, pyrexia or hypoxia (Smithard 2015).

Swallow Assessment

If there is a suspicion that there is dysphagia present, then the patient will require a SALT referral. The speech and language therapist will undertake a swallow assessment. The patient may feel anxious about this test, and the nursing associate should take time to explain what happens during the test and be available to assist prior to, during and after the test. A swallow test includes:

- An examination of the oral cavity
- An assessment of the person's ability to manipulate the many muscles utilised during swallow such as the tongue
- Listening to breathing
- Watching as the patient eats or drinks
- Videofluoroscopy – an X-ray image of swallow

If the speech and language therapist makes a diagnosis of a swallowing impairment, then they will advise of the next steps that need to be taken. This must be documented in the person's notes, and local policy and procedure must be adhered to.

Take Note

Swallow tests should only be undertaken by those who are deemed competent in the procedure.

Speech and language therapist may advise that the person has no oral diet after the initial assessment. This can be difficult for the patient and the relatives to understand. It is important that they are offered reassurance by including them in the nutritional care plan and always providing explanations underpinning the rationale for no oral diet. The person will have had an explanation from the speech and language therapist as to the danger of aspiration pneumonia and choking and, therefore, the necessity for no oral diet. The nursing team should reassure the patient that nutrition and hydration will be provided by an alternative means such as nasogastric enteral feeding and/or intravenous fluids. The person should be offered oral hygiene as without oral nutrition, the mucous membranes in the oral cavity can become dry and uncomfortable. The person will still have feelings of thirst and hunger, and it is important to ask about these and reporting them as the prescriptions for alternative nutrition may need to be changed.

The person and their family need to be reassured that there will be a continuous re-evaluation of swallow and that oral diet will be reintroduced once the danger of choking or aspiration pneumonia has passed. The speech and language therapist may advise that oral diet is permissible but that modifications are required, for example, food may have to be liquidised, pureed, minced or soft and moist and bite sized.

Fluids may have to be thickened to reduce the risk of aspiration. Thickening agents are used to achieve the correct consistency. Consistencies may be thin, slightly thick, mildly thick, moderately thick or extremely thick. These terms have been introduced as part of the International Dysphagia Diet Standardisation Initiative framework to standardise the descriptions of textures and consistency of food (NHS Improvement 2019).

The speech and language therapist may also provide the person with some exercises that are designed to help improve swallow. The diet prescribed and the exercises devised must be part of the patient's care plan.

Working in Teams

Their are many professionals involved in providing nutritional support to those who have a compromised swallow. The speech and language therapist assesses swallow and advises on the correct type of diet for people. The dietician will calculate the correct calorific intake required and prescribe oral diet, enteral nutrition or oral nutritional supplements. The doctor will prescribe intravenous fluids if there is a risk of dehydration. The nursing team will assess, plan, implement and evaluate the nutritional care plan which may include insertion of the nasogastric tube, risk assessments, assistance with eating and drinking, oral care and support for the person and their family.

Take Note

Risk assessment and safety are two important considerations when assisting people to eat and drink. The involvement of the specialist in the multidisciplinary team as well as person centred assessment can help minimise the risk of malnutrition developing.

The Care Environment

The environment is an important consideration within nutritional care, particularly where people have difficulty with concentration, for example those living with dementia. A quiet peaceful environment should be provided without music or an excess of stimulation. Eating is usually considered a social activity. Providing a room for eating rather than bedside eating is a more normal experience for people, promotes independence and encourages nutritional intake. Flexibility in when food is available ensures that people have a more consistent access to nutrition.

To reduce activity within hospital, care home and rehabilitation settings, protected mealtimes are implemented (Department of Health 2010). Protected mealtimes are an initiative which aims to reduce activities within a clinical environment when meals are served. There should be no cleaning, consultations or visitors during this period to allow people and the nursing team to focus on the nutritional needs of those in their care. This initiative allows time for food and drink to be enjoyed and eaten at the right temperature. While this initiative has been widely implemented in health care settings there are mixed reviews as to the success of the initiative (Porter et al. 2017)

The hygiene needs of people should be considered before meals are served. Offer the use of the toilet and hand hygiene before sitting down for a meal. Where possible, avoid bringing bedpans and commodes out during mealtimes.

The best position and place to eat and digest food should be considered. Dining table and chairs should be used. This allows people to sit upright when eating with utensils; drinks and napkins should be within easy reach. Being out of bed on a chair is a preferential position to eating in bed. If people have to eat in bed, and if there are no contraindications, then they should be positioned as upright as possible.

Occupational therapists can provide adapted cutlery to those who need it to promote independence with nutrition (Anderson 2017) (see Figure 31.1). Other aids such as non-slip mats, adapted cups and food guards are also useful. Special consideration must also be given to those people who may have visual challenges such as blindness or partial sightedness.

The nursing team needs to identify those people who require support with nutrition. Support can range from ensuring everything is close to hand and within easy reach, to opening packaging or identifying those who need additional assistance. The red tableware or red tray initiative is one way of identifying who needs assistance with their nutritional intake (Anderson 2017; National Health Service Scotland 2014) (see Figure 31.2).

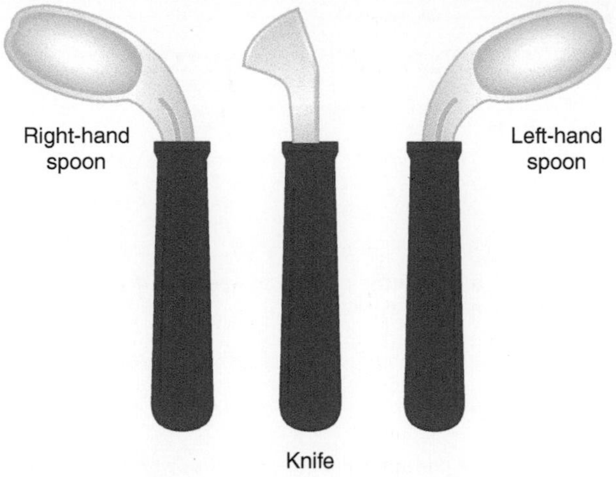

Figure 31.1 **Adapted cutlery.** ***Source:*** **Based on Anderson (2017).**

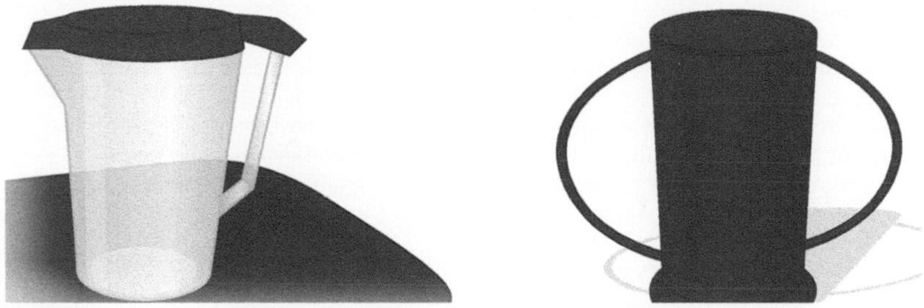

Figure 31.2 **Red Tableware can highlight people who need help.** ***Source:*** **Based on Anderson (2017).**

Orange Flag

The role of the nursing associate within an eating disorder care facility is challenging. Malnutrition risk assessments must be undertaken as the risk of malnutrition in eating disorders is high. A person-centred approach is required as goals set by the person living with an eating disorder are more likely to be more successful than those set by the team. Nursing associates will have to help set realistic goals for the person living with an eating disorder. They may have to supervise the person to ensure that they do eat and that they do not vomit after eating. Nursing associates should be encouraging at mealtimes. Mealtimes can be distressing for the person living with an eating disorder. The recommendation is to set a limit to mealtimes to reduce stress and anxiety (Walsh 2007).

Guidelines on How to Assist a Person with Eating and Drinking

Following assessment the plan of care shoud include preparing to assist a person with eating and drinking. Prepare the following equipment:

- A clean table or tray
- Equipment needed to assist the patient to eat, for example, adapted cutlery
- A serviette
- A chair for the nursing associate to sit beside or opposite the patient

The procedure to be undertaken when assisting a person to eat their meal is detailed in Box 31.1. The nursing associate must always ensure that the procedure is adapted to meet the individual needs of the people in their care. Independence should be encouraged, and it is important to assess and implement the specific assistance that is required (Anderson 2017).

Improving Safety and Quality of Care

Age Concern (2006) discusses the use of volunteers to assist patients at mealtimes. This ensures that there are enough people to help with nutritional care, and those identified as requiring assistance are not left to last. Robinson et al. (2014) recommend that volunteers undertake a training

Box 31.1 Procedure to be Undertaken to Assist a Person to Eat Their Meal

1. Explain to the person that you are going to help them with their meal.
2. Decontaminate your hands and put on an apron.
3. Assist the person to sit in an upright position:
   At a table in a dining room
   In a chair by the bed with a bedside table
   Upright in bed with a bedside table
4. Dentures should be clean and well fitting.
5. Decontaminate your hands before handing food and allow the persons to wash and dry their hands prior to their meal.
6. Protect the persons clothing with a serviette to maintain dignity.
7. Use a serviette throughout when and if needed.
8. Take a seat, at the persons' eye level, make yourself comfortable. This communicates that you have the time to help them eat and enjoy their meal.
9. Concentrate on this activity and avoid any distractions.
10. Inform them about what is on the plate.
11. Offer them seasoning or sauces; ask if they have a preferred order in which they wish to eat their meal.
12. Ask them how it is that they would like to receive their food; some people may prefer a fork, others a spoon. Ensure, where possible, that they are in control of the mealtime.
13. Do not overload the fork. Bring it up to their mouth; this eliminates the need to bend to reach the food. Ensure that there is plenty of time for the person to chew and swallow.
14. Use verbal and non-verbal skills of communications throughout.
15. For those people with a small appetite, suggest they try to eat a little of each course for a balanced nutritional intake.
16. Provide them with sips of fluid after every couple of mouthfuls.
17. When they have had enough of the main course, offer a dessert in the same way. Ensure that the spoon is the correct size, for example, using a teaspoon for yoghurt.
18. When the meal is finished, ensure that they are clean and comfortable and have had sufficient to eat and drink. People should be encouraged to eat but do not pressurise them when they have indicated that they have had enough.
19. Provide them with an opportunity to clean their teeth and dentures or, if this is not possible, perform mouth care.
20. At the end of the meal, ensure that they have a drink, being aware that those who require help with eating will need help with drinking also, and regular fluids should be offered.
21. Remove your apron, decontaminate your hands and document the patients' dietary intake.

Source: Adapted from Dougherty et al. (2015); Anderson (2017)

programme and are sufficiently supervised when assisting people with eating or drinking. The use of volunteers can improve team working and relationships as well as improve nutrition. Poor staffing levels may have an adverse effect on nutrition (Semerdzhieva & Reid 2019); therefore, the use of trained volunteers may help with nutrition in busy clinical environment.

Initiatives such as the use of volunteers, red trays or protected mealtimes have been introduced; however, their success in preventing malnutrition has not been fully evaluated. The nursing associate can be involved in the audit of these initiatives to evaluate their success.

Eating and drinking is a social activity, but people may not see it as a social activity if they are having difficulty with eating or drinking and require assistance. This can be socially isolating and add to feelings of hopelessness and depression. It is important to find out what the person's preference is in relation to eating with others; some may prefer to be with others while others may prefer to eat alone.

Blue Flag

Eating and drinking is generally enjoyed with the company of others; having a meal out and dining out are often where relations begin and where they are sustained (personal and otherwise). Dining in company can provide the opportunity for social interactions to take place.

Eating and drinking are both key to providing energy, nutrients and an adequate intake, as well as to affect physiological, psychological and social well-being and quality of life. Eating with others might encourage the people to eat more that they might normally but the nursing associate must bear in mind that some people may be self-conscious and embarrassed (for whatever reason) to eat in company.

Food should be presented in a way that is appetising, and the temperature of the food should be appropriate. The plate should not be overloaded as this can put those with a small appetite off their food.

Yellow Flag

Nursing associates should have an understanding of the cultural preferences of those that they care for. BAPEN (2018) discusses the issue of patients in hospital and care homes being presented with food that is not aligned with their cultural norm. In addition, not every culture uses knives and forks; some preferring to eat with their hands or chopsticks. It is therefore important to consider if there may be a cultural requirement to provide a different type of food or to ask family members to bring in more familiar food to stimulate appetite and prevent malnutrition.

Where assistance is required, it is important to ensure that you use portions of food that meet the patient's requirements. Consider the nature of the food; if it is very dry, then gravy or sauce could be added. Give the patient time to chew and swallow the food before being ready with the next mouthful. If there is dysphagia, the patient should be discouraged from talking as this increases the risk of aspiration. Have a drink available and allow the patient time to have some sips of water. This will help clear the oral cavity and assist with swallowing. Always refer to the patient's care plan prior to feeding or assisting with feeding and drinking.

During the process of assisting people, it is important to observe for coughing or gurgling, or anything that may indicate that they are experiencing difficulties. If this is the case, then stop feeding. A reassessment may be required by speech and language therapist. Report concerns to a more senior clinician.

People should be encouraged to eat, but pressuring them to eat when they do not want to is counterproductive and removes person-centredness from care delivery.

Touch Point

There is a plethora of information on the practical skill of helping people with eating and drinking. It is important to include the people in the planning of care and the setting of nutritional gaols. Set goals that they feel are achievable and give consideration to their preferences. This will improve the chances of delivery a balanced diet.

Monitoring Care and Promoting Health and Preventing Ill Health

The nursing associate should document on the food chart and/or the fluid balance chart the amount of food and drink that have been consumed (Dougherty et al. 2015). It is also important to report the person's subjective feeling about the food and its quality; this can help in making improvements if needed.

By participating in the nutritional care of people, nursing associates are preventing malnutrition, promoting healing and health and well-being. West (2019) discusses making every patient encounter count with regard health promotion. Nursing associates have an opportunity when caring for people to talk to them about healthy food choices. This can empower the patients to make their own decisions with regard food choices when they are well enough and on the road to recovery.

Integrated Care

The nursing associate should be knowledgeable about the team who are involved in providing nutrition and hydration to people. If volunteers are used to help at mealtimes the nursing associate should know about the training, they have had and their abilities. Documentation of the assistance required, and escalation of concerns will contribute to the onward care and safety of the people within the care environment. Within acute care environments, people are presenting with increasing complex conditions and comorbidities which can affect their ability to eat and drink. Detailed assessment of their nutritional and hydration status is required to provide person centred care.

Discharge Planning

Preparing patients for discharge is an important part of person-centred care. The nursing associate should consider how people will manage at home and involve the patient in planning care. The social circumstances of the person should be noted. Family or friends who can assist at home are important. A care package may be required for those people who do not have support at home. Important considerations include the ability of the patient to gain access to food physically. The use of online shopping is only useful if the person has a device and a good internet connection. The person has to be able to physically prepare the food. Finding out if there is someone who can help shop and prepare food is important. Some local councils offer a meal at home service delivering prepared or frozen food to people. There are also many private companies that offer this service at cost to the individual.

Violet Flag

Voluntary organisations may be able to provide people with help and support regarding nutrition. The Food Chain, for example, is an organisation that ensures people living with human immunodeficiency virus (HIV) in London can access the nutrition they need to get well, stay well and lead healthy, independent lives. The Food Chain delivers meals and groceries, offer cookery and nutrition classes and communal eating opportunities to people living with HIV in London and their dependents.

Having an understanding of such organisations can help the nursing associate help those who may need additional support.

Communication with community services including the patients' general practitioner is essential to help the people maintain their level of nutritional intake when discharged from hospital.

Conclusion

The nursing associate has an essential role to play in working with those who require assistance with feeding and drinking across a range of settings and from admission to safe discharge. Undertaking an assessment of need, implementing the care required, maintianig the safety of people by the referral for a swallow test (if appropriate) can help to ensure that nutritional needs are met.

References

Age Concern. (2006) *Hungry to be heard.* [online] Available: https://www.scie.org.uk/publications/guides/guide15/files/hungrytobeheard.pdf. Accessed 30 October 2019.

Anderson, L. (2017) Assisting patients with eating and drinking to prevent malnutrition, *Nursing Times*, 113(11): 23–25. [online] Available: https://www.nursingtimes.net/clinical-archive/nutrition/assisting-patients-with-eating-and-drinking-to-prevent-malnutrition-09-10-2017/. Accessed 30 October 2019.

BAPEN. (2018) *Introduction to malnutrition.* [online] Available: https://www.bapen.org.uk/malnutrition-undernutrition/introduction-to-malnutrition?showall=1. Accessed 30 October 2019.

British Dietetic Association. (2017) *The nutritional care of adults with a learning disability in care settings.* [online] Available: https://www.bda.uk.com/publications/professional/adults_with_ld_in_care_settings. Accessed December 2019.

Dougherty, L., Lister, S. and West-Oram, A. (2015) *The royal Marsden manual of clinical nursing procedures* (9th edn), Chichester: Wiley Blackwell.

National Health Service Scotland. (2014) *Food fluid and nutritional care.* [online] Available: file:///Users/louisemcerlean/Downloads/20141015%20FFNC_STANF_OCT2014.pdf

NHS Improvement. (2019) *Resources to assist with the transition to the international dysphagia diet standardisation initiative (IDDSI) framework.* [online] Available: https://improvement.nhs.uk/resources/transition-to-iddsi-framework/. Accessed 30 October 2019.

Nursing and Midwifery Council. (2018a) *Standards of proficiency for nursing associates.* [online] Available: https://www.nmc.org.uk/standards/standards-for-nursing-associates/standards-of-proficiency-for-nursing-associates/. Accessed December 2019.

Nursing and Midwifery Council (NMC). (2018b) The code, Professional standards of practice and behaviour for nurses, midwives and nursing associates. [online] Available: https://www.nmc.org.uk/globalassets/sitedocuments/nmc-publications/nmc-code.pdf. Accessed December 2019.

Porter, J., Pilgrim, A.L. and Truby, H. (2017) The efficacy of protected mealtimes in hospital patients: a stepped wedge cluster randomised controlled trial, *BMC Medicine*, 15:25. https://www.ncbi.nlm.nih.gov/pmc/articles/PMC5295189/pdf/12916_2017_Article_780.pdf. Accessed December 2019.

Robison, J., Pilgrim, A.L., Rood, G., Diaper, N., Marinos, E., Jackson A.A., Cooper, C., Aihie, A., Robinson S. and Roberts, H.C. (2014) Can trained volunteers make a difference at mealtimes for older people in hospital? A qualitative study of the views and experience of nurses, patients, relatives and volunteers in the Southampton mealtime assistance study, *International Journal of Older People Nursing*, 10: 136–145.

Semerdzhieva, E. and Reid, B. (2019) Getting the fundamentals right: assisting patients with eating and drinking, *Nursing and Residential Care*, 21(10): 562–565.

Smithard, D.G. (2015) Dysphagia: prevalence, management and side effects, *Nursing in practice.* [online] Available: https://www.nursinginpractice.com/dysphagia-prevalence-management-and-side-effects. Accessed 30 October 2019.

Walsh, L. (2007) Caring for patients who have eating disorders, *Nursing Times*, 103: 28–29.

West, S. (2019) *Blog: a nurse's role in promoting health and preventing ill health (from the bedside to the bingo hall).* [online] Available: https://www.nmc.org.uk/news/news-and-updates/blog-a-nurses-role-in-promoting-health-and-preventing-ill-health/. Accessed 30 October 2019.

Wright, B., Beavon, N., Branford, D., Harding, C., Howseman, T., Ramussen., J., Sandhu, S., Smith, A. and White, A. (2014). *Guideline for the identification and management of swallowing difficulties in adults with learning disability.* [online] Available: https://www.guidelines.co.uk/dysphagia/swallowing-difficulties-management-in-adults-with-learning-disability/236036.article. Accessed 30 October 2019.

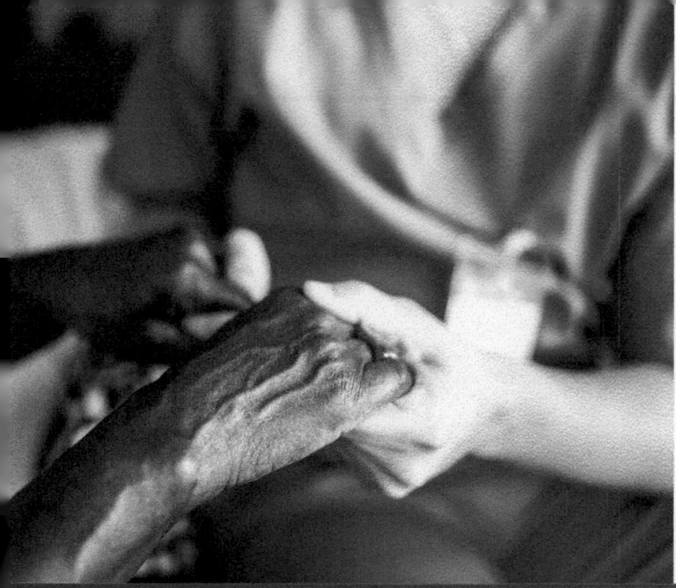

32

Fluid Balance

Louise McErlean

Department of Nursing, School of Health and Social Work, Ulster University, Northern Ireland, UK

Chapter Aim

- **To provide the reader with an understanding of the importance of fluid balance in maintaining health**

Learning Outcomes

- **The reader should be able to understand the importance of providing hydration to people.**
- **The reader should be able to understand the difficulties associated with ensuring hydration across a range of settings.**
- **The reader should be able to understand how to monitor fluid balance.**

Test Yourself Multiple Choice Questions

1. **How much of the body is composed of water?**
   A) 10%
   B) 40%
   C) 60%
   D) 90%
2. **Which of these is not a function of water?**
   A) Maintenance of blood volume
   B) Transport of nutrients
   C) Formation of the structure of the cell
   D) Processing of sensory information
3. **How much urine do the kidneys produce in health?**
   A) 0.1-0.2 mL/kg/hour
   B) 0.1-0.2 L/kg/hour
   C) 0.5-1.0 mL/kg/hour
   D) 0.5-1.0 L/kg/hour

The Nursing Associate's Handbook of Clinical Skills, First Edition. Edited by Ian Peate.

Companion website: www.wiley.com/nursingassociate

4. **Which of these statements is true?**
   A) Potassium is the main extracellular fluid cation
   B) Intracellular fluid includes intravascular fluid
   C) Extracellular fluid is fluid contained within the cells
   D) Intracellular fluid contains the largest volume of water

5. **Which of these could be described as insensible loss?**
   A) Vomit
   B) Fluid from a drain
   C) Nasogastric aspirate
   D) Sweat

Introduction

Fluid balance is the measuring of fluids entering the body and comparing them to the fluids leaving the body to determine if there is an excess or deficit. The human body is approximately 60% water (Ojo 2017); water is considered one of the essential nutrients required for health (Campbell 2014) and has many essential functions in the body including the following:

- Transportation of
  - Nutrients
  - Gases
- Regulation of body temperature
- Lubrication of
  - Joints
  - Internal organs
- Moistening of tissues
- Maintaining and giving shape to cells
- Dissolving vitamins and minerals
- Maintenance of blood volume and therefore blood pressure
- Maintenance of acid–base balance

Despite the many functions of water and the associated importance of water, dehydration remains evident in healthcare. This includes within-hospital settings and in the community (Sheills & Morrell – Scott 2018).

Green Flag

The Nursing and Midwifery Council (NMC) 2018 requires the nursing associate to have an understanding of homeostasis. As water has many important functions within the body, it is important that water balance is controlled. Osmoregulation is the name given to the maintenance of a constant osmotic pressure and the control of water and electrolyte concentrations. Monitoring of fluid balance can give an indication of how well homeostasis in relation to fluid balance is being maintained. This is particularly relevant during ill health or in conditions that affect the kidneys.

Fluid and Electrolytes in the Body

In order to consider the importance of fluid balance in the body, it is important to have a fundamental understanding of how the homeostasis of fluid is maintained.

Fluid is contained within functional spaces or compartments. Intracellular fluid (ICF) is fluid contained within the cells and accounts for two-thirds of the body's water. The remaining one-third is contained outside the cells in the extracellular compartment and is called extracellular fluid (ECF) (see Figure 32.1). Extracellular fluid includes interstitial fluid (the fluid that surrounds the cells), intravascular fluid (fluid in the blood plasma) and all of the other ECFs such as lymph, urine, sweat, saliva, fluid produced by glands, cerebrospinal fluid, pleural fluid, pericardial fluid and more (McCance et al. 2018).

Fluid contains electrolytes, for example, sodium, potassium, calcium and chloride, and nonelectrolytes, such as creatinine, urea, lipids and glucose. The electrolytes have a role in fluid balance. Small changes in electrolyte concentrations will lead to water moving between the compartments, resulting in changes in blood volume and, therefore, blood pressure.

Movement of Fluid and Electrolytes

The compartments are separated by a semi-permeable membrane. The ECF contains more sodium and less potassium. The intracellular fluid is the reverse.

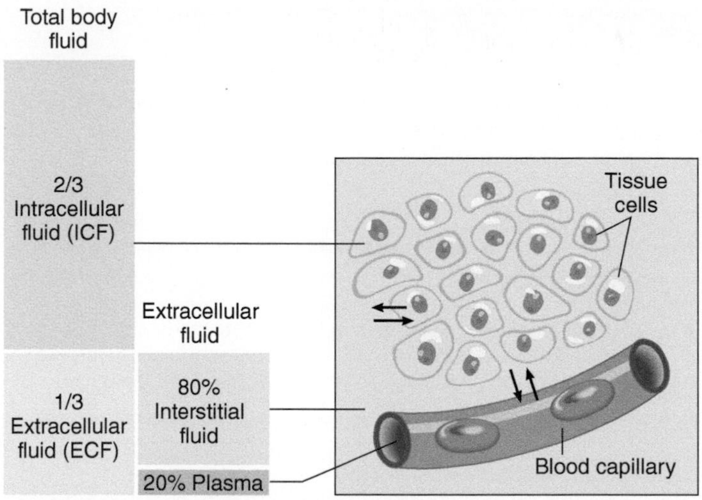

Figure 32.1 Fluid distribution. *Source:* **Peate (2017), chapter 17, figure 17.2, p. 508.**

Electrolytes move by a process called *diffusion*, moving from an area of high concentration to an area of low concentration. Water moves by a process called *osmosis*. It moves across the semi-permeable membrane from an area of low solute concentration to an area of high solute concentration until an equilibrium is established. Therefore, changes in the sodium and potassium levels will lead to water movement between the intracellular fluid and the ECF. The intracellular space contains the largest volume of water.

The Maintenance of Fluid Balance

Maintaining fluid balance means that the body must not lose more water than it takes in. The majority of fluid intake is from fluids and food ingested, but cellular metabolism accounts for about 10% of the fluid. Insensible loss describes fluid loss that it is difficult to measure and includes loss through sweat and water vapour.

Fluid leaves the body in a variety of ways:

- Urine
- Stool
- Sweat
- Water vapour

Figure 32.2 illustrates water intake and output.

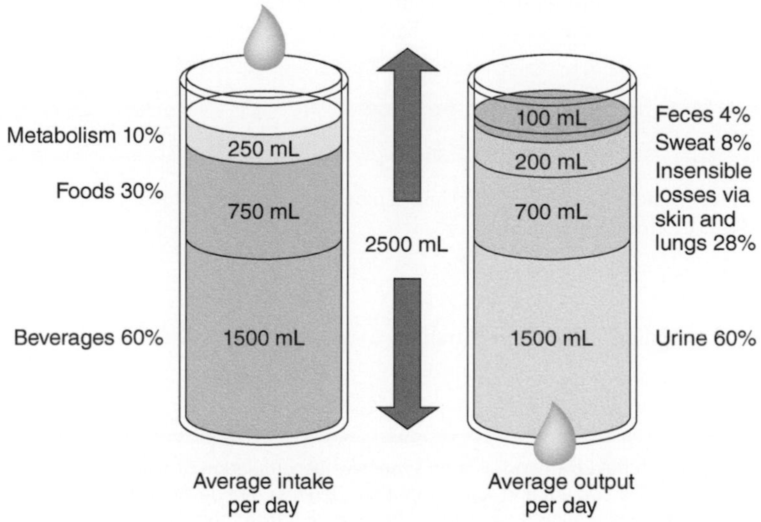

Figure 32.2 Sources of intake and output volumes. *Source:* **Redrawn from Benjamin Cummings, an imprint of Addison Wesley Longman. Inc.**

Fluid Balance

Small changes to the electrolyte content or the water content of these fluids will lead to a response to maintain homeostasis. It is important for the nursing associate to be able to recognise changes in the fluid and electrolyte balance of those who they offer care and support to and to escalate any concerns so that a treatment plan can be prescribed without delay.

Red Flag

Clostridium difficile is an infection associated with antibiotics. The spore forming bacteria is easily spread to others particularly those who are already vulnerable due to illness. The symptoms include watery diarrhoea several times a day, pyrexia, painful stomach cramps, nausea, appetite loss, weight loss. In some cases, the loss of appetite and profuse diarrhoea can quickly lead to severe dehydration. The signs of dehydration include decreased urine output, dry mouth and skin, thirst and headache. Clostridium difficile can be treated with antibiotics and dehydration is managed with fluid replacement therapy.

There are several ways that fluid balance is maintained during health.

The amount of electrolytes in the fluid determines the osmolarity of a solution. If the osmolarity increases, it is detected by the hypothalamus, and thirst is stimulated. Drinking restores the balance of water and sodium in the ECF. If a reduction in fluid in the bloodstream is detected, then less saliva is produced. This leads to a dry mouth and stimulates the desire to drink (Marieb 2017). By responding to the thirst stimulus and drinking fluid, homeostasis is maintained.

The renal and endocrine systems have a role in fluid homeostasis by reabsorbing water and electrolytes back into the blood during filtration at the kidney.

When blood volume (hypovolaemia) drops as a result of haemorrhage or dehydration from vomiting, diarrhoea or any other reason, then this causes a fall in blood pressure (hypotension). The fall in blood pressure leads to a decrease in the amount of filtrate formed at the kidneys – this is seen as a decrease in the amount of urine output. At the same time, the endocrine system becomes involved. Anti-diuretic hormone (ADH) is released from the posterior pituitary in response to the change in blood composition (less water). ADH acts on the kidneys to reduce the urine volume which increases the amount of fluid in the blood, leading to an increase in blood volume and blood pressure.

A further mechanism to restore balance is the renin angiotensin aldosterone (RAAS) system.

Renin is released in response to low blood pressure in the afferent arteriole or changes in the solute concentration in the filtrate. Renin converts angiotensin to angiotensin I, and angiotensin I is converted to angiotensin II. Angiotensin II acts on the systemic arteries, leading to vasoconstriction which increases peripheral vascular resistance. Angiotensin II also causes aldosterone to be secreted which leads to an increase in sodium and water reabsorption at the kidneys and an increase in blood volume and therefore blood pressure.

The sympathetic nervous system is stimulated in response to dehydration and leads to vasoconstriction, and this causes the blood pressure to increase. Heart rate also increases in response to sympathetic nervous system activation.

The maintenance of blood pressure is vital as the circulating blood is how the body cells receive the vital oxygen and nutrients required to carry out their function. The body therefore relies on several mechanisms to maintain this essential function.

As you can see, there are many compensatory mechanisms activated when a change in fluid status is detected within the body. This compensation can make it difficult for the nursing associate to recognise deterioration. Signs of deterioration include a drop in blood pressure. However a drop in blood pressure can be a late sign of deterioration associated with dehydration or fluid loss and therefore the nursing associate must be vigilant in undertaking patient assessment and assess not only the parameters on the National Early Warning Scoring (NEWS 2) (Royal College of Physicians 2017) observation chart but also consider the patients urine output.

There are two problems associated with the homeostasis of fluid balance, fluid overload and fluid loss.

Fluid Overload

Fluid overload occurs when there is too much fluid in the blood and can be caused by the following:

- Over infusion of intravenous fluids or blood transfusions
- Acute kidney injury
- Sepsis
- Cardiac failure
- Increased secretion of antidiuretic hormone following head trauma

Red Flag

Oedema is a sign associated with fluid overload. It is an excessive accumulation of fluid in the interstitial spaces. Oedema occurs in conditions where there is excessive sodium and water retention. Oedema can be localised or generalised. Localised oedema affects specific organs or tissue whereas generalised oedema is characterised by a more uniform fluid distribution throughout the body. Dependent oedema is where fluid gathers in areas gravity affects for example the legs and feet.

Dehydration or fluid loss

Dehydration or fluid loss occurs when fluid loss exceeds fluid intake.

It can occur for a variety of reasons:

- Inability to take fluid in
- Vomiting
- Diarrhoea
- Excessive diaphoresis
- Diabetes insipidus
- Blood loss through trauma
- Hyperglycaemia

Supporting Evidence

Acute kidney injury (AKI) is a complication associated with hypovolaemia which can occur during dehydration. National Institute for Health and Care Excellence (NICE) (2013) stresses the importance of using a track and trigger scoring system as well as measuring urine output as a means of identifying those who may be at risk of AKI and early intervention to prevent this.

Being an Accountable Professional

A failure to recognise a fluid imbalance can lead to deterioration of the patient. The nursing associate has to ensure that monitoring and reporting of any changes or concerns are communicated without delay and issues are documented.

Assessment

Patient history will reveal if there are any factors that affect fluid balance. These can include:

- Age. Older adults and babies are sensitive to small fluid changes
- Medications. Some medications can affect fluid balance, for example diuretics, non-steroidal anti-inflammatory drugs
- Long-term conditions, for example, diabetes mellitus, heart failure and chronic renal failure
- Lifestyle factors, for example, alcohol misuse

Visual assessment will include observation of the patient's oral mucosa which would appear dry if the patient is dehydrated. The patient may complain of thirst. Skin turgor can be assessed by gently pinching two folds of skin which should return to their normal position; during dehydration, the skin may take longer to return to its normal. The skin turgor test is not reliable for older adults as skin turgor takes longer to return to normal even in a healthy patient. The presence of oedema could be indicative of fluid overload.

There are many symptoms associated with dehydration. Patients may have sunken eyeballs and complain of dry eyes. Vasoconstriction as a response to dehydration means that the patient may have cool peripheries.

This will also affect the capillary refill time and it will be slower (the normal capillary refill time is 2–3 seconds). Headache and confusion can occur (McLafferty et al. 2014). Fluid and electrolyte imbalance can trigger seizures. The symptoms of dehydration in babies include:

- a sunken fontanelle
- few wet nappies
- failure to produce tears when crying
- no energy
- drowsiness
- dry mucous membranes

Children who have dehydration should be referred for urgent medical attention.

The nursing associate should complete the following vital signs as part of the National Early Warning Scoring System (see Table 32.1).

Due to the risks of developing acute kidney injury associated with hypovolaemia, a serum electrolytes blood test would usually be required.

Take Note

Venepuncture is a procedure that the nursing associate can undertake as part of monitoring a patient's condition (NMC 2018). The employer's policy on venepuncture should reflect this.

Urine

One of the symptoms associated with dehydration is a reduced urine output. The normal value for urine output is 0.5–1 mL/kg/hour. It is important to ask the patient about the last time they passed urine, and if dehydration is considered, then monitoring of all input and output, on a fluid

Table 32.1 NEWS 2 observations, including normal values and expected values during dehydration and fluid overload.

	NORMAL VALUE	EXPECTED VALUE IN RELATION TO DEHYDRATION AND FLUID OVERLOAD
Respiratory rate	12–20 breaths per minute	A high respiratory rate could occur in the presence of both fluid deficit and excess
Oxygen saturation	>96% on NEWS 2 scale 1	Oxygen saturation could be low in a patient with a fluid imbalance
Blood pressure	Patient's normal blood pressure. In the absence of the patient's normal blood pressure: 90–130/60–80 mmHg	During dehydration, the blood pressure may remain within the patient's normal range until the compensatory mechanisms fail and then it will drop. In fluid overload, the blood pressure may increase above the patient's usual normal range.
Heart rate	60-100 beats per minute	Dehydration: tachycardia. The pulse will feel weak and thready. Fluid overload: normal or tachycardia
Conscious level	Alert	Dehydration and fluid overload can affect conscious level including confusion.
Temperature	36.5–37.5°C	Dehydration: if due to infection, this can be elevated Fluid overload: normal

balance chart, will be required. Urine output may increase in the presence of fluid overload and also if the patient is taking diuretic medications. The colour of urine should be examined. Dark and strong-smelling urine could be an indication of dehydration.

Weight

Weight does not usually change by significant amounts when measured daily. Daily weights can be useful when there is dehydration, as weight may reduce, and in fluid overload, weight may increase. Discrepancies in recording a patient's body weight, as well as using inaccurate or inappropriate weighing equipment, can have a negative impact on patient outcomes.

The Fluid Balance Chart

The fluid balance chart is an assessment of the fluid intake and fluid output. In order for care to be person centred, the patient must be included in discussions around the reasons this chart is required, and they can participate in their own care by telling a member of the team when they have had a drink or used the bathroom. The privacy and dignity of the patient should be considered when emptying drainage bags such as urine or stoma bags for measuring.

Provide the patient with a cup and glass that has graduated measurements on it. If there is uncertainty about the volume a cup holds, then a measure should be taken. A measuring jug should be available to measure liquids, for example, the volume of milk taken in cereal or the volume of soup served for lunch.

Ensure the fluid balance chart has the patient's name and identification details written on it. Always check you have the correct chart for the correct patient before adding anything to the chart. The fluid balance chart must have the date (day, month and year) written on it. If available, the previous day's balance should be written on the front of the chart as well as today's target. See Figure 32.3 for an example of a fluid balance chart.

Monitoring and documenting patient fluid balance can be undertaken using digital systems. The nursing associate must ensure that they are competent with regard to using a digital/electronic recording system.

Fluid Input and Output – Measurement

See Table 32.2 for the procedure to be used to measure a person's fluid input and output. At all times, local policy and procedure must be adhere to.

Working in Teams

The patient, the nursing associate, the healthcare support workers and registered nurses complete the fluid balance charts. The fluid balance chart is a reliable assessment tool only if it is completed correctly by all of the team. Nazli et al. (2016) reported that 52% of fluid balance charts were inadequately completed. The NMC (2018) requires the nursing associate to maintain accurate and clear documentation.

Time	Input							Output								Fluid Balance
	Oral	Enteral	IV1	IV2	IV3	Hourly total	Total	Urine	NG loss	Vomit	Drain 1	Drain 2	Bowel/ stoma	Hourly total	Total	
0800																
0900																
1000																
1100																
1200																
1300																
1400																
1500																
1600																
1700																
1800																
1900																
2000																
2100																
2200																
2300																
2400																
0100																
0200																
0300																
0400																
0500																
0600																
0700																

Figure 32.3 Sample fluid balance chart.

Table 32.2 Procedure to measure fluid input and output.

1	Complete the fluid balance chart hourly
Input	
2	Consider how fluids are being taken, orally, via enteral feeding tubes or intravenously. Fluid input may be via all three routes
3	Write the volume of fluid taken in the last hour in the appropriate column.
4	Complete the total for the hour.
5	Complete the cumulative total.
Output	
6	Urine output. If the patient does not have a urinary catheter in situ, ensure that they have a supply of urine bottles or bedpans. Ask the patients to let you know when they have used the bottle or bedpan and where they are to be left. It may be useful to have an agreed identification mark on the bottle or bedpan to reduce errors. If the patient has a urinary catheter, hourly urine measurements can be made using a urometer.
7	Bowel output. It is important to measure the bowel movement, particularly if it is loose. The patient should be asked to use a bedpan, and the contents can be measured using a jug or a scale. If the bowel movement cannot be measured or weighed, the bowel movement must still be documented on the fluid output part of the fluid balance chart. If the patient has a stoma, the contents of the stoma bag should be emptied into a jug and measured or weighed.
8	Nasogastric aspirate or vomit. The patient should have a supply of sick bowls (receivers) available, and any vomit should be measured and recorded. A nasogastric tube with a drainage bag attached should be drained into a clean jug, the volume of aspirate measured and recorded on the appropriate section of the fluid balance chart.
9	Surgical drains. If the drain has an attached drainage bag which can be opened and drained, then the drainage should be measured. If the drainage bag cannot be drained, drainage should be calculated and the drain marked with time and date. The volume should be included in the fluid output chart.
10	Personal protective equipment such as gloves, aprons and goggles should be used when managing bodily fluids. Infection prevention and control practices should be maintained.
11	Fluid output should be added up hourly and a cumulative score calculated.
Calculate the fluid balance	
12	Calculate if the person is in a positive or negative balance hourly.
13	Report your findings to the registered nurse and seek help if the balance is becoming excessively positive or negative.

Source: Modified from Dougherty & Lister (2015).

Take Note

Patient history, visual observation, vital signs and fluid balance all form part of the patient assessment. The information gathered should be appropriately shared so that the most appropriate treatment plans can be created for the patient.

Complications and Management of Dehydration

Dehydration leads to a reduction in blood volume and drop in blood pressure. A fall in blood pressure will affect renal perfusion and can lead to acute kidney injury. It is important to encourage the patient to drink oral fluids, and if this is difficult, intravenous fluids may be prescribed. Reduced fluid intake leads to an increased risk of urinary tract infections and constipation, increased risk of falls (associated with a drop in blood pressure) and dizziness.

Complications and Management of Fluid Overload

Fluid overload can occur due to cardiac failure and acute kidney injury. It can also be caused by excessive intravenous fluid administration. Usually, excessive fluid intake is managed by the renal system: urine output increases and fluid homeostasis is restored. During ill health, this may not happen. Excess fluid will leak from the blood and move into tissues and will be seen as oedema. Oedema is usually seen in the lower limbs and sacrum but can progress to generalised oedema. When the excess fluid leads to pulmonary congestion within the blood vessels of the lungs, fluid moves out of the vessels and into the lungs; this is called pulmonary oedema. The patient would have respiratory symptoms such as increased respiratory rate, reduced oxygen saturation, cough and the production of pink frothy sputum. Pulmonary oedema is a medical emergency requiring urgent medical attention.

Patients at risk of fluid overload may require a fluid restriction and diuretic therapy. Strict fluid balance and patient education are key to managing fluid restrictions.

Practical Assistance

Improving fluid status is important, and the nursing associate can help patients with fluid intake by offering drinks hourly. Ensuring that drinks are placed close to the patient and can be reached and helping those who require assistance will help promote hydration in hospitals.

Violet Flag

Older adults become dehydrated easily. Reducing fluid intake is often deliberate to avoid urinary urgency and incontinence. Older adults living with physical health needs may find it difficult to drink as frequently as they did before, and this adds to dehydration. Nursing associates working in the community and visiting elderly patients should take the time to offer the patient a drink and improve the hydration status of the patient. In care homes, spending time assisting people to access drinks will help promote good hydration.

Promoting Health and Preventing Ill Health

The Scottish Urinary Tract Infection Network (Health Protection Scotland 2018) has launched a number of campaigns aimed at improving hydration and the complications associated with dehydration, for example, urinary tract infections. These include the National Hydration Campaign, the Children's National Hydration Campaign and National Urinary Catheter Passport. The British Heart Foundation (BHF) (2015) launched a campaign – the hydration challenge, the aim of which was to promote better hydration for employees.

Orange Flag

Caring for people who live with dementia can present challenges with regard to hydration. The use of poster and verbal prompts, reducing noise, offering choices of fluids to suit the person's preference, using appropriate cups that are highly coloured and ensuring that the care plan reflects preferences are some of the strategies to improve hydration (Wilson & Dewing 2019).

Touch Point

Fluid balance includes understanding fluid gain and fluid loss in normal health, understanding the patient's health issue, identifying signs of dehydration or fluid overload and escalating care appropriately.

Conclusion

Fluid balance is a complex topic and requires the nursing associate to have an understanding of when it is appropriate to restrict fluids and when fluids are to be encouraged. A knowledge and understanding of long-term health conditions such as heart failure and chronic kidney disease is a requirement.

References

British Heart Foundation (BHF). (2015) *Hydration challenge*. [online] Available: https://www.bhf.org.uk/informationsupport/publications/health-at-work/health-at-work-hydration-challenge. Accessed 3 December 2019.

Campbell, N. (2014) Recognising and preventing dehydration in patients, *Nursing Times*, 10(46): 20–21.

Dougherty, L. and Lister, S. (2015) *The royal Marsden manual of clinical nursing procedures* (9th edn), Chichester: John Wiley and Sons.

Health Protection Scotland. (2018) *National campaigns materials*. [online] Available: https://www.hps.scot.nhs.uk/web-resources-container/national-hydration-campaign-materials/. Accessed 3 December 2019.

Marieb, E.N. (2017) *Essentials of human anatomy and physiology* (12th edn), Harlow: Pearson.
McCance, K.L., Huether, S.E., Brashers, V.L. and Rote, N.S. (2018) Pathophysiology, *The biologic basis for disease in adults and children* (8th edn), St Louis: Elsevier Mosby.
McLafferty, E., Johnstone, C., Hendry, C. and Farley, A. (2014) Fluid and electrolyte balance, *Nursing Standard*, 28(29): 42–49.
National Institute for Health and Care Excellence (NICE). (2013) *Acute kidney injury: prevention, detection and management,* Clinical guideline [CG 169]. [online] Available: https://www.nice.org.uk/guidance/cg169/chapter/1-Recommendations. Accessed 30 October 2019.
NMC. (2018) *Standards of proficiency for nursing associates*, London: NMC.
Nazli, A., Brighman-Chan, F., Fernandes, M. and Anjum, A. (2016). Adequacy of fluid balance documentation on wards. *Clinical Medicine.* 16(Suppl 3): S21.
Ojo, O. (2017) The role of nutrition and hydration in disease prevention and patient safety, *British Journal of Nursing*, 26(18): 1020–1022.
Peate, I. (ed) (2017) *Fundamentals of applied pathophysiology: an essential guide for nursing and healthcare students* (3rd edn). Oxford: Wiley.
Royal College of Physicians. (2017) *National early warning score*, NEWS 2. [online] Available: https://www.rcplondon.ac.uk/projects/outputs/national-early-warning-score-news-2. Accessed 30 October 2019.
Sheills, R. and Morrell-Scott, N. (2018) Prevention of dehydration in hospital patients, *British Journal of Nursing*, 27(10): 565–569.
Wilson, K. and Dewing, J. (2019) Strategies to prevent dehydration in older people with dementia. *Nursing Older People*, 32(1): 27–33. doi: 10.7748/nop.e1208.

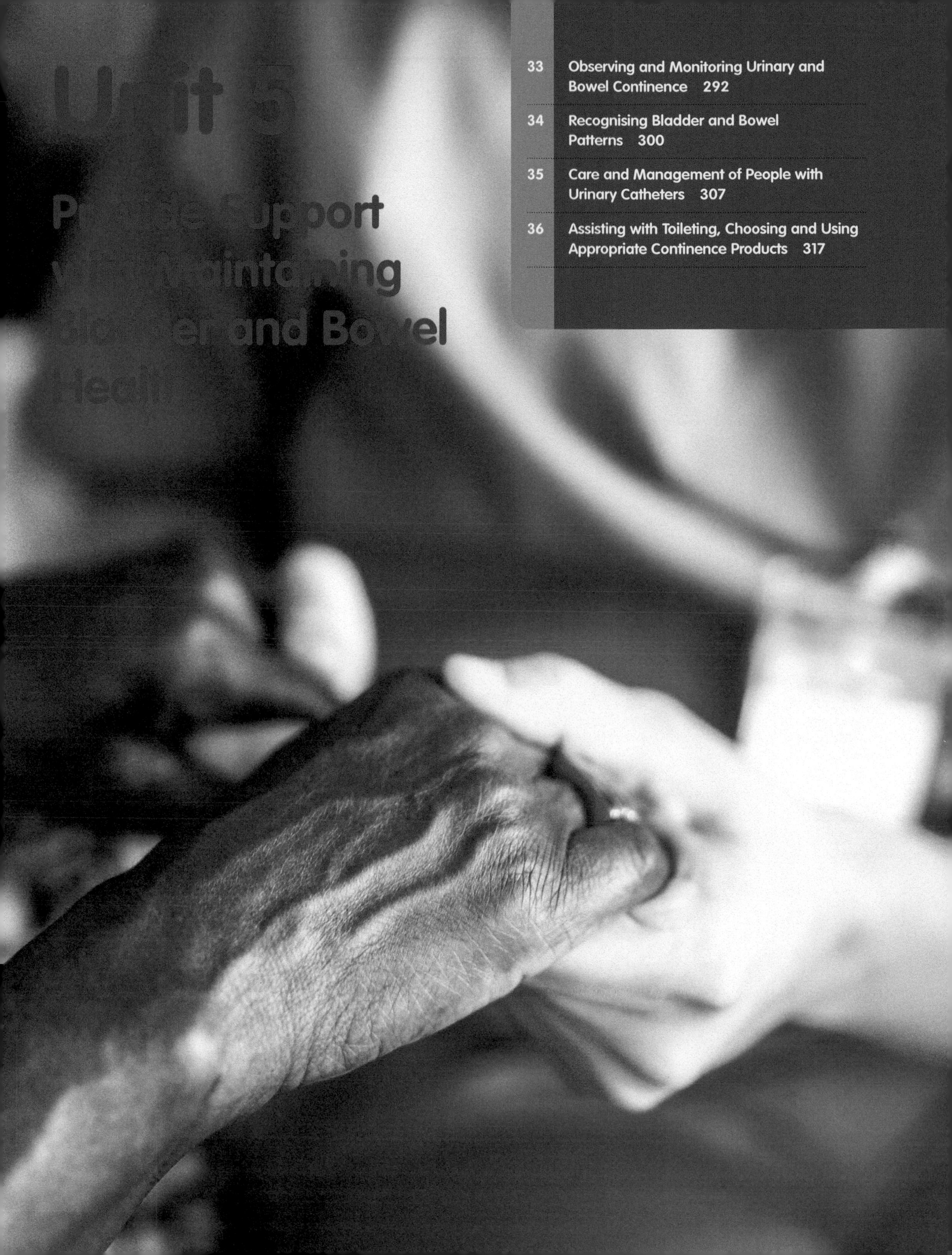

Unit 5

Provide Support with Maintaining Bladder and Bowel Health

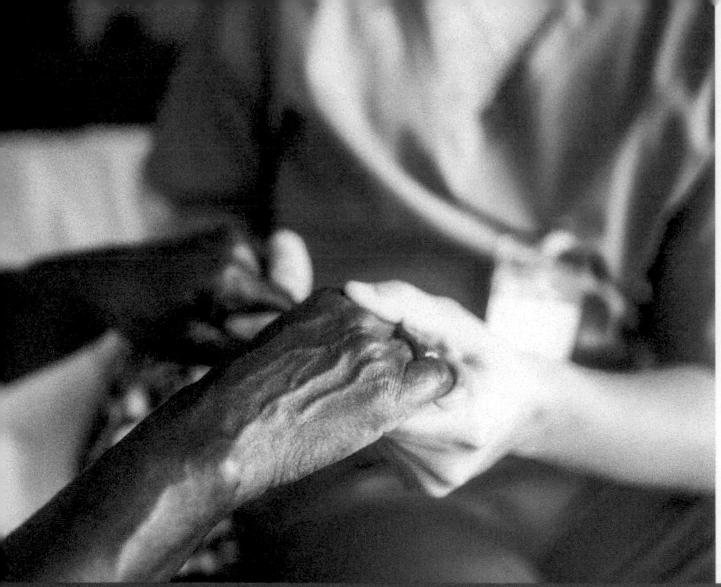

33

Observing and Monitoring Urinary and Bowel Continence

Kathy Whayman

University of Hertfordshire, UK

Chapter Aim

- **This chapter aims to develop the readers' understanding of the importance of observing and monitoring urinary and bowel continence in providing person-centred care. Good continence care begins with assessment and this chapter aims to develop the nursing associate's knowledge and skills of assessing continence, and delivery of compassionate dignified care in this vital area of clinical practice.**

Learning Outcomes

- **Examine the key issues and the nursing associate's role in observing and monitoring continence in clinical practice**
- **Explore the rationale for the assessment of continence based on current clinical guidelines and evidence**
- **Use appropriate assessment tools to enable the successful monitoring and maximising of continence in partnership with service users and their carers/families**

Test Yourself Multiple Choice Questions

1. ***Continence*** **is the term used to:**
   A) **Describe a person's ability to control their bladder or bowel emptying**
   B) **Describe a person's ability to use the toilet**
   C) **Describe the nervous control of the bladder and bowel function**
   D) **Describe involuntary leakage of urine or faeces from the bladder or bowel**

The Nursing Associate's Handbook of Clinical Skills, First Edition. Edited by Ian Peate.

Companion website: www.wiley.com/nursingassociate

2. **Problems with continence can affect:**
   A) Infants
   B) Children
   C) Adults from age 18 years onwards
   D) All ages
3. **The original meaning of continence is**
   A) Holding back
   B) Holding on
   C) Letting go
   D) Holding forth
4. **Most children learn to be continent**
   A) By the age of 2 years
   B) By the time they have started nursery
   C) By the time they have started reception
   D) At variable stages of development
5. **Which of these is a structure involved in micturition?**
   A) Kidney
   B) Ureter
   C) Cervix
   D) Pelvic floor

Introduction

Continence is the term originating from the phrase 'holding back' and is used when individuals have the ability to control when to empty their bladder by voiding urine and their bowels through defaecation. This ability is developed from early childhood and retained through to adulthood where individuals can perform their urinary or bowel function voluntarily in what they or others consider to be a socially acceptable place. Continence and the ability to control this function is an important part of a person's health and well-being, influencing physical, social and psychological health and independence (National Health Service Executive (NHSE) 2018).

Orange Flag

The main psychological effects of incontinence on people are the following:

- Stress
- Depression
- Sexual dysfunction
- Loss of self-respect and self-confidence
- Shame

Continence care is an essential component of the nursing associate's role which must be approached with sensitivity, compassion and competency to ensure the dignity and privacy of the individual is always respected (Royal College of Nursing (RCN) 2019a, 2019b). It is an essential nursing skill and the responsibility of all healthcare professionals to support people to maximise their continence (Booth 2013; Cheesley 2017).

Blue Flag

Loving, caring relationships are important for all of us, as these relationships can bring happiness and sadness, joy and disappointment, anxiety and pleasure, fulfilment and rejection. A bladder or bowel control problem is a further complication; this does not mean, however, that intimate relationships are impossible. For most people, sexual activity is a source of anxiety as well as pleasure. It is natural to worry about what can go wrong; incontinence is just another hurdle. A good way to remove some of the worries about how incontinence could affect intimacy and sexual activity is to plan ahead regarding practical problems that could happen and think about how to deal with them.

On behalf of the RCN Continence Forum, Cheesley (2017) takes this a step further and calls for continence care to be given ever greater importance: being so fundamental to care, she advocates it should be recognised as a seventh 'C' alongside the Core 6Cs of nursing (NHS Commissioning Board Chief Nursing Officer 2012). Indeed, when incontinence is experienced or when continence care and support fall short, the impact on the service users and their family can be devastating. Struggling with incontinence can have long-term implications for a person's health and well-being, often resulting in psychological morbidity, social isolation and physical disability.

Violet Flag

Stigma and misunderstanding surround invisible disabilities. People with continence issues can be subjected to discrimination just for trying to use the accessible toilet they urgently need. The RADAR key is part of the National Key Scheme that gives thousands of people with disabilities and health conditions independent access to locked public toilets around the country. It is important for those with bladder and bowel conditions to be able to have access to toilet facilities while they are out and about. Having a RADAR key can make the person feel more secure knowing that they are likely to be in close vicinity to accessible public toilet facilities. With the turn of the RADAR key, the person is granted immediate access to usable and toilet facilities.

This chapter will address the importance of assessment, observing and monitoring continence of service users in the nursing associate's care. Understanding and utilising different approaches and methods of observation, monitoring and recording of continence will enable the nursing associate to provide person-centred, safe and effective care. The proficiencies and standards set out by the NMC (Nursing and Midwifery Council 2018a) related to this chapter and the subsequent chapters will assist the nursing associate to demonstrate the knowledge, skills and ability required to meet people's needs related to bladder and bowel health.

Green Flag

Risk of faecal incontinence relates closely to several protected characteristics covered by the Equality Act 2010, including age, disability, sex and pregnancy and maternity. People at high risk of faecal incontinence include frail older people, women following childbirth (especially following obstetric anal sphincter injury), people with neurological or spinal disease/injury, those with severe cognitive impairment and people with learning disabilities.

Touch Point

- Service users and families will require good communication, consistency of care, support and provision of information to monitor continence and participate in decisions about their care to maximise well-being and when problems occur.
- Promotion of dignity, comfort and privacy is central to the nursing associate role and are of upmost importance in this sensitive and intimate area of care.

Urinary Continence

The elimination of urine from the body is a complex process involving neural pathways and signals passed between the brain, spinal cord, the bladder and associated structures (Marieb 2015), which can be seen in Figure 33.1. Fundamentally, the bladder is a smooth collapsible sac which acts as storage for urine; the release of urine is controlled by the relaxation of the urethral sphincter and pelvic floor whilst the bladder muscles contract to expel the urine (Marieb 2015). Signals are passed from the bladder wall and muscles to the brain once optimum expansion and tension is reached to inform the brain that the bladder is full and micturition needs to occur. The reader is advised to refer to anatomy and physiology textbooks (for example, Peate & Evans 2020) for a detailed description of the complex physiology and neural pathways involved in this process.

Red Flag

Bladder/muscle/sphincter weakness may be caused by a variety of factors (RCN 2019a), and it is important to identify the following as a risk factor in the continence assessment:

- surgery – particularly in men following prostate surgery
- pregnancy and childbirth
- obesity
- menopause
- chronic cough
- chronic constipation

Bowel (Faecal) Continence

Passage of faeces or stool is controlled by relaxing and contracting of the structures, as seen in Figure 33.2. The rectum is part of the large bowel involved in storage and is usually empty until just prior to defaecation. Movement of faeces into the rectum brings on the 'call to stool' which is a desire to defaecate (RCN 2019b). The anus and rectum are highly vascular, and the anus has two sphincters – ring-like muscles which control the release of stool. Neurological control involving the enteric nervous system, sympathetic and parasympathetic nerves convey information between the brain and the lower bowel when the rectum is full (Marieb 2015; RCN 2019b). The internal sphincter relaxes involuntarily, whereas

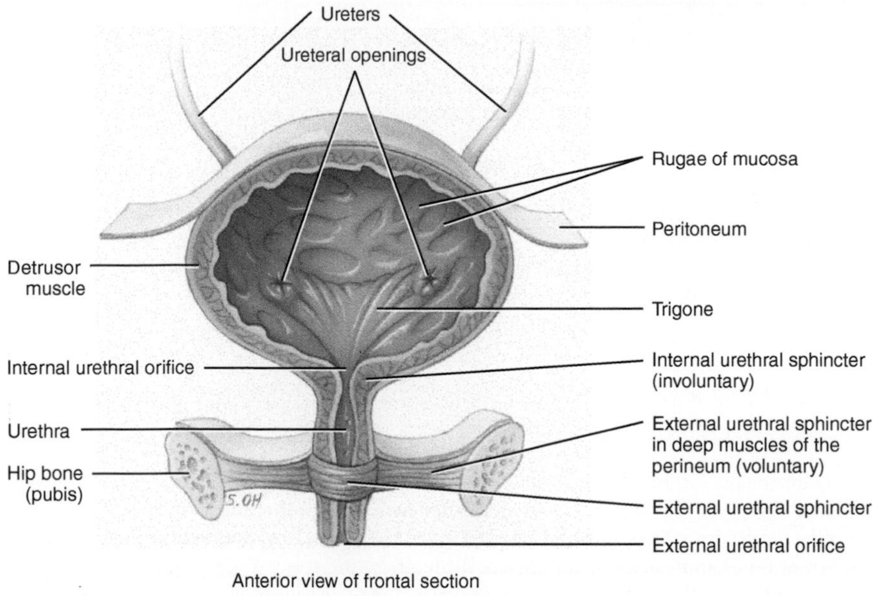

Figure 33.1 The bladder, pelvic floor, muscles and sphincters involved in elimination of urine. ***Source:*** **Peate (2017). Reproduced with permission of John Wiley & Sons, Ltd.**

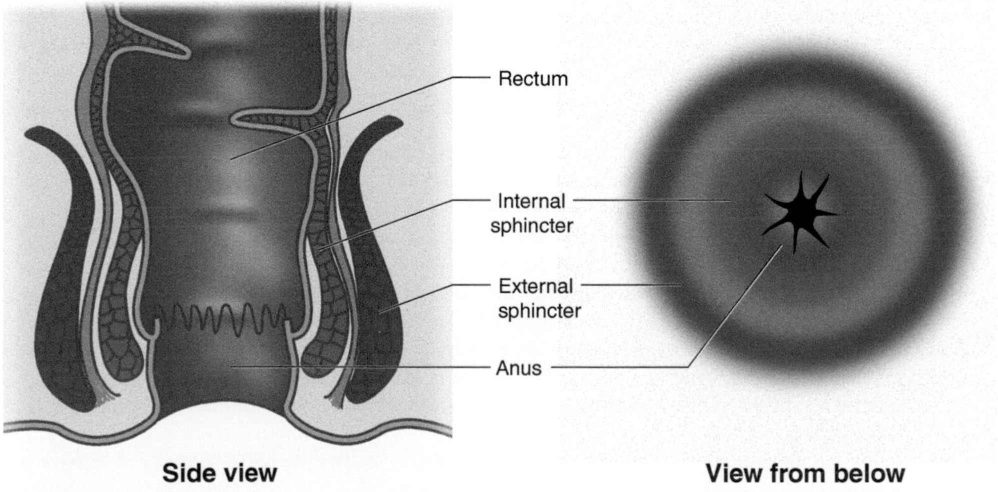

Figure 33.2 Rectal and anal muscles and sphincters involved in the elimination of faeces.

the external sphincter relaxes voluntarily and allows stool to be expelled typically when it is convenient for that person to pass the stool. Muscle tone, neural pathways, age, psychological health, hydration and consistency of stool can all affect this process and overall bowel function.

When taking a history of bowel habit, it is important for the person undertaking the review to consider any warning signs for lower gastrointestinal cancer such as rectal bleeding and change in bowel habit. A full list can be seen in Section 1.5 of the referral guidelines for suspected cancer (National Institute for Health and Care Excellence (NICE) 2017).

In an ageing population, bowel and urinary control issues are prevalent, particularly when loss of muscle or sphincter tone associated with age is a risk factor. There is a greater need to improve continence assessment and care, however, in all ages (NHSE 2018). Observing and monitoring continence is part of this assessment process and so it is important for the nursing associate to recognise that loss of bladder or bowel control an occur at any age not just the older adult. Box 33.1 outlines the continence assessment and communication skills that are required in order to provide high-quality person-centred care.

Supporting Evidence Continence resource (RCN 2019a)

This resource is a comprehensive overview of the assessment and recommended interventions which has been developed. The RCN Continence Forum and RCNi have collaborated to create this online resource for all healthcare professionals and can assist in the assessment of continence, planning and evaluating care for service users and their families/carers. Please go to https://rcni.com/hosted-content/rcn/continence/home

Box 33.1 Continence Assessment and Communication Skills

- Identifying there is a problem is the first step in promoting continence.
- This may be the first time the person has talked about issues regarding their continence since childhood, and they may be feeling a sense of shame or embarrassment in doing so.
- The actual or potential of losing control in passing urine or stools can be devastating to the individual, and it may take a person a long time to seek help.
- Active listening, demonstration of empathy, sensitive and timely communication are needed, to find out more about what has been happening.
- Encouraging the person to speak about worries they have and what support they need is an important step in the review of continence and can help that person access the right treatment to improve symptoms.

The Importance of Individualised Assessment

In order to plan and deliver care for the person in relation to their bladder or bowel function, it is very important to firstly conduct an individualised continence review. This will help the nursing associate and other members of the healthcare team understand whether the person is continent or if problems may be occurring. They can then progress to identify if any intervention is required as a result of this review (Nazarko 2013). There are different types and causes of continence difficulties, and it is very important that assumptions are not made related to any pre-existing conditions (Bladder and Bowel Foundation 2019). There may be causes which are reversible and can be easily treated, such as urinary tract infection or diarrhoea. Other causes such as nerve damage could be related to a long-term condition (Chelvanayagam & Norton 1999) where there is little or no response to simple interventions and where more invasive or complex care is required.

Take Note

Incontinence is a symptom of an underlying complaint, and a continence review is essential to identify possible causes and to plan treatment or make a referral for specialist advice. This requires a holistic review as opposed to just the person's urinary symptoms.

A full individualised continence review includes observation and details of the individual's signs and symptoms, and a physical examination may be indicated (RCN 2019b). The following four-step framework offers a full person-centred review where there is opportunity to understand the history of a person's continence and any problems (Nazarko 2013; RCN 2019a):

- **Step 1** is to conduct a simple continence review, to determine the type of incontinence if present and identify possible causes. Healthcare professionals at all levels will be able to conduct this, where good communication is essential (see Box 33.1). A few simple questions here can identify if the person has a bladder or bowel problem and identify the need for a specialist referral.
- **Step 2** can involve a more detailed assessment by a registered professional competent in continence care and includes history taking, a physical examination and other investigations such as urine testing, digital rectal examination, frequency recording, service user diaries and bladder scanning to ascertain residual urine volume after a person has voided.
- **Steps 3 and 4** involve more detailed specialist history taking and examination involving professionals such as clinical nurse specialist, nurse consultant and/or medical consultant.

The consent of the individual to an assessment and examination must be gained as per the NMC Code, and if there is any doubt about the individual's capacity, the intervention should only be undertaken in the person's best interest (RCN 2019a; Nursing and Midwifery Council 2018b).

Yellow Flag

The nursing associate can undertake a simple review but also can be involved in the undertaking of the complex history and further investigations. Fear of incontinence may be as debilitating as actual incontinence for a person, affecting their confidence and self-esteem. Supporting the service user during potentially intimate and embarrassing tests is very important, and the nursing associate has a key role in allaying people's anxiety and fear.

Once a baseline assessment has been established, the different tools outlined here are helpful in the observation and monitoring of continence and regular review of urinary or bowel function:

- Frequency volume tools (Nazarko 2013) are used to record the time of using the toilet, how much a person is drinking, how much they have voided or passed and understanding a person's overall fluid balance of input and output. In the clinical setting such as the hospital, a fluid balance chart can help with this monitoring. Pellatt (2007) identifies that assessing hydration and maintaining adequate fluid intake is essential for health, where hydration is important also for promoting good bladder and bowel function (RCN 2019a).
- Fluid balance charts, however, are often not used appropriately in clinical practice, and to be effective, these input/output monitoring tools need to be consistently completed to ensure accurate documentation, measurement and safety of care (Jeyapala et al. 2015) (see Box 33.2).
- Within hospitals but also outside in a clinic or community care setting, other frequency volume tools (Nazarko 2013) can help the healthcare professional monitor a person's intake and output, establish voiding or bowel function and also determine whether any pads or undergarments

Box 33.2 Improving Fluid Balance Monitoring

A study Jeyapala et al. (2015) conducted in one National Health Service (NHS) Trust identified that outside of the intensive care unit, accuracy of fluid balance monitoring was inadequate. Healthcare assistants, nursing staff and junior doctors were found to be inconsistent in recording fluid input and output on the charts in nearly half of all charts audited in the Trust. Poor documentation included the use of inappropriate measurements such as terms PU'd (for passing urine) and estimated or rounding up volume measurements. This does not assist in an accurate observation of bladder or bowel function let alone continence. Identification of the factors affecting this problem led to improvements in this Trust – with simple practical solutions. A 3-stage plan was implemented. Staff were able to give feedback on what they felt needed improving; education was provided and equipment as well as the charts were modified. Input and output were recorded accurately. This resulted in better commitment from staff, more appropriate chart usage, accuracy of documentation and ultimately safer care.

Source: Modified from Jeyapala et al. (2015)

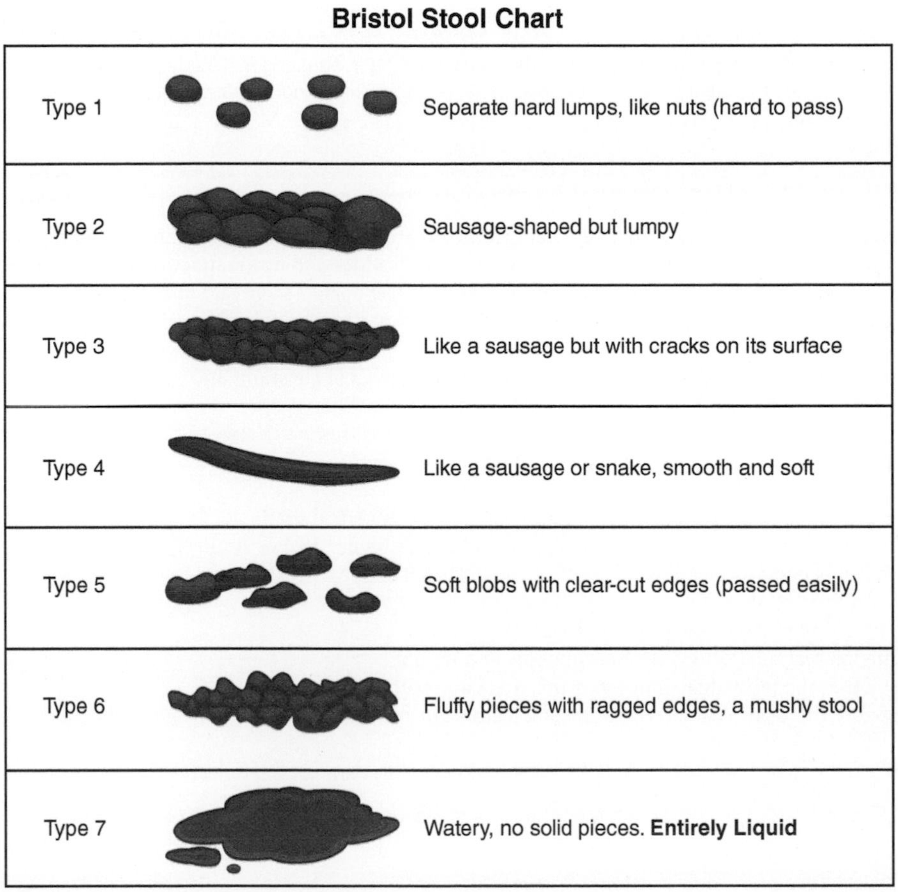
Bristol Stool Chart
Type 1
Separate hard lumps, like nuts (hard to pass)
Type 2
Sausage-shaped but lumpy
Type 3
Like a sausage but with cracks on its surface
Type 4
Like a sausage or snake, smooth and soft
Type 5
Soft blobs with clear-cut edges (passed easily)
Type 6
Fluffy pieces with ragged edges, a mushy stool
Type 7
Watery, no solid pieces. Entirely Liquid

Figure 33.3 Bristol stool scale.

are wet/soiled, or if has there been leakage when maintaining continence is a problem. Assessment tools are used over a 3-day period for assessment of urinary continence and over a 7-day period for bowel function (RCN 2019a). This is to establish a pattern to aid the planning of interventions. In the recording of bowel function, for example, information can also be provided about diet, time of bowel movement and consistency of stool.

- To establish consistency of stool, frameworks such as the Bristol Stool Scale (Lewis & Heaton 1997) can be used alongside the frequency chart (see Figure 33.3). Here, consistency, as in liquid/softness or hardness of stool, can be observed and monitored. This is particularly useful when underlying causes such as irritable bowel syndrome, diarrhoea or constipation are thought to be disrupting bowel function causing potential continence issues.
- Service users can be encouraged to complete a bladder or bowel diary (RCN 2019a, 2019b) over the assessment period: recording information such as frequency of passage/voiding, ease of passage or voiding, dietary intake, consistency of stool and other factors such as toilet facilities/environmental factors which influence bowel or bladder function.
- Other tools which may be useful are skin assessment frameworks as suggested by Nazarko (2013) and Holroyd (2018), particularly in urinary incontinence where skin excoriation can be a problem. Reviewing skin changes alongside the physical examination can help identify problems which require intervention to promote skin integrity, comfort and hygiene.

Box 33.3 Points to Consider in the Assessment of Continence

Touch Point

- Passing urine or defaecation is an intimate body function that is normally carried out in private.
- People who are limited in mobility, elderly and frail may require the assistance of others, and an individual experiencing this or family member may find this embarrassing (Nazarko 2013).

The nursing associate should at all times be mindful of this and observe and monitor continence sensitively and discreetly to provide respectful and dignified care.

Red Flag

When urine and faeces come into contact with the skin, the natural pH is changed making it alkaline; this causes the skin to become reddened and break down. This skin irritation is known as maceration, incontinence-associated dermatitis or excoriation; this can be very painful for individuals.

- All these tools can be used by the nursing associate and other healthcare professionals in partnership with service users/carers to self-assess. Used in conjunction with each other, they can help the team understand bladder and bowel function which goes beyond the simple documentation of 'passed urine' or 'bowels opened'. This can help individuals feel part of their care and participate in shared decision-making. Equally, they can be used by the nursing associate and the service user to open up a timely discussion about their urinary or bowel activity over a period of time.
- The RCN Continence Forum and NHS England have also developed a useful list of questions and points to think about when taking a simple assessment of an identified continence problem (RCN 2019a; NHSE 2018) (see Box 33.3).
- How often the person goes to the toilet to urinate and/or defecate and whether this is a change to their normal routine
- Current or previous medical history (including pregnancy and urine infections)
- Possibility of physical or sexual abuse, including female genital mutilation
- A rough estimate of the amount of urine passed unless accurate measurement is required
- Visual description of the faeces (normally based on Bristol Stool Chart (see Figure 33.3 or similar))
- If there is leakage, whether it is urine or faeces
- Information about diet and fluid intake
- Any medications being taken (prescribed and over the counter)
- Lifestyle factors, including recreational drugs, alcohol, smoking and weight
- Ability – for example, whether the individuals can eat, drink, dress and bathe on their own
- Mobility/sensory ability – are there physical or environmental factors affecting the person's ability to use the toilet? Can the person see where the facilities are?
- Capacity – does the person recognise the need to go to the toilet or do they forget where the toilet is – can they reach it/see it/remember where it is located?

Conclusion

Many people who have developed incontinence have never had the benefit of assessment (Nazarko 2013). With recent initiatives and guidance, however, it is hoped that this will change. Appropriate observation, monitoring and review of urinary and bowel continence will lead to better awareness, while education of staff, public and patients will help to break some of the social taboos (Holroyd 2018) and enable accuracy of measurement (Jeyapala et al. 2015). The use of evidence-based assessment tools, and good communication working in partnership with individuals and families/carers helps build a picture of the person's situation. Offering timely, accurate information and education (NHS Choices 2018) on continence can help the individual participate in decision-making and feel in control of their care. Getting the right treatment and support for the service-user by the right service is vital, which will lead to reduced costs for healthcare services but most importantly an improved patient experience and outcome.

References

Bladder and Bowel Foundation. (2019) *Bladder care.* [online] Available: https://www.bladderandbowel.org/bladder/. Accessed 2 January 2020.

Booth, J. (2013) Continence care is everyone's business, *Nursing Times*, 109(17–18): 12–16.

Cheesley, A. (2017) Why continence should be the seventh 'C' for all nurses, *Nursing Standard*, 31(27): 29.

Chelvanayagam, S. and Norton, C. (1999). Causes and assessment of faecal incontinence. *British Journal of Community Nursing*, 4(1), 28–35. Doi:10.12968/bjcn.1999.4.1.7522

Holroyd, S. (2018) Continence care in care homes, *Nursing and Residential Care*, 20(6): 265–272. doi:10.12968/nrec.2018.20.6.265.

Jeyapala, S., Gerth, A., Patel, A. and Syed, N. (2015) Improving fluid balance monitoring on the wards, *BMJ Quality Improvement Reports*, 4(1). doi: 10.1136/bmjquality.u209890.w4102. [online] Available: https://bmjopenquality.bmj.com/content/4/1/u209890.w4102. Accessed 2 January 2020.

Lewis, S.J. and Heaton, K.W. (1997) Stool form scale as a useful guide to intestinal transit time, *Scandinavian Journal of Gastroenterology*, 32(9): 920–924.

Marieb, E.N. (2015) *Essentials of human anatomy & physiology* (11th edn), Harlow: Essex: Pearson Education Limited.

Nazarko, L. (2013) Continence series 4: the importance of assessment, *British Journal of Healthcare Assistants*, 7(3): 118–124. doi:10.12968/bjha.2013.7.3.118.

NHS Choices. (2018) *Overview bowel incontinence.* [online] Available: https://www.nhs.uk/conditions/bowel-incontinence/. Accessed 2 January 2020.

NHS Commissioning Board Chief Nursing Officer. (2012) *Compassion in practice nursing, midwifery and care staff: our vision and strategy.* [online] Available: https://www.england.nhs.uk/wp-content/uploads/2012/12/compassion-in-practice.pdf. Accessed 02 January 2020.

NHSE. (2018) *Excellence in continence care.* [online] Available: https://www.england.nhs.uk/publication/excellence-in-continence-care/. Accessed 2 January 2020.

NICE. (2017) *Suspected cancer: recognition and referral NICE guideline [NG12].* [online] Available: https://www.nice.org.uk/guidance/ng12. Accessed 02 January 2020.

Nursing and Midwifery Council. (2018a) *Standards of proficiency for nursing associates.* [online] Available: https://www.nmc.org.uk/standards/standards-for-nursing-associates/standards-of-proficiency-for-nursing-associates/ [accessed January 2020].

Nursing and Midwifery Council. (2018b) The code, *Professional standards of practice and behaviour for nurses, midwives and nursing associates.* [online] Available: https://www.nmc.org.uk/globalassets/sitedocuments/nmc-publications/nmc-code.pdf. Accessed January 2020.

Peate, I. and Evans, S. (2020) *Fundamentals of anatomy and physiology for nursing and healthcare students* (3rd edn), Oxford: Wiley.

Pellatt, G.C. (2007) Clinical skills: bowel elimination and management of complications, *British Journal of Nursing*, 16(6): 351–355. doi:10.12968/bjon.2007.16.6.23008.

RCN. (2019a) *Continence care.* [online] Available: https://rcni.com/hosted-content/rcn/continence/home

RCN. (2019b) Bowel care, *Management of lower bowel dysfunction, including digital rectal examination and digital removal of faeces.* [online] Available: https://www.rcn.org.uk/-/media/royal-college-of-nursing/documents/publications/2019/september/007-522.pdf

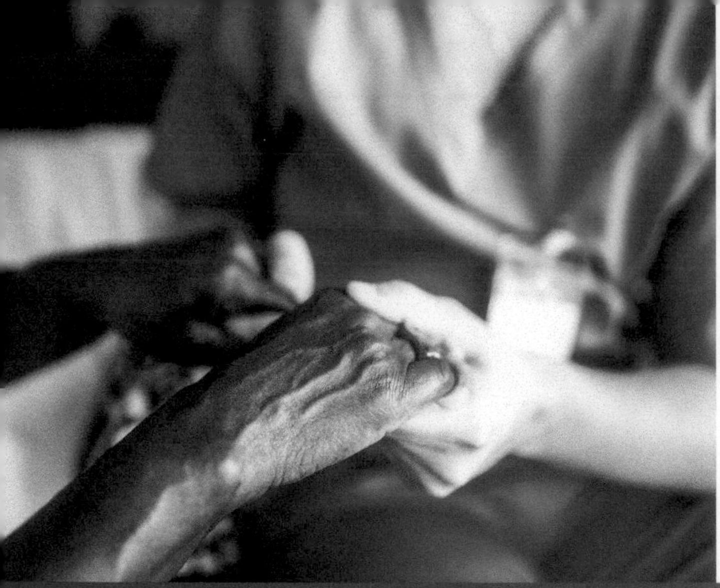

34

Recognising Bladder and Bowel Patterns

Kathy Whayman

University of Hertfordshire, UK

Chapter Aim

- **This chapter aims to develop the reader's knowledge and skills to recognise patterns in a person's bladder and bowel function. The chapter aims to build upon the reader's ability to observe and monitor urinary and bowel function to help them identify, assess and respond to problems as they arise.**

Learning Outcomes

- **Understand the key issues and the nursing associate's role in recognising the patterns of bladder and bowel function and common symptoms in clinical practice**
- **Demonstrate knowledge of the meaning of incontinence, and understand the impact this pattern of bladder and bowel function can have on the service-user and their family/carers**
- **Develop the ability to identify when incontinence has occurred and respond in a way to ensure the service user receives the right care and their dignity is preserved**

Test Yourself Multiple Choice Questions

1. ***Incontinence* is the term used to:**
   A) **Describe involuntary leakage of urine or faeces from the bladder or bowel**
   B) **Describe a person's inability to use the toilet**
   C) **Describe nerve damage involved in bladder and bowel function**
   D) **Describe the voluntary control of urine or faecal elimination**

The Nursing Associate's Handbook of Clinical Skills, First Edition. Edited by Ian Peate.

Companion website: www.wiley.com/nursingassociate

2. **Problems with incontinence can affect:**
   A) **Infants only**
   B) **Children aged 5–12 years**
   C) **Adults from aged 18 years to 75 years**
   D) **All ages**
3. **Which of these is not a 'containment aid' used when helping someone manage their incontinence?**
   A) **Urinary sheath**
   B) **Absorbent pad**
   C) **Commode**
   D) **Indwelling catheter**
4. **Post-micturition dribble affecting men is commonly caused by which of the following**
   A) **Coronary artery bypass**
   B) **Diarrhoea**
   C) **Prostate surgery**
   D) **Aging**
5. **Which of these statements is true?**
   A) **The rectum is part of the large bowel where faeces is stored just before defaecation**
   B) **There is one sphincter in the anus controlling the release of faeces from the rectum for defaecation**
   C) **Release of faeces into the rectum is controlled by a voluntary sphincter in the colon**
   D) **Incontinence occurs when the rectum is full and cannot store further faeces prior to defaecation**

Introduction

Bladder and bowel patterns are varied and very individual i.e. experienced differently from person to person. Changes to these patterns and problems such as incontinence can arise at any stage in a person's lifetime. *Incontinence* is a term that describes any accidental or involuntary loss of urine from the bladder (urinary incontinence) or bowel motion, faeces or gas (flatus) from the bowel (faecal incontinence) (RCN 2019a). This can occur at any age, and is not solely the domain of the older person (Cheesley 2017). When incontinence is experienced or when continence care and support fall short, the impact on the service users and their families can be devastating (Booth 2013). There are many factors affecting patterns of bladder and bowel function, along with incontinence, and these will be explored in this chapter. Struggling with incontinence can have long-term implications for a person's health and well-being often resulting in psychological morbidity, social isolation and physical disability (Norton and Chelvanayagam 2004; Apau 2010; National Health Service Executive (NHSE) 2018).

Caring for a person experiencing a change in their bladder or bowel pattern is an important part of the nursing associate's role, and providing such care must be approached with the upmost sensitivity, compassion and competency to ensure the dignity and privacy of the individual is always respected (Royal College of Nursing (RCN) 2019a). Helping a person maximise their continence and managing any problems arising is a fundamental nursing skill. Identifying when incontinence has occurred, responding to care needs and supporting service users and their families/carers is everybody's business: a multidisciplinary team responsibility (Booth 2013; Cheesley 2017).

Following on from a holistic review of continence as outlined in Chapter 33, this chapter will address the importance of understanding bladder and bowel function patterns and the timely identification of incontinence. This recognition and identification using different approaches and methods will enable the nursing associate to provide person-centred, safe and effective care. The proficiencies and standards set out by the NMC (Nursing and Midwifery Council (NMC) 2018a) related to this chapter and the subsequent chapters will assist the nursing associate to demonstrate the knowledge, skills and ability required to meet people's needs related to bladder and bowel health.

Touch Point

- When a person is fearful of or has experienced a loss of bladder or bowel control (even once), it can have a devastating effect on their psychological, social and physical well-being.
- Assessing and responding to incontinence requires a holistic approach, sensitive communication and a consistency care to support to enable the persons and/or their family to participate in their care as much as they wish or are able to. Promotion of dignity, comfort and privacy is central to the role of nursing associate, and they are of upmost importance in all areas of person-centred care.
- The person must be at the centre of all that is done.

Green Flag

The NMC Code (NMC 2018b) requires all registrants to uphold the tenets of the Code within the limits of their competence. While a nursing associate and nurse will play different roles in an aspect of care, both must uphold the standards in the Code within the contribution they are making to overall care. The professional pledge to work within one's competence is a key factor that underpins the principle of the Code which, given the implication and its impact on public protection, has to be upheld at all times.

Urinary Incontinence

It is estimated around 14 million people in the United Kingdom experience changes to their bladder pattern which can result in a bladder problem (Bladder and Bowel Foundation 2019). Urinary incontinence is the involuntary leakage of urine and according to the National Institute for Health and Care Excellence (NICE) causes can be categorised as follows:

Women (NICE 2015)

- Stress incontinence is the involuntary leakage of urine on effort, exertion, sneezing or coughing. This is usually caused by a weakness in the bladder neck or urethral sphincter and loss of muscle tone controlling the outflow of urine from the bladder.
- Urgency incontinence is the involuntary leakage of urine with or immediately preceded by urgency (a sudden compelling desire to urinate that is difficult to delay).
- Mixed urinary incontinence is the involuntary leakage of urine associated with both urgency and exertion, effort, sneezing or coughing.
- Overactive bladder is defined as urgency with or without urgency incontinence and usually with frequency and nocturia (night-time urination) (Figure 34.1)

Men (NICE 2010)

Lower urinary tract symptoms and altered bladder patterns in men can be categorised as voiding, storage or post-micturition symptoms as follows

- Voiding symptoms include weak or intermittent urinary stream, straining, hesitancy, terminal dribbling and incomplete bladder emptying.
- Storage symptoms include urgency to urinate, frequency sometime resulting in urgency incontinence and nocturia (night-time urination).
- Post-micturition symptoms are seen with dribbling: when men experience an involuntary loss of urine immediately after they have finished passing urine, usually after leaving the toilet.

Red Flag

A referral should be made for urgent or specialist investigation if an individual has any of the following urinary symptoms:

- haematuria (blood in the urine)
- recurrent urinary tract infections (three or more in the last six months)
- loin pain (pain in the lower back)
- recurrent catheter blockages
- hydronephrosis
- kidney stones on imaging
- biochemical evidence of renal deterioration.

Source: (NICE 2015)

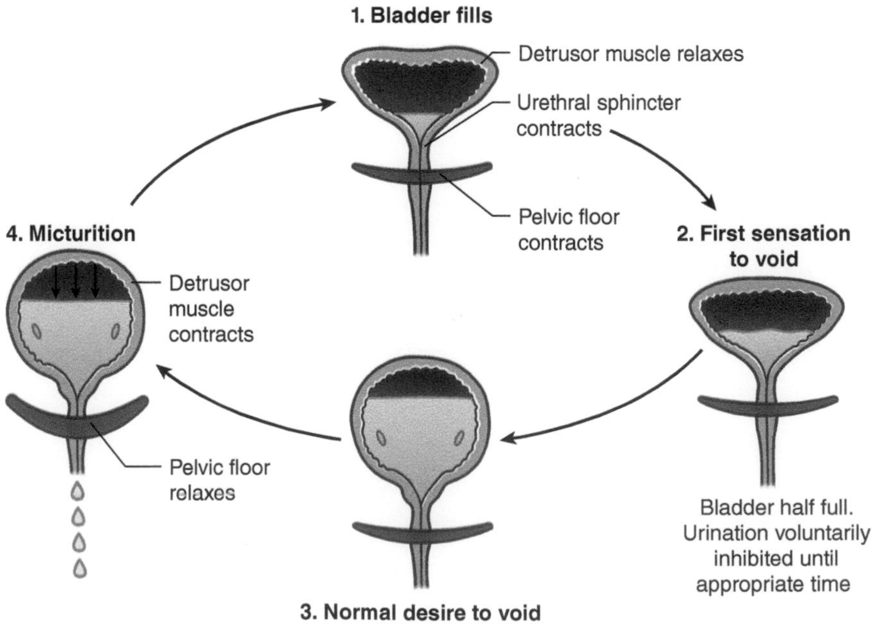

Figure 34.1 The bladder, pelvic floor, muscles and sphincters involved in elimination of urine.

Bowel Incontinence

Problematic changes in bowel patterns, and particularly bowel (faecal) incontinence is surprisingly common but underreported (Apau 2013). According to NHSE (2018), it is estimated that 1 in 10 people will be affected by bowel incontinence at some point in their life, and although it can affect people of any age, it is more common in women and older people. Bowel incontinence is an involuntary passing or leakage of stool, liquid or gas (flatus), which is usually a sign of an underlying condition (NICE 2014). Types of bowel incontinence can be categorised are as follows (RCN 2019a, 2019b):

- Urge incontinence – when the person has to rush and may not make it to the toilet in time
- Flatus (wind or gas) incontinence – when the rectum feels full, but the nerves cannot tell whether it is gas or stool
- Passive incontinence – when the rectum is full, but the person does not feel it and stool can pass without their knowledge
- Overflow incontinence – in the presence of hard faeces when liquid stool can leak – this is often mistaken for diarrhoea
- Anal and rectal incontinence – when the sphincter or muscles around cannot be controlled and the rectum is full and leakage of flatus, liquid or solid stool can occur (Figure 34.2)

Underlying Causes of Bowel Incontinence and High-Risk Groups

(NHS Choices 2018; NICE 2014; RCN 2019b):

- Commonly following childbirth or surgery which has damaged or torn the muscles or nerves used to control internal or external anal sphincters
- Severe or long-lasting constipation or diarrhoea
- Irritable bowel syndrome (IBS)
- Inflammatory bowel disease (IBD) – such as Crohn's disease or ulcerative colitis
- Severe haemorrhoids
- Neurological conditions that can affect the sacral nerves – such as diabetes, multiple sclerosis, stroke or spina bifida
- Degenerative damage to anal sphincter tone and strength due to advancing age or treatment such as radiotherapy
- Pharmacological agents can cause loss of sphincter control/tone – such as nitrates or calcium channel blockers. In addition, laxative use can produce loose stools which may be difficult to control. Some drugs such as some chemotherapy agents, metformin and digoxin can also cause diarrhoea and potential faecal leakage (Apau 2013; Nazarko 2013)
- Cognitive, physical or psychological impairment can impede ability to sense the need to defaecate or the ability to manage the environment (for example, physically locating and reaching the toilet or commode). Thorough review of the patient's environment and activities of living should be undertaken and any physical obstacles or impairment noted and rectified (NICE 2007; Apau 2013).

Touch Point

- In an ageing population, bowel and urinary control issues are prevalent, and there is a pressing need to improve assessment and person-centred continence care (NHSE 2018).
- It is important for the nursing associate, however, to recognise that the loss of bladder or bowel control can occur at any age not just the older adult, and there are many causes and subsequent impacts of incontinence whenever it occurs in the individual's lifetime.

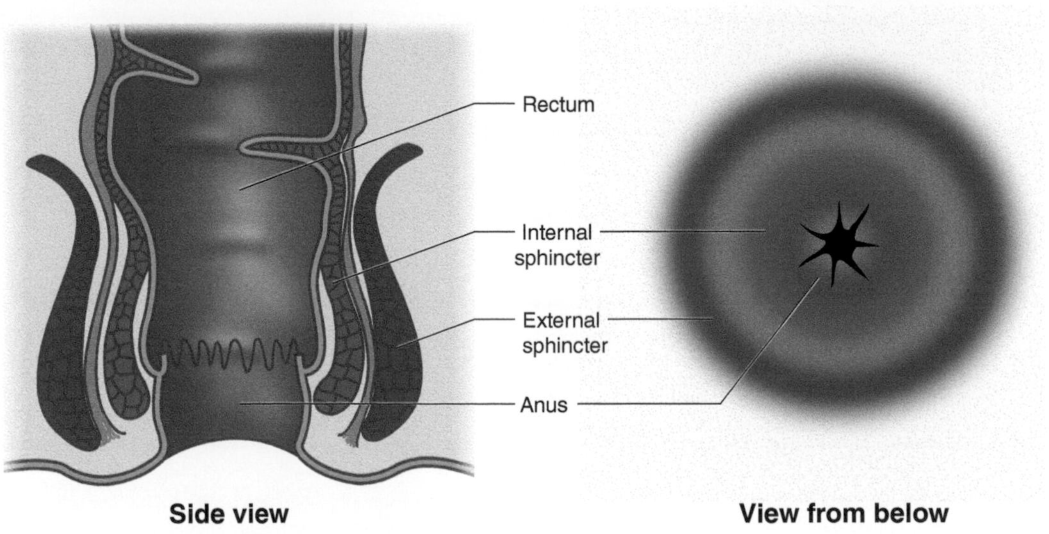

Figure 34.2 Rectal and anal muscles and sphincters involved in the elimination of faeces.

Supporting Evidence Continence resource (RCN 2019a) and Bowel Care (RCN 2019b)

These resources provide a comprehensive overview of the causes, assessment and recommended interventions which has been developed in response to the reported lack of support, embarrassment and social isolation experienced by people affected by incontinence. The Royal College of Nursing (RCN) Continence Forum, Gastrointestinal Forum and RCNi have collaborated to create this online resource and bowel care guidelines for all healthcare professionals. They and can assist in the assessment, planning and evaluating care for service users and their families/carers. Please go to https://rcni.com/hosted-content/rcn/continence/home (Continence) and https://www.rcn.org.uk/-/media/royal-college-of-nursing/documents/publications/2019/september/007-522.pdf for the Bowel Care Guidelines (RCN 2019b)

Incontinence in Children

An estimated 900,000 children in the United Kingdom are thought to be affected by bowel and bladder pattern difficulties, and they can face daily challenges in schools. Factors such as later infant toilet training, an increasing number of school-age children in nappies, poor school toilet facilities, restrictions of toilet use in lesson time and lack of teacher awareness compound the problem (Dean 2019).

Orange Flag

The stigma and impact of incontinence in children and young adulthood.

In children, bladder and bowel issues such as daytime incontinence, bedwetting, constipation and faecal soiling can impact learning, development and quality of life, as well as causing families increased stress and social isolation (Dean 2019). Children in schools experiencing continence problems are at higher risk of bullying and withdrawing from social situations (Lepkowska 2019).

Lepkowska (2019) goes on to identify that many children and young adults suffer embarrassment and stigma, and some may experience behavioural or psychological problems into adulthood accompanied with low self-esteem and poor self-image. Individual and family care needs can be complex, and support needs to be consistent and multifaceted (NHSE 2018). A holistic assessment of the child's physical, psychological, social and emotional development whilst understanding the family situation is crucial.

With the right support, guidance and education alongside, often practical simple approaches can enable people to maintain continence or manage their conditions and symptoms to lessen the impact on their health and wellbeing.

Incontinence in Adults – The Importance of Assessment

In the older adult, there is often a sense of inevitability that continence will be a problem (Nazarko 2013), particularly in hospital and care homes (Holroyd 2018). Booth (2013) identifies that observing and monitoring continence particularly in busy clinical areas often results in simply accepting 'containment' as the solution without adequate assessment of the cause – i.e. the use of aids, absorbent pads, sheaths and catheters. With careful assessment, communication and identification of the cause, many people can be helped irrespective of age to regain some or all of their continence (Nazarko 2013). One example is the rise in prevalence of urinary tract infections in older adults. Rates of emergency admissions due to urinary tract infections have almost doubled over the last 5 years, placing additional pressure on acute settings (NHSE 2018; RCN 2019a). NHSE (2018) recognise that this could often be avoided through early continence assessment and intervention.

Bowel function equally has patterns which affect emptying and continence. Following review, these can be observed, recognised and responded to (RCN 2019b). Two common patterns of bowel dysfunction are constipation and diarrhoea.

- Constipation – This is difficult to define as perceptions and experience of constipation differ widely and symptoms can often be overlooked (Norton & Chelvanayagam 2004). Symptoms include difficulty and/or infrequency in defaecating. Bowel transit can be slow and in primary constipation (i.e. no known cause) issues such as poor mobility, poor diet and pelvic floor abnormalities can be linked (RCN 2019b). There are other types of constipation such as functional and faecal impaction. This can sometimes result in leakage of liquid stool which overflows and is misinterpreted as diarrhoea (Apau 2010).
- Assessment of constipation is important – This includes investigations such as history of symptoms, medications, abdominal examination, digital rectal examination, assessment of transit or sphincter function, possible imaging and also assessment of frequency and also consistency using Bristol Stool Scale charts (Lewis & Heaton 1997) or similar (Norton & Chelvanayagam 2004). A service user's bowel function diary can also be of assistance over seven days recording of frequency (NICE 2014; RCN 2019b).

Red Flag

In constipation, particularly faecal impaction, the presence of a full colon with hard stool can result in an overflow of liquid and is often misdiagnosed as diarrhoea. This can result in incorrect treatment and worsening of the problem. Careful assessment is required.

- Diarrhoea – This is a common acute problem. This usually presents suddenly and usually resolved on its own after a few days without treatment (RCN 2019b). Symptoms often present with loose watery stool, cramping pain in the abdomen, occasionally a fever or bloody stool and sometimes is accompanied with nausea and loss of appetite (Bladder and Bowel Foundation 2020).

- The causes of diarrhoea – Commonly, these are acute infection of the gut, medications (e.g. antibiotics or overuse of laxatives), anxiety/stress or dietary issues (food poisoning or overeating of fibre; RCN 2019b). Diarrhoea can also present as a result of other conditions such as IBS (a functional disorder) or IBD (Bladder and Bowel Community (2020) and requires careful specialist multi-disciplinary team management.
- Management of diarrhoea – This can resolve on its own if short term, however needs careful assessment particularly in the older frail person (Holroyd 2018). Incontinence can be an issue, and causes which are treatable and reversible must be considered. Hydration and fluid balance monitoring is indicated and anti-diarrhoea medication may be considered and prescribed if appropriate (RCN 2019b).

Violet Flag

Social isolation and seeking help with continence

- Problems with continence often go underreported, and conditions affecting the bladder or bowel can go undiagnosed (International Continence Society 2019).
- Loss of continence, and particularly faecal incontinence, has been historically considered a taboo subject (Chelvanayagam & Norton 1999), and still is viewed by many in society as embarrassing and socially unacceptable (RCN 2019a).
- Only an estimated 40% of people affected by continence difficulties seek help (RCN 2019a). For a person affected by the loss of control of urinary or bowel function at any age, to seek help and talk about this can feel very uncomfortable and embarrassing and result in further social withdrawal and isolation (Norton & Chelvanayagam 2004).
- Service users/families or carers may express a sense of relief at being asked about bowel control and being given the opportunity to ask questions and seek help (Chelvanayagam & Norton 1999).

Touch Point

In many healthcare settings, containment aids are heavily relied upon, e.g. using pads, sheaths, washable underwear and catheters to manage incontinence.

- Overreliance without regular review can result in skin breakdown, increased urinary tract infections, complete dependence and poor self-image.
- Their use with careful selection and monitoring of effectiveness using best available evidence is appropriate, but with adequate and individualised assessment, a plan of care can be established to help a person regain some independence or (depending on the cause of the incontinence) complete control of their bladder or bowel function

Supporting Evidence

- The National Institute of Clinical Excellence (NICE) has produced evidence-based quality statements and clinical guidance on managing urinary and faecal incontinence, with flow charts and useful summaries of the evidence base. Two publications are in support in this topic: Faecal incontinence in adults: management – Clinical guideline [CG49] (NICE 2007; and Faecal incontinence in adults – Quality standard [QS54] (NICE 2014).
- This includes a series of questions for a detailed history taking of continence. The questions are holistic and consider the person's physical well-being, social and psychological welfare. The questions cover issues such as the person's ability to manage facilities, either at home or in hospital and the impact of environment on continence. They work well alongside the RCN Continence resource (2019a) list of points to consider.
- Urinary incontinence in women – Quality standard [QS77] (NICE 2015) – this publication outlines the importance of categorising the reason and nature of the continence issue to enable the person to get the correct treatment.

Source: NICE (2007, 2015)

Touch Point

- Passing urine or defaecation is an intimate body function that is considered to be by society normally carried out in private. Issues with incontinence such as damage to clothing and odour and soiling are distressing to the individual (Williams 2008).
- People who are limited in mobility, old and frail may require the assistance of others and an individual experiencing this or family member may find this embarrassing (Nazarko 2013).
- The nursing associate should at all times be mindful of this and observe and monitor continence sensitively and discreetly to provide respectful and dignified care.

Conclusion

Giving people the time and opportunity to talk about this sensitive issue is very important. The nursing associate is ideally placed to help individuals discuss their bladder or bowel patterns, identifying symptoms and to seek help. Carrying out a detailed continence assessment, the recognition that a person may be at risk of or has actual incontinence can be achieved. This is important for all ages. Recent initiatives and guidance assist the nursing associate to understand patterns of bowel and urinary function. Knowledge of common causes as well as factors impacting a person's holistic wellbeing can contribute to better awareness. Incontinence can be treated and where possible continence can be achieved for improved service user experience and outcome.

References

Apau, D. (2010) Faecal incontinence: assessment and conservative management, *Gastrointestinal Nursing*, 8(8): 18–22. doi:10.12968/gasn.2010.8.8.79161.

Bladder and Bowel Community. (2019) *Bladder care.* [online] Available: https://www.bladderandbowel.org/bladder/. Accessed 02 January 2020.

Bladder and Bowel Community. (2020) *Diarrhoea.* [online] Available: https://www.bladderandbowel.org/bowel/bowel-problems/diarrhoea. Accessed 02 January 2020.

Booth, J. (2013) Continence care is everyone's business, *Nursing Times*, 109 (17–18): 12–16.

Cheesley, A. (2017) Why continence should be the seventh 'C' for all nurses, *Nursing Standard*, 31(27): 29.

Chelvanayagam, S., Norton, C. (1999). Causes and assessment of faecal incontinence. British *Journal of Community Nursing*, 4(1), 28–35. doi:10.12968/bjcn.1999.4.1.7522

Dean, E. (2019) Support for children with bowel and bladder problems, *Primary Health Care*, 29(6): 11–11. doi:10.7748/phc.29.6.11.s13.

Holroyd, S. (2018) Continence care in care homes, *Nursing and Residential Care*, 20(6): 265–272. doi:10.12968/nrec.2018.20.6.265.

Lepkowska, D. (2019) New guidance to support children with bladder and bowel problems, *British Journal of School Nursing*, 14(9): 434–435. doi:10.12968/bjsn.2019.14.9.434.

Lewis, S.J., Heaton, K.W. (1997) Stool form scale as a useful guide to intestinal transit time, *Scandinavian Journal of Gastroenterology*, 32(9): 920–924.

Nazarko, L. (2013) Continence series 4: the importance of assessment, *British Journal of Healthcare Assistants*, 7(3): 118–124. doi:10.12968/bjha.2013.7.3.118.

NHS Choices. (2018) *Overview bowel incontinence.* [online] Available: https://www.nhs.uk/conditions/bowel-incontinence/. Accessed 02 January 2020.

NHSE. (2018) *Excellence in continence care.* [online] Available: https://www.england.nhs.uk/publication/excellence-in-continence-care/. Accessed 1 December 2019.

NICE. (2007) *Faecal incontinence in adults: management clinical guideline [CG49].* [online] Available: https://www.nice.org.uk/guidance/cg49. Accessed 02 January 2020.

NICE. (2010) *Lower urinary tract symptoms in men: management - clinical guideline [CG97].* [online] Available: https://www.nice.org.uk/guidance/cg97/chapter/Introduction. Accessed 02 January 2020.

NICE. (2014) *Faecal incontinence in adults: management clinical guideline [CG49].* [online] Available: https://www.nice.org.uk/guidance/cg49/chapter/Introduction. Accessed 02 January 2020.

NICE. (2015) *Urinary incontinence in women quality standard [QS77].* [online] Available: https://www.nice.org.uk/guidance/qs77. Accessed 02 January 2020.

NICE. (2017) *Suspected cancer: recognition and referral NICE guideline [NG12].* [online] Available: https://www.nice.org.uk/guidance/ng12. Accessed 02 January 2020.

Norton, C., Chelvanayagam, S. (2004) *Bowel Continence Nursing.* Beaconsfield: Beaconsfield.

Nursing and Midwifery Council. (2018a) *Standards of proficiency for nursing associates.* [online] Available: https://www.nmc.org.uk/standards/standards-for-nursing-associates/standards-of-proficiency-for-nursing-associates/. Accessed January 2020.

Nursing and Midwifery Council. (2018b) The code, *Professional standards of practice and behaviour for nurses, midwives and nursing associates.* [online] Available: https://www.nmc.org.uk/globalassets/sitedocuments/nmc-publications/nmc-code.pdf. Accessed January 2020.

RCN. (2019a) *Continence care.* [online] Available: https://rcni.com/hosted-content/rcn/continence/home. Accessed 02 January 2020.

RCN. (2019b) *Bowel care.* [online] Available: https://www.rcn.org.uk/-/media/royal-college-of-nursing/documents/publications/2019/september/007-522.pdf. Accessed 02 January 2020.

Williams, J. (2008) Flatus, odour and the ostomist: Coping strategies and interventions. *British Journal of Nursing*, 17(2): S10–S12.

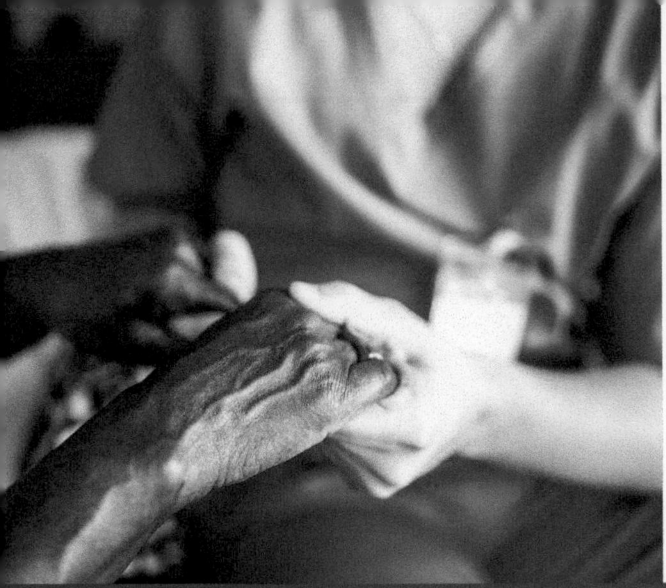

35

Care and Management of People with Urinary Catheters

Esme Elloway[1] *and Ian Peate*[2]

[1] Plymouth University, Plymouth, UK
[2] School of Health Studies, Gibraltar

Chapter Aim

- **This chapter aims to provide the reader with an overview of care required for those who need to have a urinary catheter.**

Learning Outcomes

- **Understand the fundamental urinary system anatomy**
- **Identify a patient who may require a urinary catheter**
- **Understand the potential risks involved in urinary catheter insertion**
- **Outline the care required for the safe insertion of a urinary catheter**

Test Yourself Multiple Choice Questions

1. **Men and women have the same length urethras?**
   A) **True**
   B) **False**
2. **How long can a short-term catheter stay in according to National Institute for Health and Care Excellence (NICE) (2014) guidelines?**
   A) **14 days/2 weeks**
   B) **21 days/3 weeks**
   C) **28 days/4 weeks**
   D) **42 days/6 weeks**

The Nursing Associate's Handbook of Clinical Skills, First Edition. Edited by Ian Peate.

Companion website: www.wiley.com/nursingassociate

3. **Which of these is a symptom of a catheter associated urinary tract infection according to the NHS (2017)?**
   A) Pain around groin or lower abdomen
   B) Pyrexia
   C) Increased confusion
   D) All of the above
4. **Which of these is not a common indication for a catheter?**
   A) Bladder pain
   B) For strict fluid balance monitoring
   C) Acute urinary retention
   D) Chronic urinary retention
5. **Which of the following are functions of the urinary system?**
   A) Excretion
   B) Elimination
   C) Regulation of acid base balance
   D) All of the above

Introduction

This chapter provides an introduction to urinary catheters; it explores and explains the care and management of people with urinary catheters. The care and management of catheters is complex, and this chapter cannot address all catheter-related care, rather it covers some of the common and important considerations when caring for patients who may require or already have a catheter, it does not cover troubleshooting of catheter complications, e.g. how to manage a blocked catheter. The Nursing and Midwifery Council (NMC) (2018a) requires the nursing associate to demonstrate proficiency in relation to providing bowel and bladder health, and to care for and manage catheters for all genders. This chapter is related to adult catheter care and management.

Functions of the Urinary System

Urine production is influenced by several body systems; if any of these body systems fail to function, this has the potential to alter urine production, for example a patient with chronic kidney disease may pass little or no urine. When a catheter has been inserted, these influencing factors have to be considered in the measurement of urine output and fluid intake (Royal College of Nursing (RCN) 2019).

A number of important functions are associated with the urinary system. Table 35.1. outlines some of these.

Knowledge of the anatomy and physiology of the urinary tract/renal system is vital in being able to provide safe and effective care. The organs of the renal system are shown in Figure 35.1.

Urinary Catheters

Catheters can be used for short- and long-term periods, as indicated for a wide range of conditions and circumstances. As a result of the potential complications associated with indwelling catheters, they should only be used in cases where other options are not suitable, such as intermittent self-catheterisation.

Table 35.1 Functions associated with the urinary system.

FUNCTION	DESCRIPTION
Excretion	The body removes waste material from the plasma in the blood and eliminates it from the body in the urine.
Elimination	The body eliminates waste products from organs. Water, salt, ions and drugs can be eliminated from the digestive system. Carbon dioxide, water and hydrogen can be eliminated from the respiratory system. Sodium chloride, uric acid, ammonia, water and creatinine can be eliminated from the integumentary system.
Urinary elimination	Occurs when the bladder becomes full of urine and expands, stimulating nerves in the bladder to signal a need to pass urine. As urine is passed, the brain tells the bladder muscles to tighten, causing urine to be expelled from the bladder. The internal and external sphincter muscles relax allowing urine to flow out of the bladder and down the urethra, out of the body.
Water balance	Kidney tubules regulate concentration of urine. Regulation of the acid–base balance: to maintain homeostasis and the body's pH balance.
Produce erythropoietin	Kidneys secrete erythropoietin, a hormone which helps to speed up the process of red blood cell formation.

Source: Based on Nair (2017), chapter 10, pp. 299–332.

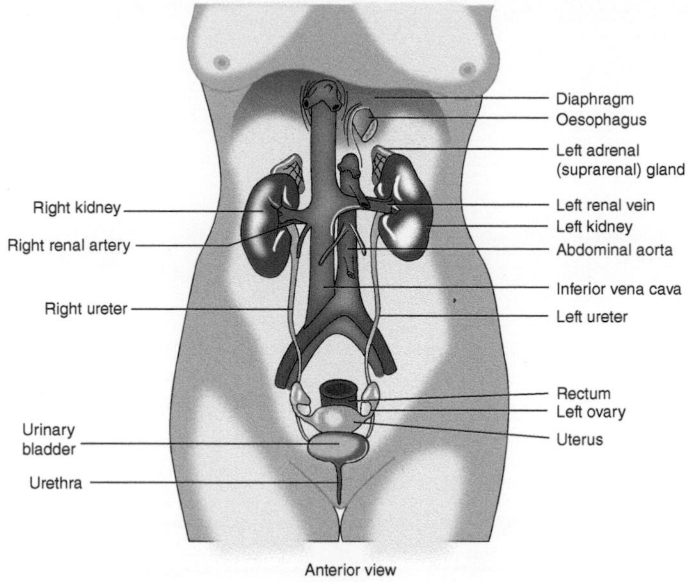

Figure 35.1 The organs of the renal system. *Source:* Peate and Nair (2017), chapter 10, figure 10.1, p. 301.

It is essential that nursing associates working in all settings are familiar with managing any complications that may be related to urinary catheters and that they know how to change the devices safely. The nursing associate has an important role to play in supporting patients to ensure that they have the information that they need to manage the catheter.

Indications for a Catheter

There are many reasons why a person may need to have urinary catheter. The procedure must be carried out using aseptic technique, and the person inserting the catheter must be adequately trained and competent to do so, they must always adhere to local policy and procedure. When the initial decision is made to insert a catheter, this must be taken by an appropriately qualified healthcare professional, and the decision has to be based on sound clinical judgement and in partnership with the patient. Prior to a urinary catheter being inserted, a comprehensive and holistic review of the patient should be undertaken, ensuring that insertion is based on the patient's individual needs (NICE 2015). Indwelling urinary catheters should not be used for the purpose of managing urinary incontinence (Geng et al. 2012) or for nursing convenience.

Green Flag

The NMCs Code of Conduct (NMC 2018b) requires that patient dignity and privacy must be maintained; this a central tenet that recurs throughout the Code.

Box 35.1 lists some of the indications for the use of urinary catheters (this is not an exhaustive list).

Box 35.1 Some Indications for the Use of Urinary Catheters

Management of acute urinary retention
Management of chronic urinary retention (this may be due to neurological disorder)
To allow irrigation of the bladder (e.g. post urological surgery)
Bladder outlet obstruction
To relieve retention of urine if all other options have been exhausted
To enable bladder function tests to be performed
To measure urinary output accurately (for example, in the case of sepsis)
Installation of drugs into the bladder (for example, chemotherapeutic agents)

Source: Dougherty & Lister (2015); Jevon & Joshi (2020).

Touch Points

Catheters can be used for short- and long-term periods, for a wide range of conditions and circumstances. Indwelling catheters should only be used in cases where other options are not suitable.

There are a variety of reasons why there is a need for a urinary catheter, and the procedure must be carried out using aseptic technique; the nursing associate must adhere to local policy and procedure.

Risks and Potential Complications of Urinary Catheterisation

Catheterisation is a common procedure; it is, however, invasive, and this brings with it many risks. Using any type of catheter brings with it associated risks. These include risk of urinary tract infections and associated life-threatening complications, for example, sepsis. For these reasons, risk assessment undertaken by an appropriate and competent healthcare professional is essential. Catheterisation should only be undertaken after considering alternative methods of management, and the person's clinical need for catheterisation should be reviewed regularly, with the urinary catheter being removed as soon as possible (NICE 2012).

Red Flag

Sepsis is a major cause of mortality and the use of urinary catheters increase the risk of severe sepsis. They should only be used if clinically indicated.

Invasive devices such as urinary catheters are necessary to help treat those who are ill. They are commonplace in most healthcare organisations and at home. Whenever an invasive device is used, there is a potential for infection, and this can include healthcare-acquired infections which can lead to sepsis.

Any patient who has a catheter inserted (long term or short term) as part of their care, will be exposed to the risks of acquiring a catheter-associated urinary tract infection (CAUTI). The RCN (2019) notes that there are some patients who are at an increased risk of acquiring a CAUTI and these include:

- Pregnant women
- Patients aged over 65 years
- Patients with diabetes
- Patients who are immunocompromised
- Patients with renal tract abnormalities or with one functioning kidney
- Patients with chronic wounds due to risk of cross infection to the bladder

In addition to the possibility of causing infection, urinary catheterisation can also cause pain and trauma. Pain can be caused by the introduction of the catheter into the urethra. The urethra is lined by transitional epithelium cells which are not lubricated and are also very sensitive. The use of sterile lubricant with anaesthetic (for example, lidocaine 2% gel) can reduce tissue damage as well as provide an anaesthetised effect to the urethra, thus helping to manage any pain or discomfort. Often, infection is caused by poor aseptic technique where microorganisms are introduced as the catheter is inserted from the gloved hands of the practitioner or from the flora of the perineum.

Take Note

Those who have a catheter inserted (long term or short term) will be exposed to the risks of acquiring a CAUTI.

Types of Catheter

Catheters come in a variety different types and are available in various materials, designs and sizes. Consideration also needs to be given to ensure that the catheter selected is appropriate and the risk of potential complications is minimised. Nazarko (2010) notes that the promotion of patient comfort and quality of life is essential when deciding on the most appropriate catheter. See Table 35.2 for a discussion on the various types of catheters.

Yellow Flag

Intermittent self-catheterisation enables patients to maintain body image and is easier for patients to engage in sexual intercourse. There is a reduced risk of pressure damage when using intermittent self-catheterisation compared to having an indwelling catheter, as the intermittent catheter is only left in long enough for the urine to drain, which minimises bacteria colonisation.

Table 35.2 Types of catheters.

TYPE OF CATHETER	DESCRIPTION
Intermittent urinary catheters (see Figure 35.2)	These catheters are inserted several times a day, just long enough to drain the bladder, then removed. The patient may be taught how to insert the catheter themselves. The sterile catheter is usually pre-lubricated, reducing the risk of discomfort during insertion. One end of the catheter is either left open-ended to allow drainage into a toilet or attached to a bag to collect the urine. The other end is guided through the urethra until it enters the bladder and urine starts to flow. When the flow of urine stops, the catheter can be removed. A new catheter is used each time.
Indwelling urinary catheters (see Figure 35.2)	An indwelling urinary catheter is inserted using aseptic technique. The catheter (often known as a Foley catheter) is left in place in the bladder, which is secured by a water-filled balloon, preventing it from falling out. Urine is drained through a tube in to a collection bag, this can be strapped to the outside of the leg or attached to a stand on the floor. Short term catheters usually need to be removed before 28 days, long term catheters usually need to be removed before 12 weeks, however all catheters should be regularly reviewed and removed as soon as possible. Please refer to manufacturer's guidance, for how long the short and long term catheter your patient has can remain in situ for.
Suprapubic catheters	A suprapubic catheter is inserted through an incision in the abdomen directly into the bladder. This procedure is initially carried out using general, epidural or local anaesthetic. A suprapubic catheter is used when the urethra is not a viable route. The catheter may be secured to the side of the body and attached to a collection bag strapped to the leg. Usually, this type of catheter is changed every 6 to 8 weeks.

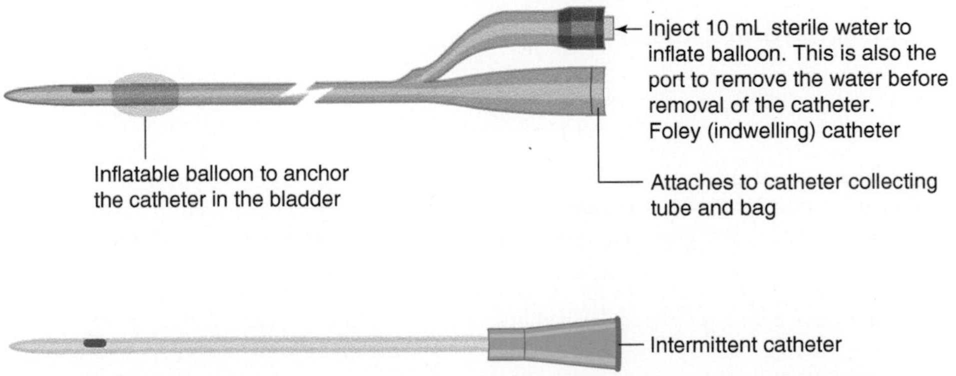

Figure 35.2 Intermittent and indwelling urinary catheter. *Source:* Lindsay et al. (2018), chapter 32, figure 32.1, p. 66. © John Wiley & Sons.

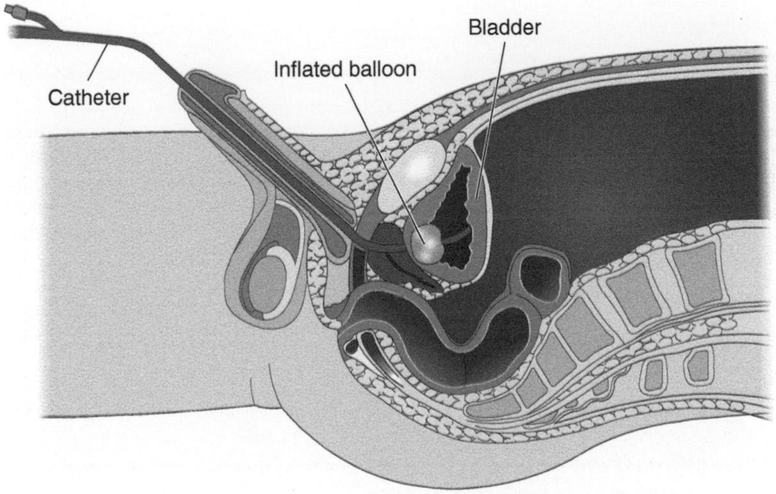

Figure 35.3 Indwelling urinary catheter.

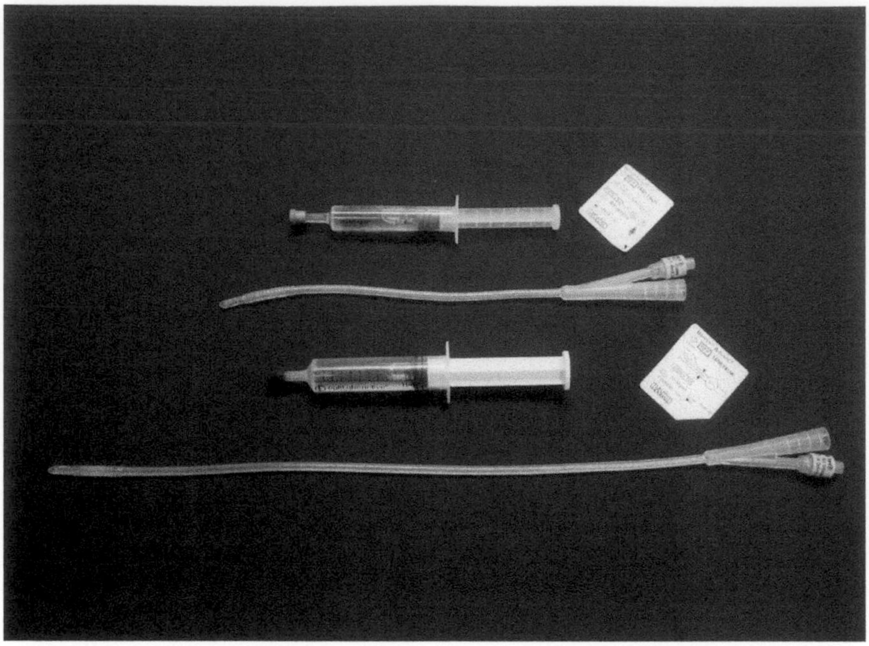

Figure 35.4 Urinary catheters and local anaesthetic gel. *Source:* Thomas (2015), chapter 31, figure 31.3, p. 78. © John Wiley & Sons.

There are two lengths of catheters: short, for female patients and long, used for males, see Figure 35.4 for examples of urinary catheter and local anaesthetic gel.

Males and females have different length urethras. Catheters used for males are longer, usually 40–45 cm in length, whereas female catheters are usually 23–26 cm long (shorter catheters for females can reduce the risk of the tube kinking, which would obstruct urine flow). Catheter size and diameter are measured in French gauge or Charrière (Ch); the average size used for adults is 12–14 Ch (Yates 2016). However, this is determined based on individual need and patient anatomy. A size 14Ch or 16Ch is usually used for a suprapubic catheter. The length for suprapubic catheters is chosen based on individual patient need and anatomy, the catheter must be able to pass through the abdominal wall.

The most common type of catheter is a Foley catheter. Three-way catheters can be used for bladder irrigation after surgery to the prostate or urinary bladder.

Catheters are made from various types of materials, for example, latex, Teflon, polytetrafluoroethylene or silicone elastomer coatings and polyvinyl chloride. Each type is chosen for a specific reason and in response to individual needs, such as allergy status.

Touch Point

Catheters are available in different types and various materials, designs and sizes. The nursing associate has to ensure that the catheter selected is effective and the possible risk of complications reduced. The promotion of patient comfort and quality of life is key when deciding on the most appropriate catheter.

Blue Flag

An indwelling urinary catheter may have a negative impact on body image, sex and sexuality. Sexual function can become compromised; altered body image due to urethral or suprapubic catheterisation may hinder the person's desire to want to engage in sexual intercourse. An indwelling catheter in the male urethra may cause trauma to the urethra on erection. Painful erections, particularly when sleeping, are complication of having an indwelling urethral catheter. Pressure damage can occur to the glans penis if a fixation device is not used. Also an unsecured catheter tube can cause bladder spasms which can lead to urine leakage outside of the catheter (bypassing) (Holroyd 2018). When the nursing associate undertakes catheter care review, consider the patient's sexual needs and plan care where possible to facilitate an individual's ability to meet these.

An active sex life can be possible with a urethral or a suprapubic catheter; it may be easier with a suprapubic or intermittent catheter than with an indwelling catheter. Prior to sex, a man can tape the urethral catheter along the shaft of the penis and cover it with a condom, a woman can tape it up along her abdomen. Please discuss with the patient's medical team before giving advice about this, as catheters should not be occluded or drainage prevented for any prolonged length of time.

Orange Flag

Logan et al. (2008) have reported that the prospect of introducing a urinary catheter into the bladder several times a day can pose physical and emotional challenges. The nursing associate who has a good knowledge of intermittent catheterisation can help patients with voiding problems to manage these issues and enhance their well-being.

Catheterisation

As per the NMC standards of proficiency for nursing associates (2018c), nursing associates can "care for and manage catheters for all genders", the NMC (2018c) future nurse: standards of proficiency for registered nurses states nurses can "select and use appropriate continence products; insert, manage and remove catheters for all genders; and assist with self-catheterisation when required". Therefore please ensure you are working within your scope of competence and proficiency as a registered nursing associate in relation to catheter care and management. Your local Trust or workplace may have catheter care policies which you should also consider when delivering catheter care. To insert a catheter you must be trained and deemed proficient to do so, different clinical areas may have different training and proficiency assessments.

Prior to catheterising a patient the professional must ensure; the person's identity has been checked, the procedure has been explained, along with any associated risks and benefits and that consent has been gained for the procedure to take place. Before inserting a catheter, ensure that the patient has been advised of why a catheter would benefit their care. The patient should also be given the opportunity to have any questions about the procedure answered.

Privacy and dignity should be maintained throughout the procedure regardless of care setting. The patient should be given the option of having a chaperone present during the procedure; a chaperone can offer reassurance to the patient and help to position the patient if needed.

Prior to catheter insertion, a bladder scan may be performed to see how much urine is in the bladder. The bladder may also be palpated or noted to be distended prior to catheter insertion. As with medicines administration, patient's identity and allergy status should be confirmed prior to the insertion of a medical device, such as a catheter.

The patient's genitals should be clean and dry before a catheter is inserted, to minimise the risk of bacterial infection. If the patient is able to wash their own genitals, this should be encouraged.

Gather all equipment needed to insert an indwelling urinary catheter. Please note that some areas may have specific catheter packs, which already have some or all of the required equipment in them, including:

- Aseptic pack, which should include a sterile field, sterile gauze and galley pot
- Sterile gloves (two pairs)
- Correct size catheter: shorter for female, longer for male
- Sterile water for injection (depending on manufacturer and local Trust policy) to inflate the catheter balloon
- Syringe to instil the sterile water into the catheter balloon
- Local anaesthetic gel (if prescribed and required)
- Lubricating gel
- Catheter bag
- Cleansing solution
- Catheter fixation device
- Towel, incontinence pad or other absorbent pads

Box 35.2 Outlines the procedure for inserting a urinary catheter; it is reiterated that at all times the nursing associate must adhere to local policy and procedure, and any deviation from this must be explained, reported and documented. Catheterisation must be performed using aseptic non-touch technique; therefore, hands must be washed (see Chapter 47 of this text, using hand hygiene techniques). An apron must also be worn during the procedure, to protect the uniform from contamination from bodily fluids.

Providing Catheter Care

The genital area can be cleaned with soap and warm water. It is important to gently pull the male foreskin back and clean underneath. Cleaning of the genitals should be in a downward motion to avoid any bacteria from entering the urethra. The genital meatus should be cleaned regularly and before catheterisation (sterile saline may be used to cleanse the area immediately prior to catheterisation). The external catheter tubing should also be cleaned regularly, and care should be taken to avoid tugging on the tubing, as this could be uncomfortable for the patient. It is important the skin is dried after washing to prevent growth of bacteria in a warm and wet environment. The skin can be patted dry with a towel.

Take Note

Catheter care (also known as perineal hygiene) is carried out daily using soap and water; this is appropriate for meatal care. Routine daily meatal cleansing with antiseptics is not recommended.

In the uncircumcised male, the area under the foreskin should be cleansed daily to remove smegma, decrease trauma and ulceration to the meatus and glans penis and reduce the risk for catheter-associated urinary tract infection.

Violet Flag

Hospitals are places where adults experiencing homelessness receive healthcare. The nursing associate has to develop an understanding of the types of support required upon discharge from hospital; this is essential especially for the person who is being discharged with a catheter in situ.

With the right support to tackle entrenched medical, personal and social problems, it is possible for those people who experience homelessness to secure positive health; this is the foundation for rebuilding more secure and stable lives (Queen's Nursing Institute 2019).

Box 35.2 Insertion of a Urinary Catheter

1. Collect equipment; move to the bedside. Wash hands. Clean the trolley, according to local policy, and adapt the process if in a community setting (for example, use a clean area) wash hands.
2. Open the sterile pack on to trolley or clean area.
3. Open the packets and empty them onto the sterile field, without touching the outside packaging of the products on the sterile field. Contents required on the sterile field: catheter, catheter tubing and bag, gauze, lubricating gel, anaesthetic gel (if using and prescribed – anaesthetic gel will take a few minutes to work and can reduce discomfort), syringe (usually 10 mL, size depends on how much fluid is required to inflate the catheter balloon, see manufacturer's guidance), sterile water to fill the catheter balloon with. Pour the cleansing solution into gallipot. The rubbish bag in the sterile pack can be used as a glove to move the contents around on the sterile field if needed. If you need an extra pair of sterile gloves, these can be opened and put on to the sterile field.
4. Fix the waste bag on to the side of the trolley, or put it open on a clean surface, if in the community.
5. If possible, raise the bed to a safe working height.
6. Assist the patient into a comfortable supine position. Remove clothes below the waist. The legs can be straight and flat if catheterising a male patient. If catheterising a female patient the legs can be bent at the knees and opened into a diamond shape (if the woman is able).
7. With clean and dry hands, put on the sterile gloves. Put apron on.
8. Place the drape under the patient's genitals.
9. If catheterising a male, hold the penis with gauze in one hand; with the other hand, soak another piece of gauze with saline, and if they have a foreskin, pull the foreskin down and clean underneath. Discard wet gauze into the waste bag. With another piece of saline-soaked gauze, clean the penis in downward movement; discard gauze after one wipe of the penis; you may need to repeat this process several times. If catheterising a female, wipe the external genitals with saline-soaked gauze in a downward motion and discard the gauze after each wipe. Ensure the genitals are dry before moving to the next stage.
10. If catheterising a male, hold the penis with a piece of gauze, and insert the tip of the anaesthetic gel syringe into the urethra. If catheterising a female, hold the labia majora open and insert the tip of the anaesthetic gel syringe into the urethra. Slowly depress the plunger until the gel has been instilled.
11. Allow time for the gel to take effect, this may vary from brand to brand. While the gel is taking effect, you may ask the male to hold his penis with a piece of sterile gauze or you may hold his penis in an upright position to prevent the gel from leaking out.
12. Once the anaesthetic gel has taken effect you should remove your gloves, wash your hands.
13. Connect the catheter tube to the sterile catheter bag.
14. Either use the pre-filled syringe or fill a syringe with the required amount of sterile water to fill the catheter balloon. Connect the syringe to the balloon inflation portal. Do not depress the syringe at this point to fill the balloon.
15. Partially remove the catheter tip from the packaging.
16. In a male, hold the penis in an upright position (see Figure 35.5). In a female, open the labia majora (see Figure 35.6). Ensure that the urethra is exposed and visualised if possible.
17. Gently insert the catheter into the urethra; pull back the packaging of the catheter tube as you insert it further into the urethra. Slowly insert the catheter tube; you should not feel any resistance in a female patient. You may feel slight resistance when passing the male prostate, you may ask the patient to cough as you pass the catheter past this point, if you are not able to pass the catheter any further past this point, gently remove it and ask another healthcare professional trained in catheterisation to insert the catheter (this is to avoid any internal damage to the patient); explain this to the patient.
18. Continue to insert the catheter until urine fills the tubing. In some instances, you may not see urine instantly in the catheter tube; continue to insert the catheter until you have inserted it nearly to the bifurcation point.
19. When urine starts to fill the catheter tube or you have inserted it until near the bifurcation point, stop inserting the catheter; and holding the catheter in place, fill the catheter balloon, this will secure the catheter in place. The balloon should be easily filled and should not be uncomfortable for the patient.
20. Gently pull the catheter back until you feel a slight resistance, ensuring the catheter is in the correct position.
21. Attach the catheter draining device, using a non-touch technique (if not already done at step 13).
22. Use the catheter fixation device to secure the catheter tubing to the patient's leg.
23. Ensure the catheter drainage device/bag is positioned below the level of the bladder; this ensures the urine can drain by gravity into the drainage device and prevents backflow of urine into the bladder. You may use straps or a sleeve to attach the catheter to the patient's leg. Or a catheter stand may be used to hold the catheter in the correct position (this is particularly useful in a bedbound or chair bound patient, as it prevents pressure damage which could be caused if leg straps are used and fastened too tightly). Alternatively, the catheter bag may be attached to the patient's bed using the hook provided with the catheter drainage device.
24. Clean the genitals to remove any excess remaining anaesthetic/lubricating gel.
25. Remove the drape. Redress the patient.
26. Discard the used materials into a clinical waste bin.
27. Make the patient comfortable. Advise the patient of whom to contact if the catheter stops draining or becomes dislodged or uncomfortable. Wash hands.
28. Start recording urine output or advise the patient how to monitor urine output; this includes volume and colour.
29. Advise the patient how to empty the catheter bag, if they are doing this themselves.
30. Document the insertion into the patient notes (for example: aseptic technique used, catheter type, volume of fluid used to inflate balloon, any problems encountered, complications noted, residual urine drained, planned removal date). Documentation and reporting must be aligned to local policy and procedure; labels/stickers may need to be saved from the catheter pack to be added to the patient's notes.

Source: Dougherty & Lister (2015); Jevon & Joshi (2020); Lindsay et al. (2018); Thomas (2017).

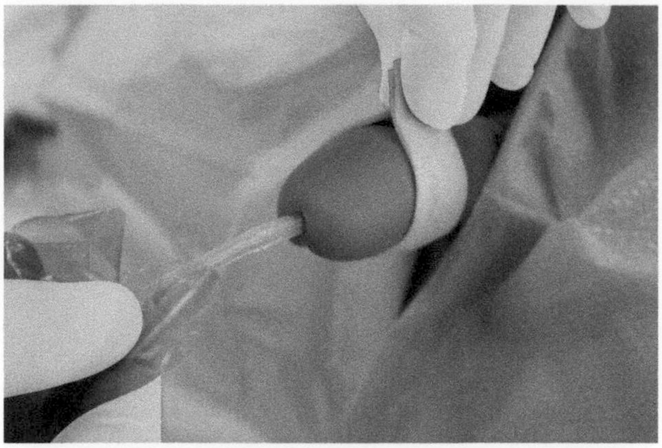

Figure 35.5 Catheter insertion into a male. *Source:* Thomas (2015), chapter 31, figure 31.5, p. 78. © John Wiley & Sons.

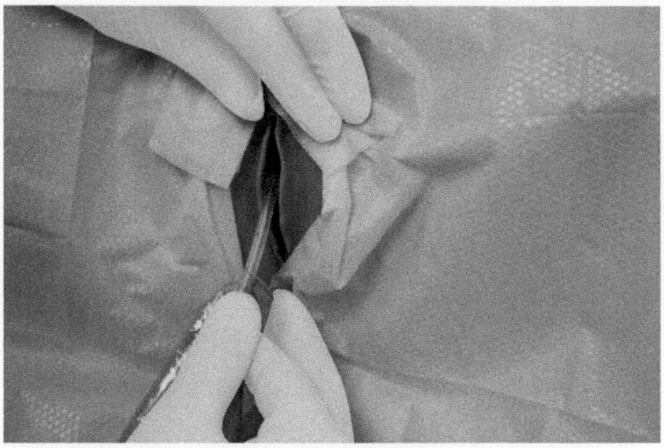

Figure 35.6 Catheter insertion into a female. *Source:* Thomas (2015), chapter 31, figure 31.6, p. 78. © John Wiley & Sons.

How to Empty the Catheter Bag

Prior to emptying the catheter bag, consider if the amount of urine produced needs to be measured. The catheter bag should be emptied before it is full; this is to avoid backtracking/backflow of urine up the tube and back into the bladder. Backtracking of urine can cause urinary infections. The catheter bag valve should be cleaned with an alcohol wipe before emptying. The catheter bag can be emptied into a urine bottle or the toilet. To empty the bag, the valve must be in the open position. When emptying the catheter bag, the bag should remain below the level of the bladder to allow for gravity to assist in the drainage of urine from the bag and to prevent backflow. Once the urine has been emptied from the bag, the valve should be closed and cleaned with a new alcohol wipe. The cleaning and closure of the valve prevents bacteria from entering the bag, if this process is not followed bacteria could enter the bladder and cause an infection. The catheter bag may be a gravity bag which may rest on a catheter stand or be attached to the side of the bed. If the patient has a leg bag, re-secure the bag to the leg if it was removed during the emptying process. Follow manufacturers' guidance and policy for how frequently the urine collection bag needs replacing.

Measuring Urine Output

Urine output may need to be measured for a number of reasons. There are a few ways to measure the amount of urine passed from the catheter. Some catheter bags may have an hourly urine capture box attached. If this is the case, the urine should be decanted hourly from the capture box into the catheter bag, as the capture box usually holds less urine than the catheter bag. Also not needed be required to be measured hourly to ensure accurate fluid input and output. In some cases, for example, after kidney transplant, the hourly urine output may need to be matched by fluid input. Other catheter bags have volume measurements clearly marked on the bag. Different catheter bags may have different volumes demarcated on the bag. A catheter bag needs to be monitored regularly to determine how full it is, and it should not be allowed to fill beyond three-quarters. However, it is not good practice to empty catheter bags too often as frequent opening and closing of the catheter bag valve can increase the risk of exposure to pathogens outside of the body. Bags should be positioned below the level of the bladder; many of them are fitted with an anti-reflux valve. When a 2L drainage bag is used, attach it to an appropriate stand and contact with the floor should be avoided. A separate clean container is to be used when emptying bags, avoiding any contact between the outlet valve and container (Loveday et al. 2014). When emptying catheter bags, contact between the outlet valve and toilet/urine bottle/other urine collection apparatus, should be avoided (Loveday et al. 2014). Drained urine may also be decanted in to a urine bottle and weighed on scales. In this instance weigh the urine bottle before filling with urine, fill with urine (not to the top), weigh the bottle containing urine and minus the bottle weight from the total to calculate the urine weight. 1 gram of urine equates to approximately 1mL.

Supporting Evidence

Loveday et al. (2014) epic3: National Evidence-Based Guidelines for Preventing Healthcare-Associated Infections in NHS Hospitals in England Journal of Hospital Infection *86S1 (2014) S1–S70*

These guidelines (epic3) provide comprehensive recommendations for preventing healthcare-associated infections in hospital and other acute care settings that are based on the best currently available evidence; they can reduce variation in practice and maintain patient safety. Clinically effective infection prevention and control practice is a key feature of patient protection. When the nursing associate incorporates these guidelines into routine daily clinical practice, then patient safety can be improved and the risk of patients acquiring an infection during episodes of healthcare settings can be minimised.

How to Remove a Catheter

Explain the procedure to the patient and gain consent to remove the catheter. Ask the patient to clean their genitals or assist them if required. Ensure privacy and dignity is maintained throughout this procedure.

- Wash hands.
- Don non-sterile gloves and apron.
- Clean the patients' genital area.
- Remove the catheter tubing from the fixation device (at this point the fixation device can also be removed).
- Using a syringe, remove the liquid from the balloon.
- Gently hold catheter tube and pull; it should easily slide out.
- Discard the catheter apparatus using local policy. Wash hands.
- Monitor the patient's urine output post catheter removal. If the patient does not pass urine within two hours, or the bladder becomes visibly distended or uncomfortable, a bladder scan may be required to ensure the patient is not in urinary retention. If a patient has been catheterised for a long period of time they may need a flip flo catheter valve prior to a trial without catheter to help them regain sphincter control.
- Document the catheter removal.

Conclusion

Urinary catheterisation is the insertion of a catheter through the urethra and into the bladder or the insertion of a suprapubic catheter through the anterior abdominal wall into the dome of the bladder undertaken for the withdrawal of urine.

Urinary catheterisation is a risk factor for the development a urinary tract infection, which can result in significant morbidity and mortality. Reducing complications will improve patient outcomes, assist with early hospital discharge and decrease community care.

References

Dougherty, L. and Lister, S. (2015) *The royal Marsden hospital manual of clinical nursing procedures* (9th edn), Oxford: Blackwell Publishing.

Geng, V., Cobussen-Boekhorst, H., Farrell, J., Gea-Sanchez, M., Pearce, I., Schwennesen, T., Vahr, S., Vandewinkel, C. (2012) *Evidence based guidelines for best practice in urological health care – catheterisation – indwelling catheters in adults*, Arnhem: European Association of Urology Nurses.

Holroyd, S. (2018) The importance of indwelling urinary catheter securement, *British Journal of Nursing*, 28(15): 976–977.

Jevon, P. and Joshi, R. (2020) *Procedural skills*, Oxford: Wiley.

Lindsay, P., Bagness, C., Peate, I. (2018) *Midwifery Skills at a Glance*. UK: Wiley-Blackwell.

Logan, K., Shaw, C. and Webber, I., Samuel, S., Broome, L.. (2008) Patients' experiences of learning clean intermit- tent self-catheterization: a qualitative study, *Journal of Advanced Nursing*, 62(1): 32–40.

Loveday, H.P., Wilson, J.A., Pratt, R.J., Golsorkhi, M., Tingle, A., Bak, A., Browne, J., Priete, J., Wilcox, M. (2014) Epic3: national evidence-based guidelines for preventing healthcare-associated infections in NHS hospitals in England, *Journal of Hospital Infection*, 86: S1, S1–S70.

Nair, M. (2017) The renal system, in Peate, I. & Nair, M. (eds.) *Fundamentals of anatomy and physiology for nursing an healthcare students Ch 10* (2nd edn), Oxford: Wiley, 299–332.

National Health Service (NHS). (2017) *Risks urinary catheter.* [online] Available: https://www.nhs.uk/conditions/urinary-catheters/risks/. Accessed 6 October 2019.

National Institute for Health and Care Excellence (NICE). (2012) *Healthcare-associated infections: prevention and control in primary and community care CG139.* [online] Available: https://www.nice.org.uk/guidance/cg139. Accessed December 2019.

National Institute for Health and Care Excellence (NICE). (2014) *Infection prevention and control.* [online] Available: https://www.nice.org.uk/guidance/qs61/resources/infection-prevention-and-control-pdf-2098782603205. Last accessed 06 October 2019.

National Institute for Health and Care Excellence (NICE). (2015) *Urinary incontinence in women: management. Clinical guideline* CG171. [online] Available: www.nice.org.uk/guidance/CG171/chapter/Key-priorities-for-implementation [accessed December 2019].

National Institute for Health and Care Excellence (NICE). (2018) *Urinary tract infection (catheter-associated): antimicrobial prescribing.* [online] Available: https://www.nice.org.uk/guidance/ng113/chapter/Recommendations#preventing-catheter-associated-urinary-tract-infections. Accessed January 2021.

National Institute for Health and Care Excellence (NICE). (2019) *Urinary retention.* [online] Available: https://bnf.nice.org.uk/treatment-summary/urinary-retention.html. Accessed 2 November 2019.

Nazarko, L. (2010) Effective-evidence based catheter management: an update, *British Journal of Nursing*, 19 (15): 948–953.

Nursing and Midwifery Council (NMC). (2018a) *Standards of proficiency for nursing associates.* [online] Available: https://www.nmc.org.uk/globalassets/sitedocuments/education-standards/nursing-associates-proficiency-standards.pdf. Accessed January 2021.

Nursing and Midwifery Council (NMC). (2018b) *The code professional standards of practice and behaviour for nurses, midwives and nursing associates.* [online] Available: https://www.nmc.org.uk/globalassets/sitedocuments/nmc-publications/nmc-code.pdf. Accessed December 2019.

Nursing and Midwifery Council (NMC). (2018c) *Future nurse: standards of proficiency for registered nurses.* [online] Available: https://www.nmc.org.uk/globalassets/sitedocuments/standards-of-proficiency/nurses/future-nurse-proficiencies.pdf Accessed January 2021.

Queen's Nursing Institute. (2019) *Homeless health programme.* [online] Available: https://www.qni.org.uk/nursing-in-the-community/homeless-health-programme/. Accessed December 2019.

Rawal, G. and Yadav, S. (2015) Green urine due to propofol: a case report with review of literature, *Journal of Clinical and Diagnostic Research*, 9(11): 2–4.

Royal College of Nursing (RCN). (2019) *Catheter care RCN guidance for healthcare professionals*, London: RCN.

Takehisa, O., Sugino, Y., Shibahara, T., Masui, S., Yabana, T., Sasaki, T. (2017) Randomized controlled study of the efficacy and safety of continuous saline bladder irrigation after transurethral resection for the treatment of non-muscle-invasive bladder cancer, *Urology Oncology*, 119(2): 276–282.

Thomas, R. (2015) *Practical Medical Procedures at a Glance.*UK: Wiley-Blackwell.

Torres, P.A., Helmstetter, J.A., Kaye, A.M., Kaye, A.D. (2015) Rhabdomyolysis: pathogenesis, diagnosis, and treatment, *The Ochsner Journal*, 15 (1): 58–69.

Tubaro, A. (2019) Acute urinary retention increases the risk of complications after transurethral resection of the prostate: a population-based study, *BJU International*, 110 (11c): 902.

Yates, A. (2016). Indwelling urinary catheterisation: What is best practice? *British Journal of Nursing (Urology Supplement)*, 25(9): S4–S13.

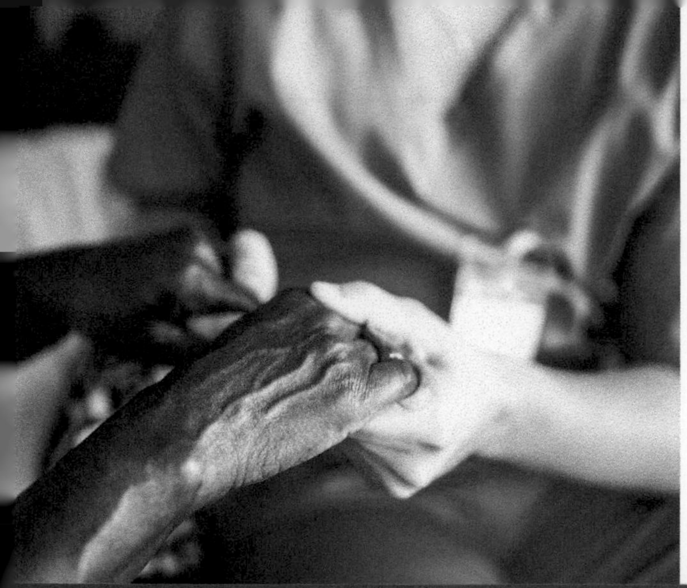

36

Assisting with Toileting, Choosing and Using Appropriate Continence Products

Ian Peate

School of Health Studies, Gibraltar

Chapter Aim

- **This chapter provides the reader with a discussion concerning the ways in which the nursing associate can assist people with their toileting needs and to consider appropriate continence products.**

Learning Outcomes

- **To help the nursing associate identify issues concerned with continence and incontinence**
- **To enhance interpersonal and therapeutic relationship skills**
- **To support the nursing associate when choosing and using appropriate continence products**
- **To reinforce the importance of the 6 'Cs' that underpin the provision of high-quality care**

Test Yourself Multiple Choice Questions

1. **Health-related shame can:**
   - A) **Have a significant impact on health**
   - B) **Have a negative impact on illness and health-related behaviours**
   - C) **Both of the above**

The Nursing Associate's Handbook of Clinical Skills, First Edition. Edited by Ian Peate.

Companion website: www.wiley.com/nursingassociate

2. The nature of incontinence means
   A) This is a part of the normal ageing process
   B) That the person accepts that they will have 'accidents'
   C) The person may feel shame and embarrassment resulting in social isolation
3. Dignity is concerned with
   A) How people feel, think and behave in relation to the worth or value of themselves and others
   B) How people feel and manage their condition
   C) How people judge others
4. A person with an overactive bladder:
   A) Needs to be taken to the toilet every hour
   B) May not have incontinence but have symptoms that significantly affect their quality of life
   C) Will have incontinence and the symptoms will significantly affect their quality of life
5. Passive incontinence occurs when:
   A) A person feels no urge to open their bowels
   B) A person defaecates and urinates involuntarily
   C) Neither of the above

Introduction

A key role of the nursing associate is to provide support to people and help them maintain their bladder and bowel health. The Nursing and Midwifery Council (NMC) (2018a) standards of proficiency require the trainee nursing associates on successful completion of their programme of study to be able to assist people with toileting, maintaining their dignity and privacy and to use appropriate continence products.

The NMC's Code (2018b) requires all registrants to put the interests of people who use or need nursing services first. The patients' care and safety are the nursing associate's main concerns, and this includes ensuring that their dignity is preserved and they are treated with kindness, respect and compassion.

The nursing associate is also required to work co-operatively; they are required to respect the skills, expertise and contributions of their colleagues, referring matters to them when appropriate – this is an important requirement, as the nursing associate may be expected to draw on the expertise of others and to make appropriate referrals.

Green Flag Health and Social Care Act 2008 (Regulated Activities) Regulations 2014: Regulation 10

The intention of this regulation is to ensure that those who use services are treated with respect and dignity at all times while they are receiving care and treatment. To adhere to this regulation, care providers must make sure that they deliver care and treatment in such a way that it ensures people's dignity and treat them with respect at all times. This includes making sure that people have privacy when they need and want it with regards to toileting and their continence needs.

This chapter provides the reader with a discussion concerning the ways in which the nursing associate can assist people with their toileting needs. These are the principles of care that can be adapted and applied where appropriate to a range of care environments and patient groups. There will also be a discussion regarding continence products.

The focus of this chapter will be on the adult. Children will have specific needs regarding their toileting needs as well as particular requirements should they need assistance with the choice of and appropriate use of continence products. In chapters 33 and 34, issues around continence and bladder and bowel patterns have been discussed along with the nursing associate's response to incontinence, diarrhoea and faecal incontinence.

Dignity is central to every task that the nursing associate is involved in. Often, dignity concerns the small things that are very important, such as maintaining hygiene and personal appearance, being able to have access to the toilet, being provided with choices and being involved in decisions.

Blue Flag

Continence problems are sometimes debilitating; they often cause embarrassment and can be life-changing. They can have a considerable psychological impact and affect personal and sexual relationships and body image.

Toileting

The British Geriatrics Society (2007), in its campaign – 'Behind Closed Doors' states that 'People, whatever their age and physical ability, should be able to choose to use the toilet in private in all care settings'. This is a standard that all professionals must adhere to it is an example of best

Table 36.1 Standards of the British Geriatrics Society.

Access	All people, whatever their age and physical ability, should be able to choose and use the toilet in private and sufficient equipment must be available to achieve this.
Timeliness	People who need assistance should be able to request and receive timely and prompt help and should not be left on a commode or bedpan longer than necessary.
Equipment for transfers and transit	Essential equipment for access to a toilet should be readily available and used in a way that respects the dignity of the patient and avoids unwanted exposure.
Safety	People who are unable to use a toilet alone safely should normally be offered the use of a toilet with appropriate safety equipment and with supervision if needed.
Choice	Patients' choice is paramount; their views should be sought and respected.
Privacy	Privacy and dignity must be preserved; people who are bed-bound need special attention.
Cleanliness	All toilets, commodes and bedpans must be clean
Hygiene	All people in all settings must be enabled to leave the toilet with a clean bottom and washed hands.
Respectful language	Discussions with people must be respectful and courteous, especially regarding episodes of incontinence.
Environmental audit	All organisations should encourage a lay person to carry out an audit to assess toilet facilities.

Source: Modified from British Geriatric's Society (2007).

practice which upholds human rights and promotes dignity. The aim of the campaign is to raise awareness of the rights of people in all care settings, whatever their age and physical ability, to choose to use the toilet in private. Table 36.1 outlines the campaign standards.

Using the toilet is a private activity. It is likely that patients will be embarrassed if others can see or hear them while using the toilet. An inadequate response to the toilet needs of those who are confined to bed, including poor continence management, is unacceptable.

Orange Flag

Health-related shame, according to Dolezal and Lyons (2017), can have a significant impact on health, illness and health-related behaviours. They suggest that its impact is sufficiently powerful for it to be considered an affective determinant of health.

Dean (2012) describes toileting as one of the fundamental elements of nursing. Failure to meet the toileting needs of patients is a common complaint by patients and their families. Toileting can also mean to provide the patient with appropriate facilities for the person to micturate or defaecate; this can be a toilet, commode, bedpan or urinal. A bedpan, urinal or commode should be provided for those who are confined to bed or are only up for short periods. Assistance to the toilet should be provided for those people who are too frail or immobile to be self-caring in relation to toileting.

For those patients unable to use the toilet independently, they will require a regular toileting programme that aims to ensure bladder emptying prior to incontinence occurring. This will differ with each patient, and the best time between visits to the toilet should be identified using a voiding chart (sometimes called a voiding record or a bladder diary). The voiding chart is the patient's record of daily bladder activity; it can capture real-time objective data on bladder activity and establish baseline function. The chart can also be used to track responses to interventions implemented. In the beginning, a short toileting time may be initiated, and this can be progressively lengthened depending on results.

Box 36.1 provides an overview of the principles underpinning toileting activities. It must be reiterated that any care offered must be tailored to meet the individual needs of the patient; care provision has to be provided based on the best available evidence.

Take Note

Some patients' may give signs about wanting to use the toilet, they can become agitated and fidgety; they may tug on clothing, wander, open doors, express the need to go outside, and touch the genital area.

The Royal College of Nursing (RCN) offers the following tips that can be used when working with people who have continence issues:

- Encourage women to sit on the toilet rather than hover; this will enable them to empty their bladders properly.
- Sit comfortably with the knees just above hip level and arms on knees to aid opening of the bowels.
- Have a well-balanced diet.

Box 36.1 The Principles of Toileting

- Get to know your patients (see Chapter 6 of this text).
- Ensure the toilet/bathroom is accessible.
- Place a call bell near them so that they can attract attention when they wish to use the toilet.
- Make sure that it is as easy as possible for them to get on to and off the toilet, for example, the provision of a raised toilet seat and grab bars.
- Take note when they give signs about needing to use the toilet; they may become agitated, fidgety, tug on clothing, wander and touch their genital area. Develop a routine and take the person to the toilet using a regular schedule; this might be every two hours. There will be a need to respond quickly if someone indicates that they need to use the toilet.
- Some people have a regular schedule, particularly for bowel movements. If this is so, remind them to go to the bathroom at the usual time; this might be, for example, straight after breakfast.
- If they need help to remove their clothes, assist them, but encourage them to help themselves. Remind them that before they sit down, they need to pull down their pants. Using clothes that are easy to remove will help.
- It is important not to rush them; give time for them to empty their bowel and bladder. It may take a little time to get started. Walk away, provide privacy, maintain safety and come back in a few minutes or stand just outside the door.
- If they are able, provide toilet paper for them to use as appropriate. You may need to help get them started. Using wet wipes can sometimes be easier than using toilet paper if you are required to wipe for them.
- Assist them as necessary to pull their pants back up. They might try to walk away without pulling pants up, beware that this is a fall hazard. Provide privacy and preserve modesty.
- Make clear where the toilet is, put a sign, with a picture, on the door to the toilet. Keep the door to the toilet open so that they can see the toilet.
- Consider using a commode or urinal by the bed at night so that they do not have to get up and walk to the toilet, which increases the risk of falls and incontinence. Use a night light if they do go to the toilet at night. If they have urgency when needing to urinate, a commode or urinal close by them can also be helpful. Beware, however, that the commode or urinal could also be a fall hazard.
- Some people will purposely reduce their fluid intake anticipating that they may not make it to the bathroom. This can result in dehydration and may lead to other problems, such as urinary tract infections. Promote hydration, however; it may be helpful to limit fluid intake at night, no or limited fluids after 20:00 hours.
- The use of caffeine and alcohol can also increase urgency with urination; these may have a diuretic effect.
- Wastepaper baskets, flowerpots and other items/containers on the floor may be mistaken by the person for a toilet. Remove them from the area they stay in and the area close to the toilet. Ensure that the path to the bathroom is kept clear of obstacles and any clutter.
- Construct an individualised programme for elimination based on their needs and personal patterns.
- The programme should be part of the care plan.
- Regularly review and evaluate the contents of this programme, particularly in terms of its effectiveness and the need for reassessment based on changes in their condition or ability to go to the toilet.

- Avoid going to the toilet 'just in case' as the bladder will become used to holding smaller volumes, developing frequency and urgency.
- Be relaxed, unhurried and maintain a safe environment when using a toilet.
- Stop smoking.
- Carry a spare set of clothes for continence issues.
- Throughout the day, drink gradually, and stay hydrated; large volumes in the evening can result in nocturnal frequency.
- Practice pelvic floor exercises.
- The use of a Radar key will allow access to all public toilets for the disabled, and information regarding this can be obtained from the local authority or online.
- Reduce weight if appropriate. Extra weight can increase intrabdominal pressure and worsen urinary incontinence.

Touch Point

Using the toilet is a private activity. Patients may be embarrassed if others can see or hear them using the toilet. The nursing associate should strive to offer the highest quality of care with regard to continence.

The very first step in providing high-quality continence care is for the nursing associate to get to know their patients. Whatever their age, regardless of the care setting and their physical ability, people have the right to use the toilet in private.

Containment Products

There are a variety of containment products available, and many agencies produce equipment. Getting the correct equipment to manage and support incontinence is vital. Assessment with a specialist nurse or occupational therapist is key to the provision to the most suitable equipment being sourced.

Supporting Evidence

Bladder and Bowel UK provides a range of resources for staff and patients with regard to continence issues. They have a range of equipment and ideas to manage incontinence in people of all ages.

Bladder and Bowel UK has a national confidential helpline that is managed by a team of Specialist Nurses and Continence Product Information Staff, who are available for advice on specialist services, product information and general advice on continence promotion.

www.disabledliving.co.uk/BladderandBowelUK/About

The choice of product(s) must be individually matched to patient needs. Absorbent pads or urine-collecting devices, such as penile sheaths, handheld urinals and faecal collectors, are products that can maintain social continence, but treatment of the incontinence must always be the preferred option. Ongoing review is required to ensure that products are fit for purpose; where independence can be recovered, a return to standard toileting should be facilitated to promote quality of life.

Red Flag

Pads are not the only product available to manage continence; there are many alternatives that should be tried first. The nursing associate needs to take into account who is using the equipment and who is available to support the individual. Consider the type of incontinence the product has to manage, availability, ease of use and cost. Is the person using the equipment without support? How much urine or faeces does the product have to cope with?

By using the right equipment, the management of continence issues can become easier.

The use of appropriate containment products can offer security and comfort helping people to continue with their normal daily activities. However, they can have an impact on people's dignity and their self-esteem; they do not offer a long-term solution unless the patient has not responded to other treatments, and they are also expensive.

Touch Point

The choice of any continence product must be appropriate and suitable to the individual's needs. Absorbent pads or urine-collecting devices, such as penile sheaths, handheld urinals and faecal collectors, can help to maintain social continence. It is key, however, that the treatment of the incontinence always be determined if at all possible.

Ongoing evaluation of care interventions is required to ensure that products are fit for purpose and remain fit for purpose.

It is recognised that indwelling urinary catheterisation can be associated with infection which can lead to illness and hospital admission (see Chapter 35 of this text). Those living with a long-term catheter may find them distressing, uncomfortable and undignified; for others, however, they can encourage independence.

Take Note

Where bowel management programmes are already in place, for example, for those patients with spinal cord injury, the RCN (ND) notes that it is essential that these are continued after admission to any care setting/hospital.

Conclusion

Living with continence problems can be challenging. Those people with continence issues may feel uncomfortable or ashamed when discussing it with others; they may be embarrassed to admit they have a problem, which can result in them not getting the support and advice that could improve their quality of life.

The nature of the condition means that the person lives with the fear of being incontinent, particularly in public; this may lead to feelings of shame and embarrassment, resulting in social isolation. The nursing associate can offer care and support with toilet training and working with the patient using appropriate continence products.

References

British Geriatric's Society. (2007) *Behind closed doors: using the toilet in private.* [online] Available: http://www.wales.nhs.uk/sitesplus/documents/1064/Behind%20Closed%20Doors%20Leaflet.pdf. Accessed December 2019.

Dean, E. (2012) Dignity on toileting, *Nursing Standard*, 26(24): 19–20.

Dolezal, L. and Lyons, B. (2017) Health-related shame: an affective determinant of health? *Medical Humanities*, 43(3): 257–263. doi:10.1136/medhum-2017-011186.

Nursing and Midwifery Council. (2018a) *Standards of proficiency for nursing associates.* [online] Available: https://www.nmc.org.uk/standards/standards-for-nursing-associates/standards-of-proficiency-for-nursing-associates/. Accessed December 2019.

Nursing and Midwifery Council. (2018b) The code, *Professional standards of practice and behaviour for nurses, midwives and nursing associates.* [online] Available: https://www.nmc.org.uk/globalassets/sitedocuments/nmc-publications/nmc-code.pdf. Accessed December 2019.

Royal College of Nursing. (ND) *Continence.* [online] Available: https://rcni.com/hosted-content/rcn/continence/impact-and-dignity. Accessed December 2019.

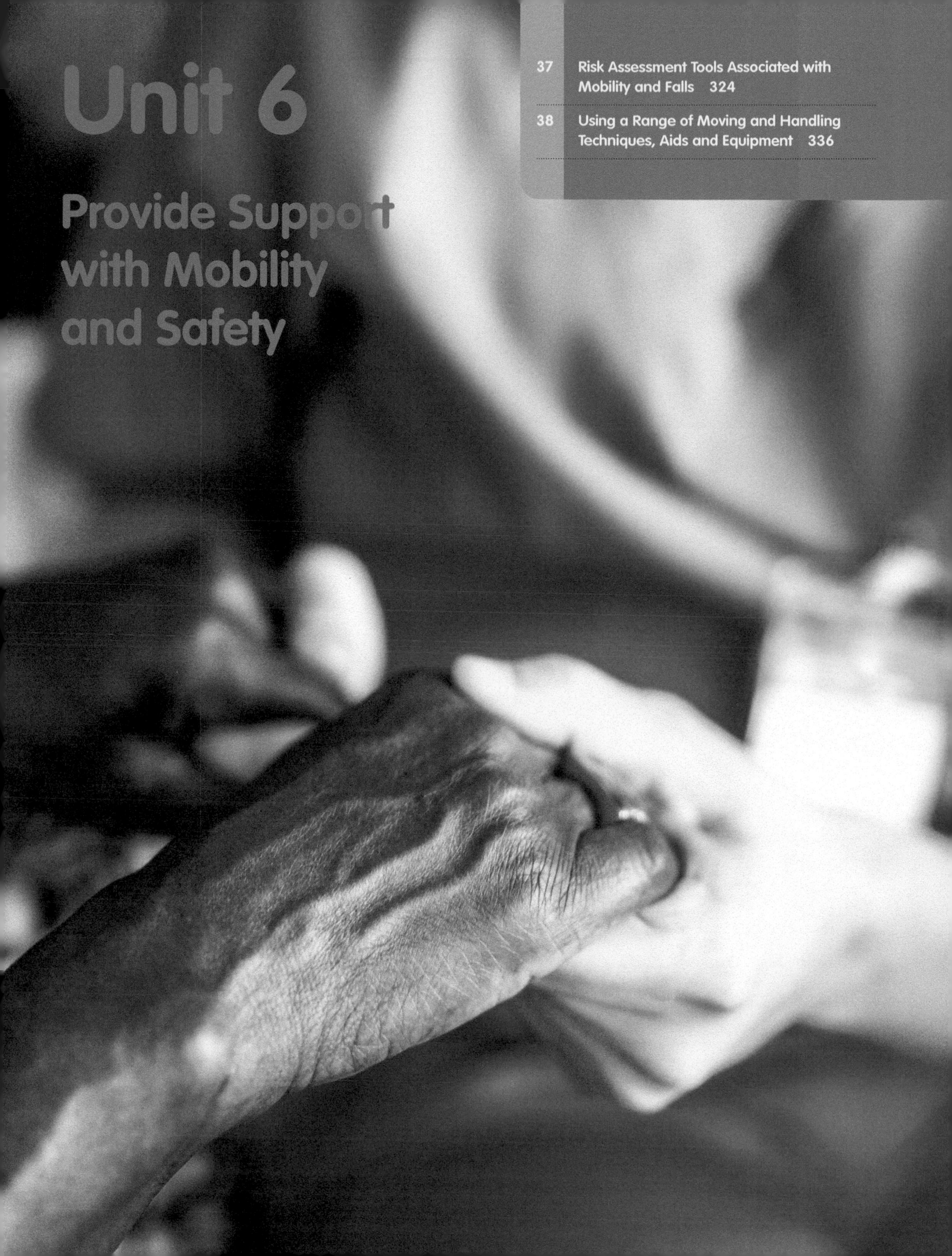

Unit 6

Provide Support with Mobility and Safety

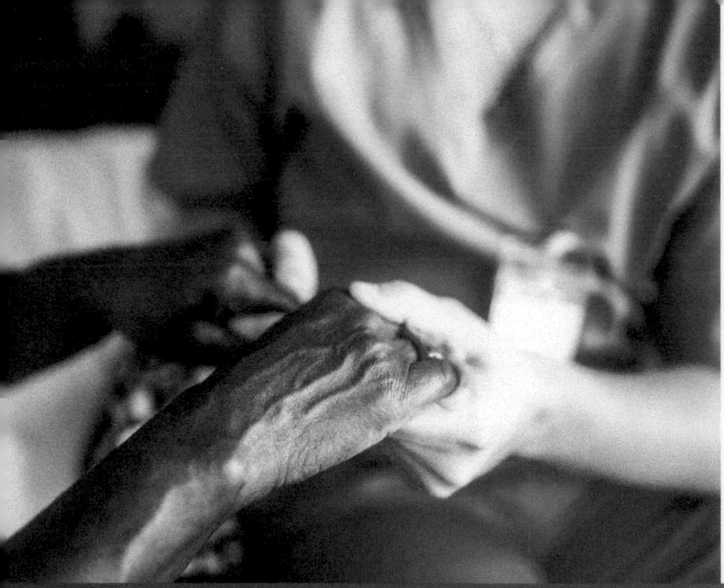

37

Risk Assessment Tools Associated with Mobility and Falls

Hamish MacGregor

Docklands Training Consultants Ltd, Portpatrick, UK

Chapter Aim

- **This chapter aims to provide the reader with an introduction to the use of assessment tools associated with mobility and falls.**

Learning Outcomes

By the end of the chapter, the reader should be able to:
- **Define which groups of people are more at risk of falls**
- **List the main causes of falls**
- **Describe the interventions that can be made to reduce the risk of falls**

Test Yourself Multiple Choice Questions

1. **The majority of falls cause:**
   A) **No harm**
   B) **Broken bones**
   C) **An admission to hospital**
2. **The causes of falls are:**
   A) **Due to a number of reasons**
   B) **Due to one specific medical condition a person suffers from**
   C) **Not really known**

The Nursing Associate's Handbook of Clinical Skills, First Edition. Edited by Ian Peate.

Companion website: www.wiley.com/nursingassociate

3. **The risk of falls increases when a person is**
   A) **Over 55 years of age**
   B) **Over 65 years of age**
   C) **Over 80 years of age**
4. **Elderly people who keep fit and healthy will**
   A) **Increase their risk of falls as they are out and about more**
   B) **Live longer**
   C) **Reduce their risk of falls as they become stronger and have better balance**
5. **A patient who is over 65 years or has a history of falls and is admitted to hospital should have**
   A) **Have bed rails put up on their bed immediately**
   B) **A falls risk assessment completed on admission**
   C) **Be kept on bed rest to prevent further falls**

Definition of a Fall

A *fall* is defined as an unintentional or unexpected loss of balance resulting in coming to rest on the floor, the ground or an object below knee level (National Institute for Health and Care Excellence (NICE) 2017a, 2017b).

In using assessment tools associated with falls and mobility, the nursing associate is practicing within platform 5 of the Nursing and Midwifery Council's proficiencies (NMC) (2018), whereby they are required to improve safety and quality of care and provide support with mobility and safety. They are required to use appropriate risk assessment tools to determine the ongoing need for support and intervention, the level of independence and self-care that an individual can manage and use appropriate assessment tools to determine, manage and escalate the ongoing risk of falls.

Statistics and Incidence

Falls and fractures are common and serious health issues faced by older people in England. People aged 65 years and older have the highest risk of falling; around a third of people aged 65 years and over and around half of people aged 80 years and over fall at least once a year. Falling is a cause of distress, pain, injury, loss of confidence, loss of independence and mortality.

Red Flag

Falls are a common problem in the elderly. Managing the immediate injuries, trying to establish the cause (or causes) of a fall, remedying these causes and limiting the harm patients will come to if they do fall are key concerns for the nursing associate.

For health services, they are both high volume and costly. In terms of annual activity and cost:

- the Public Health Outcomes Framework (PHOF) reported that, in 2017 to 2018, there were around 220,160 emergency hospital admissions related to falls among patients aged 65 years and over, with around 146,665 (66.6%) of these patients aged 80 years and over
- falls were the ninth highest cause of disability-adjusted life years (DALYs) in England in 2013 and the leading cause of injury
- unaddressed fall hazards in the home are estimated to cost the National Health Service (NHS) in England £435 million
- the total annual cost of fragility fractures to the United Kingdom has been estimated at £4.4 billion, which includes £1.1 billion for social care; hip fractures account for around £2 billion of this sum
- short- and long-term outlooks for patients are generally poor following a hip fracture, with an increased one-year mortality of between 18% and 33% and negative effects on daily living activities such as shopping and walking
- a review of long-term disability found that around 20% of hip fracture patients entered long-term care in the first year after fracture
- falls in hospitals are the most commonly reported patient safety incident with more than 240,000 reported in acute hospitals and mental health trusts in England and Wales (Public Health England (PHE) 2019)

Orange Flag

The psychological effects of falls can result in:

- Increased dependency
- Emotional distress
- Loss of confidence
- Loss of control

- Anxiety and depression
- Social isolation
- Embarrassment
- Fear of falling
- Low self-esteem

Those at Risk of Falling

Anyone can fall and, as described above, the older a person becomes, the likelihood of falls increases. Be aware that other groups can be prone to falls too. Examples could be:

- A 40-year-old person with alcohol misuse issues
- A postoperative hospital patient
- A woman after giving birth
- A 16-year-old stretching to get their phone

Consequences of a Fall

The majority of falls do not cause any harm. However, a fall can:

- Decrease a person's confidence
- Increase the fear of falling
- Increase the incidence of a further fall
- Increase dependency
- Delay hospital discharge

In the case of a severe fall, this can have huge consequences for the person and their significant other. This is particularly true when there are other medical conditions such as osteoporosis. Over 3 million people in the United Kingdom have osteoporosis, and they are at much greater risk of fragility fractures. Hip fractures alone account for 1.8 million hospital bed days and £1.9 billion in hospital costs every year, excluding the high cost of social care (PHE 2019).

> **Touch Point**
>
> A fall (in hospital or elsewhere) can be devastating. The human cost of falling can include distress, pain, injury, loss of confidence, loss of independence and increased morbidity and mortality. Falling can also have an impact on family members and other carers of people who fall impacting on quality of life and health and social care costs.

Causes of Falls

The causes of having a fall are multifactorial – a fall is the result of the interplay of multiple risk factors. These include:

- Having a history of falls
- Muscle weakness
- Poor balance
- Visual impairment
- Tiredness
- Alcohol
- Polypharmacy – and the use of certain medicines
- Foot problems or inappropriate footwear
- Environmental hazards and a number of specific conditions
- Having a condition that affects mobility or balance, such as arthritis, diabetes, incontinence, stroke, heart disease, Parkinson's disease, dementia and delirium, will increase the risk of falling

In a Person's Home

- floors are wet, such as in the bathroom, or recently polished
- the lighting in the room is dim
- rugs or carpets are not properly secured
- tripping over pets

- the person reaches for storage areas, such as a cupboard, or is going downstairs
- the person is rushing to get to the toilet during the day or at night
- Another common cause of falls, particularly among older men, is falling from a ladder while carrying out home maintenance work

When a Person is Out and About

- A person has not given time to adjust to changing light when moving outdoors
- Trip hazards such as cracked pavements
- Carrying too much heavy shopping
- Adverse weather conditions

In a Hospital or Residential Health Facility

- Disorientation due to a new environment; remember that disorientation is a normal human reaction and should not be mixed up with confusion
- Call bell not used or is not within reach
- Bed too high
- Walking aid not within reach
- Bed rails not used appropriately
- No suitable footwear available
- Falls in bathroom/toilet especially at night

Yellow Flag

There may be different ethnicity and culture-related factors that could play roles in falling among different cultures and ethnic groups. There is a need for future investigations in various ethnic populations in order to characterise the associated factors in this issue so as to develop preventive strategies for different target groups to be ethnicity and culture-specific.

Assessment and Prevention in the Community (General)

Strength and Balance Training

There are Steady and Strong Classes run by many local authorities. See an example below from Hampshire Council.

http://documents.hants.gov.uk/SteadyandStronginformationleafletforweb2017.pdf

If these types of classes are not available, the following can help prevent falls in the over-65-year-olds.

- Doing regular strength exercises and balance exercises can improve strength and balance.
- Simple activities such as walking and dancing, or specialist training programmes. This needs to be something the person enjoys so that it is not a chore.
- Many community centres and local gyms offer specialist training programmes for older people. It is important that a strength and balance training programme is tailored to the individual and monitored by an appropriately trained professional.
- There is also evidence that taking part in regular tai chi sessions can reduce the risk of falls. Tai chi is a Chinese martial art that places particular emphasis on movement, balance and co-ordination. Unlike other martial arts, tai chi does not involve physical contact or rapid physical movements, making it an ideal activity for older people.

Medication Review

People receiving long-term medication need to have their medicines reviewed annually (NHS 2018). This is particularly important if they are on four or more medicines a day. A review can possibly recommend an alternative medicine or a lower dose and, in some cases, stop the medication where the side effects may increase the risk of a fall.

Supporting Evidence

Review a person's medicines support to check whether it is meeting their needs and preferences. This should be carried out at the time specified in the provider's care plan or sooner if there are changes in the person's circumstances, such as:

- changes to their medicine's regimen
- a concern is raised
- a hospital admission
- a life event, such as a bereavement

Source: (NICE 2017a, 2017b)

Take Note

A medication review is a structured, critical examination of an individual's medicines. It should involve the person or their family members. The objective is to reach an agreement with the person about:

- treatment
- optimising medicines
- minimising medication-related problems
- reducing waste

It involves a multidisciplinary team, including a pharmacist, community matron or specialist nurse (such as a community psychiatric nurse), general practitioner (GP), member of the care home staff and practice nurse or social care practitioner.

Source: Care Quality Commission (2018).

Sight Tests

People should be encouraged to have a regular sight test as poor sight or having certain types of glasses, e.g. bifocals, can increase the risk of falling. For people with reduced mobility, there are some opticians who will make a home visit. Not all vision problems can be cured, but some problems can be treated with surgery – for example, cataracts can be removed using cataract surgery.

Foot Care

People should be encouraged to keep toenails trimmed and, if necessary, request their GP to refer them to a podiatrist for any foot problems. Wearing well-fitting shoes that are in good condition with a non-slip sole and with ankle support will also reduce the risk of falling.

Alcohol

Drinking alcohol can lead to loss of coordination and exaggerate the effects of some medicines. This can significantly increase the risk of a fall, particularly in older people. Avoiding or reducing the amount a person drinks can reduce the risk of having a fall. Excessive drinking can also contribute to the development of osteoporosis.

Assessment and Prevention – Home

Tips for preventing falls in the home include:

- Encourage a person to immediately mop up spillages
- Removal of clutter, trailing wires and frayed carpets
- Use of non-slip mats and rugs
- Use of high-wattage light bulbs in lamps and torches
- Organising the home so that climbing, stretching and bending are kept to a minimum, to avoid bumping into things
- Encourage people to get help with things that they cannot do safely on their own
- Prevent people from walking on slippery floors in socks or tights and not wearing loose fitting and trailing clothing that might trip the person up

Home Hazard Assessment

A formal home hazard assessment can be undertaken in the person's home and should be more than a 'checklist' of hazards. It is essential that the assessment explores how the actual use of the environment affects the person's risk of falling. This will be carried out by a healthcare professional with experience in falls prevention. For example, as the bathroom is a common place where falls occur, many older people can benefit from having bars fitted to the inside of their bath to make it easier for them to get in and out.

Fitting a personal alarm system may also be recommended so that the person can signal for help in the event of a fall. An alternative to this would be to recommend the person always keep a mobile phone in their pocket so they can phone for help after having a fall.

Violet Flag

Getting housing right for older people could have huge benefits for society as well as the economy. Poor housing can have a serious impact on the lives of older people. Damp, unfit and cold housing causes a number of health problems, including respiratory conditions, arthritis, heart disease and stroke as well as mental health problems, which are often caused by stress and anxiety. Hazards in the home and poor accessibility contribute to falls and accidents.

Assessment and Prevention – Hospital and Residential Health Facility

All patients who are over 65 years or who have had a fall or have a history of falls should have a multifactorial risk assessment. This may include:

- Identification of falls history
- Assessment of gait, balance and mobility, strength and muscle weakness

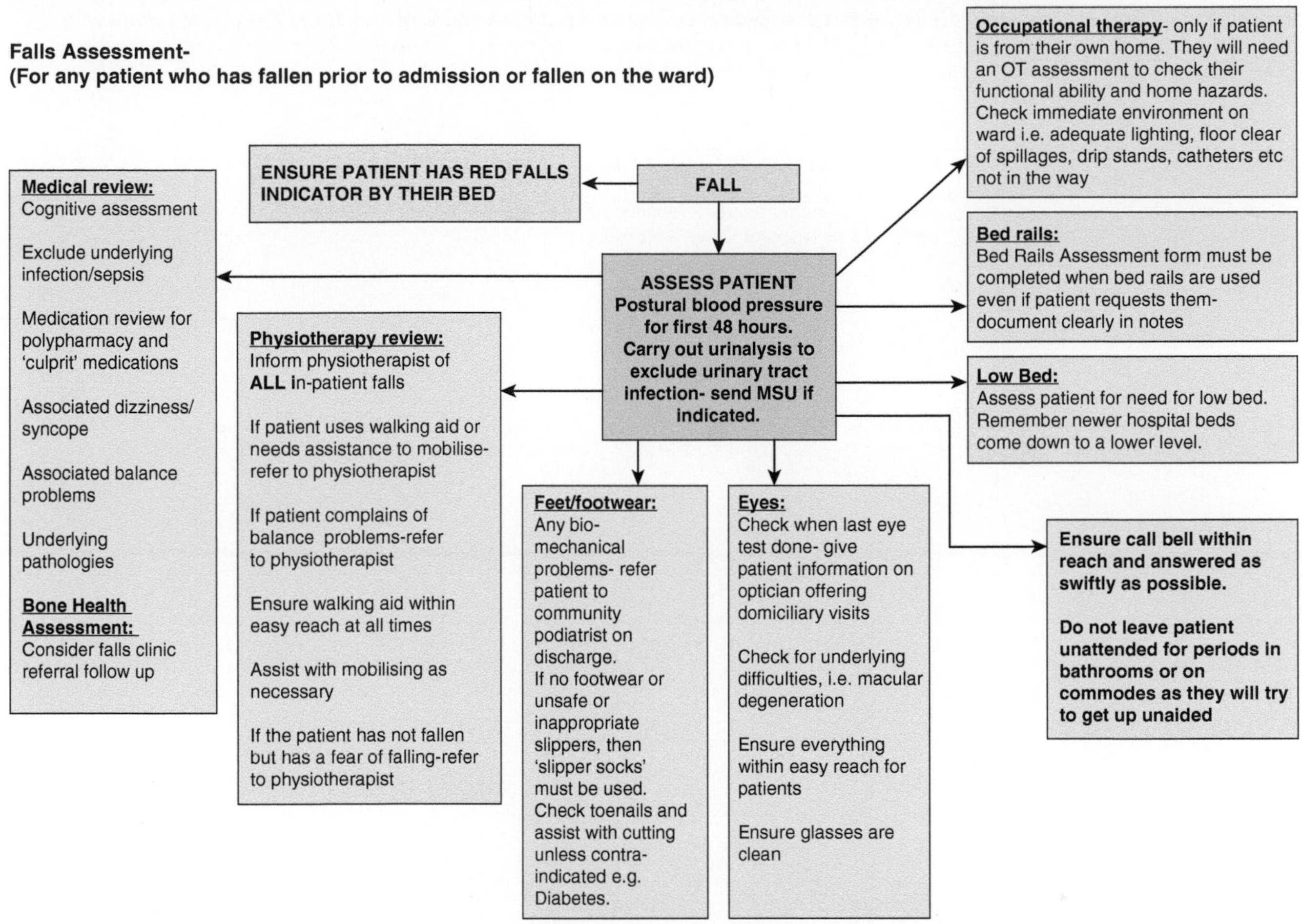

Figure 37.1 **Falls assessment.**

- Assessment of osteoporosis risk
- Assessment of fracture risk
- Assessment of perceived functional ability and fear relating to falling
- Assessment of visual impairment
- Assessment of cognitive impairment and neurological examination
- Assessment of urinary incontinence
- Assessment of home hazards
- Cardiovascular examination and medication review

See Figure 37.1 for flow chart identifying areas that needs to be covered.

The sections are as follows:

Baseline Observations

If a patient has a history of falls or has fallen, it is important that postural blood pressure observations are carried out. In addition, a urinalysis should be carried out to exclude a urinary tract infection.

Medical Review

This includes a cognitive assessment which is often carried out as part of the patient's admission to hospital. An example of this is the Abbreviated Mental Test Score (see Table 37.1).

Physiotherapy Review

This will ensure that the patient is fully assessed and walking aids, if used, are appropriate, and any balance and weakness issues are addressed. A physiotherapist can also perform specialist tests such as the timed get up and go test. This test is basically asking the patient to stand from a chair, walk three metres, turn and come back and sit down in the chair.

If this takes more than 15 seconds, then this may suggest that the patient needs to be more active and a referral to a physiotherapist who can do a full assessment and provide an exercise plan. See link below to a video from the Chartered Society of Physiotherapists.

https://www.csp.org.uk/publications/get-and-go-guide-staying-steady-english-version

Table 37.1 Abbreviated Mental Test Score (each question scores one point). A score of less than 7 suggests dementia.

QUESTION	POINT SCORED
1. Age	
2. Time to the nearest hours	
3. An address – for example, 83 Arcadia lane (N.B. to be repeated by the patient at the end of the test)	
4. Year	
5. Name of the hospital, residential institution or home address (depending or where the patient is situated)	
6. Recognition of two persons – e.g. doctor nurse, community care worker etc.	
7. Date of birth	
8. Year the second world war started	
9. Name of the present monarch	
10. Count backwards 20 to 1	
Total score	

Source: Modified from Hodkinson (1972).

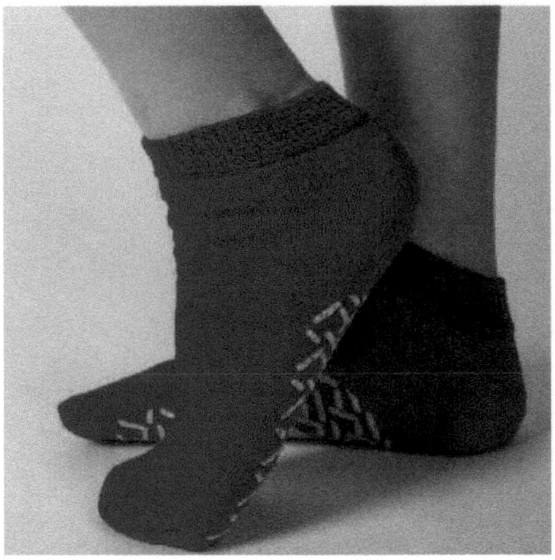

Figure 37.2 An example of footwear with a non-slip sole.

Feet and Footwear

This includes referral to podiatry if needed but also includes the provision of appropriate footwear if the patient does not have them. Footwear should have a non-slip sole; there is an example of them in Figure 37.2.

Eyes

In addition to the clinical checks described earlier, the nursing associate needs to be aware that the patients may not have their glasses on admission, or the glasses they have belong to a spouse. It is also important to ensure that the patient's glasses are clean.

> **Touch Point**
>
> A holistic approach is required in order to ensure the patient risk is assessed and interventions instigated so as to reduce any hazards.

Occupational Therapy

The occupational therapist is essential to ensure there is a smooth discharge home and will often make a home visit before discharge to assess for any equipment and adaptations that may be necessary prior to discharge.

Blue Flag

A key aspect of the role of the nursing associate concerns effective team-working and collaborative practice, multidisciplinary working and care navigation. In assessing and preventing fall, it is essential that a multidisciplinary team approach is taken.

Bedrails

All patients should be assessed prior to using bed rails. Inappropriate use of bed rails can cause serious injury to confused or restless patients, as they may climb over the rails or get trapped. The assessment assesses the patients' mental state and also their mobility. This is plotted on a chart that will give three options:

1. Bedrails recommended
2. Use bedrails with care
3. Bedrails NOT recommended

This assessment should be completed within two hours of admission and needs to be reassessed daily, if the patient's condition changes or if the patient has fallen. See Figure 37.3 for an example of this form.

Green Flag

Each nursing associate must exercise a duty of care. A duty of care is the legal obligation to always act in the best interests of individuals and others and not act or fail to act in a way that results in harm to people. The duty of care is applicable to the use of bed rails, and this must be given much consideration.

Low Beds

These are beds that will go extra low and, therefore, are useful if a patient is restless and confused and is at risk of falling out of bed. 'Crash mats' can be used at the side of the bed so that, if the patient falls, they will have a soft landing. The beds come with bed rails which are transport sides and must only be used when moving the bed with the patient in it. The bed rails must not be put up when the patient is in bed as they may climb over and fall further.

Many newer hospital beds can be lowered further than older beds and, therefore, can be used to reduce risk with the appropriate patient. Be aware that these beds do not come down as low as extra-low beds, which are a specific design.

Take Note

Please note that low beds are not only for patients who are confused but also for patients who are short in stature and need a lower bed to get in and out of it.

Falls Indicator

If a patient is at risk of a fall, it is often prudent to have a sign above the bed giving this information. This can be a sign letting staff know that the patient is a falls risk. There might be a sign for the patients that say 'Call don't fall' to remind them to use the call bell for assistance.

Call Bells

Call bells should always be tested to ensure they are working when a patient is admitted. It is also important that the call bell is within reach of the patient. Patients not only fall because they cannot call for assistance but also when they have to overreach to access the call bell.

Falls Assessment and Care Plan

Falls assessments are usually in two parts: the assessment and the care plan, both parts are completed in all patients over 65 years. Part one is a quick checklist. This covers areas such as:

- Falls history or fear of falling
- Unsteadiness
- Sight problems
- Balance problems
- Taking more than four medicines or taking medicines that increase risk of falls
- Frequency of urine or incontinence
- Is at risk of a fall
- Agitated or disorientated
- Dementia or Parkinson's

If the patient has any of these factors, then a more in-depth assessment should be carried out. This assessment covers all the above areas but with greater depth; see Figure 37.4 for an example of this type of assessment form.

Touch Point

Assessing risk in relation to mobility and falls in the community and hospital settings is a skill that the nursing associate will need to develop. There are a variety of tools available to the nursing associate. The older person who reports a fall or who is considered at risk of falling must be observed for balance and gait deficits, and they should also be considered for their ability to benefit from interventions to improve strength and balance.

A multifactorial assessment requires input from the patient, family and carers, and a multidisciplinary team approach is advocated. The assessment process must be individualised.

Patient Name: ....

Bed Rails Assessment

Complete within 2 hours of admission - Re-assess daily or if patient's condition changes or if patient has fallen.

		Mobility		
		Patient is very immobile (bedbound or hoist dependant)	patient can mobilise with assistance	Patient can mobilise without help from staff
Mental State	Patient is confused and disorientated	Use bedrails with care [A]	Bedrails NOT recommended [A]	Bedrails NOT recommended [A]
	Patient is Drowsy	Bedrails recommended [A]	Use bedrails with care [A]	Bedrails NOT recommended [A]
	Patient is orientated and alert	Bedrails recommended [A]	Bedrails recommended [A]	Bedrails NOT recommended [A]
	Patient is unconcious	Bedrails recommended [A]	N/A [A]	N/A [A]

Initial assessment
Is the use of Bedrails indicated?   **Y/N**   Reason: [ ]

Signature: .... Print name: .... Designation: .... Date & time: ....

Reassess Is the use of Bedrails indicated?   **Y/N**   Reason: [ ]

Signature: .... Print name: .... Designation: .... Date & time: ....

Reassess Is the use of Bedrails indicated?   **Y/N**   Reason: [ ]

Signature: .... Print name: .... Designation: .... Date & time: ....

Reassess Is the use of Bedrails indicated?   **Y/N**   Reason: [ ]

Signature: .... Print name: .... Designation: .... Date & time: ....

Reassess Is the use of Bedrails indicated?   **Y/N**   Reason: [ ]

Signature: .... Print name: .... Designation: .... Date & time: ....

Reassess Is the use of Bedrails indicated?   **Y/N**   Reason: [ ]

Signature: .... Print name: .... Designation: .... Date & time: ....

Reassess Is the use of Bedrails indicated?   **Y/N**   Reason: [ ]

Signature: .... Print name: .... Designation: .... Date & time: ....

Figure 37.3 **Bed rails assessment.**

Patient Name: ....

Falls Prevention and Assessment Care Plan:

To reduce likelihood of falls whilst maintaining dignity and independence

Individual problems	State specific care planned for patient:
☐ **History of falling/fear of falling** **Nurse near to nurses' station and supervise with mobilising** Identify patient at risk with falls indicator Refer patient to physiotherapist Assist patient with mobilising Ask about previous falls and injuries sustained. Ask about fear of falling Ensure bed side chair is on same side as patient gets out of bed at home	Number of falls since admission: location of patient's bed:
☐ **Postural Hypotension/postural stability syncope:** **Advise patient to stand up/get up slowly** **Postural BP for 48 hours** / as directed by ward DR Before patient gets out of bed advise them to sit on edge of bed and move their feet up and down to increase flow back up from feet Ensure optimal oral hydration. Ask patient if they fell dizzy on standing/feel off balance	I & S BP on assessment:
☐ **Eyesight:** **Ensure patient has glasses if worn, they are clean and within reach** Carry out basic eye test as below: Ask patient if they can see a pen held at end of bed/count fingers/read a newspaper headline	
☐ **Toilet use:** **ARMS reach approach-patents at risk of falling must not be left alone in the toilet/on the commode** Carry out basic continence assessment; Any urgency/Stress incontinence Frequency- report results to any of these to ward doctor Monitor bowel function to prevent constipation Regular planned visits to toilet If catheterised, apply leg bag during the day	Urinalysis on assessment:
☐ **Cognitive impairment:** **Ensure patient is on the pathway for cognitively impaired patients over 65 (to include patient identifiers on wards and 6 point checklist)** Is the cognitive impairment chronic (dementia) or acute (delirium) or acute on chronic- (delirium on top of dementia)? Refer to managing challenging behaviour in older adults with cognitive impairment policy (complete behaviour charts if required) Be aware of: 1. Ensure patient is closely monitored on the ward and assess best position for patient on the ward 2. lack of safety awareness/own limitations 3. Tries to mobilise/transfer/get up unassisted but unsteady 4. Reduce ward moves/transfers as far as possible 5. Reassure patient and speak calmly and dearly with clear instructions/ advice 6. Discuss with nurse in charge if 1 to 1 nursing is indicated	Cognitive assessment score: Delirium Assessment completed on .... (Date) Challenging Behaviour Chart completed: y ☐ / NA ☐
☐ **Mobility:** **If patient uses walking aid or is unable to get out of chair without** help or is unsteady when walking - refer to physio If patient uses a walking aid ensure the walking aid is within easy reach If in-patient fall refer to physiotherapist and OT Refer to Falls team/community rehab when planning patient discharge Ensure GP/community teams are informed if patient falls in hospital	
☐ **Footwear/ feet:** **Supply patient with slipper socks if necessary** Check footwear for secure fit. non-slip sole. no trailing laces. Give patient advice on self referral to chiropodist on discharge and referral form	
☐ **Neuromuscular Diseases:** Refer to appropriate Nurse specialist Ensure medication is given at correct time as charted	
☐ **Medication:** Check for any medication associated with falls risk i.e. anti hypertensive/ sedation. Ask doctor I pharmacist to review medication. **Following a fall inform doctor if patient is on any anti coagulation therapy or if platelet count is < 50**	
Post Fall:	
Post Falls Observations and pathway commenced: Y ☐ N ☐	CT scan: Y ☐ N/A ☐ Xray: Y ☐ N/A ☐
Post Falls care plan No: 9 commenced: Y ☐ N ☐	Falls indict tor by bed: Y ☐ N ☐
Patient reviewed by medical team: Y ☐ N ☐	Pink form and Sticker used: Y ☐ N ☐

Date: .... Signature: ....

Figure 37.4 Falls prevention and assessment.

(Continued)

Patient Name: ....

Falls Prevention and Assessment

Complete within 2 hours of admission, then weekly and after a Fall or on Transfer

Is patient over 65? Y/N

Yes = go straight to Falls Prevention Care Plan **Part 2**
No = Complete trigger questions in Part 1.
If any question = yes then go to Falls Prevention and Assessment Care plan Part 2

FALLS PREVENTION AND ASSESSMENT - PART 1

	Date and time of assessment		
	Yes	**No**	**Comments**
Admitted after a fall/history of falls?			
Tries to walk alone but unsteady/ unsafe/dizzy			
Problems with sight			
Problems with balance			
Is the patient on 4 or more medications/ or prescribed sedatives/ antipsychotics			
Incontinence or frequency affecting safety			
Are there any concerns that the patient is at risk of falls?			
Is the patient agitated/ disorientated or unaware of their safety limitations?			
Dementia/Parkinsons			Ensure patient is on dementia care pathway Inform Parkinson's disease nurse specialist of patient's admission
Signature and designation:			

FALLS PREVENTION AND ASSESSMENT CARE PLAN - PART 2

AIM: To reduce likelihood of falls whilst maintaining dignity and independence	
For all patients:	**Date & Time & Signature**
1. Explain the importance of asking for help when needed and show patient how to use call bell **(if patient is unable to use call bell/forgets to use - patient will need to be moved nearer to nurses' station and/or closely supervised)** 2. Ensure bed rails assessment carried out- bed rails not to be used on anyone with cognitive impairment who is attempting to get out of bed 3. **Leave bed at lowest height** 4. Maintain SSKIN bundle 5. Handover patient's falls risk at start of each shift and also to OT and Physio 6. Provide falls information leaflets for patient and their NOK/ family 7. Ensure falls indicator by bed if required 8. Re-assessment to be done weekly/if clinical conditions changes or patient has a fall/or if patient transferred to another ward 9. Following a fall ensure that all lacerations and bruising are entered on to the Body map	

Figure 37.4 **(Continued)**

If a Patient Has Had a Fall

There should be a local protocol to be followed in the event of the patient falling. This should include:

- Checks by healthcare professionals for signs or symptoms of fracture and potential for spinal injury before the patient is moved.
- Safe manual handling methods for patients with signs or symptoms of fracture or potential for spinal injury (community hospitals and mental health units without the necessary equipment or staff expertise may be able to achieve this in collaboration with emergency services).
- Frequency and duration of neurological observations for all patients where head injury has occurred or cannot be excluded (for example, unwitnessed falls) based on the NICE guidelines on head injury.
- Timescales for medical examination after a fall (including fast-track assessment for patients who show signs of serious injury, are highly vulnerable to injury or have been immobilised); medical examination should be completed within a maximum of 12 hours, or 30 minutes if fast-tracked.
- The timely reporting of the fall as per incident reporting procedure. This needs to include input from any persons who witnessed the fall.
- A system should be in place for staff to debrief and see if there are any learning action points that need to be taken in light of the fall.
- The post-fall protocol should be easily accessible.

Take Note

Nursing associates must make themselves familiar with local policies and procedures with regard to what to do in the event of a fall occurring.

Touch Points – Revisited

- Although most falls cause no harm for people over 65 years, the risks increase. This can cause distress, pain and injury, loss of confidence and loss of independence.
- Causes of falls are multifactorial. These need to be investigated whether the fall is at home, in the community or in hospital.
- Keeping fit and healthy will help reduce risk of falls.
- Patients on numerous medications need to be regularly reviewed to see if the side effects of their medication could be increasing their risk of falling.
- A formal home hazard assessment can reduce the risk of falls at home.
- Always complete a bedrails assessment form before using them.
- Aim to complete a falls risk assessment and care plan as soon as possible after a patient's admission to hospital.
- Simple interventions such as ensuring correct footwear and ensuring the patient's glasses are clean can reduce the risk of falls.
- Ensure that patients in bed can reach their call bell and encourage them to use it if appropriate.
- Use the skills of the whole multidisciplinary team to assess the patient's risk of falls and develop a risk-reducing plan.

References

Care Quality Commission. (2018) *Medicines reconciliation and medication review.* [online] Available: https://www.cqc.org.uk/guidance-providers/adult-social-care/medicines-reconciliation-medication-review. Accessed September 2019.

Hodkinson, H.M. (1972) Evaluation of a mental test score for assessment of mental impairment in the elderly, *Age and Ageing*, 4(1): 233–238.

NHS. (2018) *Prevention: falls.* [online] Available: https://www.nhs.uk/conditions/falls/prevention/. Accessed September 2019.

National Institute for Health and Care Excellence. (2017a) Falls in older people, *Quality standard [QS86] Published date: March 2015 Last updated: January 2017.* [online] Available: https://www.nice.org.uk/guidance/qs86/chapter/Quality-statement-1-Identifying-people-at-risk-of-falling. Accessed September 2019.

National Institute for Health and Care Excellence. (2017b) *Managing medicines for adults receiving social care in the community. [online] Available*: https://www.nice.org.uk/guidance/ng67/resources/managing-medicines-for-adults-receiving-social-care-in-the-community-pdf-1837578800581. Accessed September 2019.

Nursing and Midwifery Council. (2018) The code, *Professional standards of behaviour for nurses, midwives and nursing associates*, London: NMC.

Public Health England. (2019) *Falls: applying all our health.* [online] Available: https://www.gov.uk/government/publications/falls-applying-all-our-health/falls-applying-all-our-health. Accessed September 2019.

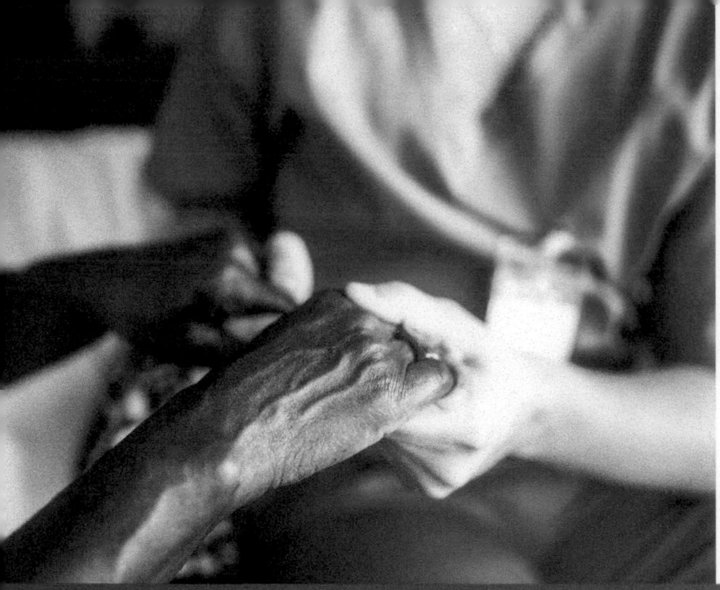

38

Using a Range of Moving and Handling Techniques, Aids and Equipment

Hamish MacGregor

Docklands Training Consultants Ltd, Portpatrick, UK

Chapter Aim

- **To provide the reader with fundamental skills in moving and handling to ensure safe evidence-based practice.**

Learning Outcomes

By the end of the chapter, the reader should be able to:

- **Understand the key pieces of legislation related to moving and handling and apply them to practice**
- **Understand the importance of good back health and the promotion of good musculoskeletal health**
- **Understand the moving and handling risk assessment**
- **Apply the safe principles of moving and handling in the patient setting**
- **To apply (after suitable and sufficient face-to-face practical moving and handling training) some safer handling techniques within a hospital, residential or community setting.**

Test Yourself Multiple Choice Questions

1. **If you are offered moving and handling training by your employer and given the time to attend, you should:**
   A) **Attend when asked**
   B) **Attend if you think you need an update**
   C) **It is up to you to decide if you need training**
2. **If you develop low back pain:**
   A) **Have bed rest until the pain eases**
   B) **Stay in work and gradually resume normal activities**
   C) **Ignore it and hope it goes away**

The Nursing Associate's Handbook of Clinical Skills, First Edition. Edited by Ian Peate.

Companion website: www.wiley.com/nursingassociate

3. **If you have back pain and it does not clear up after 6–8 weeks, you should:**
   A) **Take lots of pain killers**
   B) **See a physiotherapist or GP**
   C) **Take some time off sick**
4. **The component parts of a moving and handling risk assessment are:**
   A) **Task, Individual Capability, Load or Person, Environment, Equipment and Other Factors**
   B) **Task, Strength, Load or Person, Environment, Equipment and Other Factors**
   C) **Technique, Individual Capability, Load or Person, Environment, Equipment and Other Factors**
5. **When using a hoist to move a patient from bed to chair:**
   A) **The brakes must be ON when lifting the patient**
   B) **The brakes must be OFF when lifting the patient**
   C) **It does not matter if the brakes are OFF or ON**

Introduction

The Royal College of Nursing (2019) makes it clear that no one should routinely manually lift patients. There is equipment available that can be used as substitutes for manual lifting, for example, hoists, sliding aids and electric profiling beds. Patient manual handling, it adds, should only continue in those cases that do not involve lifting most or all of a patient's weight. A balanced approach to managing the risks from patient handling is required and these will include:

- care workers are not required to perform tasks that will put them and those they offer care and support to at risk unreasonably
- the patient's personal wishes on mobility are to be respected wherever this is possible
- the patient's independence and autonomy must be supported as fully as possible

This chapter provides the nursing associate with an overview of the fundamental aspects of moving and handling techniques, aids and equipment. It is not possible in a chapter of this size to address all issues associated with moving and handling techniques, aids and equipment. MacGregor (2016) provides a comprehensive discussion of moving and handling patients.

At all times, the nursing associate is required to ensure adherence to any local policies and procedures that pertain to manual handling. Demonstrating competence is a key aspect of the role and function of the nursing associate; this just as important when engaging in any manual lifting, moving and handing of people or loads.

The Nursing and Midwifery Council (NMC) (2018) requires nursing associates to demonstrate proficiencies in a number of spheres.

The Nursing Associate Proficiencies

The nursing associate must demonstrate proficiency in the provision of support with mobility and safety:
6.3 use a range of contemporary moving and handling techniques and mobility aids
6.4 use appropriate moving and handling equipment to support people with impaired mobility

The Law and Moving and Handling

There are a number of legal aspects that need to be addressed in relation to moving and handling. This section highlights the fundamental issues required to promote safety; many elements of legislation refer to the responsibilities of employers and employees.

Green Flag

The law surrounding manual handling is vast. Legislation dictates that all employers have a legal responsibility to ensure the health and safety at work of their staff. The Health and Safety at Work Act 1974 and other legislation place general duties on employers and employees.

The Health and Safety At Work Act 1974 (HSWA)

An umbrella Act covering much of the legal aspects and deals in general terms about moving and handling. Key areas the nursing associate must take particular note of include:

Employer requirements:

- Provide safe equipment and a safe system of work.
- Provide safety in connection with the use, storage and transport of loads (including people) and substances hazardous to health.
- Provide information, instruction, training and supervision.

- Maintain a safe working environment.
- Provide a written health and safety policy statement.

Employee requirements:

- Take reasonable care of their own health and safety, and of others who may be affected by their acts or omissions. If a moving and handling technique is unsafe, the nursing associate should say no and ask for a further moving and handling assessment to be carried out.
- Not damage or disable equipment.
- Be willing to receive training. If offered moving and handling training and given the time to attend, you must, as far as is reasonably practical, attend that training.

The Management of Health and Safety at Work Regulations 1999 (MHSWR)

- Risk assessments are required to be carried out by a competent person.
- In order to carry out the risk assessments, hazardous activities in the workplace need to be identified.
- Hazard is defined as something with the potential to cause harm.
- Risk is defined as the chance or likelihood that harm will occur.
- Risk needs to be reduced to: 'so far as is reasonably practicable'.

Manual Handling Operations Regulations 1992 as Amended in 2002 (MHOR)

This is an important piece of legislation and encompasses clearly where this legal requirement affects your moving and handling practice.

The *employer* has a duty to:

- Avoid manual handling tasks so far as is reasonably practicable. Avoid manual handling in relation to patient care; encourage the patients to do as much for themselves as possible. This increases independence, promotes dignity and well-being and can reduce a hospital stay.

Yellow Flag

Ensure at all times when assisting the person with moving and handling activities that the person's dignity is maintained, paying particular attention to individual values and beliefs, respecting and responding to fears and anxieties.

- Assess all handling tasks where there is a perceived risk. As a nursing associate, you may be asked to assist the employer in completing formal risk assessments and patient handling plans. It is important to realise that in your role as a nursing associate, you carry out informal risk assessments all the time as you interact with a patient. The more experience gained as a nursing associate will fine-tune these skills.
- Reduce the risk as far as is reasonably practicable. The legislation talks of reducing risk not removing risk. Every time we move and handle a patient, there is a risk to them and us, however small that may be. If you think that risk is still unreasonably high, you need to ask for a further risk assessment.
- Review all assessments as changes take place and/or at regular scheduled intervals. In acute areas, patients' conditions tend to change more rapidly; therefore, the assessment process is dynamic. If the patient is in a longer stay area such as nursing home or receiving domiciliary care their condition may not fluctuate from day to day; therefore, having a set time to carry out a reassessment needs to be decided upon. This should allow the care team, the patient and their significant other's input into the risk assessment process.

The *employee* has a duty to:

- Follow appropriate systems provided for the handling of loads by the employer, adhering to risk assessment and their associated moving and handling plans. If you disagree with this, then based on your or a colleague's risk assessment, you may choose to take another course of action. Under the HSWA, you are responsible for your own health and safety and that of your colleagues.
- Report accidents and near-miss events. In health and social care, we are skilled at reporting accidents but less good at reporting 'near misses'. A near miss could be that the patient nearly fell when they were being mobilised. If this is reported and the hazard that nearly caused the fall, e.g. a broken tile on the floor is identified, this might prevent an actual fall occurring with another patient.

Touch Point

We all have a role to play in ensuring that the law, local policy and procedure are adhered to when we engage in moving and handing.

Lifting Operation and Lifting Equipment Regulations 1998 (LOLER) and the Provision and Use of Work Equipment Regulations 1998 (PUWER)

Both pieces of legislation apply to equipment. LOLER applies to equipment whose primary function is to lift, and PUWER applies to other equipment; for example, an electric profiling bed will lift a patient but its primary function is a bed not a lifting device, whereas a hoist is a lifting device.

Supporting Evidence

The Health and Safety Executive website document *How the Lifting Operations and Lifting Equipment Regulations apply to health and social care* provides further information.
http://www.hse.gov.uk/pubns/hsis4.pdf

Lifting Operation and Lifting Equipment Regulations 1998 (LOLER)

- Lifting equipment should have adequate strength and stability for its proposed use
- Risk from positioning and installing lifting equipment be minimised as far as is reasonably possible
- Equipment has to be marked indicating its safe working load
- Equipment which lifts people to be examined by a competent person at six monthly intervals

Provision and Use of Work Equipment Regulations 1998 (PUWER)

- Ensure work equipment is used for operations for which it is suitable
- Is maintained efficiently and a maintenance log is kept up

Take Note

It is a legal requirement that equipment is maintained and that there is evidence that maintenance has taken place.

Keeping Your Back, Neck and Shoulders Healthy

Working in health care involves using good moving and handling techniques. Most people worldwide will experience back pain during their lifetime. It can be disabling and worrying, but it is very common and rarely dangerous; the spine is a strong, stable structure and not easily damaged; so, in most instances, this is a simple sprain or strain. According to research, 98% of people recover reasonably quickly, and many do so without treatment (Charted Society of Physiotherapists 2017). Some people experience repeat episodes, which can be distressing, but these are rarely dangerous.

If you do develop back pain, avoid bedrest, stay in work and gradually resume normal activities. Scientific studies now indicate prolonged rest and avoidance of activity for people with low back pain actually leads to higher levels of pain, greater disability, poorer recovery and longer absence from work. In the first few days of a new episode of low back pain, avoiding aggravating activities may help to relieve pain (Charted Society of Physiotherapists 2017). However, staying as active as possible and returning to all usual activities gradually is important in aiding recovery – this includes staying in work where possible. While it is normal to move differently and more slowly in the first few days of having back pain, this altered movement can be unhealthy if continued in the long term.

Some Ways of Keeping the Back, Neck and Shoulders Healthy

Exercise and Activity Reduce and Prevent Back Pain

Exercise is shown to be very helpful for tackling back pain and is also the most effective strategy to prevent future episodes. Start slowly and build up both the amount and intensity of what you do, and do not worry if it is sore to begin with – you will not be damaging your back. No one type of exercise is proven to be more effective than others, choose an exercise you enjoy, that you can afford to maintain in the long term and that fits in with your daily schedule.

Get Good Quality Sleep

The importance of sleep in tackling back pain has become increasingly clear in recent years. This is because it reduces stress and improves overall well-being, making you less susceptible to the triggers of pain in the first instance and helping you to cope when it does occur. It is important to know that there is no best position or type of mattress – whatever feels most comfortable for you is best.

You can have Back Pain Without Any Damage or Injury

Many physical or psychological factors can cause back pain and often a combination of these are involved.

They could be:

- Physical factors, such as 'protecting' the back and avoiding movements, or a simple strain.
- Psychological factors, including a fear of damage or not getting better, feeling down or being stressed.

- More general health and lifestyle factors, like being tired and rundown, not getting enough good quality sleep, being overweight or not getting enough physical activity.
- Social triggers, such as difficult relationships at work or home, low job satisfaction or stressful life events, such as a bereavement or illness. All pain is 100% real, and it is never 'all in your head', even when factors such as stress or mood are involved.

Each of the factors can turn up the volume of pain, and gaining a greater understanding of when that can happen puts you in a stronger position to recognise them and learn how to turn down the dial again.

- If it does not clear up, seek help but do not worry.
- If back pain does not clear up after 6–8 weeks, see the GP or physiotherapist.
- Physiotherapists provide expert advice, guidance and treatment for back pain.
- This is to help reduce your chances of future episodes, while improving your overall health and well-being.
  Symptoms to be aware of:
  These symptoms are very rare, but you should contact a doctor if you experience any of them:
- Difficulty passing urine or having the sensation to pass urine that is not there
- Numbness/tingling in genitals or buttocks
- Loss of bladder or bowel control
- Impaired sexual function, such as loss of sensation during intercourse
- Loss of power in legs
- Feeling unwell with back pain, such as a fever or significant sweating that wakes you from sleep

Supporting Evidence

For further information on back care, see the following link to two short videos giving current thinking on good back care: http://www.pain-ed.com/blog/2019/08/30/myths-about-back-pain/

Touch Point

- It is essential to know about safe moving and handling so that you do not hurt yourself or the person you are looking after.
- The most common injuries carers get are back injuries. Injuring your back can limit your movement and your ability to care for someone.
- If you do develop back pain, avoid bedrest, stay in work and gradually resume normal activities.
- Lifting someone incorrectly can also damage fragile skin, cause shoulder and neck injuries, increase existing breathing difficulties or cause bruising or cuts.

Key Safe Principles of Moving and Handling

These principles must underpin all moving and handling practice.

- Avoid moving and handling if it is at all practicable to do so. In relation to patient handling, encourage the patient to do as much for themselves as possible.
- Keep the spine in line. This is keeping the spine in its natural curves and keeping it in a neutral position. It does not mean that you keep your spine 'poker straight', nor does it mean you cannot bend or stretch. The back loves to move and is strong but avoid end of range movements where you may be twisting and holding a load for a lengthy period of time.
- Hold the load close. This is keeping the load, and, in some circumstances, this may be a patient, as close to your body as possible. As we hold a load away from us, it effectively gets heavier. A weight held at arm's length can feel as much as five times as heavy.
- Having a stable mobile base with soft flexible knees.

Take Note

There are a number of principles that must underpin all moving and handling practice.

The nursing associate should ensure they stand with the feet shoulder-width apart, one foot slightly in front of the other with soft flexible knees. When this stance is adopted, this permits the handler to transfer their weight back and forth making use of their quadriceps and gluteal muscles.

Risk Assessment

There are six component parts in a moving and handling risk assessment:

1. The task
2. The individual capability
3. The load or person
4. The environment
5. The equipment that is being used
6. Other influencing factors

Task

The application of the safe principles of moving and handling is fundamental to any moving and handling task. If you are unable to keep your spine in line, the load close and adopt a mobile stable base with soft flexible knees, then the task may need closer scrutiny.

Consideration need to be given to the following:

- Task redesign
- Introduction of equipment
- Increase in staffing levels
- Re-training staff

Individual Capability

All individuals who handle loads and/or people are different; therefore, the handlers are a key element of the risk assessment process. We all have different levels of fitness and stamina affecting the ability to perform throughout the day.

Factors to address are, does the job:

- Require a certain level of fitness?
- Present a risk to those who have pre-existing health problems?
- Constitute a hazard to those who are pregnant?
- Require specialised training?
- Require a certain level of knowledge, skills and competency?
- Become more risky at certain times of the day?

Blue Flag

Employers should reduce very heavy physical activities and lifting for pregnant workers where possible, particularly in late pregnancy. However, if a pregnant worker who has been informed of the possible risk wishes to continue, then there are insufficient grounds to impose restrictions against her will.

Source: Royal College of Physicians (2009).

Load or Person

The Manual Handling Operation Regulations (1992) provide guidelines for when an inanimate load needs to be risk assessed based on weight and its position in relation to the body. People are complex; *therefore, remember there are no safe working loads.*

Factors that may need to be considered in relation to loads:

- Heavy?
- Bulky?
- Difficult to grasp?
- Unstable or have an uneven weight distribution?
- Potentially harmful, for example, hot?

Factors that may need to be considered in relation to patient handling:

Many of the previous load factors can be applied to people. In addition, consider the following:

- Medical conditions that will affect handling
- Level of understanding
- Level of cooperation
- Conscious level
- Pain
- Attachments: intravenous lines, catheters, drains and so on

Environment

Consider the following factors:

- Is there enough space?
- Type of flooring?
- Are stairs to be negotiated?
- Is there a good ergonomic layout?
- Are obstacles in the way?
- Is the temperature conducive to the work being carried out?
- Is there sufficient lighting?

Violet Flag

When caring for people in their own homes or when working in environments that may have limited space, for example, the back of an ambulance, a police or prison custody cell, the nursing associate must consider the environment and determine the best way to ensure that the activity they are undertaking is safe for the person being cared for and for themselves. There may be a need to engage other members of the emergency services if needed.

Equipment

Factors that may need to be considered:

- Is it appropriate for the task?
- Has the safe working load been identified?
- Is it in good working order and free from damage?
- Has it been serviced/checked in accordance with legal requirements, for example LOLER?
- Do the staff require any special training to operate the equipment?

Other Influencing Factors

The areas below can be relevant to the risk assessment process:

- Levels of stress or other psychosocial factors
- Poor staffing levels or staffing levels supplemented by high numbers of temporary staff
- Pressures of work or at home
- Organisational policies

Practical Moving and Handling

The handling techniques described below are some of the more common techniques used, but this is not an extensive list. It is important that the nursing associate receives suitable and sufficient training from a moving and handling practitioner before carrying out any techniques. For extensive guidance, see MacGregor (2016). There are four techniques now described:

1. Assessing a patient before standing them up from a chair
2. Safely helping a patient to stand from a chair while maintaining a good posture
3. Inserting two flat slide sheets underneath a patient in bed from the top of the bed
4. To move a patient up the bed who is unable to do so with two flat slide sheets

1. **Assessing a patient before standing them up from a chair**

Prior to the assessment

1. Consult any handling plans relating to this patient. Check that they are clear, up-to-date and regularly reviewed.
2. If there is no written plan, ask your colleagues if they have relevant information relating to this patient.
3. Communicate with the patient and tell them what you plan to do. Ensure that they understand and obtain their consent.

Orange Flag

Before the nursing associate or anyone else looking after a person's health treats the person, that person must give their consent. That means the person must agree, and they need to understand the likely benefits and possible risks before agreeing. This respects the person's physical and mental health.

4. Ensure that the patient has suitable footwear before they attempt to stand, for example, flat enclosed shoes.

During the assessment

1. Get down to the side of the patient's chair. Be careful to ensure that you have a good posture.
2. Ask if you can put the edge of your hand on their knee and ask if they can lift their knee up against your hand (Figure 38.1). This will allow you to test if the patient has strength in their quadriceps. Do not use the flat of the hand as this can appear invasive and for some patients compromise their dignity.

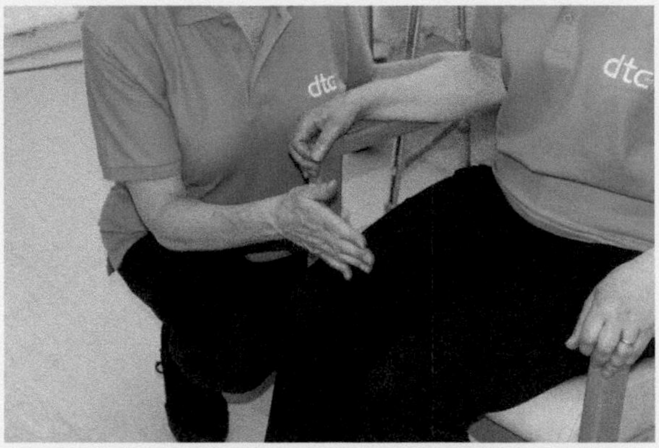

Figure 38.1 Testing strength in patient's legs. *Source:* MacGregor (2016), figure 14.1, p. 30. © John Wiley & Sons.

3. Ask the patient to straighten their leg and place your hand so that patient can aim for it (Figure 38.2).

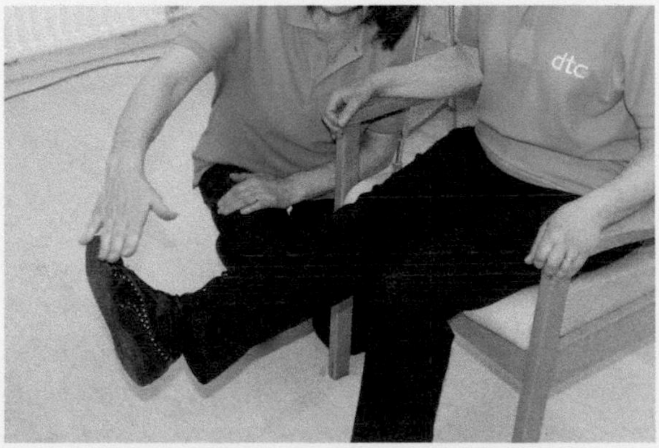

Figure 38.2 Testing range of movement in patient's legs. *Source:* MacGregor (2016), figure 14.2, p. 30. © John Wiley & Sons.

The patient needs to be able to fully straighten their leg. As the patient brings their leg down, put your hand underneath the patient's calf and feel the resistance on the way down (Figure 38.3).

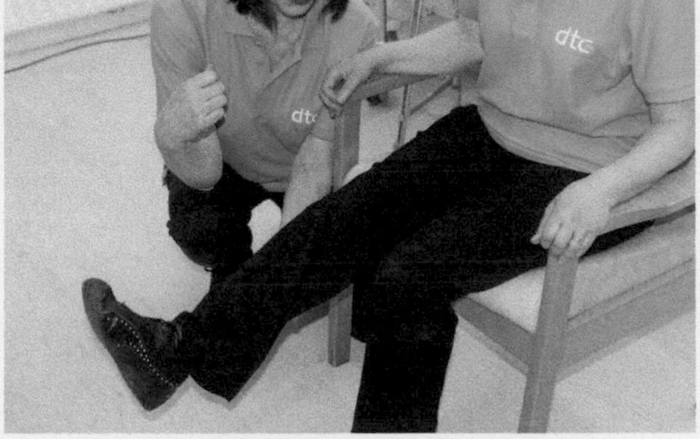

Figure 38.3 Testing strength and range of movement in patient's legs. *Source:* MacGregor (2016), figure 14.3, p. 30. © John Wiley & Sons.

4. Move round to the other side of the chair and repeat the procedure. Note: If there are two handlers, it is important only one does the assessment of both legs.
5. Stand in a stable base in front of the patient and get them to push gently down on your hands. Check that the arm strength is equal (Figure 38.4). Note: Stand with your feet shoulder-width apart, one foot slightly in front of the other with flexed knees and your weight balanced between them.

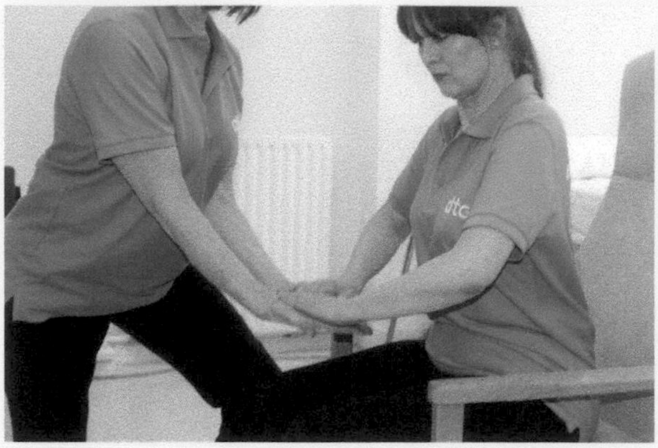

Figure 38.4 Testing strength in patient's arms. *Source:* MacGregor (2016), figure 14.4, p. 30. © John Wiley & Sons.

6. Ask the patient to shuffle forward in the chair, holding on to the arms of the chair (Figure 38.5).

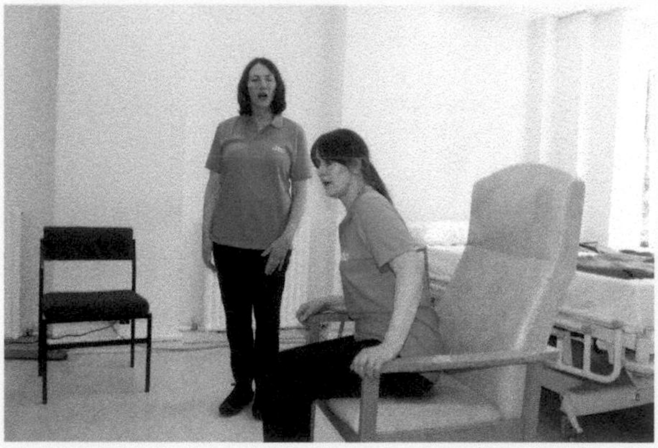

Figure 38.5 Encouraging the patient to move forward in the chair. *Source:* MacGregor (2016), figure 14.5, p. 30. © John Wiley & Sons.

7. Once the patient is forward in the chair, ask the patient to put their hands on their knees. This will allow you to assess if they have any sitting balance. Patients may cover up poor balance by keeping hold of the arms of the chair (Figure 38.6).

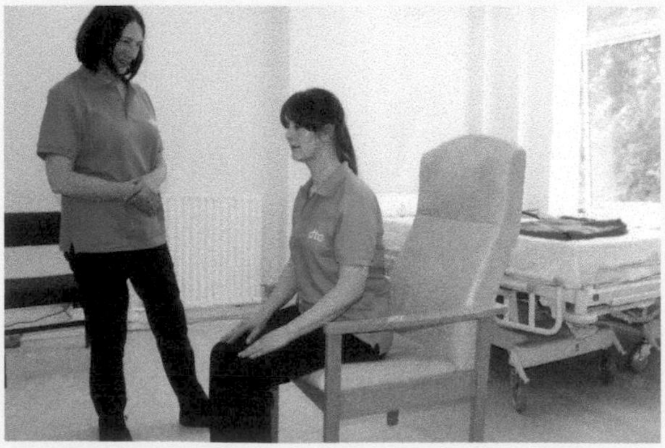

Figure 38.6 Checking the patient's sitting balance. *Source:* MacGregor (2016), figure 14.6, p. 30. © John Wiley & Sons.

	8. During this task, you will also be able to assess whether the patient has good cognition, as they will have had to follow instructions.
After the assessment	**1.** Check that the patient has no pain and/or discomfort. **2.** Ensure that they are far enough forward in the chair to stand. **3.** 3. If the patient uses any walking aids, ensure that they are at hand, and the patient can reach them easily when preparing to stand up.

2. To safely stand a patient from a chair whilst maintaining a good posture	
Prior to the handling task	**1.** Consult any handling plans relating to this patient and check that it is clear, up-to-date and regularly reviewed. **2.** If there is no written plan, ask your colleagues if they have relevant information relating to this patient. **3.** Ensure a suitable and sufficient assessment has been carried out beforehand. See the preceding point titled 'Assessing a patient before standing them up from a chair'. **4.** Ensure that the patient has suitable footwear before they attempt to stand, that is, flat enclosed shoes. **5.** Communicate with the patient and tell them what you plan to do. Ensure that they understand and obtain their consent. **6.** Make a final check that the patient cannot do this for themselves before continuing with the task. **7.** Ensure that they are at the front of the chair.
During the task	**1.** Stand at the side of the patient's chair in a walk stance position with your feet in the direction you are facing, with your inside leg back and outside leg in front. **2.** Ask the patient to put one foot in front of the other. If the patient has a weakness on one side, check again if it is safe to stand them, and if so, ensure their strong leg is placed back and the weak leg is placed forward. You will need to stand on the weak side. If necessary, get the help of another handler to stand on the opposite side. **3.** Place your hand nearest the patient in the centre of their lower back below the waistline (Figure 38.7) or, if it does not involve too much stretching, put your hand on the opposite iliac crest (Figure 38.8).

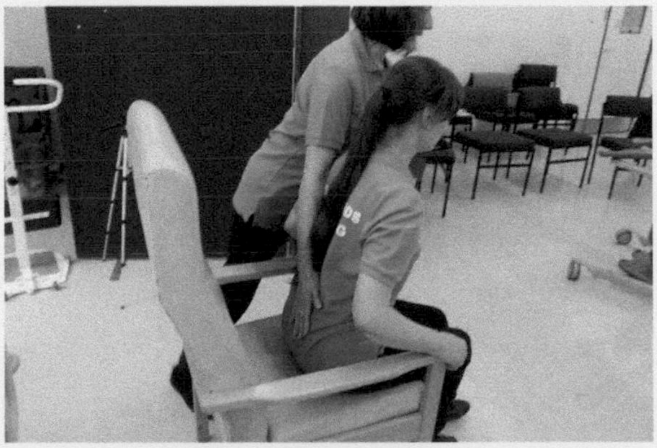

Figure 38.7 Place your hand nearest the patient on their lower back. *Source:* MacGregor (2016), figure 16.1, p. 34. © John Wiley & Sons.

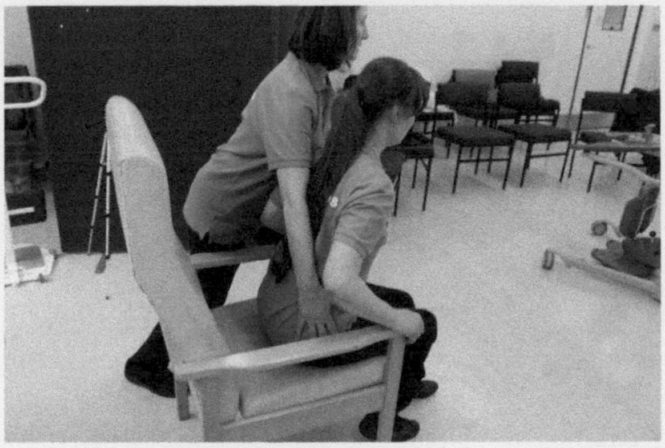

Figure 38.8 Alternatively place your hand on the patient's iliac crest. *Source:* MacGregor (2016), figure 16.2, p. 34. © John Wiley & Sons.

4. Place your hand furthest away from the patient, in front of the patient's shoulder (Figure 38.9).

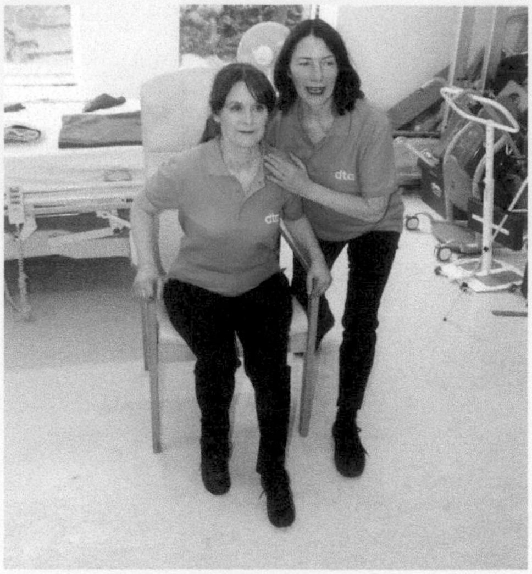

Figure 38.9 **Place your other hand on the patient's shoulder.** *Source:* MacGregor (2016), figure 16.3, p. 34. © John Wiley & Sons.

5. Using the clear verbal instructions of 'Ready, Steady, Stand', ask the patient to stand up, bringing their head forward with their nose coming over their toes and pushing with their arms on the side of the chair. The patient should be leading the move with you guiding. Do not rock the patient unless it has been identified in the risk assessment that this is necessary (Figure 38.10.). Avoid using '1, 2, 3', as the patient may be unsure if they move on the '3' or the imaginary '4'. An exception to this may be with a patient who has stood successfully at home on '1, 2, 3', with carers but due to problems of cognition, such as dementia or learning disability, it may be difficult to learn new commands. In this case it is incumbent on the handlers to find out if the patient stands on '3' or the imaginary '4'. This then needs to be documented in the patient's handling plan and communicated to the rest of the team.

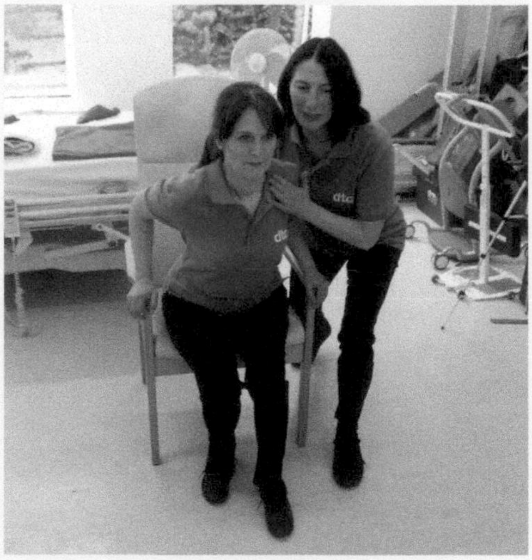

Figure 38.10 **Encourage the patient to stand using clear instructions.** *Source:* MacGregor (2016), figure 16.4, p. 34. © John Wiley & Sons.

6. When the patient has stood up, stay close by them, keeping your hand around their back and your hand on the shoulder until they are steady (Figure 38.11).

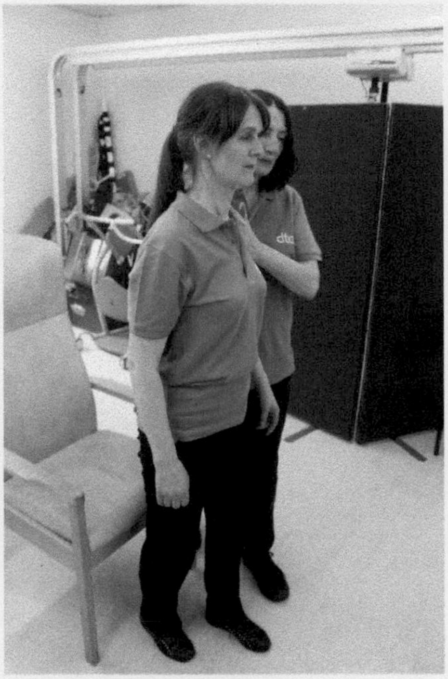

Figure 38.11 Stay close to the patient when the stand. *Source:* MacGregor (2016), figure 16.5, p. 34. © John Wiley & Sons.

7. Offer them your hand that is on their shoulder in a palm to palm grip with thumbs tucked in (Figure 38.12).

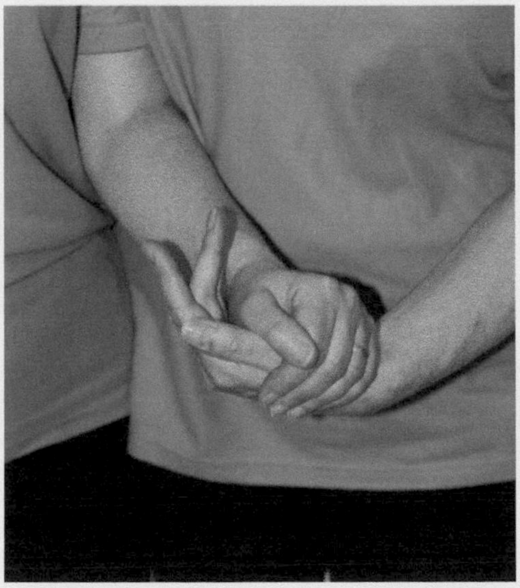

Figure 38.12 Use a palm to palm grip with thumbs tucked in. *Source:* MacGregor (2016), figure 16.6, p. 34. © John Wiley & Sons.

8. If appropriate, hand the patient their walking frame or aid. If using a walking frame, ensure it is in good condition and is the correct height for the patient.

After the task

1. Check that the patient is safe and comfortable.
2. 2. Document if the patient experiences any dizziness, light-headedness or other symptoms that may put them at risk.

3. Inserting two flat slide sheets underneath a patient in bed from the top of the bed

Purpose	Insertion of slide sheets to enable a dependent patient to be moved in bed who is unable to do so.
Prior to the handling task	**1.** Consult any handling plans relating to this patient and check that they are clear, up-to-date and regularly reviewed. **2.** If there is no written plan, ask your colleagues if they have relevant information relating to this patient. **3.** Communicate with the patient and tell them what you plan to do. Ensure that they understand and obtain their consent. **4.** Make a final check that the patient cannot do this for themselves before continuing with the task. **5.** 5. Ensure that the bed is at the correct height, that is, at waist height of the shorter handler.
During the task	**1.** With the handlers at either side of the bed, fold the slide sheet over the patient with the handles of each slide sheet being up on the top sheet and down on the bottom sheet. • The folds should be about one hand width apart (Figures 38.13 and 38.14).

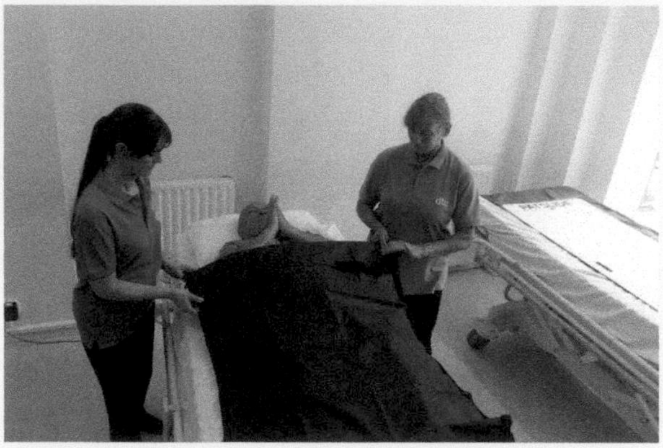

Figure 38.13 Fold slide sheet together with handles facing outwards. *Source:* **MacGregor (2016), figure 33.1, p. 68. © John Wiley & Sons.**

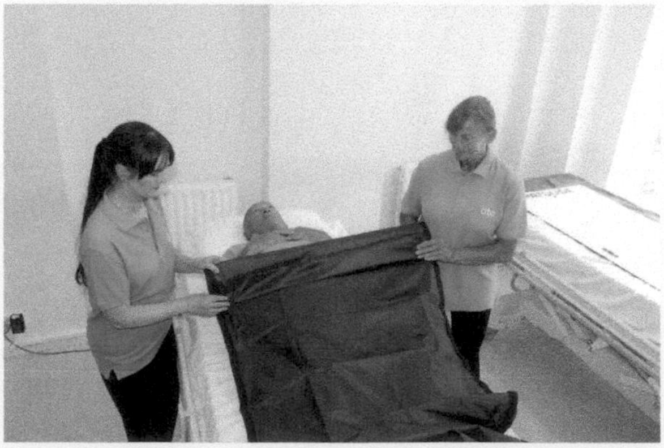

Figure 38.14 Fold both slide sheets together and place under the patient's pillow. *Source:* **MacGregor (2016), figure 33.2, p. 68. © John Wiley & Sons.**

- If you are unable to fold the slide sheet on top of the patient, find another suitable surface to carry out this task.
- If you are in hospital or other care facility, this should not be on another bed, as this will contravene infection control protocols.

2. Place the folded slide sheets under the patient's pillow with the open end at the top. This should be gently manoeuvred under the patient's shoulders.

3. Both handlers should face the head of the bed and have their inside hand palm up and thumb tucked in (Figure 38.15).

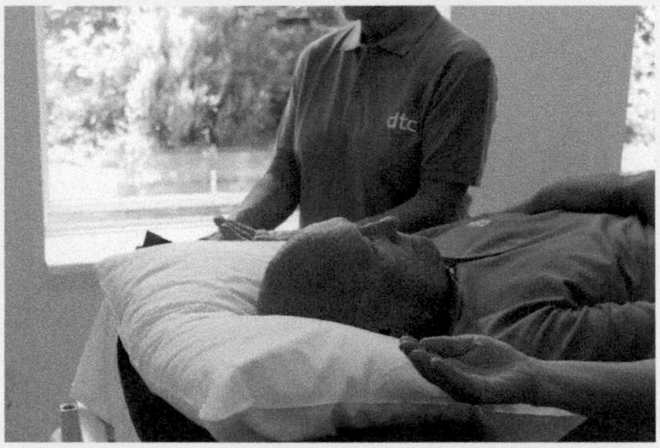

Figure 38.15 **Both handlers face the head of the bed with palms facing upwards.** ***Source:*** **MacGregor (2016), figure 33.3, p. 68. © John Wiley & Sons.**

4. The handlers place their inner hands under the slide and grip the bottom section. The handler's outer hand should take hold of the top part of the folded slide sheet and keep it in position (Figure 38.16).

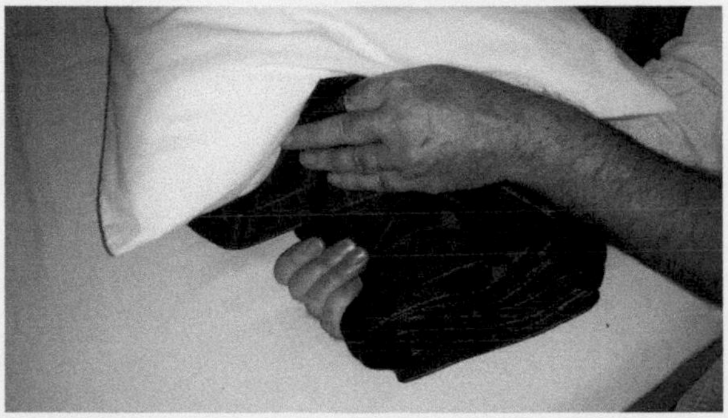

Figure 38.16 **Inner hand goes under the slide sheet with the outer hand on top.** ***Source:*** **MacGregor (2016), figure 33.4, p. 68. © John Wiley & Sons.**

5. Adopting a walk stance position, the bottom sections of the slide sheets should be pulled down underneath the patient. The handlers must keep their elbows on the bed as this will prevent them from pulling the slide sheet up instead of down towards the bottom of the bed (Figures 38.17 and 38.18).

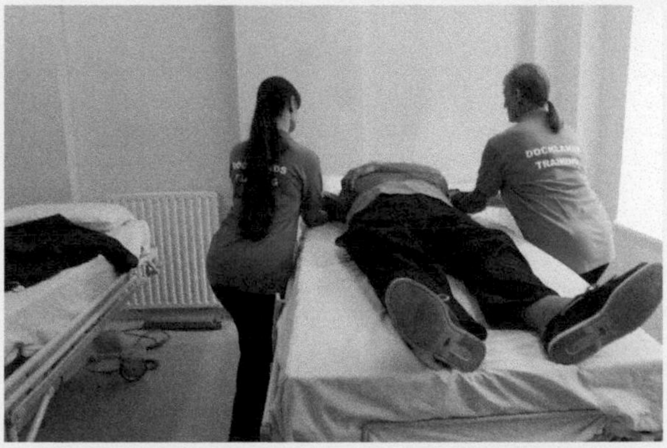

Figure 38.17 **Adopting a walk stance position pull the bottom section of the slide sheet down. Keep elbows on the bed.** ***Source:*** **MacGregor (2016), figure 33.5, p. 68. © John Wiley & Sons.**

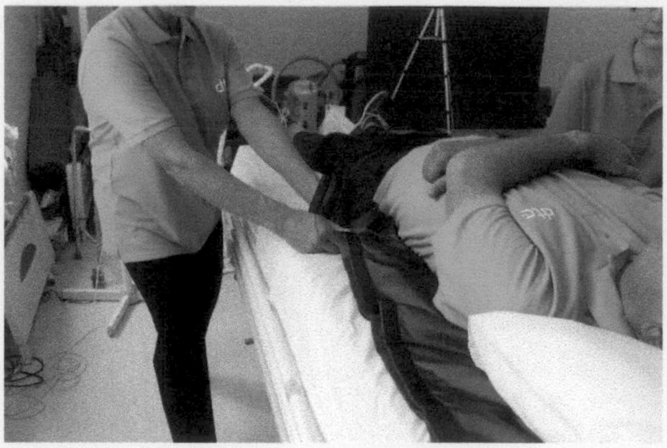

Figure 38.18 **Both handlers work in unison as the slide sheet is unravelled.** *Source:* MacGregor (2016), figure 33.6, p. 68. © John Wiley & Sons.

6. The handlers must communicate with each other as they unravel the slide sheets. Using verbal prompts, such as 'Ready, Steady, Pull', will ensure that both handlers are working together.

This needs to be continued until the slide sheet is fully under the patient. Once the slide sheet is under the patient's back, the handlers can remove their outer hand and adopt a better posture. The slide sheet will remain in position as it is anchored by the patient (Figure 38.19).

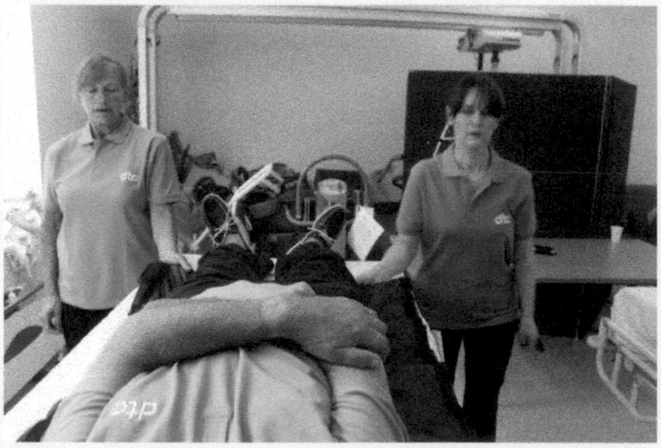

Figure 38.19 **As the slide sheet goes under the patient the handler's outer hand is removed.** *Source:* MacGregor (2016), figure 33.7, p. 68. © John Wiley & Sons.

7. If the slide sheet gets stuck under the lumbar curve of the patient's back:
  a. pull the slide sheet to one side while the other handler keeps hold of their side. This 'see-saw' action can help the slide sheet to go under the patient's hips;
  b. push down on the mattress at the hips as the slide sheet is pulled under the patient;
  c. bring the slide sheet from the feet rather than the shoulders.
  d. Be careful here as the slide sheet can get caught in the patient's clothing if this method is adopted.

After the task	**1.** Check that the patient has no pain and/or discomfort. **2.** 2. Prepare to move the patient in bed as necessary.

To move a patient up the bed who is unable to do so with two flat slide sheets

Prior to the handling task	**1.** Consult any handling plans relating to this patient and check that they are clear, up-to-date and regularly reviewed. **2.** If there is no written plan, ask your colleagues if they have relevant information relating to this patient. **3.** Communicate with the patient and tell them what you plan to do. Ensure that they understand and obtain their consent. **4.** Make a final check that the patient cannot do this for themselves before continuing with the task. **5.** Ensure that the bed is at the correct height, that is, at waist height of the shorter handler.

During the task

1. The handlers should then stand at the head of the bed facing the bottom of the bed. Adopting a walk stance position with the hand closest to the bed taking hold of the top part of the slide sheet in an overhand grip (Figure 38.20).

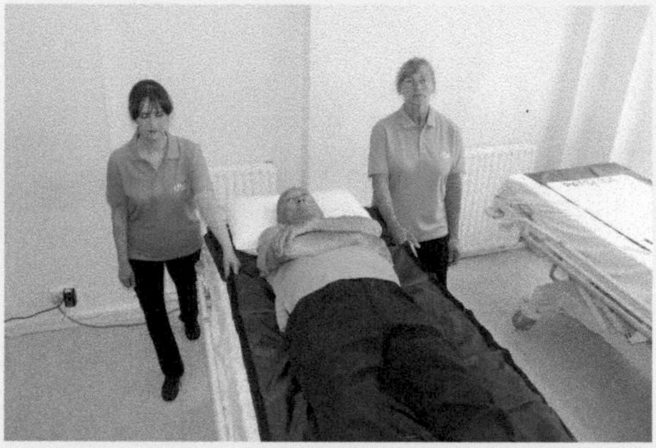

Figure 38.20 **Adopting a walk stance position hold the top slide sheet with your inner hand.** *Source:* MacGregor (2016), figure 38.1, p. 78. © John Wiley & Sons.

2. On the command of 'Ready, Steady, Move', both handlers weight transfer and slowly move the patient up the bed no more than 2 cm (1 inch) (Figure 38.21).

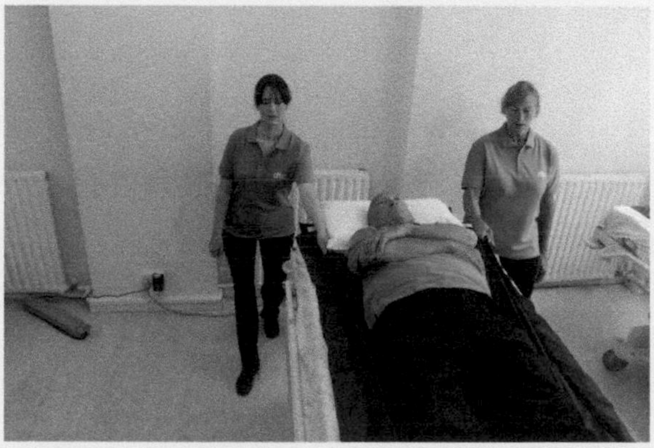

Figure 38.21 **In a coordinated way move the patient up the bed using a weight transfer.** *Source:* MacGregor (2016), figure 38.2, p. 78. © John Wiley & Sons.

3. The handlers continue to do this until the patient has reached the desired position in the bed (Figure 38.22).

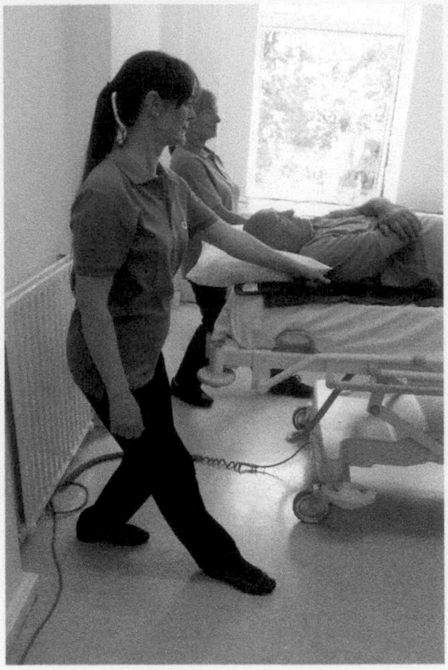

Figure 38.22 **Continue until the patient is in the desired position.** *Source:* MacGregor (2016), figure 38.3, p. 78. © John Wiley & Sons.

4. Alternative method 1: If the head of the bed can be removed, the handlers can stand at the head of the bed and adopting a walk stance position move the patient up the bed using the technique described previously (Figure 38.23).

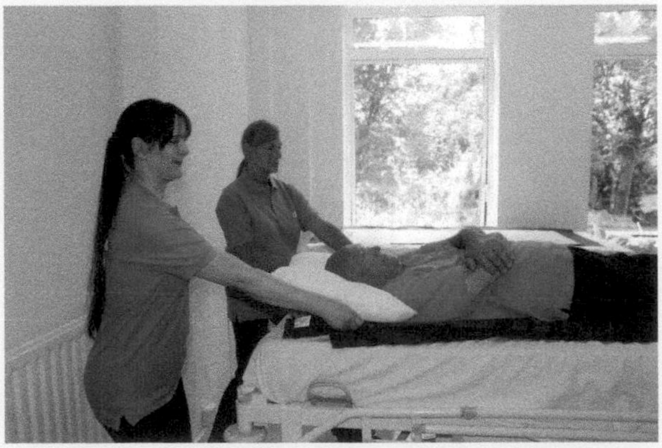

Figure 38.23 **Alternatively if the bed head can be removed stand at the top of the bed.** *Source:* MacGregor (2016), figure 38.4, p. 78. © John Wiley & Sons.

5. Alternative method 2: The handlers can use both hands in an overhand grip at the patient's hip and shoulders, then move the patient up the bed as described previously (Figure 38.24).

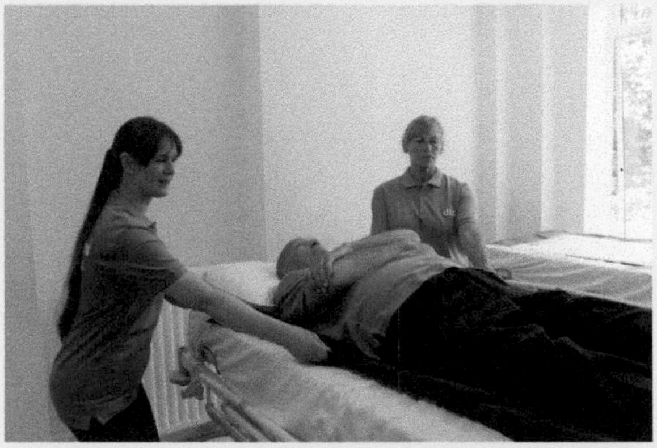

Figure 38.24 Alternatively using both hands grip the top slide sheet at the patient's hips and shoulders. *Source:* MacGregor (2016), figure 38.5, p. 78. © John Wiley & Sons.

If this method is employed, the handlers must look at the bottom of the bed diagonally opposite (Figure 38.25).

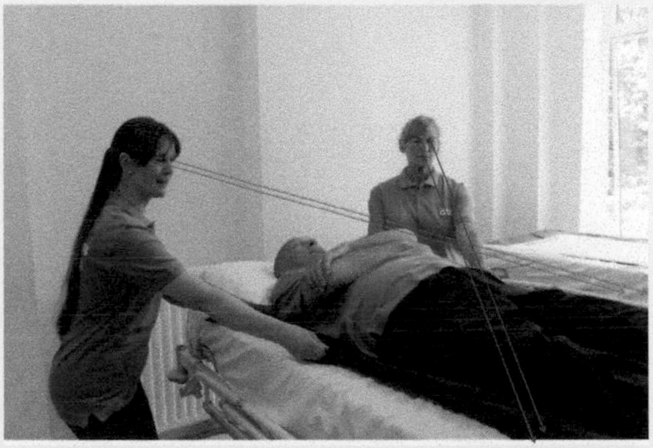

Figure 38.25 If using both hands you must look at the opposite corner of the bed. *Source:* MacGregor (2016), figure 38.6, p. 78. © John Wiley & Sons.

6. Remove the slide sheets by each handler going to the foot of the bed and taking the opposite corner of the slide sheet and pulling it underneath. This will ensure that the slide sheet slides on itself and does not damage the patient's skin (Figure 38.26).

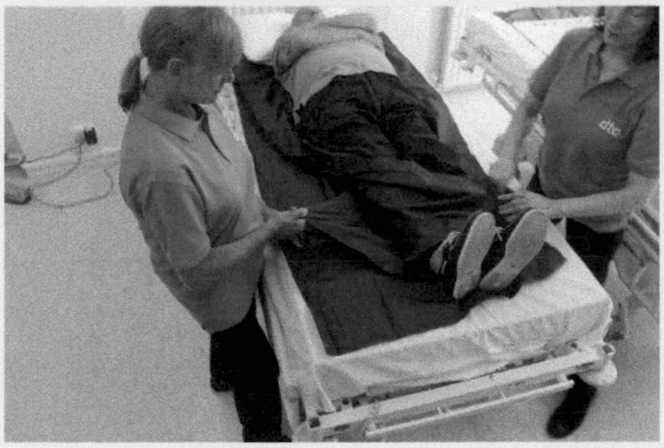

Figure 38.26 Remove the slide sheets by pulling under from opposite corners. *Source:* MacGregor (2016), figure 38.7, p. 78. © John Wiley & Sons.

7. Each handler adopts a walk stance position and using their body weight pulls the slide sheet towards them. This must be done in unison and using verbal prompts such as 'Ready, Steady, Pull' will ensure that this happens. The handlers must keep their hands close to the patient to ensure that the slide sheets slide under each other (Figure 38.27).

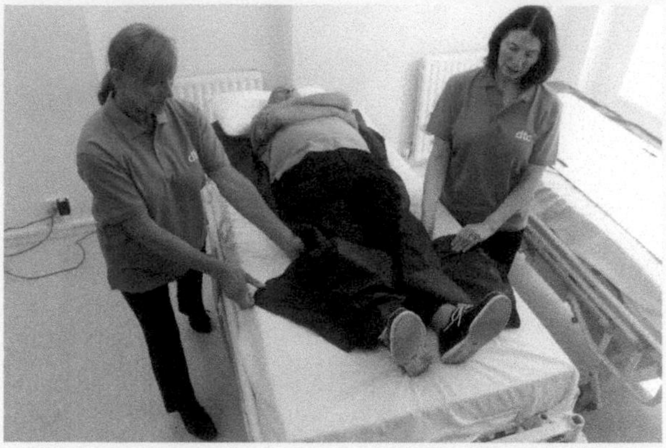

Figure 38.27 **Keep your hands close to the patient as the slide sheet is removed.** *Source:* MacGregor (2016), figure 38.8, p. 78. © John Wiley & Sons.

8. The handlers walk up the bed and steadily pull out the slide sheet. This is done with slow steady pulls, not by short sharp pulls. This is continued until both slide sheets are removed from under the patient (Figure 38.28).

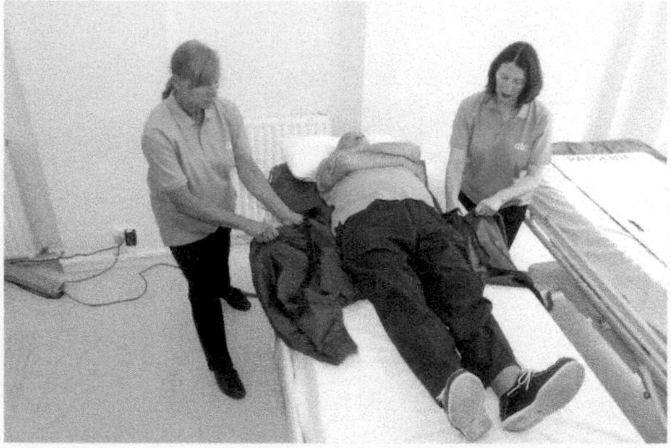

Figure 38.28 **Remove the slide sheets in unison.** *Source:* MacGregor (2016), figure 38.9, p. 78. © John Wiley & Sons.

After the task

1. Check that the patient has no pain and/or discomfort and is in the correct position in the bed.
2. Raise the bed rails if indicated in the handling plan ensuring there has been an up-to-date bed rails assessment form completed.
3. 3. Put the bed at a height that is safe for the patient.

Touch Points

Regardless of the task, the nursing associate must always give consideration to issues and circumstances prior to the handling task, during the task and after the task.

It is essential to document all care activities aligned to local policy and procedure.

Use of Hoist and Slings

It is vital that you have had suitable and sufficient training and you have been deemed competent in using a hoist before you use one. All hoist and slings are different, and the guidance below addresses safe principles. The text below relates to mobile hoist which are most common. In addition to these, you may come across other types such as ceiling tracking and gantry hoists.

Red Flag

Using a hoist to move a patient can be a hazardous manoeuvre for both nurses and patients.
Unsafe use, poor maintenance or the use of inappropriate or defective hoists or slings can be the cause of potentially fatal accidents.

Hoist and Sling Checks

Hoist

- Is the safe working load (SWL) of the hoist suitable for the patient? (See Figures 38.29–38.31 for examples of where this may be found.) If the patient's weight is near to the working capacity of the hoist or exceeds it, you will need to source a hoist with a bigger SWL. Standard mobile bariatric (plus size) hoists will have a SWL of 320 kg.
- Has the hoist been checked/serviced in the last six months? Do not use a hoist that is out of date (see Figure 38.29 and 38.30 for examples of where this may be found).
- Where is the emergency stop button? This often acts as part of the ON/OFF function of the hoist; therefore, you need to know where this is located (see Figure 38.32 for an example of where this may be found).
- Where is the emergency lower? This is often in different places on different hoists; therefore, you must find out where it is before using the hoist, as in the unlikely event of there being a hoist failure, you must know how to lower the patient safely to the bed or chair (see Figure 38.33 for an example of where this may be found).
- Is the battery sufficiently charged to carry out the lift? This must be checked prior to use. Most modern hoists have an indicator of the amount of charge left in the battery. This can be on the hoist itself or on the handset (see Figure 38.34 for an example of where this may be found). You also need to know how to charge the hoist either directly from the mains (it must be unplugged to use) or if there is a removable battery, how to remove it and where it is charged.
- Does the spreader bar and the feet of the hoist move smoothly? Ensure that you know where the buttons for these are located and how to use them. These are on the handset, but with some hoists, they are replicated on the hoist itself (see Figure 38.34).
- Are the wheels moving smoothly?
- Do the brakes work? Note that the brakes are only used when the hoist is parked; at all other times, they must be off.

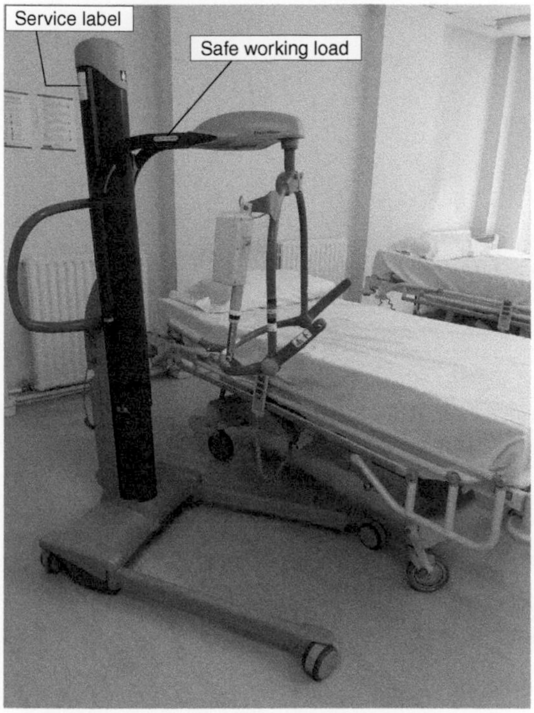

Figure 38.29 Hoist showing SWL and service label.

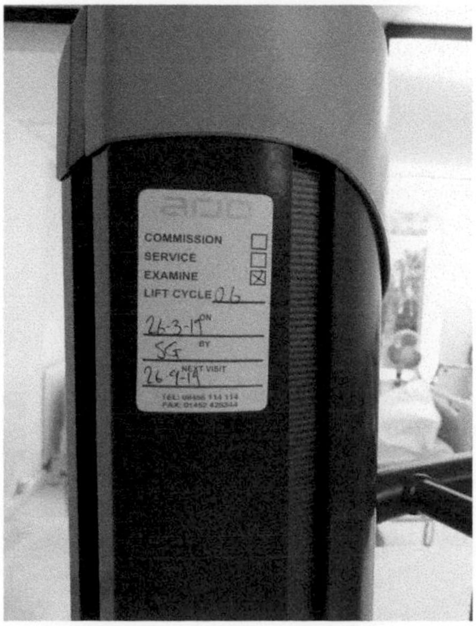

Figure 38.30 Hoist showing service label in detail.

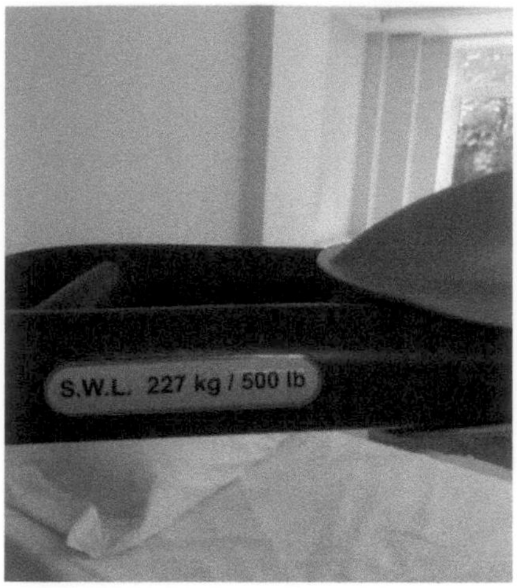

Figure 38.31 **Hoist showing SWL in detail.**

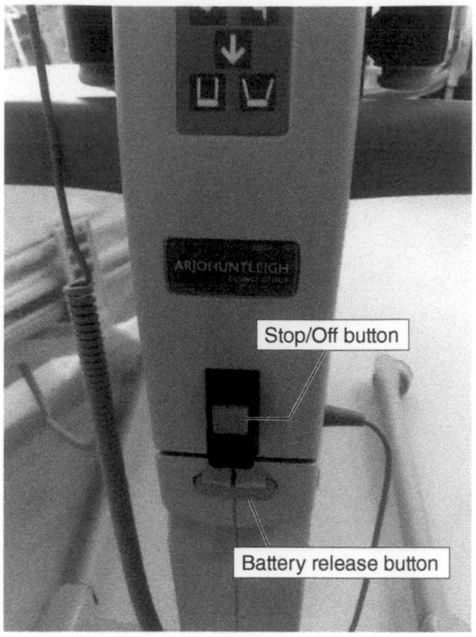

Figure 38.32 **Hoist showing Stop button and batter release button.**

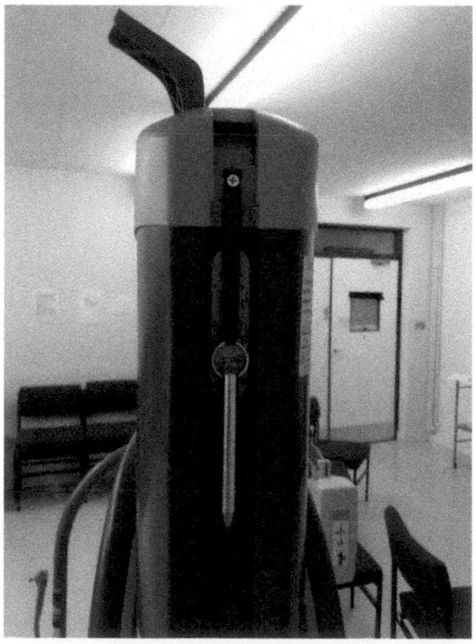

Figure 38.33 **Hoist showing emergency lower mechanism.**

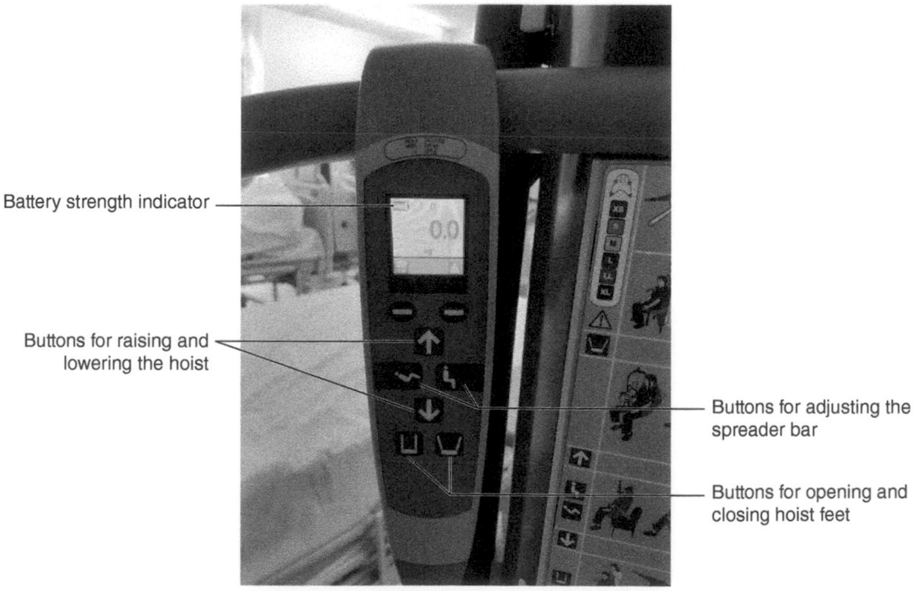

Figure 38.34 **Hoist showing handset in detail.**

Slings

Slings come in all sizes from some for small children through to bariatric patients. In addition to checking the maximum weight of the patient for the sling, the sling needs to be the correct size for the patient. A sling that is too large will allow the patient's hips to slide through the aperture, and a sling that is too small will be painful as it crushes the patient. Measuring the correct size of sling is a skilled task and should not be undertaken without having achieved the correct level of competence. This can only be achieved with face-to-face training. Most sling manufacturers provide guidance on how to measure for their particular sling.

Loop slings and clip slings. These describe the way that the sling is attached to the spreader bar of the hoist. Figure 38.35 is a loop type sling, and Figure 38.36 is a clip type sling. Figures 38.37 and 38.38 illustrate both types of spreader bar. Loops go with loops, and clips go with clips.

If it is a disposable sling, ensure that it is the patient's allocated sling and that their name is on it. Check that it has not been wet and that the safety label is intact.

If it is a reusable sling, check that it has been LOLER (Lifting Operation and Lifting Equipment Regulations (1998)) checked.

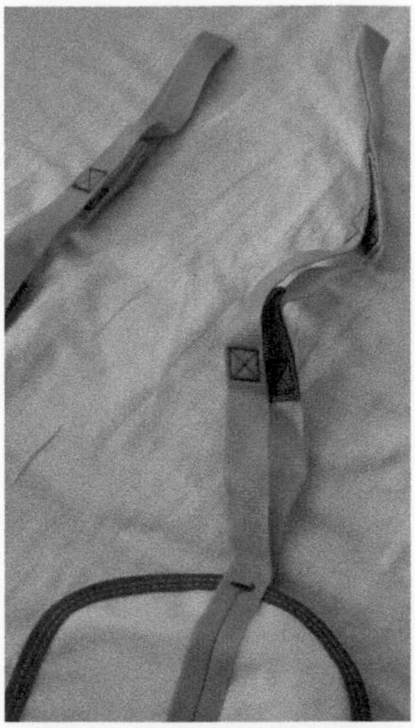

Figures 38.35 **Loop type sling.** *Source:* MacGregor (2016), figure 43.1, p. 88. © John Wiley & Sons.

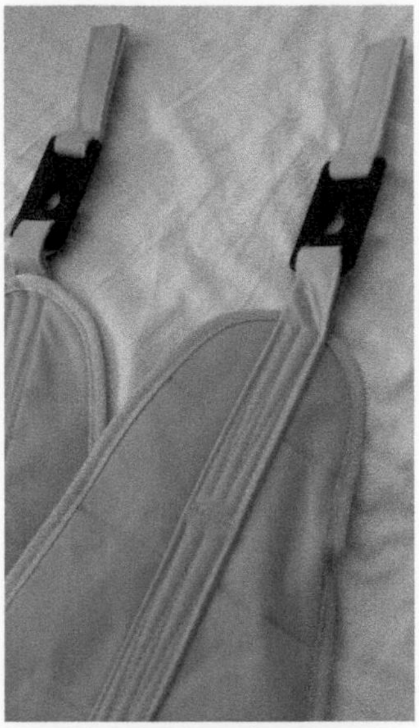

Figure 38.36 **Clip type sling.** *Source:* MacGregor (2016), figure 43.2, p. 88. © John Wiley & Sons.

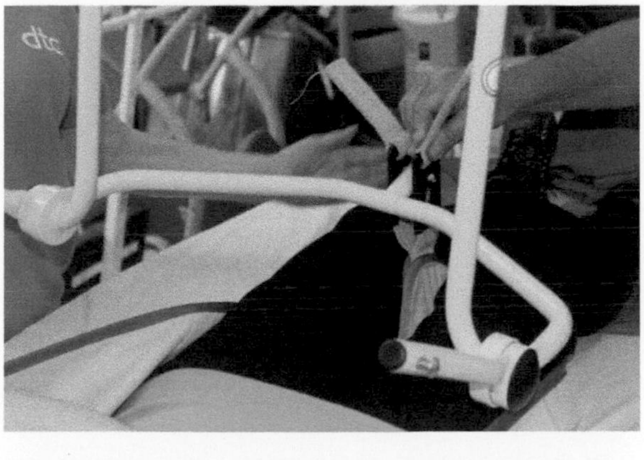

Figure 38.37 **Clip type spreader bar.** *Source:* MacGregor (2016), figure 43.3a, p. 88. © John Wiley & Sons.

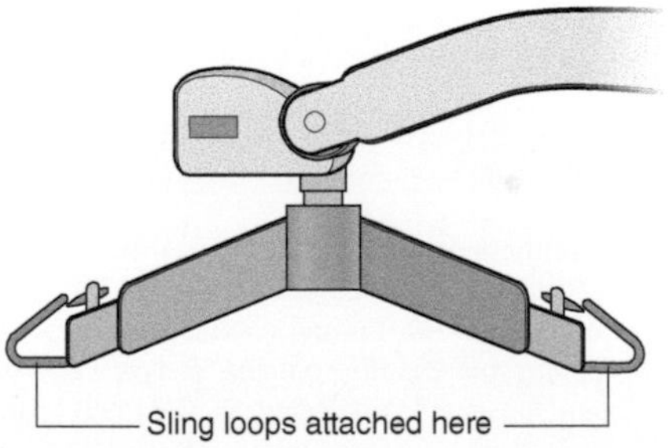

Figure 38.38 **Loop type spreader bar.** *Source:* MacGregor (2016), figure 43.3b, p. 88. © John Wiley & Sons.

There are many types of specialist slings such as amputee and in-situ. Ensure that you know how to use any specialist slings before hoisting a patient. If in doubt, don't.

Other Equipment Used for the Safe Moving and Handling of Patients

There are many types of moving and handling equipment. Two of the most common examples are standing and raising aids. These can be motorised (see Figure 38.39) or non-motorised (Figure 38.40).

Touch Points Revisited

- The Nursing and Midwifery Council (NMC) requires the nursing associate to provide support to people with their mobility and safety needs
- There is a range of legislation that guides employers and employees with appropriate moving and handling activities
- Risk assessment is essential in order to protect patient and staff
- An evidence-based approach to manual patient handling and mobilisation is required, and the nursing associate is required to embrace appropriate technology to keep preserve safety and minimise harm
- Techniques and the use of equipment (for example, slings and hoists) can help ensure that patient outcomes are positive and health and well-being is enhanced for all
- Achieving early patient mobility and safe handling requires a deliberate focus on the person being cared for being offered support to; staff education and full engagement are the cornerstone of care provision

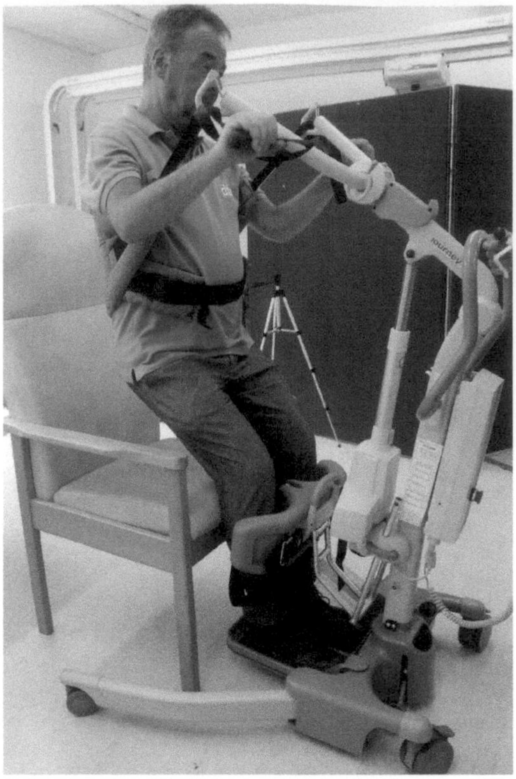

Figure 38.39 Motorised standing and raising aid.

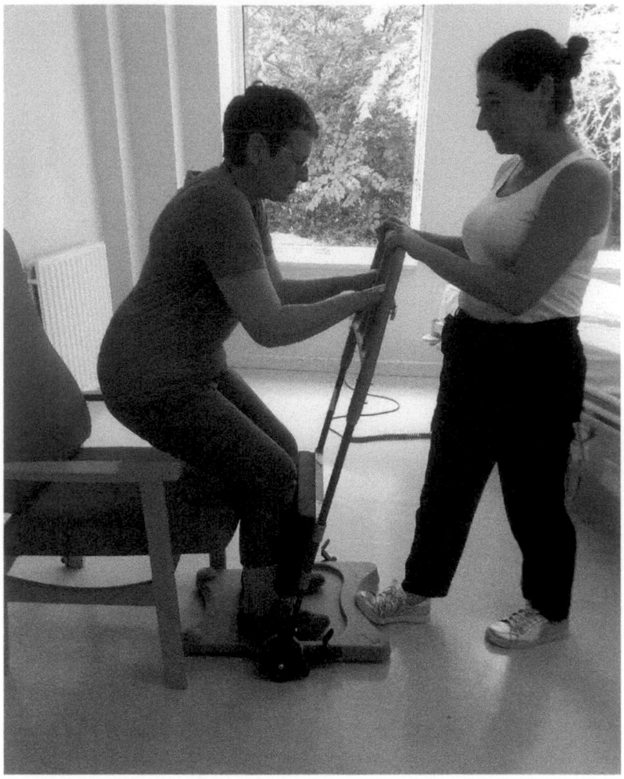

Figure 38.40 Non-motorised standing and raising aid.

References

Chartered Society of Physiotherapists. (2017) *10 things you need to know about your back.* [online] Available: https://www.csp.org.uk/publications/10-things-you-need-know-about-your-back. Accessed October 2019.

Health and Safety at Work Act. (1974) [online] Available: http://www.hse.gov.uk/legislation/hswa.htm. Accessed October 2019.

MacGregor, H. (2016) *Moving and handling patients at a glance*, Oxford: Wiley.

Management of Health and Safety at Work Regulations. (1999) [online] Available: http://www.legislation.gov.uk/uksi/1999/3242/contents/made. Accessed September 2020.

Manual Handling Operations Regulations. (1992) *As amended 2002.* [online] Available: http://www.hse.gov.uk/pubns/books/l23.htm. Accessed October 2019.

Nursing and Midwifery Council. (2018) The code, *Professional standards of behaviour for nurses, midwives and nursing associates*, London: NMC.

Royal College of Nursing. (2019) *Moving and handling.* [online] Available: https://www.rcn.org.uk/get-help/rcn-advice/moving-and-handling. Accessed October 2019.

Royal College of Physicians. (2009) *Physical and shift work in pregnancy*, London: RCP.

Unit 7

Provide Support with Respiratory Care

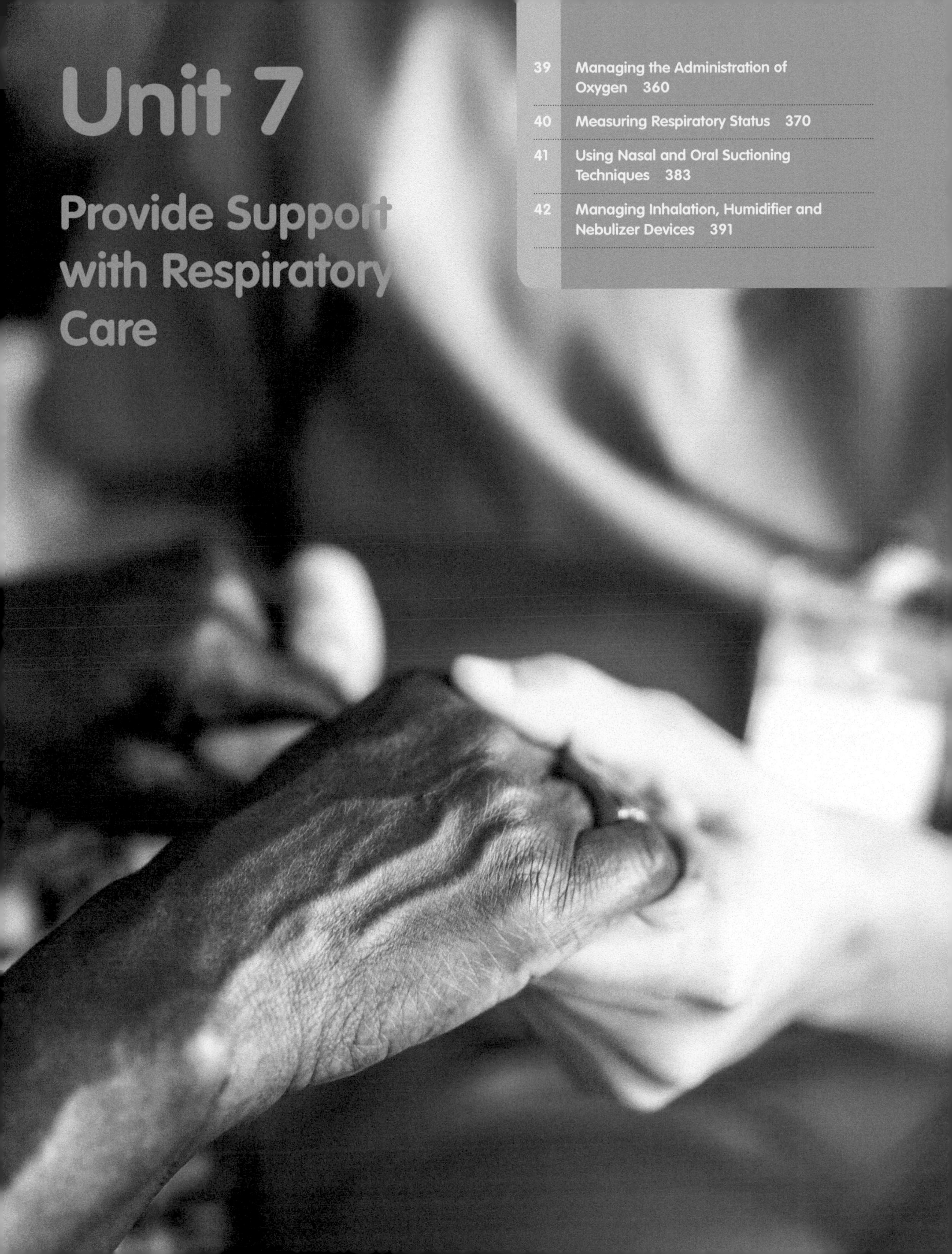

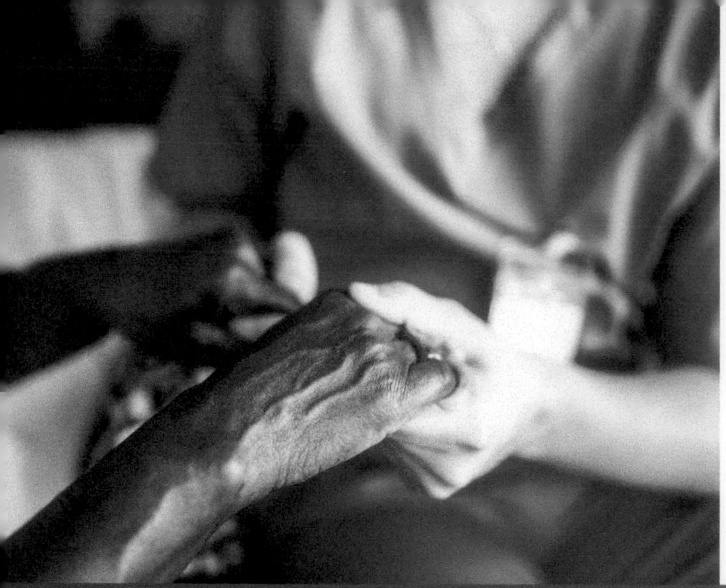

39

Managing the Administration of Oxygen

Barry Hill

Northumbria University, UK

Chapter Aim

- **This chapter aims to provide the reader with an insight into recognising and acting upon the management of the administration of supplementary oxygen therapy.**

Learning Outcomes

- **To understand the different types of supplementary oxygen therapy.**
- **Identify the common indications and contraindications for supplemental oxygen therapy.**
- **Describe the management of supplement oxygen therapy, including selection of adjunct and titration of oxygen.**

Test Yourself Multiple Choice Questions

1. **Normal oxygen saturations for patients with COPD are:**
   A) **88–92%**
   B) **84–88%**
   C) **Above 90%**
   D) **Above 94%**
2. **Hypoxemia is:**
   A) **an abnormally low level of oxygen in the blood**
   B) **an abnormally low oxygen saturation**
   C) **an abnormally high level of oxygen in the blood**
   D) **an abnormally high oxygen saturation**

The Nursing Associate's Handbook of Clinical Skills, First Edition. Edited by Ian Peate.

Companion website: www.wiley.com/nursingassociate

3. **Haemoglobin is a large protein made up of:**
   A) **1 protein chains**
   B) **2 protein chains**
   C) **3 protein chains**
   D) **4 protein chains**
4. **Indications for oxygen therapy in acute illness:**
   A) **Cardiac/respiratory arrest or peri-arrest**
   B) **Hypoxaemia**
   C) **Shock, sepsis, major trauma and anaphylaxis**
   D) **Carbon monoxide poisoning**
   E) **All the above**
5. **Normal oxygen saturations for adult patients with healthy lungs should be:**
   A) **94–98%**
   B) **Above 90%**
   C) **Above 96%**
   D) **Above 88%**

Introduction

This chapter will introduce the nursing associate to the principles of managing supplementary oxygen for patients with altered oxygen saturations. In applying clinical decision-making and proficiency in the use of managing supplementary oxygen therapy, the nursing associate with be working towards the following standards of proficiency for nursing associate's platforms (NMC 2018):

- *Platform 3* 'Provide and monitor care'
- *Platform 5* 'improving safety and quality care'

Oxygen treatment is used to save lives (National Institute for Health and Care Excellence (NICE) 2019; O'Driscoll et al. 2017). Emergency oxygen is used around two million times a year by ambulance services in the United Kingdom, equivalent to around 34% of all ambulance journeys, and around 18% of hospital inpatients in the United Kingdom are treated with oxygen at any one time (Dhruve et al. 2015).

Some of the typical indications for oxygen are for respiratory failure, in which there is inadequate oxygenation or elimination of carbon dioxide from mixed venous blood and to treat severe hypoxaemia resulting from ischaemic heart disease, sepsis or trauma. Management of the hypoxaemic patient requires continuous evaluation and treatment of the underlying cause of the hypoxaemia. It is extremely important that the nursing associate recognises that oxygen therapy relieves hypoxaemia, but not treat or resolve the underlying cause of hypoxaemia.

Hypoxaemia is an abnormally low level of oxygen in the blood. More specifically, it is oxygen deficiency in arterial blood and has many causes; often, respiratory disorders can cause tissue hypoxia, as the blood is not supplying enough oxygen to the body.

Oxygen

Oxygen is a non-metal element and is found naturally as a molecule. Each molecule of oxygen is made up of two oxygen atoms that are strongly joined together. Oxygen has low melting and boiling points, so it is in a gas state at room temperature, and therefore is invisible and is not really thought about by the average person going about their daily life. Oxygen is one of the essential elements for life and survival of all things on the earth. When mammals breathe in (inspire), oxygen molecules enter the lungs and pass through the lung walls into the circulating blood volume. Within this circulating blood, there are red blood cells (RBCs) containing haemoglobin (Hb), which carry oxygen to the cells.

Oxygen in the Blood

Hb is a large protein made up of four protein chains. At the centre of each chain, there is a haem group, containing iron. Oxygen binds to each of the four iron ions of the Hb molecule and circulates the body. Hb's ability to bind oxygen is known as oxygen saturation (SO_2) and can be measured directly from an arterial blood sample (Dhruve et al. 2015).

Medical Oxygen

Medical oxygen is classified as a medicinal product, but according to the legal status in the United Kingdom, it is a General Sales List (GSL) product and, therefore, does not require a prescription. However, the use and supply of oxygen is similar to all other GSL medicines when administered in a healthcare setting: it should be documented on a prescription chart alongside all other medicines. The prescription chart should be completed when oxygen therapy is initiated (see Figure 39.1). An appropriate delivery system and flow rates should be specified on the patient's chart, and it should also be indicated whether the patient is having continuous oxygen or oxygen as required (O'Driscoll et al. 2017).

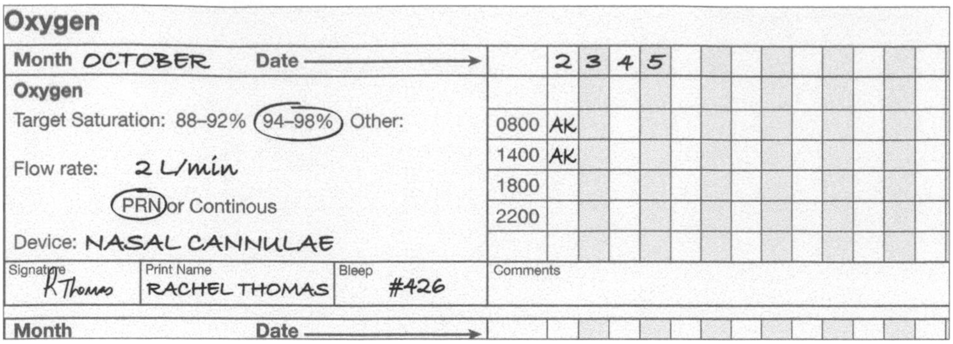

Figure 39.1 Oxygen prescription on a medication card. *Source:* Thomas (2015), chapter 21, figure 21.5, p. 52. © John Wiley & Sons.

Red Flag

Oxygen is the most common drug used in medical emergencies. It should be prescribed initially to achieve a normal or near-normal oxygen saturation; in most acutely ill patients with a normal or low arterial carbon dioxide ($PaCO_2$), oxygen saturation should be 94–98% oxygen saturation. However, in some clinical situations, such as cardiac arrest and carbon monoxide poisoning, it is more appropriate to aim for the highest possible oxygen saturation until the patient is stable. A lower target of 88–92% oxygen saturation is indicated for patients at risk of hypercapnic respiratory failure (National Institute for Health and Clinical Excellence (NICE) 2019).

High Concentration Oxygen Therapy

High concentration oxygen therapy is safe in uncomplicated conditions such as pneumonia, pulmonary thromboembolism, pulmonary fibrosis, shock, severe trauma, sepsis, or anaphylaxis (NICE 2019). In such conditions, low arterial oxygen (PaO_2) is usually associated with low or normal arterial carbon dioxide ($PaCO_2$), and, therefore, there is little risk of hypoventilation and carbon dioxide retention.

In acute severe asthma, the arterial carbon dioxide ($PaCO_2$) is usually subnormal, but as asthma deteriorates, it may rise steeply (NICE 2019). These patients usually require high concentrations of oxygen, and if the arterial carbon dioxide ($PaCO_2$) remains high despite other treatment, intermittent positive-pressure ventilation needs to be considered urgently.

Low Concentration Oxygen Therapy

Low concentration oxygen therapy (controlled oxygen therapy) is reserved for patients at risk of hypercapnic respiratory failure (NICE 2019; O'Driscoll et al. 2017), which is more likely in those with:

- chronic obstructive pulmonary disease;
- advanced cystic fibrosis;
- severe non-cystic fibrosis bronchiectasis;
- severe kyphoscoliosis or severe ankylosing spondylitis;
- severe lung scarring caused by tuberculosis;
- musculoskeletal disorders with respiratory weakness, especially if on home ventilation;
- an overdose of opioids, benzodiazepines or other drugs causing respiratory depression.

Red Flag

Until blood gases can be measured, initial oxygen should be given using a controlled concentration of 28% or less, titrated towards a target oxygen saturation of 88–92% (NICE 2019).

Oxygen Requirements

Oxygen is required by all tissues to support cell metabolism: in acute illness, low tissue oxygenations (hypoxia) can occur because of a failure in any of the systems that deliver and circulate oxygen (Preston & Kelly 2017). Box 39.1 lists the indications for oxygen therapy. Oxygen is only prescribed for hypoxaemic patients to increase alveolar oxygen tension and decrease the work of breathing. The concentration of oxygen

Box 39.1 Indications for Oxygen Therapy in Acute Illness

- Cardiac/respiratory arrest or peri-arrest
- Hypoxaemia
- Shock, sepsis, major trauma, anaphylaxis
- Carbon monoxide poising

Source: Preston & Kelly (2017). © John Wiley & Sons

required depends on the condition being treated; the administration of an inappropriate concentration of oxygen can have serious or even fatal consequences (NICE 2019). Any prescriptions made for oxygen should include the target range for oxygen saturation (O'Driscol et al. 2017), and the patient's response to any supplementary oxygen therapy requires regular monitoring (NICE 2019; O'Driscol et al. 2017; RCP 2017a, 2017b, 2017c, 2017d, 2017e).

The Different Types of Oxygen Therapy

It is important to note that there are several different types of oxygen therapy (British Lung Foundation (BLF) 2019), and the nursing associate must be able to Identify the need for supplementary oxygen therapy with support from a registered nurse. It is necessary to learn about the different types of therapy in relation to the various patient groups.

- Long-term oxygen therapy (LTOT) – used to stabilise oxygen levels for 15 hours and more a day
- Nocturnal oxygen therapy (NOT) – used to improve oxygen levels when patients are sleeping
- Ambulatory oxygen therapy (AOT) – used to improve oxygen levels when patients are active
- Palliative oxygen therapy (POT) – used to manage severe breathlessness that does not respond to other treatments in patients who are dying.

Identifying the Need for Supplementary Oxygen Therapy

Oxygen therapy is indicated in patients with oxygen saturations below the target saturation range. It is not indicated for the treatment of breathlessness in patients with adequate oxygen saturations, apart from certain patients with carbon monoxide poisoning and with pneumothorax (O'Driscoll et al. 2017).

Supplemental oxygen therapy is recommended for all patients who are acutely hypoxaemic and for many patients who are at risk of hypoxaemia. While considered a life-saving intervention, as a medical treatment, initial and ongoing review and re-evaluation is vital to ensure its use is safe and effective, because oxygen therapy can be detrimental to a patient's health (Olive 2016).

Red Flag

Oxygen is a treatment for hypoxaemia, not breathlessness. Oxygen has not been proven to have any consistent effect on the sensation of breathlessness in non-hypoxaemic patients (O'Driscoll et al. 2017).

Take Note

Nursing associates need to ensure that they have an understanding of the knowledge and skills of correct oxygen prescribing or of oxygen delivery devices.

Nursing associates have a responsibility to ensure that oxygenation is optimised at pulmonary and cellular levels as part of their duty of care to patients. This requires knowledge of respiratory and cardiac physiology, as well as selection of the appropriate equipment and delivery method for supplemental oxygen therapy. Ongoing reassessment and evaluation of patients is required to ensure that the treatment is safe and effective, preventing further deterioration and a medical emergency.

Oxygen should be started immediately and prescribed as soon as possible in emergency situations (Dhruve et al. 2015). In all other situations, oxygen should be prescribed in accordance with a legal prescription. All healthcare professionals who administer oxygen therapy should be fully trained and follow local or national protocols to ensure safe prescribing and administration of oxygen.

Oxygen saturation should be checked by pulse oximetry (supplemented by arterial blood gases tests where necessary) for at least five minutes after starting oxygen therapy and within 30 minutes after initiation. If oxygen saturation falls below the target saturation and the patient is unstable, treatment should be reviewed. If oxygen saturation is above the target range and the patient is stable, the delivery system and oxygen flow rate should be reduced accordingly (O'Driscoll et al. 2017).

Vital Signs

Vital signs, such as pulse, blood pressure, temperature and respiratory rate should be checked, documented (Figures 39.2, 39.3 and 39.4) and reported on using NEWS2 (Royal College of Physicians (RCP) 2017a, 2017b, 2017c, 2017d, 2017e), as these can affect the oxygen saturation levels. Once a patient is stable with satisfactory SO_2, oxygen should be reduced and discontinued. Oxygen saturations should be reviewed regularly during a stay in hospital as an inpatient and by the home oxygen service if a patient is discharged while on oxygen.

Reproduced from: Royal College of Physicians. National Early Warning Score (NEWS) 2: Standardising the assessment of acute-illness severity in the NHS. Updated report of a working party. London: RCP 2017.

Reproduced from: Royal College of Physicians. National Early Warning Score (NEWS) 2: Standardising the assessment of acute-illness severity in the NHS. Updated report of a working party. London: RCP 2017.

Reproduced from: Royal College of Physicians. National Early Warning Score (NEWS) 2: Standardising the assessment of acute-illness severity in the NHS. Updated report of a working party. London: RCP 2017.

Orange Flag

As a nursing associate working with adults, it is likely that you will care for patients with a variety of respiratory disorders. When completing vital signs, it is very important to integrate both physical and mental health assessment observations in order to provide a true patient-centred care. Find out how the patient is feeling? A patient with a long-term respiratory disorder who uses LTOC may always be breathless due to fibrotic (hardening) lung tissue. How does being constantly short of breath make them feel? Have they got support at home? What are their coping strategies? Can they be referred for cognitive behavioural therapy (CBT) to support their mental health?

Physiological parameter	Score 3	2	1	0	1	2	3
Respiration rate (per minute)	≤8		9–11	12–20		21–24	≥25
SpO_2 Scale 1 (%)	≤91	92–93	94–95	≥96			
SpO_2 Scale 2 (%)	≤83	84–85	86–87	88–92 ≥93 on air	93–94 on oxygen	95–96 on oxygen	≥97 on oxygen
Air or oxygen?		Oxygen		Air			
Systolic blood pressure (mmHg)	≤90	91–100	101–110	111–219			≥220
Pulse (per minute)	≤40		41–50	51–90	91–110	111–130	≥131
Consciousness				Alert			CVPU
Temperature (°C)	≤35.0		35.1–36.0	36.1–38.0	38.1–39.0	≥39.1	

Figure 39.2 The NEWS2 Scoring System. *Source:* RCP (2017c).

NEW score	Clinical risk	Response
Aggregate score 0–4	Low	Ward-based response
Red score Score of 3 in any individual parameter	Low–medium	Urgent ward-based response*
Aggregate score 5–6	Medium	Key threshold for urgent response*
Aggregate score 7 or more	High	Urgent or emergency response**

* Response by a clinician or team with competence in the assessment and treatment of acutely ill patients and in recognising when the escalation of care to a critical care team is appropriate.

**The response team must also include staff with critical care skills, including airway management.

Figure 39.3 NEWS2 thresholds and triggers. *Source:* RCP (2017d).

NEWS key	FULL NAME	
0 1 2 3	DATE OF BIRTH	DATE OF ADMISSION

Parameter	Left label	Score	Right label
	DATE		DATE
	TIME		TIME
A+B Respirations Breaths/min	≥25	3	≥25
	21–24	2	21–24
	18–20		18–20
	15–17		15–17
	12–14		12–14
	9–11	1	9–11
	≤8	3	≤8
A+B SpO_2 Scale 1 Oxygen saturation (%)	≥96		≥96
	94–95	1	94–95
	92–93	2	92–93
	≤91	3	≤91
SpO_2 Scale 2† Oxygen saturation (%) Use Scale 2 if target range is 88–92%, eg in hypercapnic respiratory failure	≥97 on O_2	3	≥97 on O_2
	95–96 on O_2	2	95–96 on O_2
	93–94 on O_2	1	93–94 on O_2
	≥93 on air		≥93 on air
	88–92		88–92
	86–87	1	86–87
†ONLY use Scale 2 under the direction of a qualified clinician	84–85	2	84–85
	≤83%	3	≤83%
Air or oxygen?	A=Air		A=Air
	O_2 L/min	2	O_2 L/min
	Device		Device
C Blood pressure mmHg Score uses systolic BP only	≥220	3	≥220
	201–219		201–219
	181–200		181–200
	161–180		161–180
	141–160		141–160
	121–140		121–140
	111–120		111–120
	101–110	1	101–110
	91–100	2	91–100
	81–90	3	81–90
	71–80	3	71–80
	61–70	3	61–70
	51–60	3	51–60
	≤50	3	≤50
C Pulse Beats/min	≥131	3	≥131
	121–130	2	121–130
	111–120	2	111–120
	101–110	1	101–110
	91–100	1	91–100
	81–90		81–90
	71–80		71–80
	61–70		61–70
	51–60		51–60
	41–50	1	41–50
	31–40	3	31–40
	≤30	3	≤30
D Consciousness Score for NEW onset of confusion (no score if chronic)	Alert		Alert
	Confusion	3	Confusion
	V	3	V
	P	3	P
	U	3	U
E Temperature °C	≥39.1°	2	≥39.1°
	38.1–39.0°	1	38.1–39.0°
	37.1–38.0°		37.1–38.0°
	36.1–37.0°		36.1–37.0°
	35.1–36.0°	1	35.1–36.0°
	≤35.0°	3	≤35.0°
NEWS TOTAL			TOTAL
	Monitoring frequency		Monitoring
	Escalation of care Y/N		Escalation
	Initials		Initials

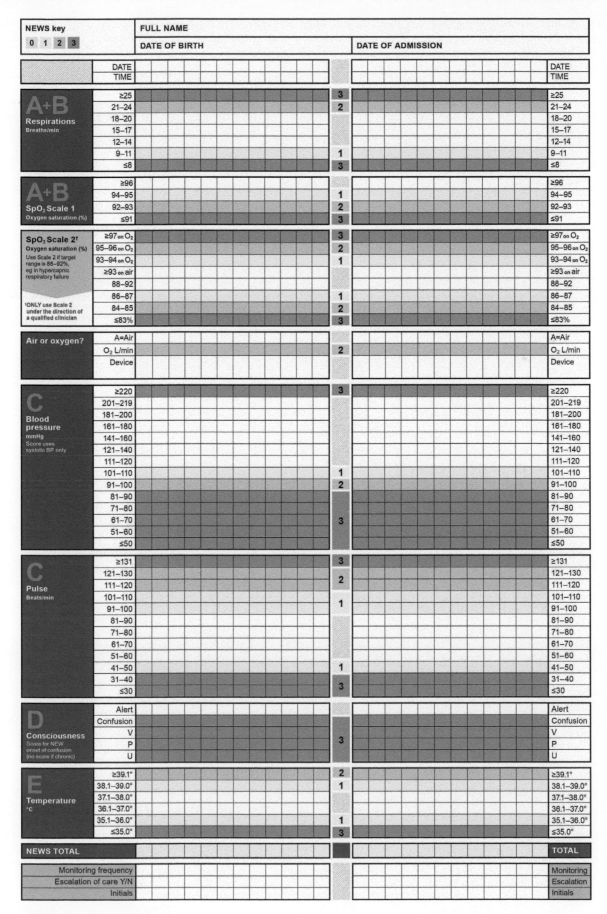

Figure 39.4 NEWS2 Chart. *Source:* RCP (2017e).

Failure to administer oxygen appropriately can result in serious harm to the patient (O'Driscoll et al. 2017). Excessive oxygen administration in some patients who are at risk of hypercapnia, for example, those with chronic obstructive pulmonary disease (COPD), morbid obesity or cystic fibrosis, may result in respiratory failure and possibly death.

Violet Flag

Clinical hazards associated with the practical aspects of supplemental oxygen therapy in the home and other care environments:

- Combustion and potentially dangerous when in contact with sources of ignition and flammable material
- Inability of healthcare practitioners to set flow correctly on oxygen cylinders
- Incorrect use of valve, for example, if it is not opened correctly, causing failure to obtain or maintain oxygen flow
- Incorrect selection of cylinder, for example, using the incorrect gas or cylinder size
- Unsafe storage, for example, in areas which are not secure, inadequately ventilated or at risk of extremes of temperature

Yellow Flag

With regard to the safe use and efficacy of oxygen therapy, some healthcare professionals have deep rooted cultural beliefs that may have a detrimental impact on positive patient outcomes. These beliefs and cultures need to be challenged at all levels.

Source: Kelly & Maden (2015).

Potential Complications of Oxygen Therapy

Complications of oxygen therapy can vary including complications such as a dry or bloody nose, skin irritation from the nasal cannula or face mask, or fatigue and morning headaches. The complications can be more serious; however, there may be adverse effects such as absorptive atelectasis, a collapse of parts of the lung making gas exchange more difficult.

Where a patient is exposed to high levels of oxygen, there is a serious risk of oxygen toxicity occurring. This can affect the central nervous system, the pulmonary system and the eyes. Early signs of central nervous system involvement will include twitching of the small muscles of the hand. Later signs may include vertigo, nausea, altered behaviour, clumsiness and finally convolutions. Longer exposure to 100% oxygen can produce tissue injury within the lungs. There will be intense, carinal irritation on deep inspiration which will eventually lead to uncontrolled coughing and finally chest pain and dyspnoea. Within the eyes, there may be a constriction of the peripheral field of vision, and delayed cataract formation can occur.

Touch Point

Knowing when to start patients on oxygen therapy has the potential to save lives; ongoing assessment and evaluation is essential and must be carried out to ensure the treatment is safe and effective.

Methods of Oxygen Delivery

There are several ways of delivering oxygen to a patient.

- Nasal cannulae
- Face mask
- Venturi mask
- Non-rebreathe mask

Nasal Cannulae

One of the simplest ways of delivering oxygen is via a nasal cannula (see Figure 39.5). This is a plastic tubing with nasal prongs that sits in the vestibule of each nostril. For reasons of patient comfort and because the oxygen delivered can dry the mucosal membranes quickly, it is not appropriate to deliver more than 3L to 4L of oxygen via nasal cannulae. Consequently, this method of delivery will only treat mild hypoxaemia.

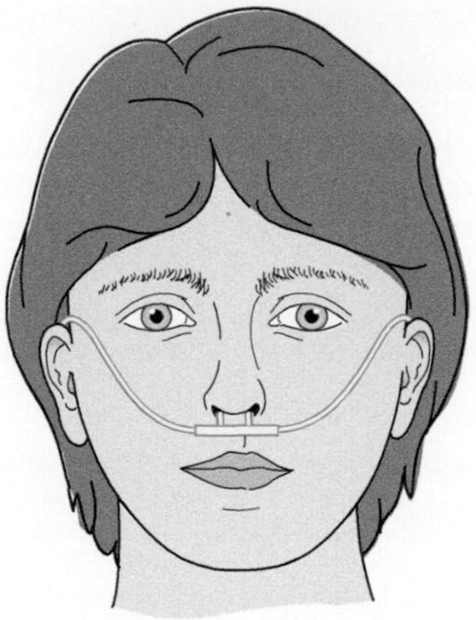

Figure 39.5 **Nasal Canulae.** *Source:* Preston & Kelly (2017), chapter 46, figure 46.4, p. 98. © John Wiley & Sons.

However, if it is only mild hypoxaemia that is being treated, then patients tend to tolerate this method of delivery well; it also enables them to eat and drink freely.

Facemask

Flow rates as high as 15L per minute can be delivered via these masks, but there is only a small reservoir, this being a plastic mask. At low flow rates, there is a risk of carbon dioxide retention with this type of mask. A maximum oxygen concentration of between 60 and 70% depending upon the patient's respiratory rate is achievable. As the patient breathes quicker, so the concentration will fall. Also, unlike the nasal cannula, it is not possible for the patient to eat and drink without removing the mask and sometimes speaking becomes difficult also. This sometimes means that the patient is less tolerant of this type of mask.

Take Note

High oxygen requirement is a sign of severity and the person may require frequent monitoring, assessment of arterial blood gasses and senior clinical input.

Venturi Mask

This relies on a well-understood physical principle whereby oxygen passes through a small hole which entrains air to a predictable dilution. These masks come with several different coloured valves which can be changed according to the percentage of oxygen which needs to be delivered. The percentage and the consequent flow rates are clearly marked on them (see Figure 39.6). It is possible due to the venturi effect to deliver quite high flow rates to the patient using this mask.

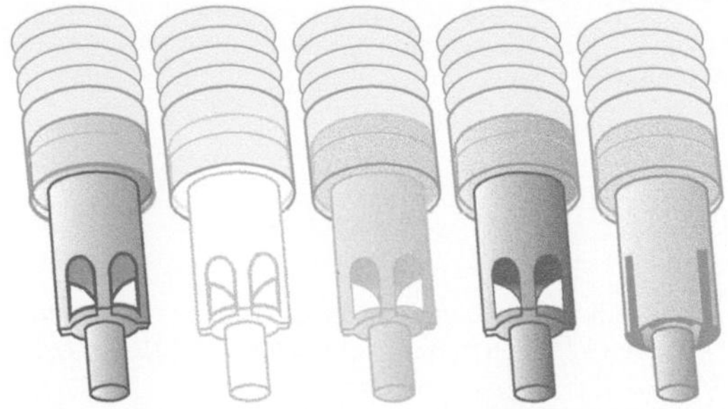

Figure 39.6 **Venturi valves.** *Source:* Preston & Kelly (2017), chapter 46, figure 46.5, p. 98. © John Wiley & Sons.

Reservoir Masks (Non-Rebreathe Mask)

If the patient has become very hypoxic, then it may be appropriate to use the non-rebreathe mask (Figure 39.7). This is similar to a face mask, with the addition of a bag underneath which forms a reservoir. Between the bag and the oxygen mask is a one-way valve which ensures that when the patient exhales the carbon dioxide will leave the mask and when they inhale the oxygen which is in the reservoir bag will be the only thing they breathe in. As a result, high concentrations of oxygen can be delivered via this method. The non-rebreathe mask would be the mask of choice when one is concerned about the patient's oxygen levels. In such a circumstance, one should turn the flow rates up to 15L per minute, occlude the valve with a finger or thumb, thereby allowing the back to fill and only then place the mask over the patient's mouth and nose.

Preparing the Patient for Oxygen Therapy

The patient should be informed what equipment is to be used, such as a mask or nasal cannula, and the importance of keeping the apparatus in place. The patient should know about the flammability of oxygen and the dangers of any naked flames. The nurse should instruct the patient make known any increasing distress, air hunger, nausea, anxiety, dry nasal passages or sore throat (Dougherty et al. 2015).

Table 39.1 outlines a procedural guideline for oxygen therapy. The nursing associate must ensure that they always adhere local policy and procedure.

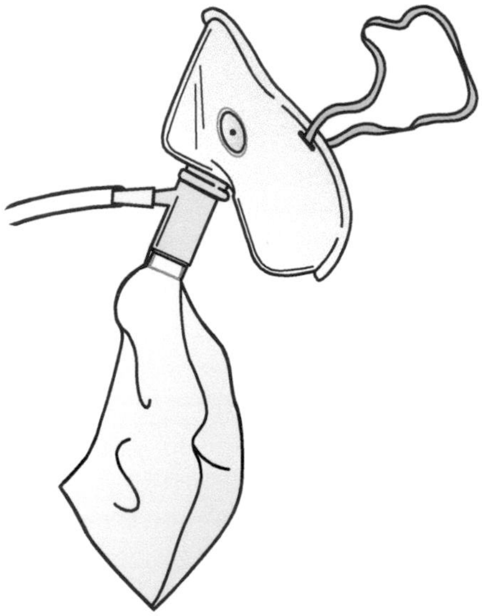

Figure 39.7 Reservoir mask. *Source:* Preston & Kelly (2017), chapter 46, figure 46.2, p. 98. © John Wiley & Sons.

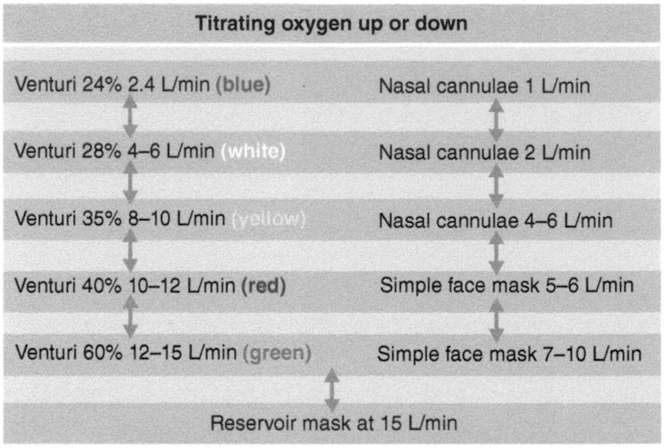
Titrating oxygen up or down
Venturi 24% 2.4 L/min (blue)
Nasal cannulae 1 L/min
Venturi 28% 4–6 L/min (white)
Nasal cannulae 2 L/min
Venturi 35% 8–10 L/min (yellow)
Nasal cannulae 4–6 L/min
Venturi 40% 10–12 L/min (red)
Simple face mask 5–6 L/min
Venturi 60% 12–15 L/min (green)
Simple face mask 7–10 L/min
Reservoir mask at 15 L/min

Figure 39.8 Titration guideline. *Source:* Preston & Kelly (2017), chapter 46, figure 46.1, p. 98. © John Wiley & Sons.

Table 39.1 Oxygen therapy. Procedural guideline.

Essential equipment	• Piped/wall oxygen and medical air • Oxygen flow meter/regulator • Oxygen cylinders for transportation • Ambu-bag for emergencies • Nasal cannulae • Selection of oxygen masks • Oxygen tubing, varying lengths and types • Oxygen analysers
Optional equipment	• Non-invasive equipment in non-critical care areas (essential within critical care environments) • High-flow O_2 and medical air mixers for use in high dependency unit (HDU) setting • Humidification equipment • Cold water bubble humidifiers medicinal products • Asthma inhalers or nebulisers • Oxygen as prescribed for the patient • Nicotine patches to aid smoking cessation

***Pre-procedure* action**	• Review the patient's condition and level of oxygen therapy required, e.g. facemask, humidified oxygenation and nasal cannulas. The rationale is to ensure that the appropriate method for delivery of oxygen is chosen to suit the patient's condition. • Ensure oxygen is prescribed with clear target oxygen saturations for oxygen therapy titration; medical oxygen is a drug. The intentions of the clinician who initiates oxygen therapy must be communicated clearly to the person administering oxygen and an accurate record must be kept of what has been administered. • Explain to the patients why they require oxygen therapy and the benefits and problems thereof; this can help to minimise patient anxiety. • Attach oxygen tubing to the port on the wall oxygen unit or cylinder (and not to the medical air port). This ensures accurate oxygen delivery and prevents hypoxia.
Procedure	• Set oxygen flowmeter to required setting (L/min); check oxygen is flowing through system by using fingertips. This ensures that the system is working. • Either apply a nasal cannula by gently placing the nasal prongs of the cannula into the patient's nostrils draping the tubing over the patient and sliding the fit connector up under the chin to hold the tubing securely in place, or apply an oxygen mask by placing the mask over the patient's mouth and nose, then pull the elastic strap over the head and adjust the strap on both sides, securing the mask in a position that seals it against the face.
Post procedure:	• Check the patient is comfortable • Record that oxygen therapy has been commenced; document time and flow rate; maintain accurate records. • Provide continued reassurance to the patient and the opportunity to ask questions; this can minimise apprehension and anxiety and improve understanding of treatment

Source: Dougherty et al. (2015).

Touch Points Revisited

- Nursing associates have an important role to play in the use of supplemental oxygen therapy in acute settings.
- They must understand the theoretical, practical and evidence-based principles of oxygen administration.
- Understanding these key issues enables the nursing associate to recognise and reduce potential hazards and complications ensuring the care they provide is safe and effective.

References

British Lung Foundation. (2019) *Why is oxygen therapy used?* [online] Available: https://www.blf.org.uk/support-for-you/oxygen/what-is-it. Accessed 25 September 2019.

Dhruve, H., Davey, C. and Pursell, J. (2015) Respiratory disease: oxygen therapy: emergency use and long-term treatment, *Clinical Pharmacist*. [online] Available: https://www.pharmaceutical-journal.com/learning/learning-article/oxygen-therapy-emergency-use-and-long-term-treatment/20068717.article?firstPass=false. Accessed 6 October 2019.

Dougherty, L., Lister, A. and West-Oram, A. (2015) Oxygen therapy procedural guideline, *Royal Marsden manual of clinical nursing procedures*, Wiley, 385.

Kelly, C.A. and Maden, M. (2015) How do health-care professionals perceive oxygen therapy? A critical interpretative synthesis of the literature Chronic, *Respiratory Disease*, 12 (1): 11–23. doi: 10.1177/1479972314562408

NICE. (2019) *Oxygen*. [online] Available: https://bnf.nice.org.uk/treatment-summary/oxygen.html. Accessed 11 October 2019.

NMC. (2018) *Standards of proficiencies for nursing associates*. [online] Available: https://www.nmc.org.uk/globalassets/sitedocuments/education-standards/nursing-associates-proficiency-standards.pdf. Accessed 10 October 2019.

O'Driscoll, B.R., Howard, L.S., Earis, J. on behalf of the BTS Emergency Oxygen Guideline Development Group, et al. (2017) British thoracic society guideline for oxygen use in adults in healthcare and emergency settings, *BMJ Open Respiratory Research*, 4: e000170. doi: 10.1136/bmjresp-2016-000170.

Olive, S. (2016) Practical procedures: oxygen therapy, *Nursing Times*, 112 (1–2): 12–14.

Preston, W. and Kelly, C. (2017) *Respiratory nursing at a glance*, UK: Wiley Blackwell.

RCP. (2017a) *NEWS2*. [online] Available: https://www.rcplondon.ac.uk/projects/outputs/national-early-warning-score-news-2. Accessed 10 October 2019.

RCP. (2017b) *NEWS2*. [online] Available: https://www.rcplondon.ac.uk/projects/outputs/national-early-warning-score-news-2. Accessed 11 October 2019.

RCP. (2017c) *The NEWS2 scoring system*. [online] Available: https://www.rcplondon.ac.uk/projects/outputs/national-early-warning-score-news-2. Accessed 11 October 2019.

RCP. (2017d) *NEWS2 thresholds and triggers*. [online] Available: https://www.rcplondon.ac.uk/projects/outputs/national-early-warning-score-news-2. Accessed 11 October 2019.

RCP. (2017e) *NEWS2 chart*. [online] Available: https://www.rcplondon.ac.uk/projects/outputs/national-early-warning-score-news-2. Accessed 11 October 2019.

Thomas, Rachel K. (2015) *Practical medical procedures at a glance*. UK: Wiley-Blackwell.

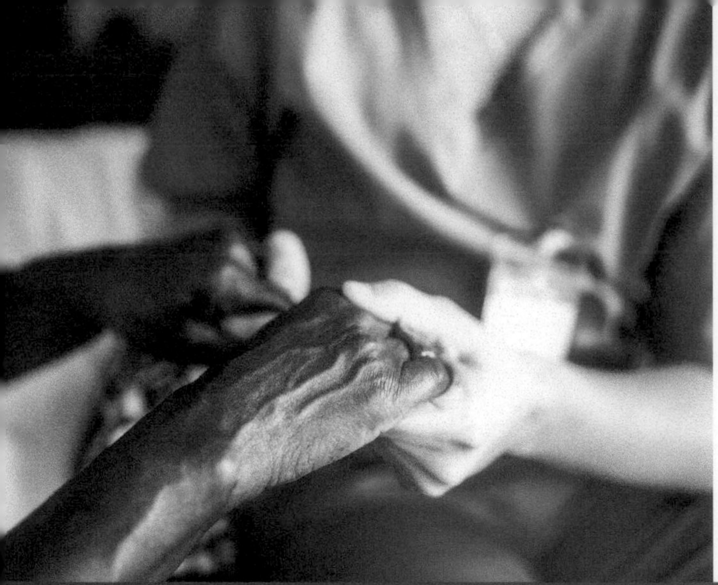

40

Measuring Respiratory Status

Barry Hill

Northumbria University, UK

Chapter Aim

- **This chapter aims to provide readers with an insight into measuring respiratory status and oxygen saturations using pulse oximetry and peak expiratory flow rate (PEFR).**

Learning Outcomes

- **Understand the clinical relevance of pulse oximetry monitoring.**
- **Demonstrate the correct use of pulse oximetry to monitor oxygen saturations.**
- **Understand the clinical relevance of PEFR in asthma management.**
- **Demonstrate the correct use of a peak flow meter to monitor the PEFR.**

Test Yourself Multiple Choice Questions

1. **Which of the following blood cells contain haemoglobin (Hb)?**
   A) **Red blood cell**
   B) **White blood cell**
   C) **Platelets**
   D) **Plasma**
2. **What are the factors that can affect pulse oximetry readings?**
   A) **Anaemia**
   B) **Hypotension**
   C) **Nail varnish or false nails**
3. **Special considerations that might affect a patient's respiration and breathing are:**
   A) **Pregnancy**
   B) **Age**
   C) **Skin colour**

The Nursing Associate's Handbook of Clinical Skills, First Edition. Edited by Ian Peate.

Companion website: www.wiley.com/nursingassociate

4. **Which of the following is a contraindication for PEF?**
   A) **Patients with severe breathlessness**
   B) **Patients who are pregnant**
   C) **Patients with reduced mobility**
5. **Which of the following are indications for PEFR?**
   A) **To detect possible lung obstruction or restriction due to inflamed airways**
   B) **To help diagnose asthma**
   C) **To help diagnose hypoxia**

Introduction

Both pulse oximetry and peak expiratory flow (PEF) provide important information for the review of patients who present with respiratory symptoms. Nursing associates should typically consider the use of pulse oximetry in patients who present with respiratory symptoms, such as shortness of breath, changes in respiratory pattern (such as agonal and abdominal breathing), an abnormal respiratory rate (below 12 or above 20 breaths per minute) (British Thoracic Society (BTS) 2016; Royal College of Physicians (RCP) 2017), or when observing patients who present with blue lips and/or fingers, indicating peripheral and central cyanosis (a lack of oxygen in the red blood cells). Pulse oximetry and PEFR are mainly used for those who have respiratory symptoms and those with respiratory disease.

When the nursing associate applies clinical decision-making and proficiency in the use of oxygen saturation and PEFR measurements and using clinical skills, you are practising within the Nursing and Midwifery Council's (NMC's) proficiencies and in particular platform 2 'providing and monitoring care' and platform 5 'improving safety and quality of care' (NMC 2018). The nursing associate is required to demonstrate proficiency in identifying normal peak flow and oximetry measurements.

Oxygen Saturation

Haemoglobin was discovered within the red blood cell in 1840 by Friedrich Ludwig Hunefeld, a member of the German Biochemistry Association. One molecule of Hb can carry up to four molecules of oxygen after which it is described as being 'saturated' with oxygen (the World Health Organisation (WHO) 2019). If all the binding sites of the Hb molecule are carrying oxygen, the Hb is said to have a saturation of 100%. Most of the Hb in blood combine with oxygen as it passes through the lungs. A healthy individual with normal lungs, breathing air at sea level, will have an arterial oxygen saturation of 94%–98% (BTS 2016). Extremes of altitude will affect these numbers. Venous blood that is collected from the tissues contains less oxygen and normally has a saturation of around 75% (WHO 2019).

Arterial blood looks bright red, while venous blood looks dark red (Gibson & Waters 2017). The difference in colour is due to the difference in Hb saturation. When humans' Hb is well saturated, this is evident in their tongues and lips appearing as a pink colour; when they are desaturated, they can appear blue. This is called cyanosis (WHO 2019). It can be difficult to see cyanosis clinically, particularly in people with darker skin tones. Nursing associates may not notice this sign until the oxygen saturation is less than 90% (BTS 2017). Detecting cyanosis is even more difficult in poorly lit environments. Cyanosis is only visible when the deoxygenated Hb concentration is greater than 5 g/dL (WHO 2019). A severely anaemic patient may not appear cyanosed even when extremely hypoxic (see Box 40.1) as there is very little Hb circulating through the tissues. In healthy patients who have no respiratory disease, oxygen saturation should always be 94–98% (BTS 2017). If the oxygen saturation is 94% or lower, the patient is mildly hypoxic and needs to be treated quickly. This may be repositioning or deep breathing exercises and some physiotherapy at first (depending on the patient's individual and holistic needs) (Nursing and Midwifery Council (NMC) 2018). A saturation of less than 90% is a clinical emergency (WHO 2019).

Red Flag

It is difficult to detect cyanosis clinically until the saturation is less than 90%. Cyanosis is therefore considered a critical test of clinical ability to be able to appropriately identify and if present, treat with supplemental oxygen. It is, however, a difficult clinical sign to elicit visually, and recognition can be complicated by several factors including room lighting, skin pigmentation and anaemia. Clinical assessment skills, including inspection, palpation, percussion and auscultation (known as APPA), is an objective way to undertake a review of patients in a systematic way (Bickley 2016).

Pulse Oximetry

Introduction to the Pulse Oximeter

According to Potter (2009), the pulse oximeter has become a well-used tool in modern practice of emergency medicine and is being increasingly used in general practice. It monitors the percentage of Hb which is saturated with oxygen (SaO2). Pulse oximeters work on the principle of spectral analysis, that is, the detection and quantification of components by their unique light absorption characteristics. Oxygenated and reduced Hb have different absorption spectra, with arterial blood appearing red and venous blood, blue (see Figure 40.1). Together in solution, their relative ratios are determined from the ratio of the light absorbed at two different wavelengths.

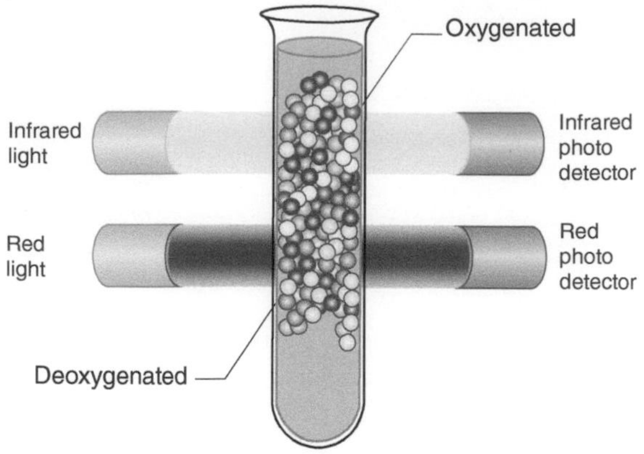

Figure 40.1 Red and infrared light absorption by oxygenated and deoxygenated haemoglobin. *Source:* Preston & Kelly (2017), chapter 19, figure 19.2, p. 38. © John Wiley & Sons.

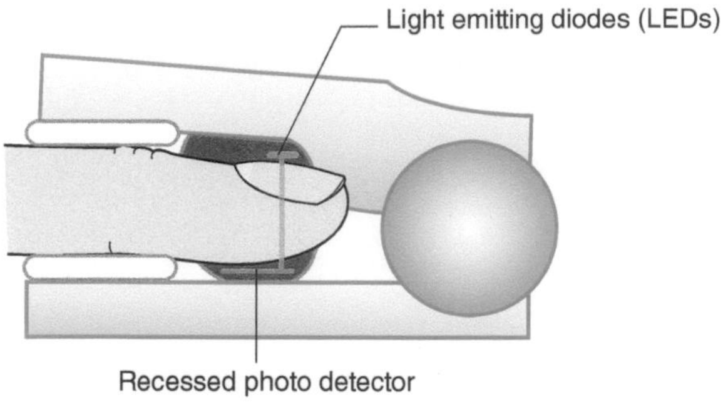

Figure 40.2 Pulse oximeter. *Source:* Preston & Kelly (2017), chapter 19, figure 19.1, p. 38. © John Wiley & Sons.

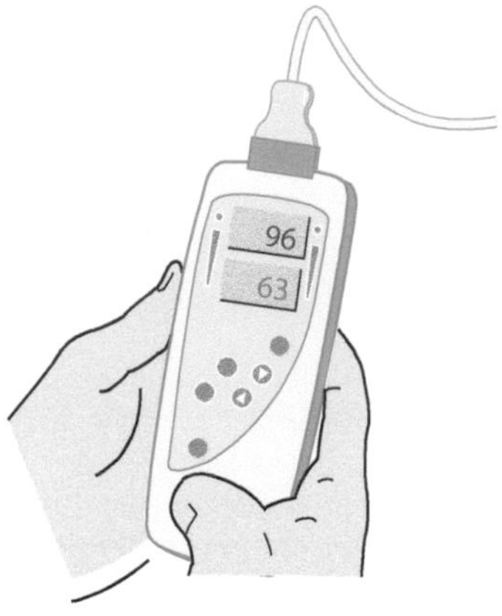

Figure 40.3 Pulse oximeter showing pulse detector and amplitude indicators. *Source:* Preston & Kelly (2017), chapter 19, figure 19.3, p. 38. © John Wiley & Sons.

The pulse oximeter possesses two light-emitting diodes which each emits light of a specific wavelength, one red and one infrared, through a cutaneous vascular bed, and a photodiode at the other side derives the oxygen saturation from the intensity of transmitted light at each wavelength. Absorption is measured at one point of the pulse wave and compared with absorption at another so that the difference between the values is due to arterial blood alone, hence eliminating the effect of absorption by other tissue and blood components (see Figure 40.2).

The pulse oximeter consists of a probe which is attached to the patient's finger or ear lobe and a computerised unit which displays the percentage oxygen saturation of Hb (see Figure 40.3).

What a Pulse Oximeter Measures

The World Health Organisation states that there are two numerical values obtained from the pulse oximeter monitor:

1. The oxygen saturation of Hb in arterial blood. The value of the oxygen saturation is given together with an audible signal that varies in pitch depending on the oxygen saturation. A falling pitch indicates falling oxygen saturation. Since the oximeter detects the saturation peripherally on a finger, toe or ear, the result is recorded as the peripheral oxygen saturation, described as SpO2.
2. The pulse rate in beats per minute, averaged over 5 to 20 seconds. Some oximeters display a pulse waveform or indicator that illustrates the strength of the pulse being detected. This display indicates how well the tissues are perfused. The signal strength falls if the patient's circulation becomes inadequate.

Red Flag

A pulse oximeter is not only a quick and practical task to measure oxygen saturations, it contributes to the Early Warning Score (RCP 2017) and therefore is considered an early-warning device. A pulse oximeter continuously measures the level of oxygen saturation of Hb in the arterial blood. It can detect hypoxia much sooner than the clinician can see clinical signs of hypoxia such as cyanosis. This ability to provide an early warning has made the pulse oximeter essential for safe care provision.

Box 40.1 Definitions of Terms Related to Oxygenation and Respiratory Failure

- Hypoxaemia – low partial pressure of oxygen in the blood (PaO2). Hypoxaemia can also be measured in relation to oxyhaemoglobin saturation or oxygen saturation within the arterial blood (SaO2). It occurs when PaO2 is less than 8kPa or SaO2 less than 90%.
- Hypoxia – occurs when oxygen supplies are insufficient to meet oxygen demands in a particular compartment, for example, alveolar or tissue hypoxia. Supplemental oxygen therapy can only correct hypoxia resulting from hypoxaemia.
- Hypercapnia – occurs when partial pressure of carbon dioxide (PaCO2) is above the normal range of 4.6–6.1kPa. Patients with hypercapnia are considered to have type II respiratory failure, even if their oxygen saturation is within the normal range.
- Type I respiratory failure – hypoxaemia in the absence of hypercapnia.
- Type II respiratory failure – hypoxaemia with hypercapnia.
- Hyperoxia – high oxygen content to the tissues and organs. The lung is designed to manage concentrations of 21% of oxygen; when given in higher concentrations, this may result in oxygen toxicity.

Source: Allibone et al. (2018).

The measurement of oxygen saturations via pulse oximetry (SpO2) is considered a fundamental vital sign and is often referred to as the 'fifth vital sign' (O'Driscoll et al. 2017). It should be performed on all patients who are breathless, those receiving supplementary oxygen and/or those who are acutely unwell with poor oxygenation and respiratory failure.

For definitions of terms relayed to oxygenation and respiratory failure, *see Box* 40.1. The British Thoracic Society recommends that oxygen saturations should be measured by trained staff using pulse oximetry (O'Driscoll et al. 2017).

Pulse oximeters are medical devices that monitor the level of oxygen in a patient's blood and alert the healthcare worker if oxygen levels drop below safe levels, allowing rapid intervention. These devices are essential in any setting in which a patient's blood oxygen level requires monitoring like operations, emergency and intensive care and treatment and recovery in hospital wards (WHO 2019).

Green Flag

Oxygen is a drug, and as such, it must be prescribed except in life-threatening emergencies when it must be started immediately. Emergency oxygen should not be withheld because of the absence of a prescription.

Nursing associates must familiarise themselves with local policy and procedure regarding the administering of emergency oxygen.

Take Note

The nursing associate may need to calibrate the pulse oximeter and undertake internal checks prior to taking a reading. In order to ensure that the reading is accurate, the manufacturer's guidelines must be followed.

Orange Flag

As a nursing associate working with older adults, it is likely that you will care for patients with long-term respiratory conditions such as chronic obstructive pulmonary disease (COPD). Therefore, to provide holistic and patient-centred care for your patient (NMC 2018), you must be mindful to incorporate physical and psychosocial care. Did you know that anxiety in patients with COPD is often associated with clinical depression? And studies indicate that patients who are depressed with COPD have a sevenfold risk of suffering from comorbid clinical anxiety compared with nondepressed patients with COPD (Tselibis et al. 2016).

Take Note

Patients receiving supplemental oxygen therapy should undergo regular SpO2 monitoring, as determined by the oxygen prescriber and in accordance with local and national guidelines. These patients should have their SpO2 monitored for at least five minutes after commencing supplemental oxygen therapy (BTS 2016). The frequency of subsequent SpO2 measurements will depend on the patients' condition and their stability, as well as the nurse's clinical judgement (BTS 2016). For example, patients who are critically ill should have their SpO2 monitored continuously and recorded every 15 minutes, whereas patients with mild breathlessness may require monitoring hourly or as indicated by a track-and-trigger system score such as the National Early Warning Score 2 (Royal College of Physicians 2017).

Pulse oximetry readings can be affected by several factors, as outlined in Box 40.2. For example, in patients with anaemia, oxygen saturation of the available Hb will be normal, even when the amount of Hb in the blood is reduced. Therefore, the patient may be hypoxaemic despite having normal oxygen saturations (O'Driscoll et al. 2017). The presence of carbon monoxide may falsely elevate SpO2 measurements, since oxygen is displaced from Hb by carboxyhaemoglobin, but this registers falsely as adequate oxygen saturation.

Box 40.2 Take Note 1: Factors That Can Affect Pulse Oximetry Readings

- Anaemia
- Critical illness
- Hypotension
- Malposition of the pulse oximeter probe
- Nail varnish or false nails
- Patient motion
- Peripheral vasoconstriction
- Presence of carbon monoxide in the blood, for example, resulting from smoke inhalation or car exhaust fumes
- Readings become inaccurate once the patient's oxygen saturation drops below 80%
- Reduced cardiac output or hypovolaemia
- Skin pigmentation, for example, jaundice
- Site used to undertake pulse oximetry; the optimal sites are the fingertips or earlobes

Source: Margereson & Withey (2012); Beasley et al. (2015); O'Driscoll et al. (2017).

Preparation and Equipment

Before undertaking the oxygen saturation procedure, the nursing associate should ensure that they are familiar with the manufacturer's instructions for use, and the functions of the oximeter to be used, to ensure safe and effective use. They should understand pulse oximetry and the physiology and technology involved, as well as ensure the necessary equipment is available, that it has been calibrated and is in working order (Peate 2019).

The equipment and paperwork required to undertake pulse oximetry is:

- Pulse oximeter
- Probes
- Cleaning wipes
- Nail polish remover, if required
- Care plan
- Patient documentation

Procedure

1. Begin by introducing yourself to the patient, before confirming their identity and explaining the procedure to obtain valid consent.
2. Ensure the patient is comfortable and request that they keep still during the procedure.
3. Ensure the oximetry probe is cleaned (decontaminated) using a locally approved cleaning wipe. Ensure the probe is in optimal working order, for example, that the hinges form a clip that will keep the probe in place, that the rubber shield is intact and functioning and the light source is illuminated. Ensure that there are no small wires protruding from the connectors.
4. Decontaminate your hands to reduce the risk of transferring microorganisms to the patient.
5. Choose a suitable area for the probe (usually the patient's fingertip).
6. Ensure the correct size of probe is being used, for example, that for an adult or child. The area chosen should have an optimal blood supply, for example, the fingertip or ear lobe, and should be warm to the touch and well perfused (good circulation of blood in the area).
7. Review any potential barriers to a clear reading, such as dirt, dried blood, intravenous dyes, poor perfusion, nail polish, acrylic nails, burns, contaminants such as oils, and oedema, as these may interfere with the transmission of the oximeter's light signals, causing inaccurate results.
8. Remove any barriers that you have identified, for example, clean the patient's finger and remove any nail polish.
9. Place the probe (usually on the index finger of the patient's nondominant hand) and secure it as directed by the manufacturer's instructions.
10. Explain to the patient that you are going to switch the oximeter on. Ensure that the probe sensor is detecting the patient's pulse. This is usually indicated by a 'beeping' noise, which sounds in time with each detected pulse, or by a graphic indication of the pulse (wave form) on the display screen, while the pulse oximeter is on the patient's finger. The numerical and graphical results are usually available within seconds, and the reading can be taken when the numerical display stops rising.
11. When the oxygen saturation monitoring procedure is complete, inform the patient, remove the probe and ensure that the patient is comfortable.
12. There may be a requirement to use pulse oximetry continually (for an hour or more), for example, to undertake sleep studies or to provide long-term monitoring and if required, this should be explained to the patient. If continuous pulse oximetry is required, the HCP and AP should set and check alarms as per local policy and inspect the sensor site every four hours in case of tissue irritation or pressure from the sensor.

13. You should decontaminate your hands following the procedure.
14. Inform the patient of the results and record them in their notes. Record the flow/concentration of any current oxygen therapy in litres per minute.
15. Explain the results to the patient and inform a registered healthcare professional, who may change the patient's care plan, if required.
16. If the reading falls outside the patient's normal parameters, check the equipment is correctly attached to the patient. You should also check if the equipment is working properly and that there is no artefact (unexpected movement that could affect the reading); for example, shivering can interfere with an accurate reading.
17. If the reading falls outside of the patient's parameters and you have performed all necessary checks, explain to the patient that you are seeking further advice from a more senior colleague. You must then report the reading immediately using local guidelines for reporting concerns and seek further advice and guidance.
18. Document any actions in the patient's notes.
19. Decontaminate the equipment using a locally approved cleaning wipe.
20. Document findings either within the patients notes (in community settings), or on a NEWS2 chart for adults in adult care, or a PEWS chart in children's departments. If an abnormality is recorded, the nursing associate must escalate their concern to the registered nurse, outreach team or a medical professional.
21. Wash hands.

(NMC 2018; RCP 2017; Peate 2019).

In patients who are acutely unwell, an arterial blood gas analysis should be undertaken, which is considered the gold standard in assessing respiratory failure. Arterial blood gas analysis enables a more accurate reading of oxygen saturations within the arterial blood (SaO2) compared with SpO2 and also measures the partial pressure of oxygen (PaO2), partial pressure of carbon dioxide (PaCO2), pH or hydrogen level and, in some devices, Hb and electrolytes (Dutton & Finch 2018; Gibson & Waters 2017). Arterial blood gas analysis enables diagnosis of respiratory or metabolic acidosis or alkalosis, which may further guide the supplemental oxygen therapy required, as well as any additional interventions (Gibson & Waters 2017).

Assessing the Need for Supplemental Oxygen Therapy

Respiratory review of a patient enables healthcare practitioners to determine if there is adequate gas exchange, that tissues are effectively oxygenated and that carbon dioxide is being excreted. Therefore, respiratory assessment/review is essential in determining if the patient has a clinical need for supplemental oxygen therapy and can also assist with evaluating the effects of the intervention. Reviewing the patient's external respiration includes recording their respiratory rate, pattern, depth and effort. Review of the patient's internal respiration involves examining their skin colour for signs of cyanosis, measuring SpO2 and checking organ function, for example, assessing for any neurological impairment.

Where possible, taking the patient's medical and social history is important in a respiratory review/assessment to identify any long-term illnesses or factors affecting their respiratory function, such as smoking. It is also important for the nursing associate to be aware of any existing oxygen requirements that the patient has, for example, home oxygen and/or non-invasive ventilation. Before nursing associates begin the review, they should identify any special considerations that might be affecting the patient's respiration and breathing, such as those listed in Box 40.3.

Box 40.3 Special Considerations That Might Affect a Patient's Respiration and Breathing

- **Pregnancy** – Changes in oestrogen and progesterone cause fluid retention and affect respiratory function. LoMauro & Aliverti (2015) identified that the progressive uterine distension is the major cause of lung volume and chest wall changes during pregnancy, which comprise elevation of the diaphragm and altered thoracic configuration. The enlarging uterus increases the end-expiratory abdominal (gastric) pressure (Pga), thereby displacing the diaphragm upwards, with two consequences. First, the negative pleural pressure (oesophageal pressure (Poes)) increases, leading to an earlier closure of the small airways with consequent reduction of functional residual capacity and expiratory reserve volume. Secondly, the chest height becomes shorter, but the other thoracic dimensions increase in order to maintain constant total lung capacity.
- **Obesity** – Obesity causes mechanical compression of the diaphragm, lungs and chest cavity, which can lead to restrictive pulmonary damage. Furthermore, excess fat decreases total respiratory system compliance, increases pulmonary resistance and reduces respiratory muscle strength (Mafort et al. 2016).
- **Circulatory issues** – Heart failure, pulmonary oedema and anaemia may inhibit effective gas exchange.
- **Environment** – Factors such as room temperature may influence assessment, for example, a cold environment might cause shivering. The environment in which the assessment takes place could also increase the patient's anxiety and cause changes in their breathing, for example, if it is noisy or busy.
- **Trauma, particularly chest trauma** – If the patient is experiencing pain, they may find it challenging to take deep breaths. A pneumothorax (collapsed lung) may be present, and, therefore, a thorough review is required.
- **Known allergies** – If an allergy causes anaphylaxis, the patient's airway may swell, causing breathing difficulties.
- **Abdominal distention** – for example caused by ascites or bowel obstruction. This may prevent full inflation of the lungs.

Source: Adapted from Moore (2009).

Violet Flag

When offering care and support to people in their own homes who are receiving home oxygen therapy, the nursing associate must ensure the patient and their family are safe.

Oxygen is a fire hazard, and precautions need to be taken if oxygen is used at home. The following precautions should be taken and explained to the patient and, if appropriate, their family:

- Never let anyone smoke while oxygen is being used
- Oxygen should be kept at least 2 metres away from flames or heat sources, such as gas cookers and gas heaters
- Never use flammable liquids, such as cleaning fluid, paint thinner or aerosols, while oxygen is in use
- Do not use oil-based emollients, such as Vaseline, when using oxygen
- Tested and working fire alarms and smoke detectors should be installed in the home
- The local fire brigade should be informed that the patient is using oxygen at home
- Always ensure that oxygen cylinders are kept upright to prevent them being damaged

Supporting Evidence

British Thoracic Society (BTS): Guidelines. https://www.brit-thoracic.org.uk/quality-improvement/guidelines/

Royal College of Physicians (RCP) *The national early warning score 2 (NEWS2)* https://www.rcplondon.ac.uk/projects/outputs/national-early-warning-score-news-2

Touch Point

Measurement of oxygen saturation, using a pulse oximeter probe, is routinely undertaken as part of patients' vital signs during diagnosis and ongoing monitoring. Oxygen saturation readings are a key component of the National Early Warning Score (NEWS2).

Peak Flow

PEF is an objective test to measure lung function and to support a review of airway obstruction or inflammation. It is recorded using a peak flow meter (see Figure 40.4).

Readings will vary from person to person and will depend on factors such as height and age and on how constricted the patient's airways are. PEFR is mainly used to support respiratory assessments particularly used with conditions such as asthma and COPD.

Although there is no single diagnostic test for asthma, measurement of PEFR plays an important role in the diagnosis and management of the condition (British Thoracic Society and Scottish Intercollegiate Guidelines Network (BTS and SIGN) (2016); National Institute for Health and Care Excellence (NICE) 2017). Figure 40.5 illustrates the effect that asthma has on the airway.

Yellow Flag

Dyspnoea (difficulty in breathing) can be very frightening for patients (and also for nursing associates) and can result in increased anxiety; this can cause the patient to become more breathless. Interventions implemented by the nursing associate can break this cycle. The nursing associate should take time with breathless patients, talk to them in a calm and reassuring manner, encouraging them to breathe slowly; breathing with the individual can be a very effective tactic.

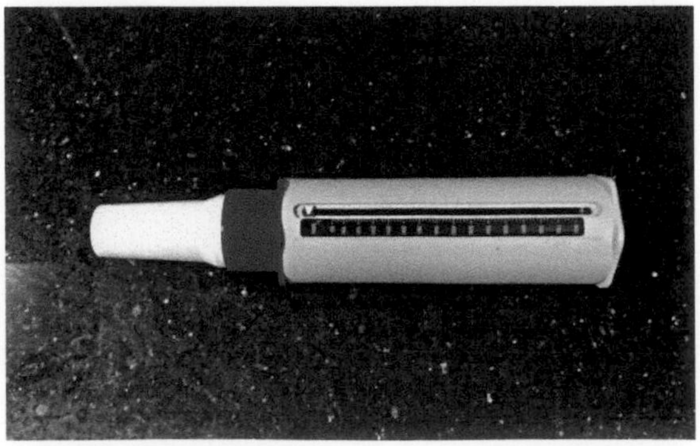

Figure 40.4 A peak flow meter. *Source:* Lindsay et al. (2018), chapter 60, figure 60.1, p. 124. © John Wiley & Sons.

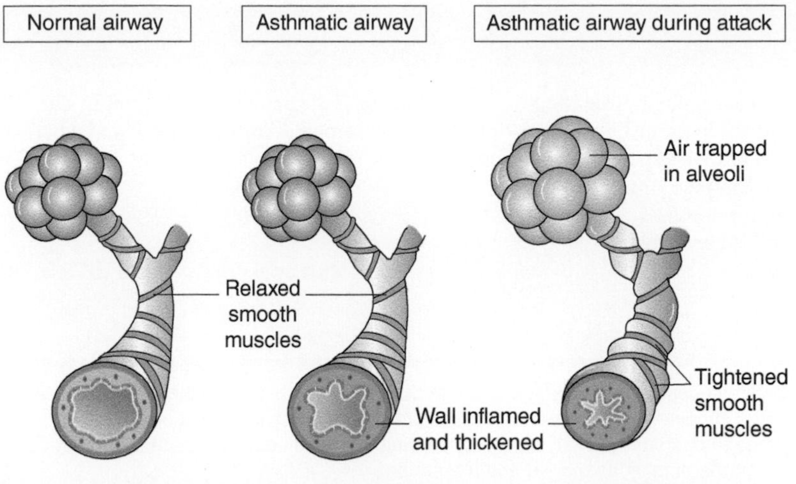

Figure 40.5 The airways and asthma. *Source:* Preston & Kelly (2017), chapter 24, figure 24.1, p. 50. © John Wiley & Sons.

PEFR is defined as the highest flow achieved on forced expiration from a position of maximum lung inflation and is expressed in litres per minute (Dougherty et al. 2015). It will indicate how narrow or open the airways are.

PEFR should be recorded as the best of three forced expirations from full lung capacity, with a maximum pause of 2 seconds before blowing (BTS & SIGN 2016). The patient can be seated or standing, and any subsequent test (if possible) should mirror the previous, i.e. the patient should be seated if this was the previous position, so it is important to record how PEFR was taken. For example, PEFR was measured in a seated position.

In the United Kingdom, there is currently no consensus about what a normal adult PEFR rate should be. As noted above, the readings will depend on a range of demographic factors, including the person's age, height, gender, ethnicity and severity of disease; it may also vary with time of day. However, according to the Royal College of Nursing (RCN) (2019), adults should achieve readings of 400 to 700 litres per minute, with men generally higher. Readings tend to be lower in the morning and will be affected by how recently the person has taken his or her inhaler to expand the airways.

Healthcare professionals tend to look for trends in peak flow readings rather than sudden and dramatic changes between readings, although they can happen. Nursing associates should report any reading they think is unusually low (or high) to the registered nurse in charge. A drop of around 20% from the normal would be cause for concern, but a drop of 50% would be alarming and would require immediate medical attention (RCN 2019). Ongoing monitoring and twice daily PEFR measurement (morning and night) will enable the healthcare team to establish each patient's own baseline.

Take Note

Incorrect technique, patient concordance and effort are major factors in accurate measurement of peak expiratory flow rate.

According to Dougherty et al. (2015), in healthy individuals without any pathological conditions of the airways, factors that determine PEFR include:

- The quality of the large airways
- The volume of the lungs
- The elastic properties of the lungs (ability to stretch and recoil)
- The power and coordination of the expiratory muscles
- The resistance of the instrument used to measure PEF

In patients with respiratory diseases and other conditions, the ability of the respiratory system to work effectively will be impeded, which will affect PEFR.

Red Flag

Conditions that may affect the respiratory system may include neuromuscular disease, cardiac failure, vascular disease, musculoskeletal deformity and infections such as sepsis.

Some people may develop occupational asthma from substances inhaled at work: those working in, for example, bakeries, zoos, carpentry workshops, hospitals and hairdressers and on farms may be exposed to workplace allergens and irritants (Asthma UK 2019).

Presentation

Nursing associates should only treat a patient presenting with acute asthma if the patient is well enough. They should not exacerbate a patient's condition, and must refer the patient to a registered nurse, outreach team or medical professional if and when necessary. If the patient is stable, the nursing associate may (if part of their expected responsibilities):

- Take a history of the patient's respiratory problems
- Record any seasonal changes in symptoms
- Find out if the patient has noticed any triggers
- Ask whether there is a personal or family history of atopic disease (i.e. eczema or allergic rhinitis) (BTS & SIGN 2016; NICE 2017).

Blue Flag

One of nursing associate's most intangible assets is that of trust, and when people are ill, they need to know that they can trust the nursing associate. Trust impacts nursing associates' ability to form meaningful relationships with patients, and this connection will positively impact on health outcomes. Trust, as one of nursing's core values, can result in patient cooperation and honest transparent communication between the nursing associate and the patient.

If there are strong indications to suspect asthma, PEFR should be undertaken. If an adult patient's symptoms are better at weekends, on days off work or on holiday, there is a possibility that they may have occupational asthma (NICE 2017). These patients should be referred to an occupational asthma specialist.

Red Flag

Patients presenting with acute symptoms should be treated immediately. If possible, PEFR tests should be undertaken on presentation or, if the patient is too unwell, once the symptoms have eased.

Frequency of PEFR Recording

For patients diagnosed with asthma, Asthma UK (2016) recommends recording PEFR twice a day. Patients should be advised to do this when they are well and unwell to identify patterns. The nursing associate can explain the importance of recording PEFR to the patient, demonstrate how to use a peak flow meter and check that the patient has a good technique.

Recording PEFR is helpful to obtain a baseline and can be subsequently used to monitor patients when they feel their condition has deteriorated, as well as at their annual asthma review.

When to Record PEFR

Outpatients should be advised to record their PEFR in a diary, and in the case of inpatients, their readings will be recorded on a PEFR chart in their notes (see Figure 40.6).

Patients with a diagnosis of asthma should be advised to record their peak flow in the morning and at night to monitor their condition. The score will indicate whether their asthma is getting worse, help determine if their medication is working and indicate if they are having an asthma attack (NHS website 2018).

Indications for PEFR

There are several reasons why the nursing associate may be required to undertake a PEFR:

- Detect possible lung obstruction or restriction due to inflamed airways
- Help diagnose asthma
- Identify asthma control strategies
- Identify triggers and exacerbating factors
- Monitor the progression of respiratory disease
- Evaluate the effectiveness of inhalers or other treatment

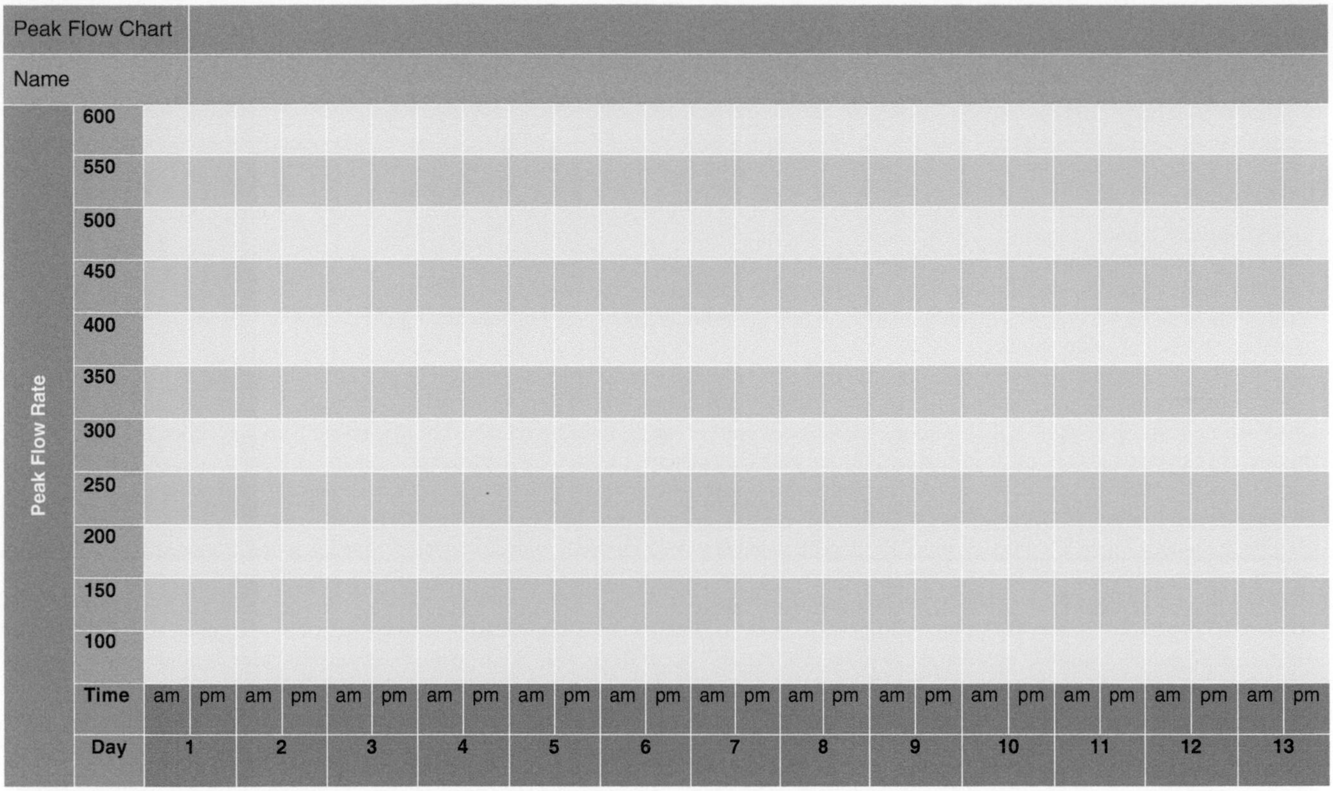

Figure 40.6 An example of a peak flow chart. *Source:* Lindsay et al. (2018), chapter 60, figure 60.3, p. 124. © John Wiley & Sons.

Contraindications for PEFR

- Patients with severe breathlessness
- Patients who are unable to inspire effectively (this will lead to an inaccurate PEFR)
- Patients who are unable to understand or lack capacity to perform the procedure independently
- Patients who have recently undergone thoracic, abdominal or cranial surgery

Advantages of PEFR

Repeated measurement and charting of PEFR have long been used to diagnose asthma. The advantages of using peak flow measurement as part of diagnosing asthma are low cost and the availability of equipment, as well as the ease with which peak flow measurement and periods of peak flow monitoring can be repeated. If a patient presents with acute symptoms, measurements can be taken at once (Keeley 2017).

Patients can keep track of their peak flow scores by recording their PEFR in between their annual asthma reviews to identify and record any triggers or allergies that could be making their asthma worse and to monitor the difference that medication adherence and concordance makes to the condition of the airways.

In addition, PEFR may provide early warning signs that a patient's airways are compromised so that prompt action can be taken, such as the use of inhalers, to avoid progression to an asthma attack.

How to Measure PEFR

Preparation and Equipment

The nursing associate should ensure the appropriate equipment is available, including:

- Peak flow meter
- Disposable mouthpiece
- Observation chart to record the readings

The nurse should explain the procedure to the patient and include a demonstration if necessary. It is important to ensure patient understanding, promote concordance and obtain valid consent for the investigation. The nurse should assist the patient into a comfortable standing or sitting position, because patient discomfort can affect respiratory effort.

Procedure

1. Decontaminate hands.
2. Use a clean peak flow meter with a new disposable mouthpiece to prevent cross infection.
3. Check that the peak flow meter pointer has returned to zero to ensure an accurate reading.
4. Ensure the peak flow meter is held horizontally and that the patient's fingers are not obstructing the pointer, which might prevent it from moving, or result in a false reading.
5. Ask the patient to take a deep breath in, to close their lips around the mouthpiece, making a tight seal, and to exhale as hard and fully as possible into the mouthpiece, with a sudden, sharp blow (huff) (Branch & Coffey 2009). A full inspiration is required to review airflow obstruction. Ensuring a tight seal around the mouthpiece prevents air from escaping, which might result in an inaccurate reading. When the patient exhales, a piston inside the cylinder of the peak flow meter is pushed down, progressively exposing a slot in the top of the meter until the piston reaches a position of rest. The piston position is indicated by a pointer on a scale from 60–800L per minute.
6. Record the reading and return the pointer to zero.
7. Ask the patient to repeat the process twice more. The peak expiratory flow rate should be recorded as the best of three forced expiratory exhalations from total lung capacity. After the patient has taken a full inspiration, there should be a maximum pause of 2 seconds before exhalation. This improves the reliability of the final recording.
8. Record the highest expiratory flow rate reading, and ensure documentation is completed in accordance with local policy and includes the time, date and an indication of any nebulised or inhaled therapy. Accurate records of any assessments/reviews are a fundamental aspect of nursing care.
9. Discard the used mouthpiece, clean the peak flow meter according to local policy and wash your hands to reduce the risk of cross infection.
10. A wide variation, such as a sudden drop in the expected value compared with the previous personal best value, could indicate deterioration in the patient's condition. If the procedure was performed in a hospital, inform medical staff of any concerns. If the procedure was performed in the community, follow the previously agreed individual patient protocol for management (Myatt 2017).

Monitoring and Documentation

If the patient maintains an accurate record of their peak expiratory flow rate measurements in their peak flow diary, fluctuations in respiratory effort can be observed over time. A historical record of lower readings during symptomatic episodes, as compared with asymptomatic periods, provides objective confirmation of symptoms. This information can be used to identify early changes in the patient's condition that require treatment to help evaluate responses to changes in therapy and to provide a quantitative measure of impairment. The peak expiratory flow rate can also be used to assess reversibility and variability in patients with asthma (Myatt 2017).

Take Note Advice to patients

Individuals should be advised to develop the following good habits to record their PEF, which the nursing associate should reinforce as part of patient education: The nursing associate should recommend that patients:

- Use a good technique and procedure – this can be demonstrated by the nursing associate.
- Maintain a regular routine, writing down exactly when they are going to take their peak flow measurement and make sure they adhere to it. Advise them to keep their peak flow meter on their bedside table as this can help them remember to record their peak flow as soon as they wake up in the morning and at night before going to bed.
- Record their readings in a peak flow diary, in the morning and at night, so they can monitor patterns. It may help them get a clearer picture of when their asthma medicines are working, to determine if the condition is getting worse and when they need to take preventative action.
- Use their peak flow diary alongside a written asthma action plan so they can be confident they know what to do if their peak flow readings drop below a certain level. Patients can write this in their action plan.
- Record their peak flow score before they use their preventer inhaler.
- Record symptoms alongside their peak flow reading to keep an eye on their asthma. If their symptoms change, but their peak flow score is the same, they still need to book an appointment with their asthma nurse or GP.
- At their asthma review, ask their asthma nurse or GP to check that they are taking their readings correctly to make sure that they are obtaining accurate measurements.
- Always use the same peak flow meter (different meters may give different readings).
- Clean their meter regularly by soaking the mouthpiece and tube in warm water mixed with mild detergent; finish by rinsing in clean water and shaking gently to remove excess water. They should not scrub inside the tube because this could damage it. Clean it at least once a month to keep it in good condition.
- Store the meter somewhere safe so it does not become damaged, such as a bedside table drawer, bathroom medicine cabinet or in a special pouch or case.

Box 40.4 Supporting Evidence Box

Supporting Evidence Box

NICE. (2017) *Asthma: diagnosis, monitoring and chronic asthma management*. [online] Available: https://www.nice.org.uk/guidance/ng80/resources/asthma-diagnosis-monitoring-and-chronic-asthma-management-pdf-1837687975621

Asthma.org. (2016) *Peak flow*. [online] Available: https://www.asthma.org.uk/advice/manage-your-asthma/peak-flow/

Take Note

- It is important that nursing associates are aware of NICE (2019) guidance and evidence-based practice when treating adult patients with asthma. In contemporary nursing practice, especially when caring for patients with chronic lung conditions, it is vital to ensure they 'live well' with their condition and that they are encouraged to live life and enjoy it.
- It is part of the nursing associate's role to support patients by providing health promotion and educating patients about how to monitor and treat their asthma.
- Nursing associates should also raise awareness about the importance of good psychological well-being to enable patients to maintain a healthy and positive outlook and prevent them being defined by their condition.

Touch Points Revisited

- Measuring respiratory status with pulse oximetry and peak flow is a key activity that the nursing associate must be able be perform proficiently with a variety of patients in a range of care settings.
- The nursing associate has a key role to play in monitoring a patient's vital signs, and monitoring pulse oximetry and peak flow can be seen as vital signs.
- Pulse oximetry is a non-invasive technique for measuring the oxygen saturation in the blood. A probe is attached to a part of the body with an optimal blood supply, such as the fingertip or the ear lobe.
- Undertaking safe pulse oximetry in an effective and person-centred way will require the nursing associate to be able to demonstrate insight, understanding and appropriate preparation.
- This activity must be carried out using local policy and procedure. Peak flow meters are inexpensive; they are handheld devices that measure how well air is expired from the lungs. It is one of several tests used to assess lung function and help diagnose conditions such as asthma.
- Nursing associates should ensure that they understand and are able to perform good PEFR technique to coach patients regarding how to take their own readings to ensure that these are reliable and accurate. It is vital that patients record PEFR to establish their baseline which should enable recognition of when their PEFR is low.
- If the nursing associate has any concerns regarding the observations noted by pulse oximetry or PEFR, then this must be reported immediately and documented according to policy and procedure.

References

Allibone, E., Soares, T. and Wilson, A. (2018) Safe and effective use of supplemental oxygen therapy, *Nursing Standard*, doi: 10.7748/ ns.2018.e11227.

Asthma.org. (2016) *Peak flow*. [online] Available: https://www.asthma.org.uk/advice/manage-your-asthma/peak-flow/. Accessed 02 September 2019.

Asthma UK. (2013) Asthma and me, *A guide to living with asthma*. [online] Available: https://tinyurl.com/y2qtj3cm. Accessed 10 July 2019.

Asthma UK. (2016) *Peak flow test*. [online] Available at: https://tinyurl.com/y2ravblb. Accessed 10 July 2019.

Asthma UK. (2019) *Occupational asthma*. [online] Available: https://tinyurl.com/yx9m9nxz. Accessed 10 July 2019.

Beasley, R., Chien, J., Douglas, J. et al. (2015) Thoracic Society of Australia and New Zealand oxygen guidelines for acute oxygen use in adults: 'swimming between the flags'. *Respirology*, 20(8): 1182–1191. doi: 10.1111/resp.12620.

Bickley, L. (2016) *Bates' guide to physical examination and history taking* (12th edn), Wolters Kluwer.

British Thoracic Society (*BTS*). *(2016)* BTS guideline for oxygen use in adults in healthcare and emergency settings. [online] Available: https://thorax.bmj.com/content/72/Suppl_1/ii1. Accessed 28 August 2019.

British Thoracic Society (*BTS)* and Scottish Intercollegiate Guidelines Network (SIGN). (2019) *British guideline on the management of asthma: a national clinical guideline*. [online] Available: https://www.brit-thoracic.org.uk/quality-improvement/guidelines/asthma/. Accessed 28 August 2019.

Dougherty, L., Lister, S. and West-Oram, A. (eds.). (2015) *The royal Marsden manual of clinical nursing procedures* (9th edn), London: Wiley-Blackwell, 530

Dutton, H. and Finch, J. (2018) *Acute and critical care nursing: at a glance*, UK: Wiley Blackwell.

Gibson, V. and Waters, D. (2017) *Respiratory care*, UK: Tayler and Francis.

Keeley, D. (2017) Peak flow monitoring and microspirometry as aids to respiratory diagnosis in primary care, *Primary Care Respiratory Update 2017*, 4(1): 25–28.

Lindsay, P., Bagness, C. and Peate, I. (2018) *Midwifery skills at a glance – at a glance (nursing and healthcare)*, UK: Wiley-Blackwell.

LoMauro, A. and Aliverti, A. (2015) Respiratory physiology of pregnancy: physiology masterclass, *Breathe (Sheff)*, 11(4):297–301. doi:10.1183/20734735.008615.

Mafort, T.T., Rufino, R., Costa, C.H. and Lopes, A.J. (2016) Obesity: systemic and pulmonary complications, biochemical abnormalities, and impairment of lung function, *Multidisciplinary Respiratory Medicine, (2016)* 11: 28.

Margereson, C. and Withey, S. (2012) *The patient with acute respiratory problems.* In: Peate, I., Dutton, H. (Eds) *Acute Nursing Care: Recognising and Responding to Medical Emergencies* (pp. 81–106). Taylor and Francis: Oxford.
Moore, T. (2009) *Oxygen therapy.* In: Woodrow, P., Moore, T. (Eds) *High Dependency Nursing Care: Observation, Intervention and Support for Level 2 Patients* (pp. 174–184), 2nd edition. Routledge: London.
Myatt, R. (2017) Measuring peak expiratory flow rate: what the nurse needs to know, *Nursing Standard*, 31(20): 40–44.
National Institute for Health and Care Excellence. (2017) *Asthma: diagnosis, monitoring and chronic asthma management [NG80].* [online] Available: https://www.nice.org.uk/guidance/ng80. Accessed 10 July 2019.
NHS. (2018) *Peak flow test.* [online] Available: https://tinyurl.com/y2npb6jr. Accessed 10 July 2019.
Nursing and Midwifery Council. (2018) *The code, Professional standards of behaviour for nurses, midwives and nursing associates,* London: NMC.
O'Driscoll, B.R., Howard, L.S., Earis, J. and Mak, V. on behalf of the BTS Emergency Oxygen Guideline Development Group. (2017) *British thoracic society guideline for oxygen use in adults in healthcare and emergency settings.* [online] Available: https://bmjopenrespres.bmj.com/content/4/1/e000170. Accessed 28 August 2019.
O'Driscoll, B.R., Howard, L.S., Earis, J. et al. (2017) BTS guideline for oxygen use in adults in healthcare and emergency settings. *Thorax.* 72(Suppl 1), ii1–ii90. doi:10.1136/thoraxjnl-2016-209729.
Peate, I. (2019) Tests, scans and investigations, 13. How to undertake pulse oximetry, *British Journal of Health Care Assistants*, 12(5): 214–217.
Potter, V. (2009) Pulse oximetry in general practice: How would a pulse oximeter influence patient management? *European Journal of General Practice*, 13(4): 216–220.
Preston, W. and Kelly, C. (eds) (2017) *Respiratory nursing at a glance*, UK: Wiley Blackwell.
Royal College of Nursing (RCN). (2019) *Peak flow.* [online] Available: https://rcni.com/hosted-content/rcn/first-steps/peak-flow-testing. Accessed on 2 September 2019.
Royal College of Physicians (RCP). (2017) *National early warning score 2 (NEWS2).* [online] Available: https://www.rcplondon.ac.uk/projects/outputs/national-early-warning-score-news-2. Accessed 28 August 2019.
Tselibis, A., Pachi, A., Ilias, I., Kosmas, E., Bratis, D., Moussas, G. and Tzanakis, N. (2016) Strategies to improve anxiety and depression in patients with COPD: a mental health perspective, *Neuropsychiatric Disease and Treatment*, 2016, 12: 297–328. doi:10.2147/NDT.S79354.
WHO. (2019) *Pulse oximetry.* [online] Available: https://www.who.int/patientsafety/safesurgery/pulse_oximetry/en/. Accessed 2 August 2019.

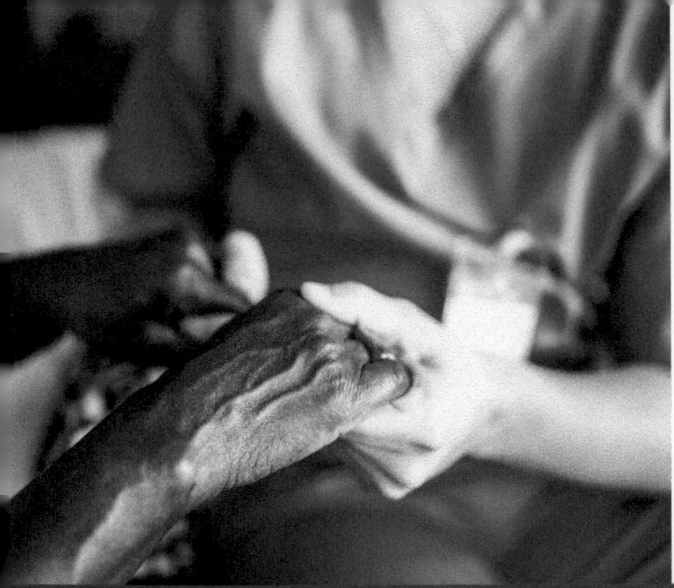

41

Using Nasal and Oral Suctioning Techniques

Barry Hill

Northumbria University, UK

Chapter Aim

- **This chapter aims to provide the reader with insight into using nasal and oral suctioning techniques**

Learning Outcomes

- **To understand the different nasal and oral suctioning techniques**
- **Describe the use of nasal and oral suctioning techniques**
- **Identify the common indications and contraindications for nasal and oral suctioning**

Test Yourself Multiple Choice Questions

1. **Airway suctioning is a common practice in the treatment of patients with a variety of respiratory conditions.**
   A) **True**
   B) **False**
2. **Suction should be considered if a patient's breathing is compromised by excessive secretions which can be assessed visually or by auscultation (listening) of the patient's chest using a stethoscope.**
   A) **True**
   B) **False**

The Nursing Associate's Handbook of Clinical Skills, First Edition. Edited by Ian Peate.

Companion website: www.wiley.com/nursingassociate

3. **Suctioning is a procedure used to remove substances from the:**
   A) **Trachea**
   B) **Pharynx**
   C) **Nose**
   D) **Mouth**
   E) **All of the above**

4. **Oral suctioning is used to remove secretions from the mouth and should be performed using a yankauer suction catheter.**
   A) **True**
   B) **False**
5. **The primary indication for suctioning the patient is the patient's inability to adequately clear the airway by independently coughing.**
   A) **True**
   B) **False**

Introduction

This chapter introduces the nursing associate to the principles of nasal and oral suctioning techniques. When using nasal and oral suctioning techniques, the nursing associate will be working towards achieving the following proficiencies (NMC 2018a): platform 3 to provide and monitor care and platform 5 to improving safety and quality care.

Airway suctioning is a common practice in the treatment of patients with a variety of respiratory conditions. Sometimes, some patients cannot remove secretions effectively; therefore, these secretions may be removed by suction.

Green Flag

Only appropriately trained staff should perform suctioning in line with their scope of clinical competence and awareness of their limitations. It is essential the nursing associate adheres to the tenets of the Code of Conduct (NMC 2018b).

Suction should be considered if a patient's breathing is compromised by excessive secretions which can be determined visually or by auscultation (listening) of the patient's chest using a stethoscope (Bickley 2016). The aim of airway suctioning is to clear secretions, thereby maintaining a patent airway and promoting adequate ventilation. Removal of these secretions also minimises the risk of atelectasis (collapse of lung tissue preventing the exchange of carbon dioxide and oxygen as part of normal respiration) (Woodrow 2018).

Touch Point

Airway suctioning aims to clear secretions with the intention of ensuring a patent airway and assisting with ventilation, gas exchange, adequate oxygenation and alveolar ventilation.

Suctioning

Suctioning is a procedure used to remove substances from the trachea, pharynx, nose or mouth through a natural orifice (nose or mouth) (Overend et al. 2009). Physiotherapists, registered nurses and doctors (especially anaesthetists) will use suctioning to promote secretion clearance (pulmonary hygiene) and/or maintain a patent airway. The technique is used in patients along the continuum of care from the critically ill to individuals living in the community.

Violet Flag

When offering care and support to people in non-clinical settings, for example, when working in the criminal justice sector or transferring a patient from one place of care to another, and if suction is needed, the nursing associate needs be competent and confident in using the suctioning equipment. The equipment should be checked regularly and used according to the manufacturer's instructions and local policy and procedure adhered to.

Take Note

Suctioning can cause complications such as hypoxia, injury to the airway, nosocomial infections and cardiac dysrhythmias; if in a hospital setting, it is important to review the patient before, during and after the suctioning procedure.

The Different Types of Oral and Nasal Suctioning

The portion of the airway that requires suctioning and whether the patient has an artificial airway determine the type of suctioning that is required. The most common types are:

- **Oral suctioning** – to remove secretions from the mouth and should be performed using a yankauer suction catheter (see Figure 41.1).
- **Oropharyngeal suctioning** – extends from the lips to the pharynx (see Figure 41.2). It can be performed for patients who are breathing spontaneously but are unable to maintain an open airway. Oropharyngeal suctioning requires the insertion of a suction catheter through the mouth to the pharynx.

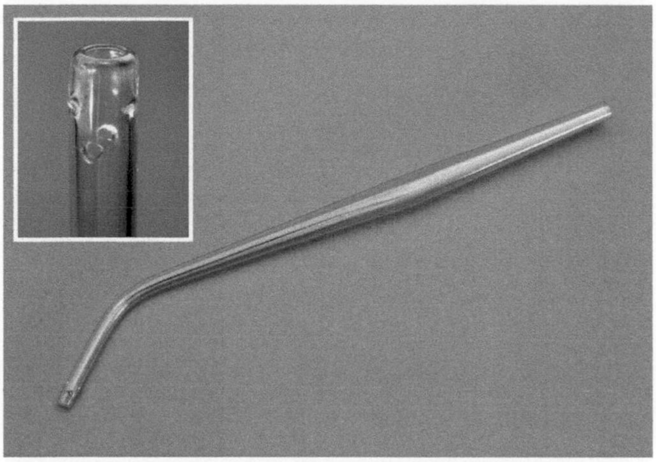

Figure 41.1 Oral suctioning. *Source:* Dougherty et al. (2015), figure 9.42, p. 417.

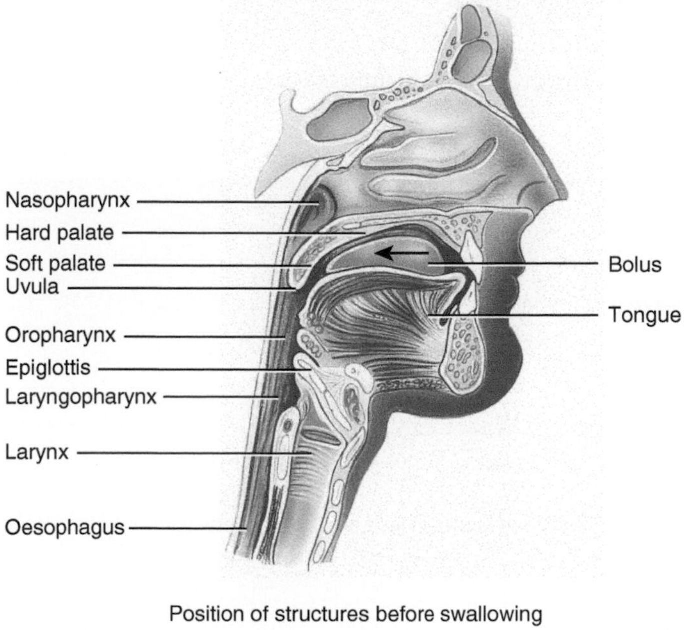

Figure 41.2 Key structures associated with suctioning. *Source:* Peate & Nair (2016), figure 9.5a, p. 264.

- **Nasal suctioning** – to remove secretions from the nares (nostrils) and should be performed using a yankauer suction catheter.
- **Nasopharyngeal suctioning** – extends from the tip of the nose to the pharynx (see Figure 41.2). The suction catheter is gently inserted through the nostrils into the pharynx. Airway adjuncts (e.g. guedal) can be used if the patient is unable to tolerate suction without their use or is in an unconscious state.

Indications for Suctioning

The primary indication for suctioning is the patient's inability to adequately clear the airway by independently coughing. The patient may exhibit some or all the following signs. The suctioning technique will depend on the patient's needs:

- More frequent or congested sounding cough
- Bubbly (wet saturated vocal sound)
- Rattling or coarse expiratory crackles (rales)
- Visible secretions
- Indication by the patient that suctioning is necessary
- Suspected aspiration of gastric or upper airway secretions
- Dyspnoea
- Decreased oxygen saturations thought to be related to mucus plugging
- End-of-life patients who are distressed by upper respiratory secretions and is unable to self-expectorate
- An increased inspiratory pressure on the ventilator
- The need to obtain a sputum specimen to identify pneumonia, other pulmonary infection or for sputum cytology

Orange Flag

There are a number of physical benefits associated with suctioning. Oral suctioning, for example, can also enhance self-esteem when used as part of oral hygiene maintenance.

Contraindications for Suctioning

Suctioning is a necessary procedure for patients unable to maintain a patent airway. Most contraindications are relative to the risks of a worsening clinical condition. There is no absolute contraindication to suctioning as the benefits almost always outweigh the risk to the patient. One absolute contraindication is if the patient refuses the procedure.

The decision to abstain from suctioning in order to avoid a possible adverse reaction may worsen the condition of the patient considerably. However, routine or scheduled suctioning, with no indication of need, is not recommended.

For patients requiring end-of-life care, drug treatment (such as hyoscine which dries copious secretions (National Institute for Health and Care Excellence (NICE) 2019) plus oropharyngeal suction can be used and only then in unconscious people, as it may be uncomfortable (see Table 41.1).

Complications of Suctioning

- Hypoxia
- Trauma to the nasal, oropharyngeal or tracheal mucosa
- Cardiac arrest/respiratory arrest
- Bronchoconstriction/bronchospasm

Table 41.1 Excessive respiratory secretion in palliative care.

By subcutaneous injection • **For Adult** 400 micrograms every 4 hours as required; hourly use is occasionally necessary, particularly in excessive respiratory secretions.
By continuous subcutaneous infusion • **For Adult** 1.2–2 mg every 24 hours.

Source: NICE (2019).

- Pneumothorax
- Pulmonary haemorrhage
- Incomplete secretion clearance
- Micro-atelectasis
- Raised intracranial pressure
- Hypotension/hypertension laryngospasm
- Sepsis
- Cardiac arrhythmias

Oral and Oropharyngeal Suctioning

The purpose of oral and oropharyngeal suctioning is to maintain a patent airway and improve oxygenation by removing mucous secretions and foreign material such as vomit or gastric secretions, from the mouth and throat (oropharynx). Oral suction is the use of a rigid plastic suction catheter, known as a yankauer (see Figure 41.1), to remove pharyngeal secretions through the mouth (Doyle & McCutcheon 2015). The suction catheter has a large hole for the thumb to cover to initiate suction, along with smaller holes along the end, through which mucous enters when suction is applied. The oral suctioning catheter is not used for those with a tracheotomy due to its large size. Oral suctioning is useful to clear secretions from the mouth in the event a patient is unable to remove secretions or foreign matter by effective coughing. Patients who benefit the most include those with cerebrovascular accident, drooling, impaired cough reflex related to age or condition or impaired swallowing (Doyle & McCutcheon 2015). The procedure for oral suctioning can be found in the checklist in Table 41.2.

Naso and Nasopharyngeal Suctioning

Suctioning can be a potentially hazardous procedure and should only be performed when there are clear indications that excessive pulmonary secretions are affecting the patency of the patient's airway or effective ventilation of the patient. Suctioning should maximise removal of secretions with minimal tissue damage and hypoxia. This is an essential procedure is determined by the patients' clinical condition. The frequency of suctioning should be determined for each patient on an individual basis and should only be carried out when the patient is unable to clear vtheir own airway effectively. It should not be performed as a matter of routine. An appropriate review must be undertaken to establish the need for suction.

Red Flag

Evidence of retained secretions will be shown by one or more of the following:

- Visible, audible or palpable secretions
- Decreased oxygen saturation levels
- Increased oxygen requirements
- Coughing
- Poor cough/inability to generate effective spontaneous cough
- Reduced movement/breath sounds of the chest
- Signs of distress due to retained secretions i.e. increased work of breathing (nasal flaring/tracheal tug/costal recession), increased respiratory rate, tachycardia/bradycardia and change of colour

Take Note suctioning asepsis

All routine oral and nasopharyngeal suction should be treated as aseptic non-touch technique. When performing nasotracheal suctioning, it is important to use surgical asepsis (sterile technique); the trachea is considered sterile. If a patient requires suctioning of both the trachea and mouth or oropharynx, suction the mouth last since it is considered clean, not sterile. In addition to gloves, be sure to wear other personal protective equipment (PPE), such as eye goggles and/or a face shield. Local policy and procedure must be adhered to at all times.

Yankauer (Tonsil Tip) Suction Catheter

A yankauer (tonsil tip) suction catheter helps clear secretions from the mouth. Patients who require this type of suctioning can cough effectively but cannot swallow or expectorate secretions. Wear clean gloves when using a yankauer suction catheter and use it multiple times for the same patient before discarding the device.

Table 41.2 Checklist: Oral Suctioning.

STEPS	ADDITIONAL INFORMATION
1. Undertake a review of patient need for suctioning	Baseline respiratory appraisal, including an O_2 saturation level, can alert the healthcare provider to deterioration in condition. Signs and symptoms include obvious excessive secretions; weak, ineffective cough; drooling; gastric secretions or vomit in the mouth; or gurgling sounds with inspiration and expiration. Pooling of secretions may lead to obstruction of airway. Suctioning is required with alterations in oxygen levels and with increased secretions.
2. Explain to patient how the procedure will help clear out secretions and will only last a few seconds. If appropriate, encourage the patient to cough.	This allows the patient time to ask questions and increase concordance with the procedure. Minimises fear and anxiety. Encourage the patient to cough to bring secretions from the lower airways to the upper airways.
3. Position patient in semi-Fowler's position with head turned to the side.	This facilitates ease of suctioning. Unconscious patients should be in the lateral position.
4. Perform hand hygiene, gather supplies and apply non-sterile gloves. Apply an eye shield if there is a risk of bodily fluids splashing into your eyes, and wear PPE as required, and in line with local organisational policy.	Wash hands and apply non-sterile gloves. This prevents the transmission of microorganisms. Supplies include a suction machine or suction connection, connection tubing, non-sterile gloves, yankauer, water and a sterile basin, PPE and clean towel. Suctioning may cause splashing of body fluids.
5. Fill basin with water.	Water is used to clear connection tubing in between suctions. Fill basin with enough water to clear the connection tubing at least three times.
6. Attach one end of connection tubing to the suction machine and the other end to the yankauer.	This prepares equipment to function effectively.
7. Turn on suction to the required level. Test function by covering hole on the yankauer with your thumb and suctioning up a small amount of water.	Suction levels for adults are 100–150 mmHg on wall suction and 10–15 mmHg on portable suction units. Always refer to local policy for suction levels.
8. Remove patient's oxygen mask if present. Nasal prongs may be left in place. Place towel on patient's chest.	Always be prepared to replace the oxygen if patient becomes short of breath or has decreased O_2 saturation levels. The towel prevents patient from coming in contact with secretions.
9. Insert yankauer catheter and apply suction by covering the thumb hole. Run catheter along gum line to the pharynx in a circular motion, keeping yankauer moving. Encourage the patient to cough.	Movement prevents the catheter from suctioning to the oral mucosa and causing trauma to the tissues. Insert yankauer and apply suction by covering the thumb hole Coughing helps move secretions from the lower airways to the upper airways. Apply suction for a maximum of 10 to 15 seconds. Allow patient to rest in between suction for 30 seconds to 1 minute.
10. If required, replace oxygen on patient and clear out suction catheter by placing yankauer in the basin of water.	Replace oxygen to prevent or minimize hypoxia. Clear suction tubing with water. Clearing out the catheter prevents the connection tubing from plugging.
11. Reassess and repeat oral suctioning if required.	Compare pre- and post-suction assessments to determine if intervention was effective.
12. Reassess respiratory status and O_2 saturation for improvements. Call for help if any abnormal signs and symptoms appear.	This identifies positive response to suctioning procedure and provides objective measure of effectiveness.
13. Ensure patient is in a comfortable position and the call bell is within reach. Provide oral hygiene if required.	This promotes patient comfort.
14. Clean up supplies, remove gloves and wash hands. Document the procedure according to hospital policy.	Cleaning up prevents the transmission of microorganisms. Documentation provides accurate details of response to suctioning and clear communication among the healthcare team.

Source: Adapted Doyle & McCutcheon (2015).

Procedure

Prior to providing any activities on patients, the nursing associate must provide verbal information to support the patient to consent to their suctioning procedures. Steps 1–7 are good examples of the explanations that would allow the patient to give informed consent.

Blue Flag

When people are involved in care decisions and treatment options, the nurse–patient relationship is strengthened. When given appropriate and sufficient information, people feel that they are being treated with dignity and respect.

Informed Consent

Reason for the selected suctioning procedure

1. Explanation of the equipment involved
2. Explanation of the practical procedure proposed
3. Explanation of any techniques used in conjunction with the suctioning procedure, e.g. postural drainage and vibrations
4. Discussion of relevant precautions/contraindications
5. Explanation of cleaning and equipment maintenance (may not need to be discussed before obtaining consent but will be covered by the end of the first treatment session; see individual procedures)
6. Informed consent will be obtained in initial assessment
7. Patients should be encouraged to give a signal to the nursing associate to stop suctioning

The following procedure for oral and nasopharyngeal suction should be followed and repeated until excess saliva/mucus has been removed:

Safety Considerations

- Avoid oral suctioning on patients with recent head and neck surgeries.
- Use clean technique for oral suctioning.
- Know you patients well enough so that you understand the patients who are at risk of aspiration. These patients are unable to clear secretions because of an impaired cough reflex. Keep supplies readily available at the bedside and ensure suctioning equipment is functioning in the event oral suctioning is required immediately.
- Know appropriate suctioning limits and the risks of applying excessive pressure or inadequate pressure.
- Avoid oral sutures, sensitive tissues and any tubes located in the mouth or nares if this is possible. This will not be possible if the person has an endotracheal tube (ETT) of nasal tube.
- Avoid stimulating the gag reflex.
- If pertinent, perform a pre- and post-respiratory review (such as respiratory rate, depth, rhythm and oxygen saturations) to monitor the patient for improvement and evaluate care interventions.
- Consider other possible causes of respiratory distress, such as pneumothorax, pulmonary oedema or equipment malfunction.
- If an abnormal side effect occurs (e.g., increased difficulty in breathing, hypoxia, discomfort, deterioration in vital signs or bloody sputum), notify appropriate healthcare provider.

Yellow Flag

When the nursing associate spends time in explaining and if appropriate showing equipment (and also demonstrating how the suction machine sounds) to the patient (and family), this can help to alleviate fears or anxieties. Taking time to do this can encourage the parent (and family) to ask questions and raising concerns.

Touch Point Revisited

- Nursing associates have an important role to play when suctioning oral and nasal secretions
- They must understand the theoretical, practical and evidence-based principles of suctioning secretions
- Understanding these key issues enables them to recognise and reduce potential hazards and complications ensuring the care they provide is safe and effective
- At all times, they must adhere to local policy and procedure

References

Bickley, L. (2016) *Bates' guide to physical examination and history taking* (12th edn), Wolters Kluwer.

Dougherty, L., Lister, S. and West-Oram, A. (2015) *The royal Marsden manual of clinical procedures* (9th edn/student edn). UK: Wiley-Blackwell.

Doyle, G.R. and McCutcheon, J.A. (2015) Clinical procedures for safer patient care, *Chapter 5. Safe oxygen therapy. 5.8 oral suctioning*. [online] Available: https://opentextbc.ca/clinicalskills/chapter/5-7-oral-suctioning/. Accessed 13 October 2019.

NICE. (2019) *Hyoscine butylbromide*. [online] Available: https://bnf.nice.org.uk/drug/hyoscine-butylbromide.html. Accessed 4 November 2019.

Nursing and Midwifery Council (NMC). (2018a) *Standards of proficiency for nursing associates*. [online] Available: https://www.nmc.org.uk/standards/standards-for-nursing-associates/standards-of-proficiency-for-nursing-associates/. Accessed 5 November 2019.

Nursing and Midwifery Council (NMC). (2018b) The code, *Professional standards of practice and behaviour for nurses, midwives and nursing associates*. [online] Available: https://www.nmc.org.uk/standards/code/. Accessed 4 November 2019.

Overend, T.J., Anderson, C.M., Brooks, D., Cicutto, L., Keim, M., McAuslan, D. and Nonoyama, M. (2009) Updating the evidence-base for suctioning adult patients: a systematic review, *Canadian Respiratory Journal*, 16(3): e6–e17. doi:10.1155/2009/872921.

Peate, I. and Nair, M. (2015) *Fundamentals of anatomy and physiology: for nursing and healthcare students* (2nd edn). UK: Wiley.

Woodrow, P. (2018) *Intensive care nursing: a framework for practice*, London and New York: Routledge.

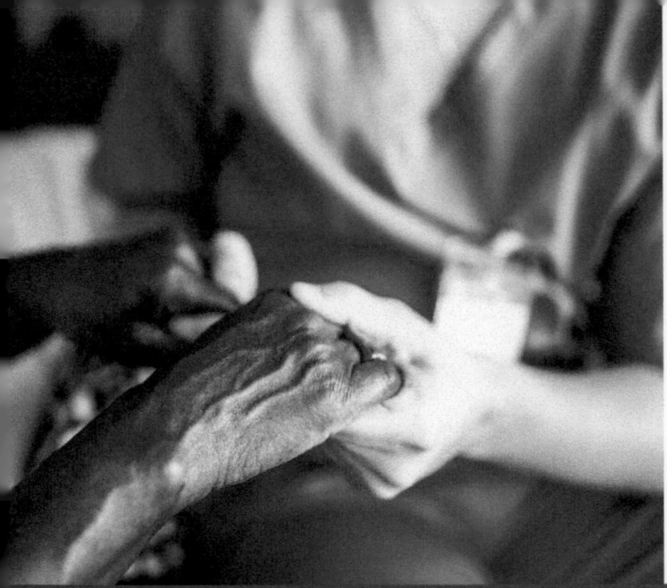

42

Managing Inhalation, Humidifier and Nebuliser Devices

Barry Hill

Northumbria University, UK

Chapter Aim

- **This chapter aims to provide the reader with an insight into the management of inhalation, humidifier and nebuliser devices.**

Learning Outcomes

- **To understand the different types of devices used to aid inhaled respiratory therapy**
- **To identify the common indications and contraindications for such devices**
- **To describe the use of inhalation, humidification and nebuliser devices**

Test Yourself Multiple Choice Questions

1. **Choosing the correct inhalation therapy device should be led by a registered healthcare professional (with agreement from the patient).**
   A) **True**
   B) **False**
2. **The best device to select is always the one the patient will use and can use correctly.**
   A) **True**
   B) **False**
3. **If a patient is unable to master the required inhalation technique for a specific delivery device, there are usually other choices for inhalers delivering equivalent drug doses and providing the same clinical efficacy.**
   A) **True**
   B) **False**

The Nursing Associate's Handbook of Clinical Skills, First Edition. Edited by Ian Peate.

Companion website: www.wiley.com/nursingassociate

4. **Dry powder inhalers are NOT important for the treatment of chronic lung disease, including asthma and chronic obstructive pulmonary disease (COPD).**
   A) **True**
   B) **False**
5. **Nebulisation involves the passage of air or oxygen driven through a solution of a drug. It creates a mist that is then inhaled into the lung tissue.**
   A) **True**
   B) **False**

Introduction

This chapter introduces the nursing associate to the principles of managing inhalation, humidifier and nebuliser devices. Platform 3 'Provide and monitor care' and platform 5 'improving safety and quality care' of the Nursing and Midwifery Council's (NMC) (2018) nursing associate proficiencies require you to apply clinical decision-making and proficiency in the use of managing inhalation, humidifier and nebuliser devices.

Drug delivery via inhalation is the mainstay of treatment for many respiratory diseases, most commonly asthma and COPD (British Thoracic Society (BTS) and Scottish Intercollegiate Guidelines Network (SIGN) 2009, National Institute for Health and Care Excellence (NICE) 2010; Preston & Kelly 2016).

Inhalers

Inhalers are small handheld devices used to administer medications to the airways in patients with asthma and COPD (Thomas 2015).

Take Note

Compared with other routes of administration, inhalation offers several advantages in the treatment of these diseases. For example, via inhalation, a drug is directly delivered to the lungs, conferring high pulmonary drug concentrations and low systemic drug concentrations. Consequently, drug inhalation is typically associated with high pulmonary efficacy and minimal systemic side effects (Borghardt et al. 2018).

Choosing the Correct Inhaler

Choosing the correct inhalation therapy device should be led by a registered healthcare professional (with agreement from the patient). The nursing associate maybe involved in this process. Sometimes, the choice of device is determined by the choice of drug. The best device to select is always the one the patient will use and can use correctly (Preston & Kelly 2016). If a patient is unable to master the required inhalation technique for a specific delivery device, there are usually other choices for inhalers delivering equivalent drug doses and providing the same clinical efficacy.

Take Note

The NICE guideline on COPD (NICE 2019) recommends inhalers should be prescribed only after people have received training in using the device and have demonstrated satisfactory technique. In addition, people should have their ability to use an inhaler device regularly assessed by a competent healthcare professional and, if necessary, should be retaught the correct technique.

Green Flag

The Code (NMC 2018) is clear that the nursing associate must treat people as individual, offer them individual choice and prioritise their needs.

The most common types of inhaler device available are:

1. Dry powder inhalers (DPI) (Figure 42.1)
2. Pressurised metered dose inhalers (MDI or pMDI) (Figure 42.2)
3. Breath-actuated MDI (BApMDI) (Figure 42.3)
   Aerosol holding chamber (commonly called a 'spacer' is often prescribed for use with pMDI inhalers, especially with inhaled steroid medications (ICS medicines)) (Figure 42.4)

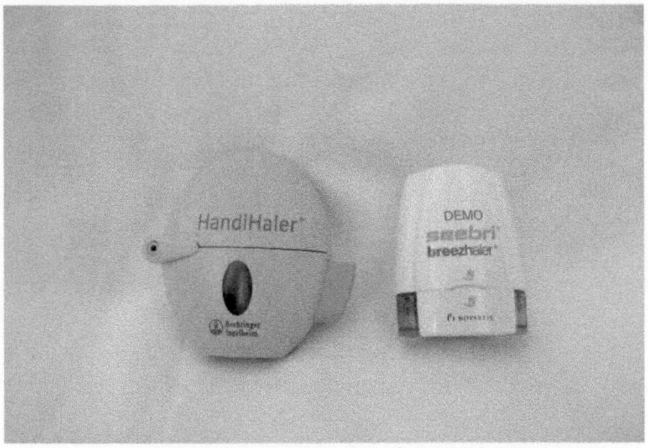

Figure 42.1 Dry powder inhaler. *Source:* Preston & Kelly (2016), figure 44.5.

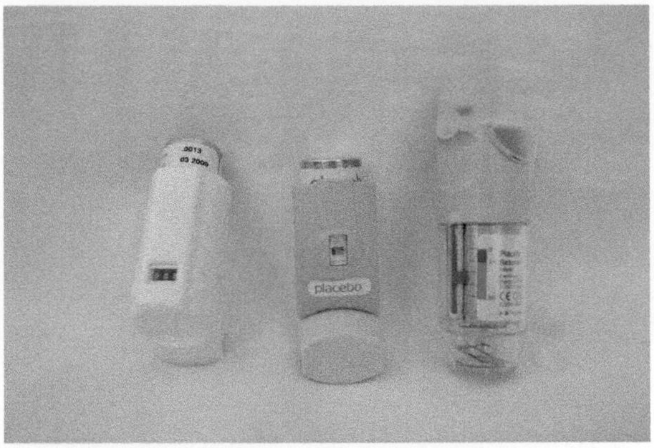

Figure 42.2 Pressurised metered dose inhalers (MDI or pMDI). *Source:* Preston & Kelly (2016), figure 44.1.

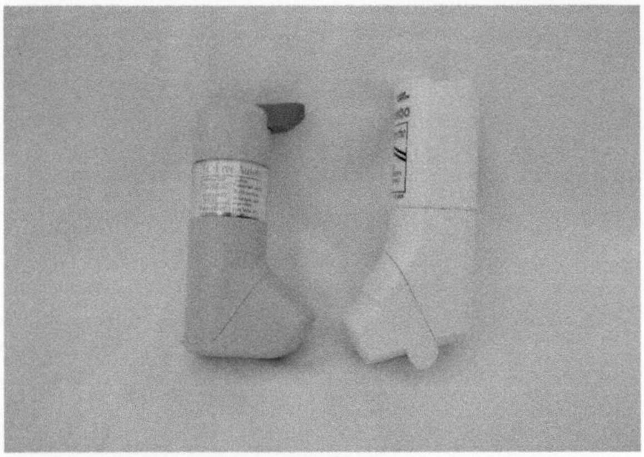

Figure 42.3 Breath-actuated MDI (BApMDI). *Source:* Preston & Kelly (2016), figure 44.2.

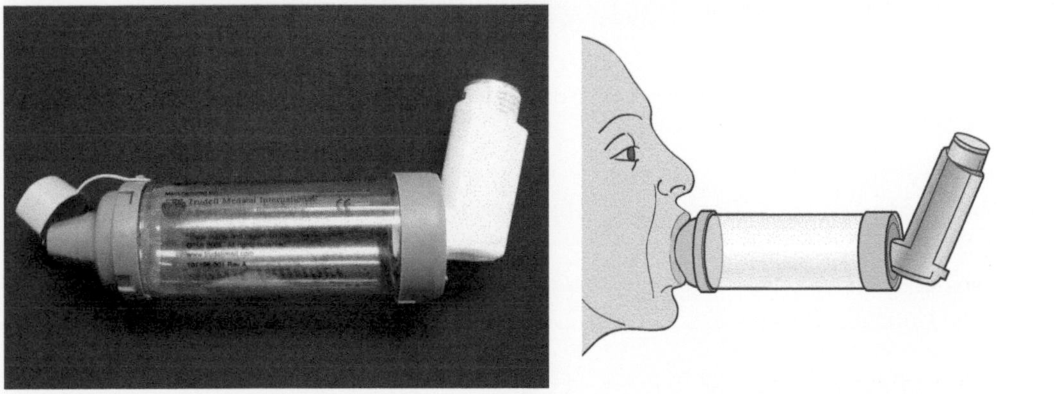

Figure 42.4 Aerosol holding chamber (commonly called a 'spacer'). *Source:* Thomas (2015), figures 22.4a and b.

Dry Powder Inhalers

Dry powder inhalers are important for the treatment of chronic lung disease, including asthma and COPD. A variety of medications are available in DPIs; they consist of a plastic device used to inhale powdered medication. The DPIs are breath activated. This means when the patient inhales, the device automatically releases the medication. Since the medicines are dry powder, they should always be delivered in a special inhaler. DPIs contain no propellant, requiring the patient to have enough inspiratory flow to obtain the dose from the device. As most patients breathe in forcefully when using all inhalers, a DPI will be suitable for most patients.

Take Note

The basic technique for using a dry powdered medication is that the patient should:

1. Exhale away from device
2. Place the mouthpiece in their mouth
3. Breathe in quickly

Pressurised Metered Dose Inhalers (MDI or pMDI)

The MDI is important for the treatment of chronic lung disease, including asthma and COPD. The development of the first commercial pMDIs was carried out by Riker Laboratories in 1955 and marketed in 1956 as the first portable, multidose delivery system for bronchodilators. Since that time, the pMDI has become the most widely prescribed inhalation device for drug delivery to the respiratory tract to treat obstructive airway diseases such as asthma and COPD (Lavorini 2013). A variety of medicines are available in an MDI. The MDI consists of a pressurised canister of medicine in a plastic case with a mouthpiece. A holding chamber consists of a plastic tube with a mouthpiece, a valve to control mist delivery and a soft sealed end to hold the MDI. The holding chamber (spacer) assists delivery of medicine to the lungs. Generally used for infants or small children, this type uses a standard MDI with a spacer. In children, a face mask can be used which attaches to the spacer. It fits over the nose and mouth to make sure the right dose of medication reaches the lungs.

Breath-Actuated MDI (BApMDI)

These comprise a small plastic construction carrying a metal aerosol canister, often containing 200 doses; branded and generic press-and-breathe pMDIs are available. The inhaler is prepared by shaking. Users should remove the mouthpiece cap, breathe out, then take a slow deep breath through the mouth, actuating the device (i.e. pressing the canister) as inhalation begins and then hold their breath.

Individuals may experience several problems with press-and-breathe pMDIs that can affect adherence (this is sometimes called concordance) to therapy and adequacy of delivery of drug to the lungs and, therefore, effectiveness. It is estimated that at least 50% of press-and-breathe pMDI users have less than optimal technique. However, it is suggested that BApMDIs are easier to use than pMDIs (Lavorini 2013). Problems affecting adherence include difficulty in co-ordinating device actuation and inhalation, oropharyngeal deposition of the drug and, in the case of chlorofluorocarbons (CFC) devices, the 'cold freon effect', when the temperature of the propellant causes some individuals to briefly stop inhaling.

Aerosol Holding Chamber (Spacer)

Use and care of spacers (BTS/SIGN 2016)

- All pMDIs should be used via a spacer, as this ensures the best drug deposition to the lung and minimises risk of oral candidiasis.
- The spacer should be compatible with the pMDI being used.
- The drug should be administered as a single actuation of the MDI into the spacer, followed by inhalation and with at least 15 seconds before the next dose is released into the spacer.
- There should be minimal delay between pMDI actuation into the spacer and inhalation.
- Tidal breathing is the preferred technique (5 breaths in and out).
- All spacers should be cleaned weekly as per manufacturer's recommendations, or performance is adversely affected.
- A Volumatic should be washed in detergent and allowed to dry in air. The mouthpiece should be wiped clean of detergent before use.
- The AeroChamber Plus Flow Vu can be washed in the dishwasher (on the top shelf). Drug delivery via the Volumatic may vary significantly due to static charge.
- Plastic spacers should be replaced at least every 12 months, but some may need changing at six months.

Inhaler Technique

Good inhaler technique is extremely important; it ensures the patients receive an effective dose of their required medication. Unfortunately, evidence shows that many patients continue to experience symptoms unnecessarily, and poor inhaler use and compliance is one of the main reasons for this. If it is an allocated role of the nursing associate working in general practice or community nursing teams, it is imperative to check whether patients have mastered the correct use of their inhaler prior to their first prescription for any type of inhaler. The patient's inhaler technique needs to be re-checked at each periodic disease review (this is usually an annual check), especially if there is poor symptom control. If there is poor symptom control, the periodic review must be scheduled as urgent.

Supporting Evidence

A systematic review by NICE (2016) found that around 30% of people using inhalers had 'poor' inhaler technique and that no appreciable change in this has occurred over the last 40 years. Correct use of inhalers is important because misuse is associated with asthma instability, increased hospital visits and increased short-acting b2-agonist (i.e. salbutamol) use.

Orange Flag

Nursing associates must take patient preference into account when choosing the appropriate inhaler device. It is important that a regimen is simple for the patient to follow, and it is not good practice to mix inhaler device types. Steroid inhaler choice is most important, because of the narrower therapeutic window, so it is recommended to start with this inhaler if more than one inhaler is being prescribed (Kaplan & Price 2018).

Choosing Inhaler Types

The benefit gained from inhaled therapy is a unique combination of the drug, device and the individual (i.e. physical, cognitive, psychological and lifestyle characteristics). Consequently, the following factors require consideration when choosing a device.

Inhaler technique – Poor technique, resulting either from poor training or from choosing a device poorly suited to the patient, can significantly reduce the amount of drug delivered to the lungs and result in poor asthma control. Some adults and children (especially the younger ones) may have difficulty with actuation–inhalation co-ordination with a press-and-breathe pMDI, while others may have inconsistent inspiratory flow, which causes problems in using a DPI, or find the automatic actuation of some breath-actuated devices off-putting.

Adherence to treatment – Even where good technique is possible, patients may not use their devices appropriately. Device use may be influenced by a range of factors, including convenience, ease of device use, portability, the stigma of having asthma and personal or peer preference for a specific device. The relative importance of these factors changes over time; therefore, the choice of inhalation device should be reviewed frequently.

Yellow Flag

Emotions can trigger asthma and as such the need to use an inhaler. These emotions include joy, anger and excitement. Depression, panic attacks and grief are linked to asthma symptoms. Positive emotions such as laughter can be a main trigger for asthma symptoms.

Availability of drugs – Some drugs are only available in particular device

Table 42.1 will support the nursing associate in understanding the pros and cons of each type.

Comparing Inhaler Types

To be a safe and accountable practitioner, nursing associates must utilise their clinical decision-making skills and, in this case, understand the differences between the three main types of inhaler. Features of the inhaler can be seen in Table 42.1.

The procedure guideline for administration of inhalation by metered dose inhaler can be seen in Table 42.2.

Blue Flag

Relationship building is important. The notion of trust is vital in healthcare because health and healthcare can involve an element of uncertainty and risk for the patient who may be vulnerable and reliant on the competence and confidence of the nursing associate.

When there are high levels of trust, this brings with it many benefits, including a perception of better care, greater acceptance to recommended treatment and adherence to the treatment as well as a reduction in anxiety associated with treatment taken.

Table 42.1 Features of Asthma inhalers.

METERED DOSE INHALER	METERED DOSE INHALER WITH A SPACER	DRY POWDER INHALER
Small and convenient to carry.	Less convenient to carry than a metered dose inhaler without a spacer.	Small and convenient to carry.
Does not require a deep, fast, inhaled breath.	Does not require a deep, fast, inhaled breath.	Requires a deep, fast, inhaled breath.
Accidently breathing out a little is not a problem.	Accidently breathing out a little is not a problem.	Accidently breathing out a little can blow away the medication.
Some inhalers require co-ordinating the breath with medication release.	A spacer makes it easier to co-ordinate the breath with medication release.	Does not require co-ordinating the breath with medication release.
Can result in medication on the back of the throat and tongue.	Less medication settles on the back of the throat and tongue.	Can result in medication on the back of the throat and tongue.
Some models do not show how many doses remain.	Some models do not show how many doses remain.	It is clear when the device is running out of medication.
Requires shaking and priming.	Requires shaking and priming and correct use of the spacer.	Single-dose models require loading capsules for each use.
Humidity does not affect medication.	Humidity does not affect medication.	High humidity can cause medication to clump.
Use of a cocking device generally is not necessary.	Use of a cocking device generally is not necessary.	May require dexterity to use a cocking device.

Nebuliser Therapy

Nebuliser therapy is frequently prescribed for management of asthma and COPD (Alhaddad et al. 2015). An illustration of a nebuliser can be seen in Figure 42.5.

Nebulisation involves the passage of air or oxygen driven through a solution of a drug. It creates a mist that is then inhaled into the lung tissue (Lister et al. 2020). Many drugs can be inhaled via nebuliser, such as bronchodilators (to prevent wheeze by dilating the bronchioles), steroids (to reduce inflammation of the airways), some antibiotics (to fight respiratory infections) and inotropes such as epinephrine (also known as adrenaline) (in emergency cases of stridor or upper airway bleeding).

According to Preston & Kelly (2016), a nebuliser is a device that converts a liquid into an aerosol suitable for inhalation. In respiratory medicine, this allows drugs, usually at higher doses than standard inhalers, to be converted to an aerosol that can be delivered to the lungs. Administration via this route increases speed of effect, requires lower doses of drug than if given systemically and, therefore, usually causes fewer side effects.

The amount of deposition of the drug is dependent on the condition of the lungs, the pattern of breathing and the particle size of the medication. In order to reach the airways, the particle size needs to be 1–5 μm in diameter; for alveolar deposition, a diameter of 1–2 μm is necessary. Deposition of the medication varies, and around 10% of the particles reach the necessary part of the airway. The remaining solution is left in the chamber as residual volume, in the tubing or mouthpiece (Preston & Kelly 2016). An illustration of particle deposition in the airways and lungs can be seen in Figure 42.6.

Touch Point

About half of the patients who remain breathless despite high-dose bronchodilators delivered by pressurised metered dose inhalers (pMDIs) or dry powder inhalers (DPIs) gain benefits from nebuliser therapy.

Violet Flag

Patients with COPD using nebulisers at home experienced problems at all stages, including problems prior to nebulisation: setting up equipment, lack of instructions, manual dexterity and time required. Problems during medication administration: inhalation technique, duration of nebulisation and understanding how to achieve optimal efficacy. Problems post administration: inadequate cleaning of nebuliser components, access to accessories and the use of damaged parts or self-repairs. Other problems included noise, weight and nonportability of equipment. Healthcare providers should be aware of these problems to effectively support patients with COPD with the use of their nebulisers at home.

Table 42.2 The procedure guideline for administration of inhalation by metered dose inhaler. Procedure guideline 12.7 Medication: administration by inhalation using a metered dose inhaler.

Essential equipment

- MDI device
- Spacer device

PRE-PROCEDURE	
ACTION	**RATIONALE**
1 Wash hands with bactericidal soap and water or bactericidal alcohol handrub.	To minimize the risk of cross-infection (DH 2007, **C**; Fraise and Bradley 2009, **E**).
2 Explain and discuss the procedure with the patient.	To ensure that the patient understands the procedure and gives their valid consent (Griffith and Jordan 2003, **E**; NMC 2013, **C**; NMC 2015, **C**).
3 Correct use of inhalers is essential (see manufacturer's information leaflet) and will be achieved only if this is carefully explained and demonstrated to the patient. If further advice is required, contact the hospital pharmacist.	Incorrect use may result in most of the dose remaining in the mouth and/or being expelled almost immediately. This renders treatment ineffective (Watt 2003, **E**; manufacturer's instructions, **C**).
PROCEDURE	
4 Sit the patient in an upright position if possible in the bed or a chair.	To permit full expansion of the diaphragm. **E**
5 Before administering any prescribed drug, look at the patient's prescription chart and check the following. **a.** The correct patient **b.** Drug **c.** Dose **d.** Date and time of administration **e.** Route and method of administration **f.** Diluent as appropriate **g.** Validity of prescription **h.** Signature of prescriber **i.** The prescription is legible	To ensure that the correct patient is given the correct drug in the prescribed dose using the appropriate diluent and by the correct route (DH 2003b, **C**; NMC 2010a, **C**). To protect the patient from harm (DH 2003b, **C**; NMC 2010a, **C**).
If any of these pieces of information are missing, are unclear or illegible then the nurse should not proceed with administration and should consult with the prescriber.	To expose the area for use. **E**
6 Remove mouthpiece cover from inhaler.	To prevent any errors occurring. **E**
7 Shake inhaler well for 2-5 seconds.	To ensure mixing of medication in canister (Potter 2011, **E**).
8 *Without a spacer device:*	
Ask patient to take a deep breath and exhale completely, open lips and place inhaler mouthpiece in mouth with opening toward back of throat, closing lips tightly around it.	Prepares airway to receive medication and directs aerosol towards airway (Potter 2011, **E**).
With a spacer device:	
Insert MDI into end of the spacer device. Ask the patient to exhale and then grasp spacer mouthpiece with teeth and lips while holding inhaler.	To enable the medication to reach the airways instead of hitting the back of the throat. The spacer improves delivery of correct dose of inhaled medication. **E**
9 Ask the patient to tip head back slightly, inhale slowly and deeply through the mouth whilst depressing canister fully.	To allow medication to be distrubted to airways during inhalation. **E**
10 Instruct the patient to breathe in slowly for 2-3 seconds and hold their breath for approximately 10 seconds, then remove MDI from mouth (if not using spacer) before exhaling slowly through pursed lips.	To enable aerosol spray to reach deeper branches of airways (Chernecky et al. 2002, **E**).

(Continued)

Table 42.2 (Continued)

11 Instruct the patient to wait 20-30 seconds between inhalations (if same medication) or 2-5 minutes between inhalations (if different medication). Always administer bronchodilators before steroids.	To ensure that the medication has optimum effect and minimal side-effects. **E**
12 If steroid medication is administered, ask the patient to rinse their mouth with water approximately 2 minutes after inhaling the dose.	To remove any medication residue from oral cavity area. Steroids may alter the normal flora of the oral mucosa and lead to development of fungal infection (Lilley et al. 2007, **E**).
POST-PROCEDURE	
13 Clean any equipment used and discard all disposable equipment in appropriate containers.	To minimize the risk of infection (Fraise and Bradley 2009, **E**).
14 Record the administration on appropriate charts.	To maintain accurate records, provide a point of reference in the event of any queries and prevent any duplication of treatment (NMC 2010a, **C**; NMC 2010b, **C**; NPSA 2007c, **C**).

Source: Dougherty et al. (2015), p. 611.

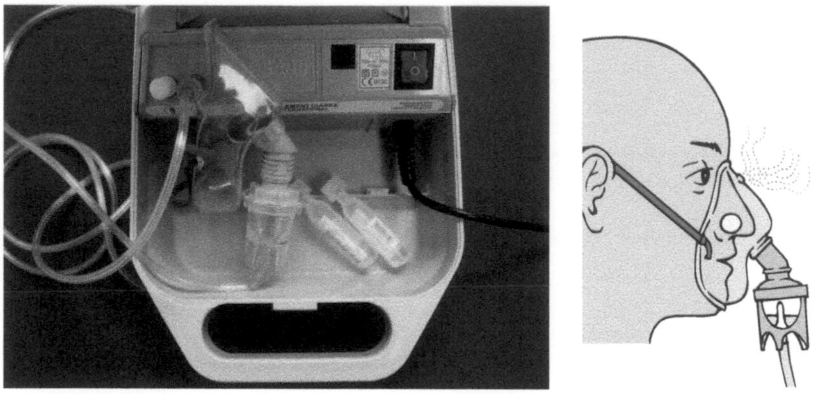

Figure 42.5 Nebuliser. *Source:* Thomas (2015), figures 22.5a and b.

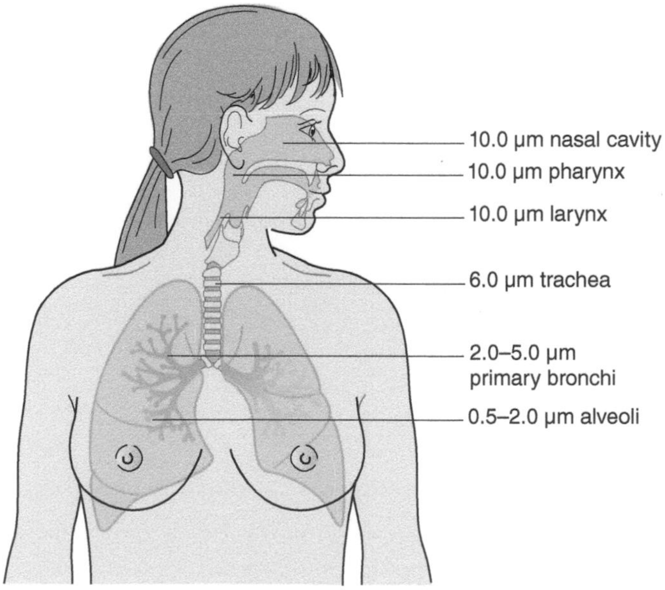

Figure 42.6 Particle deposition in the airways and lungs. *Source:* Preston & Kelly (2016), figure 45.1

Box 42.1 Inhaled Therapy: Indications, Contraindications and Complications

Indications
Disease requiring medication to be delivered to the airways

Contraindications
Patient refusal
Allergy to medication

Complications
Local – discomfort
Systemic – medication specific, *for example:*
Clinical warning sign – anaphylaxis, if there is an allergy
Clinical warning sign – tachycardia (a heart rate above 100 beats per minute) from the effects of salbutamol.

Touch Point

Nebuliser therapy may be valuable for older patients who may have difficulties with handheld inhalers, critically unwell patients who require high treatment doses of bronchodilators or steroids or for patients who have comorbidities (Alhaddad et al. 2015).

The procedure guideline for nebulisation can be seen in Table 42.3.

Red Flag

Bronchodilators can cause side effects, although these are usually mild or short-lived. Common side effects can include:

- feeling shaky
- tachycardia (for a short while but, no chest pain)
- headaches
- muscle cramps

Serious side effects:

- muscle pain or weakness, muscle cramps or a heartbeat that does not feel normal
- very bad dizziness or passing out
- chest pain, especially with a fast heartbeat or heartbeat does not feel normal
- a very bad headache

Serious reactions:

- it is possible to have a serious allergic reaction (anaphylaxis) to salbutamol

Touch Point Revisited

- Nursing associates have an important role to play in the use of inhaled therapy devices.
- They must understand the theoretical, practical and evidence-based principles of inhaled therapy devices.
- Understanding these key issues enables them to recognise and reduce potential hazards and complications ensuring the care they provide is safe and effective.

Table 42.3 The procedure guideline for nebulisation. Procedure guideline 12.8 Medication: administration by inhalation using a nebulizer.

Essential equipment • Facemask or mouthpiece • Nebulizer and tubing	*Medicinal products* • Medication required
PRE-PROCEDURE	
ACTION	RATIONALE
1 Wash hands with bactericidal soap and water or bactericidal alcohol handrub.	To minimize the risk of cross-infection (DH 2007, **C**; Fraise and Bradley 2009, **E**).
2 Explain and discuss the procedure with the patient.	To ensure that the patient understands the procedure and gives their valid consent (Griffith and Jordan 2003, **E**; NMC 2013, **C**; NMC 2015, **C**).
3 Sit the patient in an upright position if possible in the bed or a chair.	To permit full expansion of the diaphragm and facilitate effective inhalation (Jevon et al. 2010, **E**).
4 Before administering any prescribed drug, look at the patient's prescription chart and check the following. **a.** The correct patient **b.** Drug **c.** Dose **d.** Date and time of administration **e.** Route and method of administration **f.** Diluent as appropriate **g.** Validity of prescription **h.** Signature of prescriber **i.** The prescription is legible	To ensure that the correct patient is given the correct drug in the prescribed dose using the appropriate diluent and by the correct route (DH 2003b, **C**; NMC 2010a, **C**). To protect the patient from harm (DH 2003b, **C**; NMC 2010a, **C**).
If any of these pieces of information are missing, are unclear or illegible then the nurse should not proceed with administration and should consult with the prescriber.	To prevent any errors occurring. **E**
PROCEDURE	
5 Administer only one drug at a time unless specifically instructed to the contrary.	Several drugs used together may cause undesirable reactions or may inactivate each other (Jordan et al. 2003, **E**).
6 Assemble the nebulizer equipment as per manufacturer's instructions.	To ensure correct administration (manufacturer's instructions, **C**).
7 Measure any liquid medication with a syringe. Add the prescribed medication and diluent (if needed) to the nebulizer.	To ensure the correct dose (DH 2007, **C**).
8 Attach the mouthpiece or facemask via the tubing to medical piped air or oxygen as prescribed.	To ensure it is ready to use when switched on. **E**
(a) If a patient has a clinical need for supplementary oxygen therapy, oxygen therapy must *not* be discontinued whilst the nebulizer is in progress. In this situation the drug should be nebulized with oxygen therapy. The patient should receive continuous pulse oximetry for at least the duration of the nebulizer treatment.	To ensure patient maintains their target saturation (Jevon et al. 2010, **E**).
(b) If a patient is hypercapnic or acidotic (e.g. COPD) the nebulizer should be driven by medical air, not oxygen.	To avoid worsening hypercapnia (NICE 2010, **C**).
9 Ask the patient to hold the mouthpiece between the lips or apply the facemask and take a slow deep breath.	To promote greater deposition of medication in the airways (Potter 2011, **E**).
10 After inspiration, the patient should pause briefly and then exhale.	Improves effectiveness of medication. **E**
11 Turn on the piped air/O_2 and ensure sufficient mist is formed. A minimum flow rate of 6-8 litres per minute is required.	To ensure effective nebulization of the medication (Downie et al. 2003, **E**; Jevon et al. 2010, **E**).

(Continued)

Table 42.3 (Continued)

12 The patient should continue to breathe as above until all the nebulized medication is completed (0.5 mL will remain in chamber).	To ensure all medication has been received. **E**
13 Optimal nebulization of 4 mL takes approximately 10 minutes.	To ensure it is effective. **E.**
POST-PROCEDURE	
14 If appropriate and prescribed, recommence oxygen therapy at the appropriate dose.	To continue with patient's required therapy (Jevon et al. 2010, **E**).
15 Clean any equipment used and/or discard all single-use disposable equipment in appropriate containers.	To minimize the risk of infection (DH 2007, **C**; Fraise and Bradley 2009, **E**; Jevon et al. 2010, **E**).
16 Record the administration on appropriate charts.	To maintain accurate records, provide a point of reference in the event of any queries and prevent any duplication of treatment (NMC 2010a, **C**; NMC 2010b, **C**).

Source: Dougherty et al. (2015), p. 612.

References

Alhaddad, B., Smith, F.J., Robertson, T., Watman, G. and Taylor, K.M.G. (2015) Patients' practices and experiences of using nebulizer therapy in the management of COPD at home, BMJ *Open Respiratory Research*, 2(1):e000076. doi:10.1136/bmjresp-2014000076.

Borghardt, J.M., Kloft, C. and Sharma, A. (2018) *Inhaled therapy in respiratory disease: the complex interplay of pulmonary kinetic processes, Canadian Respiratory Journal,* 2018: 2732017. [online] Available: https://doi.org/10.1155/2018/2732017. Accessed 12 November 2019.

BTS/SIGN. (2016) *British guideline on the management of asthma.* [online] Available: https://www.brit-thoracic.org.uk/document-library/guidelines/asthma/btssign-asthma-guideline-2016/. Accessed 12 November 2019.

Dougherty, L., Lister, S. and West-Oram, A. (2015) The royal Marsden manual of clinical procedures (9th edn/student edn). UK: Wiley-Blackwell.

Kaplan, A. and Price, D. (2018) Matching inhaler devices with patients: the role of the primary care physician, *Canadian Respiratory Journal*, 2018: 9473051. doi:10.1155/2018/9473051.

Lavorini, F. (2013) The challenge of delivering therapeutic aerosols to asthma patients, *ISRN Allergy*, 2013:102418. doi:10.1155/2013/102418.

Lister, S., Hofland, J. and Grafton, H. (2020) *The royal Marsden manual of clinical nursing procedures (royal Marsden manual series).* Oxford, UK: Wiley Blackwell.

NICE. (2019) *Guideline for COPD.* [online] Available: https://www.nice.org.uk/guidance/ng115. Accessed 12 November 2019.

Preston, W. and Kelly. C. (2016) *Respiratory nursing at a glance*, Oxford: Wiley.

Thomas, R. (2015) *Practical medical procedures at a glance*, Oxford: Wiley.

Unit 8

Preventing and Managing Infection

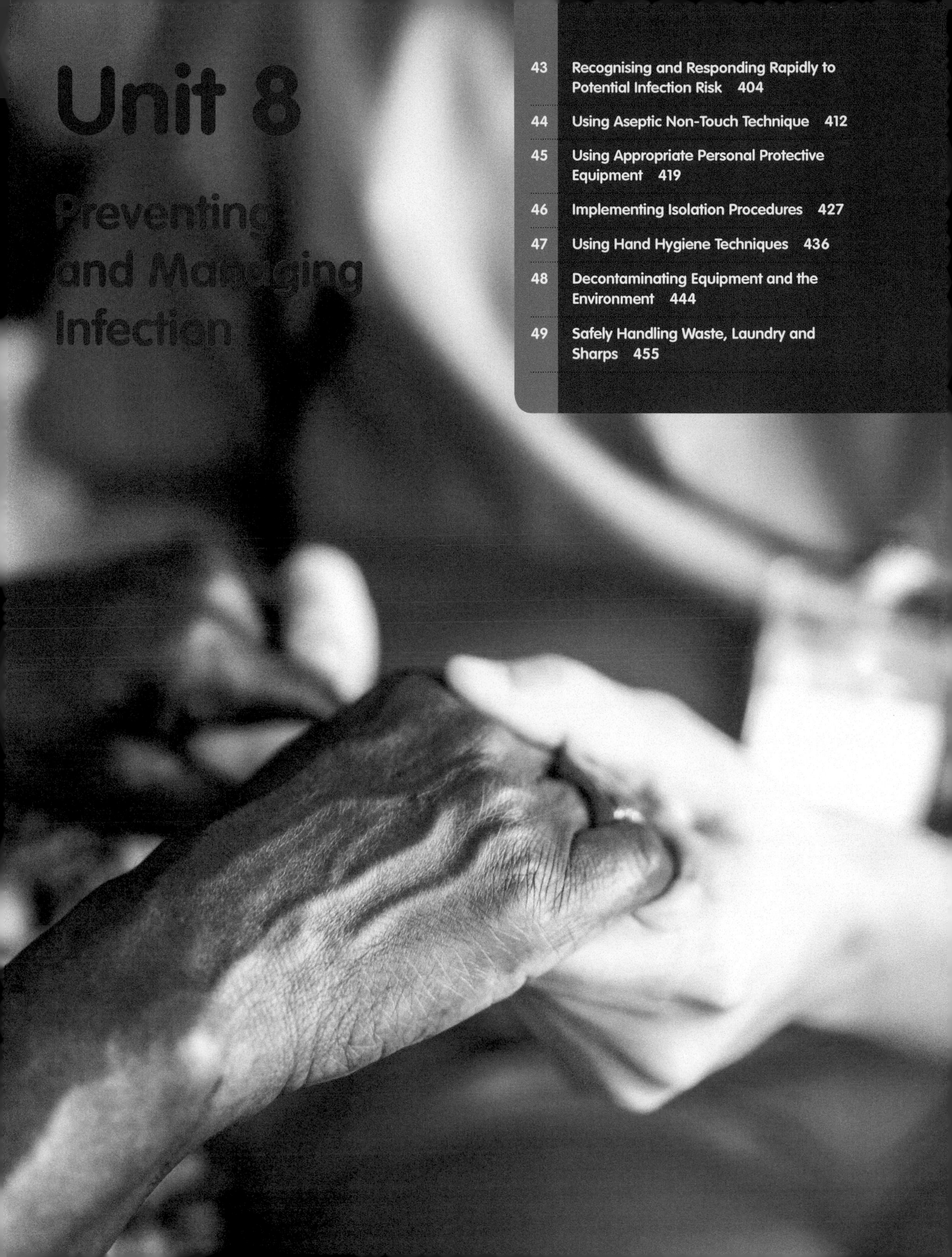

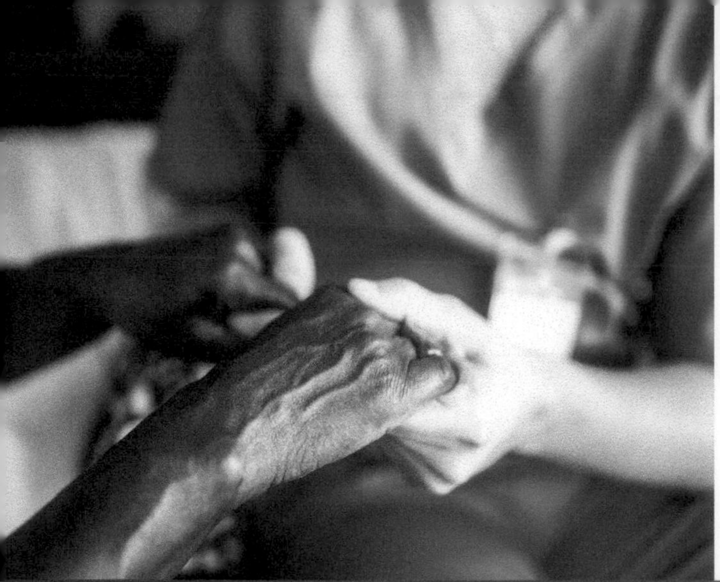

43

Recognising and Responding Rapidly to Potential Infection Risk

Nigel Davies

University of East London, UK

Chapter Aim

- **This chapter discusses how you can recognise potential infections, prevent their occurrence and control and respond rapidly.**

Learning Outcomes

- **Describe some of the tests and screening processes used to detect infection or infectious diseases.**
- **Discuss specimen collection in relation to MRSA screening.**
- **Outline the ways in which the nursing associate can contribute to prevention and control of the transmission of infection and the use of standard precautions.**

Test Yourself Multiple Choice Questions

1. **Which of the following is not a common sign or symptom of a wound infection?**
   A) **Pyrexia**
   B) **Pus oozing from around the wound**
   C) **Redness**
   D) **Abdominal cramps**
2. **Who might be your first choice to consult to gain advice about a suspected outbreak of food poisoning?**
   A) **Consultant microbiologist**
   B) **Infection control clinical nurse specialist**
   C) **Director of infection prevention and control (DIPC)**
   D) **Any of the above**

The Nursing Associate's Handbook of Clinical Skills, First Edition. Edited by Ian Peate.

Companion website: www.wiley.com/nursingassociate

3. **MRSA is the abbreviation for?**
   A) **Meticillin-resistant *Staphylococcus aureus***
   B) **Multi-resistant *Staphylococcus aureus***
   C) **Meticillin-sensitive *Staphylococcus aureus***
   D) **Meticillin-resistant *Streptococcus aureus***

4. **Prophylaxis refers to:**
   A) **Treatment or care given to deal with an infection**
   B) **A type of drug designed to have no therapeutic effect**
   C) **A type of drug which promotes wound healing**
   D) **Treatment or care given as a preventative measure**
5. **Certain procedures, for example, the use of personal protective equipment, should be applied across all healthcare settings. What are these procedures now called?**
   A) **Universal precautions**
   B) **Routine precautions**
   C) **Standard precautions**
   D) **Worldwide precautions**

Introduction

The nursing associate has a key role to play in recognising and responding rapidly to potential infection risk, using standard precautions and related protocols. There are a number of key skills that have to be learnt, honed and applied when working with others to prevent and control infection.

The nursing associate proficiencies and platforms (Nursing and Midwifery Council (NMC) 2018a) require the nursing associate to protect the health of people they have the privilege to care for. They can do this by ensuring they are able to demonstrate proficiency in infection prevention and control and ensuring that the patient is always at the centre of all that is done. Annexe B of the NMC proficiencies requires you to be able to carry out a range of procedures that are evidence based, patient centred and in a proficient manner.

Recognising and Responding to Infection Risks

Recognising an existing or emerging infection or infectious disease is a key skill not only to help promote a patient's healthcare or recovery but also to ensure other patients, staff and your own safety. Being aware of the common signs and symptoms of infection will help you recognise and respond effectively. These are:

- Pyrexia (which is the medical term for fever);
- feeling tired or fatigued;
- swollen lymph nodes in the neck, axillae (armpits) or groin;
- headache; and
- nausea or vomiting.

Depending on the site of infection, other signs and symptoms (summarised in Figure 43.1) may also be seen. In some cases, it may be difficult to differentiate between the signs for infections and other illnesses. For example, distinguishing between pneumonia, other respiratory infections, congestive cardiac failure and chronic obstructive pulmonary disease can be difficult, especially in a community care setting without access to full diagnostic options (Moreton 2019). Equally, older people do not always exhibit all the symptoms, for example, in the case of urinary tract infection (UTI), which makes identification more complex (Bardsley 2017). During the Covid-19 pandemic it became apparent that loss of the sense of smell (known as asnosia) was a symptom of the disease for many people and that in the frail older people often the first sign of Covid-19 infection was delirium (Zazzara et al. 2020). These complexities will often mean that a number of diagnostic tests need to be performed, or restrictions put in place as a precautionary measure, which you may need to explain to patients and their families.

Violet Flag

The nature of the environment within prisons and places of detention will vary widely with regard to their age, design, construction and availability of healthcare facilities.

In addition to this, the operational integrity of prisons and places of detention with regard to cell-sharing, staffing levels and access to healthcare services can present a challenge in the prevention and control of communicable diseases.

All staff are expected to take part in the prevention and control of infection. Every prison and place of detention has the responsibility to ensure that effective arrangements are in place for prevention and control of infection as well as the control of communicable diseases among prisoners, staff (including volunteers) and visitors.

Take Note

It can be difficult to differentiate between the signs for infections and other illnesses. A holistic approach to patient care is advocated.

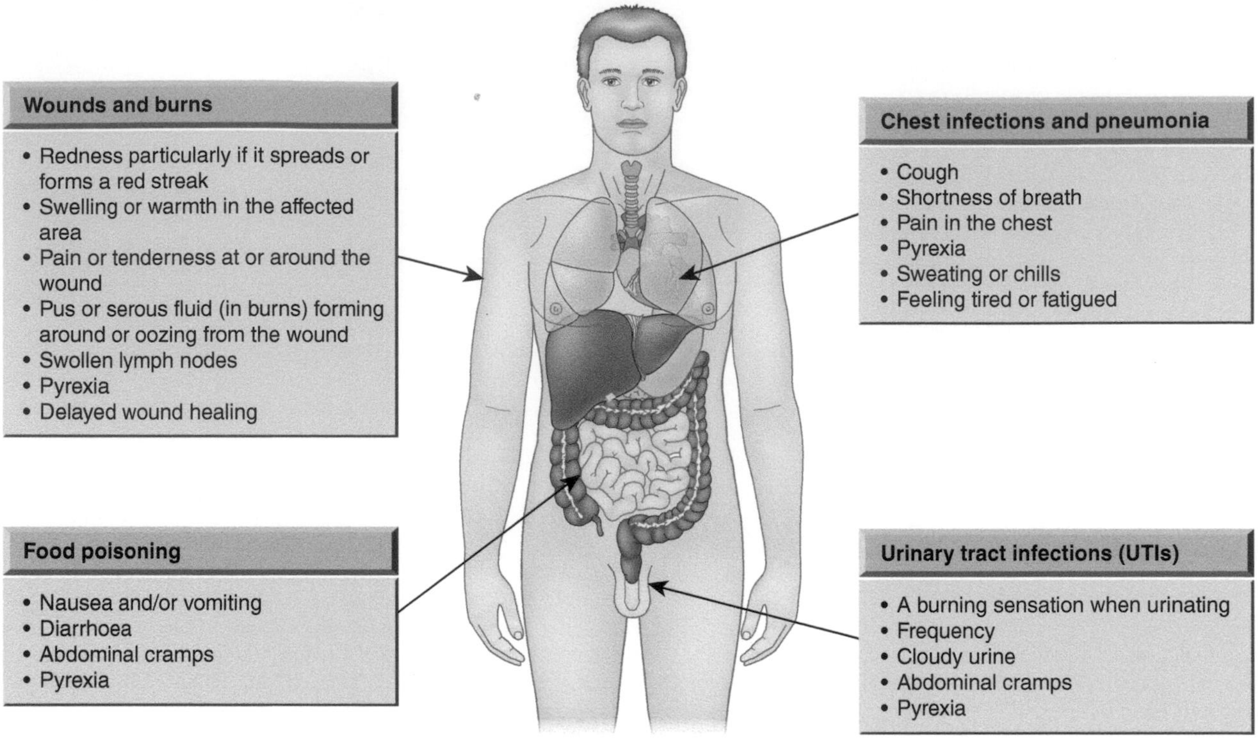
Wounds and burns
• Redness particularly if it spreads or forms a red streak
• Swelling or warmth in the affected area
• Pain or tenderness at or around the wound
• Pus or serous fluid (in burns) forming around or oozing from the wound
• Swollen lymph nodes
• Pyrexia
• Delayed wound healing
Chest infections and pneumonia
• Cough
• Shortness of breath
• Pain in the chest
• Pyrexia
• Sweating or chills
• Feeling tired or fatigued
Food poisoning
• Nausea and/or vomiting
• Diarrhoea
• Abdominal cramps
• Pyrexia
Urinary tract infections (UTIs)
• A burning sensation when urinating
• Frequency
• Cloudy urine
• Abdominal cramps
• Pyrexia

Figure 43.1 **Common signs and symptoms of infection.**

Table 43.1 Sources of Infection Control Advice.

Acute care settings • Registered nurse (e.g. staff nurse, ward manager, infection control link nurse) • Infection control clinical nurse specialist, who can also access further team members including consultant microbiologists • Medical staff with specialist knowledge, for example, an infectious diseases doctor	***Mental health settings*** • Nursing associate colleague or a registered nurse nominated as ward or unit infection control lead (often referred to as the infection control link) • Infection control clinical nurse specialist (most trusts employ specialist nurses who will have links with other local trusts and the public health teams)
Primary care • General practice nurse • District nurse or other community nurse • General practitioner	***Nursing and residential care homes*** • Home manager • System or company patient safety or infection control lead • Visiting community nurses • Public Health England advisors

For this reason, it is also important to have a good understanding of the principles of infection control. Working in partnership, collaborating with patients or service users, leads to much greater compliance from patients and their family, friends and visitors if the reasons for treatment are understood. This will often require you to explain the rationale for these policies and procedures and adapt often complex information in a meaningful way. If you are unfamiliar with a potential infection, the associated tests or treatment, then you should seek more specialist advice and consider referring or handing over the patient to another healthcare practitioner. Table 43.1 suggests different people you might consult for this advice depending on the setting you are working in.

Blue Flag

The role of the Infection Prevention and Control Team is to ensure that the risk of infection to patients, visitors and staff is minimised through a variety of prevention and control processes. The team works closely to monitor infection rates and undertake audits in order to maintain consistently high standards.

Touch Points

Differentiating between an infection and other illness or conditions requires much skill that the nursing associate will develop.

Having an understanding of the principles of infection control and working in partnership with others will lead to improved healthcare outcomes for service users (and if appropriate, their families) if the reasons for treatment are explained. The nursing associate may be required to explain the rationale for policies and procedures using their skills to adapt sometimes complex information in a meaningful way.

Policies and Procedures to Prevent and Control Infection

In healthcare settings, such as hospitals, GP practices and in residential and nursing homes, policies and protocols are often laid down to guide nursing and care staff to prevent or treat infections. These polices are written using current evidence and research with three main aims in mind:

1. to provide the best treatment for patients and service users;
2. to prevent the spread of the infection to other patients or clients; and
3. to protect staff members who care for either infected or potentially infected patients.

Sometimes, in diseases that can be particularly serious or transmitted easily to others, the policies are laid down in law, and patients are required to follow the treatment regimen, for example, in cases of tuberculosis (TB) or during the Covid-19 pandemic. These diseases have to be reported to a national database and are known as 'notifiable' diseases (Weston et al. 2017). If you suspect that someone you are caring for may have an infectious disease, you should obtain more specialist advice (see Table 43.1).

Green Flag

The four countries of the United Kingdom have various regulations and laws that are related to the notification of infectious diseases.

'Notification of infectious diseases' is the term used to refer to the statutory duties for reporting notifiable diseases in the Public Health (Control of Disease) Act 1984) and the Health Protection (Notification) Regulations 2010.

Standard Precautions

Standard precautions (previously referred to as universal precautions) should be applied across all healthcare settings to prevent direct contact and hence the transmission of blood-borne and other infections in body substances where potentially infectious materials are present (Loveday et al. 2014).

These precautions are dealt with in greater detail in the other chapters of this text and include:

- Routine use of barriers (such as gloves and/visors) when anticipating contact with blood or body fluids (see Chapter 45 on the use of personal protective equipment);
- Ensuring infectious patients are kept apart or away from others (see Chapter 46 on implementing isolation procedures);
- Washing hands and other skin surfaces immediately after contact with blood or body fluids (see Chapter 47 on using hand hygiene techniques);
- Cleaning equipment and surfaces to remove potentially infectious substances (see Chapter 48 on safely decontaminating equipment and the environment); and
- Careful handling and disposing of equipment during and after use (see Chapter 49 on safely handling waste, laundry and sharps).

Although these are standard precautions and as such should be undertaken in all healthcare environments in some settings, for example, emergency departments, urgent care centres and mental health settings, there may be a need to adapt the approach taken and thought given to where equipment is stored and accessed. Hughes et al. (2011) discuss some of the challenges to providing infection prevention and control measures within mental health settings which are also relevant in other settings such as children's wards and departments. The recommendations include the need to prevent items being used for self-harm or as potential weapons and include:

- Personal protective equipment (PPE – see Chapter 45) may need to be stored away from patients or not in public areas so it is not accessible to patients.
- Care needs to be taken regarding the placement of hand decontamination items, such as soap dispensers, so they cannot be used as ligature points or alcohol gel ingested.
- Secure storage is needed for chemicals used to disinfect body fluid spillages.
- The potential for sharps containers to be used for self-harm or used as weapons needs to be remembered.

Orange Flag

Obsessive–compulsive disorder presents itself in many ways and goes far beyond the common misconception that it is merely a little hand washing or checking light switches.

The fear of being dirty and contamination is the obsessional worry; often, fear is that contamination could cause harm to the individual or a loved one. The common compulsions might be to wash or clean or avoid. Common contamination obsessive worries and compulsions include:

The cleaning or washing is frequently carried out multiple times often accompanied by rituals of repetitive hand or body washing until the person 'feels' it is clean, rather than people without obsessive–compulsive disorder who will wash or clean once until they 'see' they are clean.

Take Note

The nursing associate is responsible in ensuring that any equipment used in infection prevention and control is stored safely, preventing items being used for self-harm or as potential weapons.

Detecting Infection – Diagnostic Tests

There are many diagnostic tests and treatment approaches used by infection control practitioners to identify the cause of infection and determine the best treatment. Diagnostic tests frequently involve a specimen being obtained, which is frequently either a nursing task you will need to perform or, if the patient is self-caring, you will need to explain.

Microbiology and virology laboratories in hospitals carry out different tests. Increasingly some tests can now be performed outside the laboratory using equipment that enables 'near-patient testing'. This is very helpful in clinical settings such as walk-in centres, emergency departments and sexual health clinics where diagnoses and decisions about treatment such as whether isolation is needed can be made more rapidly. Examples of near-patient testing for infection control can range from simple urine 'dip stick' test for the presence of protein, suggesting a UTI, to finger-prick blood tests for HIV.

Tests may be carried out either on an individual basis because signs or symptoms of infection are noted or through screening which refers to routine testing of all patients.

Specimens frequently need to be obtained to help detect the cause of the infection and also to help determine the best treatment. Chapter 14 provides further details about specimen collection.

Touch Point

Policies and protocols are provided to offer guidance to nursing and care staff in order to prevent or treat infections. All polices should be written using current evidence and research to provide the best treatment.

Standard precautions must be applied across all healthcare settings in order to prevent direct contact and as such the transmission of blood-borne and other infections.

Diagnostic tests and treatment approaches are used by infection control practitioners to identify the cause of infection and determine best treatment, frequently involving a specimen being obtained a nursing duty the nursing associate will be expected to perform. Increasingly, 'near-patient testing' is being performed outside of the laboratory setting.

MRSA Screening and Suppression

One very common infection control screening procedure is for MRSA (meticillin-resistant *Staphylococcus aureus*). This is a strain of bacteria which is resistant to a powerful antibiotic called *meticillin*. It is an organism that colonises the skin, particularly the nose, skin folds, hairline, perineum and navel. It commonly survives in these areas without causing infection – a state known as colonisation. A patient becomes clinically infected if the organism invades the skin or deeper tissues and multiplies.

Screening people to detect whether they are carriers of MRSA has been commonplace in all UK hospitals for the past decade. Typically, screening consists of taking swabs (see Chapter 14) from the nostrils (nares) and groin. If the patient has a urinary catheter, intravenous lines or wounds, then these are also swabbed. In babies, the umbilicus is often swabbed.

Take Note

When a swab is sent to the laboratory, the nursing associate should specify if it is a routine admission screen for MRSA or for the investigation of a suspected infection.

If a patient is found to carry MRSA, then this can be suppressed (sometime referred to as decolonisation) to help prevent infection occurring. Complete eradication of MRSA is not always possible, but a decrease in carriage can reduce the risk of transmission to others and the risk of wound infection to the patients themselves (Coia et al. 2014).

Suppression usually takes the form of two treatments typically including a nasal ointment and hair/body washes. You should follow the protocol for your institution with the products either being prescribed for the individual patient, or as part of a patient group direction. The choice of product may depend on whether the patient is being decolonised before admission or is already a patient; and whether they have any skin sensitivities or are resistant to certain products. The products (nasal ointments and skin washes) are described in more detail in Figure 43.2.

Touch Point

MRSA can be suppressed (or decolonisation) to help prevent infection occurring. It is not always possible to completely eradicate of MRSA; a decrease in carriage can reduce the risk of transmission.

Public health infection control measures might take the form of the whole population, for example, in nationwide immunisation programmes for all children to prevent infectious diseases such as measles, mumps and rubella (MMR).

<table>
<tr><th>General guidance</th><th>Products</th></tr>
<tr><td rowspan="2">

Nasal ointment

The ointment should be applied to the anterior nares of both nostrils. A small amount about the size of a match head is applied using a clean cotton bud for each nostril.

Squeeze the nose gently after applying to help spread the cream inside the nose.

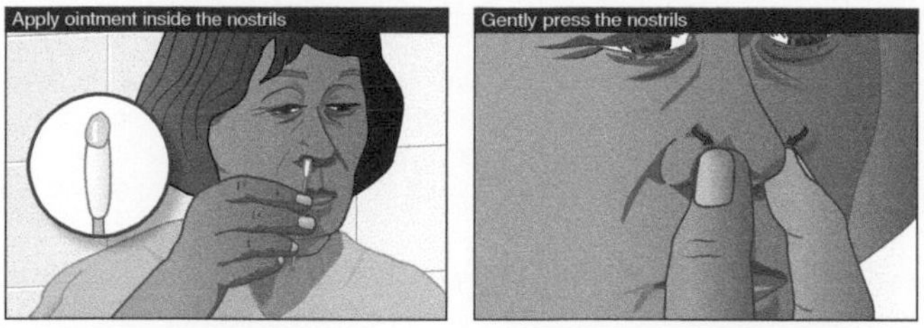

</td><td>

Mupirocin (often referred to by its trade name of Bactroban®)

Applied 2–3 times daily for 5 days

</td></tr>
<tr><td>

Neomycin (often referred to by its trade name of Naseptin®) is used in people who are resistant to mupirocin. It is applied 4 times a day for 10 days.

</td></tr>
<tr><td rowspan="3">

Body and hair washes

The manufacturer's instructions should be followed as they vary slightly between products. Patient should be told to pay particular attention to washing the axillae, groin and skin folds.

The lotions are typically applied for 5 days and hair should also be washed with the lotion 2–3 times during this period too.

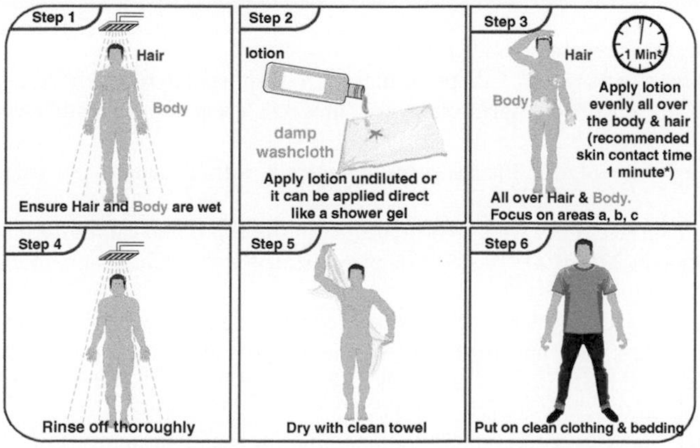

</td><td>

Chlorhexidine (Hibiscrub®) 4% skin wash/shower, daily for 5 days.

Skin should be moistened with water before applying the chlorhexidine to reduce the likelihood of reactions.

Hair should be washed at least 3 times during the 5 days, if possible. A normal shampoo can be used after the chlorhexidine each time

</td></tr>
<tr><td>

Octenisan® is similarly applied in as a lotion.

It is also available as hand-mittens/wipes which can be used by patients who are unable to shower/bathe.

Hair should be washed twice during the five days.

</td></tr>
<tr><td>

Prontoderm foam

This is a 'leave on' product.

Patients should shower or be assisted to wash as usual paying particular attention to axillae, groin and skin folders and dry with a clean towel.

The foam is then applied. It should also be combed through the hair and not washed off.

May be an easier option for bedridden elderly patients or patients with sensitive irritated skin.

</td></tr>
<tr><td colspan="2">Treatment should be prescribed or follow a patient group direction, and you should note the most recent guidance in the British National Formulary (BNF 2019). Record in the patient's notes and medicines administration record.</td></tr>
</table>

Figure 43.2 MRSA suppression.

Public Health Approaches to Prevent Infection

Public health infection control measures are concerned with a population-based approach. This might take the form of the whole population, for example, in nationwide immunisation programmes for all children to prevent infectious diseases such as measles, mumps and rubella (MMR) (Davies 2018). Alternatively, the population targeted might be a vulnerable subgroup, like the elderly or people with long-term conditions as is the case with the annual flu (influenza) vaccination campaign or during the Covid-19 pandemic when older people and those who were considered clinically extremely vulnerable where asked to 'shield' or isolate themselves for a 12-week period (Brooke & Clarke 2020). Other approaches include campaigns to promote safer sex and the provision of free condoms or PrEP (Pre-Exposure Prophylaxis) by sexual health services (Brady et al. 2019).

Red Flag

MMR is a safe and effective combined vaccine that protects against three separate illnesses – measles, mumps and rubella – in a single injection. The full course of MMR vaccination requires two doses.

Measles, mumps and rubella are highly infectious conditions that can have serious, potentially fatal complications, including meningitis, encephalitis and deafness.

In these cases, the aim is to gain sufficient take-up of the public health intervention so that the likelihood of the infection spreading in a population is diminished. This is often referred to as 'herd immunity'. Uptake can vary across the different social groups and a multifaceted approach is needed to encourage confidence (Kraszewski 2017).

Yellow Flag

Organisational culture can have a tremendous impact on the success of infection and prevention control initiatives. It is not uncommon for infection prevention and control interventions to be successful in one area (for example, a hospital); however, in another healthcare institution, they may fail, or will have significantly less success, when implemented. There are organisational factors that may be a major reason. There has been an increasing drive in recent years to understand and address organisational culture and its impact on improving healthcare performance.

Supporting Evidence

Hviid et al. (2019) strongly supports that MMR vaccination does not increase the risk for autism; it does not trigger autism in susceptible children and is not associated with clustering of autism cases after vaccination. This study adds to previous studies through significant additional statistical analysis and by addressing hypotheses of susceptible subgroups and clustering of cases.

Infection Control Glossary

These terms are frequently used in healthcare practice associated with infection prevention and control:

Bacteria are microorganisms typically a few micrometres in length and have a wide range of shapes, ranging from spheres to rods and spirals. Large numbers of bacteria can be found on the skin and as gut flora with most being harmless. Some, however, are pathogenic and cause infection.

Colonisation describes when bacteria grow on body sites exposed to the environment or in the gastrointestinal tract, without causing any infection. The patient is therefore asymptomatic.

Coronaviruses are named as such because of the crown-like spikes on their surface. They were first identified in the 1960s and can cause mild illness like the common cold. A new or novel coronavirus causing disease in 2019 (COVID-19) was responsible for the global pandemic in 2020.

Decolonisation is the process of eradicating or reducing the asymptomatic carriage of bacteria, often associated with the eradication of MRSA.

Herd immunity (also called *community immunity*) occurs when a large percentage of a population has become immune to an infection, thereby providing a measure of protection for individuals who are not immune. Chains of infection are likely to be disrupted, which stops or slows the spread of disease.

Infection: The invasion and multiplication of microorganisms such as bacteria, viruses and parasites that are not normally present within the body. Microorganisms that live naturally in the body are not considered infections.

Infectious diseases are caused by pathogenic microorganisms, such as bacteria, viruses, parasites or fungi; the diseases can be spread, directly or indirectly, from one person to another. Sometimes, they are referred to as *communicable diseases*.

M, C and S: Microscopy, culture and sensitivity (M, C and S) is the term often used when sending samples or swabs to the laboratory. It refers to the sample being viewed under a microscope, then grown (or cultured) to enable further identification of an organism. The sensitivity or resistance of the organism to specific antibiotics is also tested.

Microbiology is the study of living organisms that are too small to be seen with the naked eye. This includes bacteria, viruses, fungi, prions, protozoa and algae, collectively known as 'microbes'.

Pathogens are bacteria, viruses or other microorganisms that are harmful or can cause disease.

Prophylaxis refers to when treatment or care is given as a preventative measure.

Staphylococcus aureus is a Gram-positive, round-shaped bacterium found frequently without causing harm on the skin but can also cause more serious infections, often abbreviated and referred to 'Staph' or *S. aureus*.

Virology is the branch of science that deals with the study of viruses and viral diseases.

Viruses are sub-microscopic, infectious agents contained in a protein coat that replicate only inside the living cells of other organisms. Common examples include chicken pox and the flu influenza.

Touch Points Revisited

- The nursing associate has a key role to play in recognising and responding rapidly to potential infection risk, using standard precautions and protocols.
- Having an understanding of the principles of infection control and working in partnership with others has the potential to lead to improved healthcare outcomes for service users (and if appropriate, their families).
- Evidence-based policies and protocols offer guidance to nursing and care staff in order to prevent or treat infections.
- It is essential that standard precautions are applied across all healthcare and social care settings so to prevent direct contact and the transmission of blood. In order to identify the cause of infection and determine best treatment, diagnostic tests and treatment approaches are used by infection control practitioners often involving a specimen being obtained.
- MRSA can be suppressed helping prevent infection occurring; it is not always possible to completely eradicate of MRSA.
- The nationwide immunisation programmes for all children to prevent infectious diseases such as measles, mumps and rubella (MMR) are an example of a public health approach to infection prevention and control.

References

Bardsley, A. (2017) Diagnosis, prevention and treatment of urinary tract infections in older people, *Nursing Older People*, 29(2): 32–38.

Brady, M., Rodger, A., Asboe, D., et al. (2019) BHIVA/BASHH guidelines on the use of HIV pre-exposure prophylaxis (PrEP) 2018, *HIV Medicine*, 20: s2–80. doi: 10.1111/hiv.12718.

BNF. (2019) *British national formulary*. [Online] Available: https://bnf.nice.org.uk/. Accessed 19 October 2019.

Brooke, J., Clark, M. (2020) Older people's early experience of household isolation and social distancing during COVID-19, *Journal of Clinical Nursing*, 29(21–22): 4387–4402. doi: 10.1111/jocn.15485.

Coia, J.E., Leanord, A.T. and Reilly, J. (2014) Screening for methicillin resistant *Staphylococcus aureus* (MRSA): who, when, and how? *British Medical Journal*, 348(7948): 35–37. doi: 10.1136/bmj.g1697.

Davies, N. (2018) Measles: what you can do, *British Journal of Nursing*, 27(3): 116. doi: 10.12968/bjon.2018.27.3.116.

Hviid, A., Vinsløv, H., Frisch, M. and Melbye, M. (2019) Measles, mumps, rubella vaccination and autism: a nationwide cohort study, *Annals of Internal Medicine*, 170(8): 513–520. doi: 10.7326/M18-2101.

Hughes, J., Blackman, H., McDonald, E.M., Hull, S. and Fitzpatrick, B. (2011) Involving service users in infection control practice, *Nursing Times*, 107(25): 18–19

Kraszewski, S. (2017) Improving immunisation uptake in babies and toddlers, *Practice Nursing*, 28(7): 300–306. doi: 10.12968/pnur.2017.28.7.300.

Loveday, H., Wilson, J., Pratt, R., Golsorkhi, M., Tingle, A., Bak, A., Browne, J., Prieto, J.A. and Wilcox, M. (2014) Epic3: national evidence-based guidelines for preventing healthcare-associated infections in NHS hospitals in England, *Journal of Hospital Infection*, 86(Suppl. 1): S1–70.

Moreton, T. (2019) Challenges of diagnosing and managing pneumonia in primary care, *Nursing Times*, 115(9): 34–38.

Nursing and Midwifery Council. (2018). *Standards of proficiency for nursing associates*. [online] Available: https://www.nmc.org.uk/standards/standards-for-nursing-associates/standards-of-proficiency-for-nursing-associates/. Accessed October 2019.

Weston, D., Burgess, A. and Roberts, S. (2017) *Infection prevention and control at a glance*, Chichester: Wiley/Blackwell.

Zazzara, M.B., Penfold, R.S., Roberts, A.L., et al. (2020) Probable delirium is a presenting symptom of COVID-19 in frail, older adults: a cohort study of 322 hospitalised and 535 community-based older adults, *Age and Ageing*, 50(1): 40–48. doi: 10.1093/ageing/afaa223.

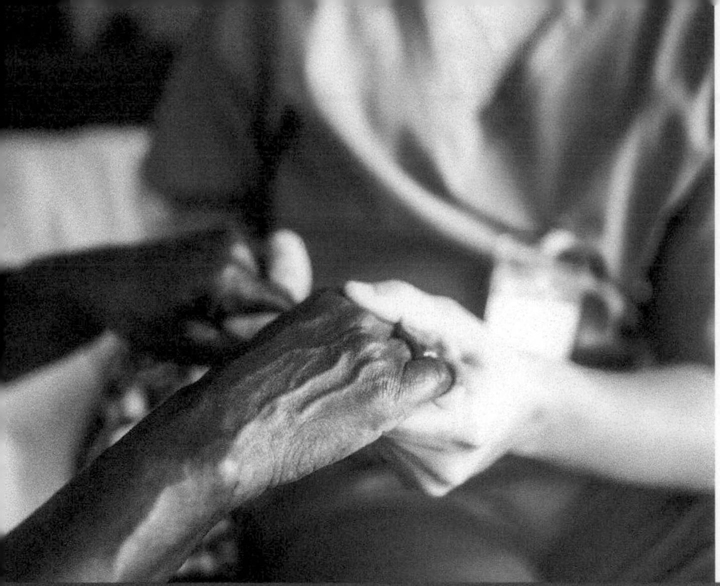

44

Using Aseptic Non-Touch Technique

Hazel Ridgers

Researcher and Lecturer in Nursing and Public Health

Chapter Aim

- To provide the meaning of asepsis and the evidence base for the use of aseptic non-touch technique
- To establish the principle behaviours required when using aseptic non-touch technique and consider how to apply them
- To provide a list of proficiencies that require the use of aseptic non-touch technique and explore the importance of person-centred care when undertaking these

Learning Outcomes

By the end of this chapter, you should be able to:

- Explain the term asepsis and describe why aseptic non-touch technique is vital to ensure safe, evidence-based practice.
- Describe what is expected at the point of registration regarding the use of aseptic non-touch technique.
- Demonstrate understanding of the principles of aseptic non-touch technique and give examples of when aseptic non-touch technique should be used.
- Demonstrate an understanding of why person-centred and culturally competent care is vital to undertaking this skill.

Test Yourself Multiple Choice Questions

1. What is asepsis?
   A) A type of dressing
   B) The absence of potentially pathogenic microorganisms
   C) A type of medication
2. Why do nursing associates need to know about asepsis?
   A) They do not
   B) Nursing associates are required to demonstrate an understanding of asepsis and to assure asepsis as part of standard infection control precautions
   C) To enable correct delegation of tasks requiring asepsis to other members of their team

The Nursing Associate's Handbook of Clinical Skills, First Edition. Edited by Ian Peate.

Companion website: www.wiley.com/nursingassociate

3. **What is aseptic non-touch technique?**
   A) The use of sterile gloves to do a dressing
   B) The use of tweezers to ensure you don't touch the patient
   C) The application of asepsis using a set of principles and practices that prevent transfer of potentially pathogenic microorganisms
4. **When should aseptic non-touch technique be used?**
   A) For all procedure involving exposure to body fluids
   B) Whenever a procedure will breach a patient's natural defences
   C) When the care plan prescribes it
5. **Is there a standardised approach to aseptic non-touch technique used across all healthcare settings?**
   A) Yes
   B) No but healthcare organisations are expected to have a standardised approach that all staff follow
   C) It depends on whether you work in a hospital or community setting

Introduction

Aseptic non-touch technique seeks to prevent potentially infectious microorganisms from entering a susceptible body site, for example, a wound. Asepsis reduces the risk of an infection developing as a result of the procedure being undertaken (Royal College of Nursing (RCN) 2017). This chapter provides an understanding of asepsis in relation to nursing associate proficiencies and describes why aseptic non-touch technique is key to ensuring safe, evidence-based practice.

Asepsis and Aseptic Non-Touch Technique

Asepsis means an absence of potentially pathogenic microorganisms. The principles of asepsis are central to standard infection control precautions (SICP). It is widely accepted that the adoption of SICP reduces the incidence of healthcare-associated infection (HAI) (Department of Health 2008; Loveday et al. 2014; National Institute of Health and Care Excellence (NICE) 2012).

Whilst asepsis applies to both medical and surgical procedures, medical and surgical asepsis have different requirements. Surgical asepsis is used in operating theatres and for invasive procedures (Loveday et al. 2014). The focus for this chapter is medical asepsis and how to assure it.

Aseptic non-touch technique is the application of asepsis. The term aseptic non-touch technique is used to describe a set of principles and practices used to achieve asepsis and prevent the transfer of potentially pathogenic microorganisms to a susceptible site on a patient's body (such as a wound) or to a sterile device (such as a needle) that will breach a patient's natural defences (Loveday et al. 2014). This is because any procedure that breaches the body's natural defences presents a risk of introducing a potentially pathogenic microorganism into the patient's body and may result in HAIs.

Take Note Asepsis

Asepsis means the absence of potentially pathogenic microorganisms. Aseptic non-touch technique is the application of asepsis using a set of principles and practices designed to prevent the transfer of potentially infectious microorganisms to a vulnerable site on a patient's body.

Natural defences are physical and chemical barriers that protect the body from pathogens. They include:

- Skin
- The normal outflow of urine
- Mucus membranes
- Stomach acid

Needle insertion for venepuncture, the injection of medication and wound care are examples of procedures that breach natural defences. Urinary catheters also breach natural defences by impeding the natural flushing action of urine through the urinary tract. Therefore, procedures such as sampling urine through a catheter port require aseptic non-touch technique to prevent the introduction of potentially infectious pathogens into the urinary tract via the catheter.

Green Flag

Nursing associates are required to apply the principles of aseptic non-touch technique when undertaking any procedure that breaches the patient's natural defences and to be able to do so wherever care is provided. They must be able to demonstrate an ability to undertake aseptic non-touch technique at the point of registration and show ongoing competence to remain on the Nursing and Midwifery Council (NMC) register (NMC 2018a, 2018b).

Touch Point Aseptic non-touch technique to prevent infection

Aseptic non-touch technique is the application of asepsis using a set of principles and practices applied to any procedure breaching the body's natural defences. The aim is to prevent the transmission of pathogenic microorganisms via the nursing associate's hands or contaminated equipment.

The Principles of Aseptic Non-Touch Technique

The principle behaviours of aseptic non-touch technique aim to minimise risks of contamination and prevent the transfer of potentially pathogenic microorganisms to the patient. The transfer of pathogenic microorganisms has been shown to occur via the hands of healthcare workers to the patient, from a device to the patient or between susceptible sites within the same patient (NICE 2012; Loveday et al. 2014).

Red Flag

It is the healthcare provider (the nursing associate) who is the main infection risk to patients when undertaking a procedure that breaches a patient's natural defences.

Table 44.1 highlights each principle behaviour and corresponding rationale. These principles are evidence-based and apply to all healthcare settings including hospital, community and home settings. Nursing associates must adopt all principles on each occasion aseptic non-touch technique is undertaken to ensure safe and effective practice.

Table 44.1 The principles of aseptic non-touch technique.

PRINCIPLE	RATIONALE
1. **Use aseptic non-touch technique for any procedure breaching the body's natural defences.**	Natural defences such as intact skin act as a barrier to the invasion of potentially pathogenic microorganisms. Breaching any of the body's natural defences increases the risk of inoculating the patient with potentially pathogenic microorganisms, e.g. via contaminated hands or equipment.
2. **Always employ SICP including the appropriate use of personal protective equipment (PPE) and hand hygiene techniques.**	To protect the patient from the transfer of potentially pathogenic microorganisms that may cause HAIs.
3. **Always maintain an aseptic area/field,** i.e. use of sterile drapes. Appropriately decontaminated blue trays can be used if key parts of equipment are protected with caps and covers. Areas of air movement should be avoided, i.e. near bed making, vacuuming or open windows.	To prevent contamination of equipment or the area immediately around equipment. Air movement can transfer potentially infectious organisms onto an aseptic field resulting in contamination.
4. **Avoid touching key parts of sterile invasive equipment or devices.** See Figure 44.1 for an example of key parts. Sterile equipment that will breach natural defences must not be touched. Caps and covers help prevent contamination that can occur via touch or contact with non-sterile surfaces, e.g. appropriately decontaminated blue trays. See Figure 44.2 for an example of use of caps and covers. Where touch/contact with sterile equipment cannot be avoided, use sterile gloves/drapes.	To prevent contamination of equipment that breaches the body's natural defences.
5. **Avoid touching susceptible sites** such as wounds, or re-palpating needle insertion sites following cleansing.	To prevent the transfer of potentially pathogenic microorganisms that may cause HAIs.
6. **Always review the task first and choose sterile gloves if a non-touch technique cannot be assured,** for example for more complex tasks.	Non-sterile (clean) gloves can be worn if a non-touch technique is achievable. If non-touch is not achievable, sterile gloves should be worn to prevent transfer of potentially pathogenic microorganisms to key parts or susceptible sites.

Source: Adapted from Loveday et al. (2014)

Violet Flag

It is essential that provision is made to reduce the risk of transmission of infectious microorganisms wherever healthcare is provided, for example, primary and community care settings, including places of detention (prisons). Key aspects of infection prevention and control within the prison environment must be deployed to protect staff and the patient/prisoner. This includes the undertaking of aseptic non-touch technique according to the principles highlighted in Table 44.1 wherever required.

Chapter 43 gives more information on SICP. For more information on appropriate use of PPE, see Chapter 45. For more on hand hygiene techniques, see Chapter 47.

Take Note The principles of aseptic non-touch technique

1. Use aseptic non-touch technique for any procedure that breaches the body's natural defences.
2. Always use SICP, including appropriate PPE and hand hygiene techniques.
3. Always maintain and aseptic area/field.
4. Avoid touching key parts. Use caps and covers to help prevent contamination.
5. Avoid touching susceptible sites.
6. The technical difficulty of a task should always be assessed. Where points 5 and 6 cannot be assured, use sterile gloves.

Source: Adapted from Loveday et al. (2014).

Key Parts

Key parts are areas of sterile equipment that make direct or indirect contact with the susceptible sites on a patient's body or with other key parts, for example, the syringe tip, needle hub and needle. Figure 44.1 shows equipment used for administration of injections with key parts highlighted.

Areas of sterile equipment that make direct or indirect contact with the susceptible sites on a patient's body include needles (for venepuncture, injection or aspirating urine samples from catheter ports), sterile swabs and wound cleansing agents. They must not be touched or make contact with non-sterile fields in order to prevent contamination with potentially infectious microorganisms. Where appropriately decontaminated re-usable fields are used, for example, blue trays, caps and covers for equipment such as needles or swabs must be kept in place until they make deliberate contact with the patient. In Figure 44.2, equipment is laid out safely in an appropriately decontaminated blue tray. Caps and covers remain in place to prevent contamination of key parts. Caps and covers are only removed immediately prior to contact with the patient.

Take Note Applying principles to ensure safe care

Nursing associates must apply a set of evidence-based principles to ensure safe and effective aseptic non-touch technique. They must apply these principles when undertaking any procedure that breaches the body's natural defences. All principles must be observed whenever and wherever the procedure takes place to prevent the transfer of potentially pathogenic microorganisms that may cause HAIs.

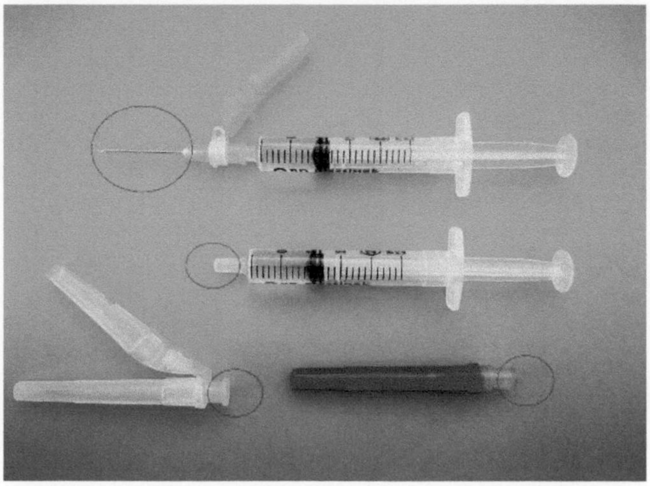

Figure 44.1 Key parts of sterile equipment are circled. Key parts identified include a needle, syringe tip and needle hubs.

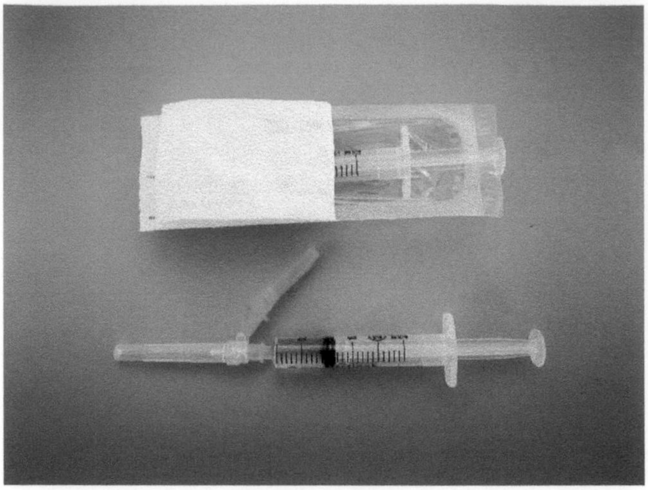

Figure 44.2 **Equipment laid out safely in blue tray using caps and covers to protect key parts.**

Nursing Associate Proficiencies Associated with Aseptic Non-Touch Technique

The list of clinical procedures requiring an aseptic non-touch technique given here are specific to the scope of practice of nursing associates. The list reflects current evidence-based recommendations (NPSA 2007; NICE 2012; Loveday et al. 2014) and the NMC (2018a) standards of proficiency for nursing associates. This is not therefore an exhaustive list of when aseptic non-touch techniques should be used in healthcare.

Nursing associates' use of aseptic non-touch technique should include the following procedures:

- care of wounds and surgical incisions
- preparation and administration of injectable medications
- administration of enteral medications
- venepuncture
- management of a catheter that requires access to key parts or susceptible sites, e.g. use of a sampling port (NPSA 2007; NICE 2012; Rowley & Clare 2011; Loveday et al. 2014)

Green Flag

The Health and Social Care Act (Department of Health 2008) requires healthcare providers to train staff to use a standardised aseptic technique and to undertake audit to ensure standardised practice.

Variations in Standardised Practice

Evidence-based guidelines on infection prevention highlight the importance of a standardised approach to undertaking aseptic non-touch technique to prevent HAIs, but the evidence does not currently support one approach over another (NICE 2012; Loveday et al. 2014). As a result, there is variation in how aseptic non-touch technique is undertaken between healthcare organisations (Loveday et al. 2014). NICE (2012) suggests that the ANTT® (Aseptic Non-Touch Technique®) practice framework provides a possible structure for developing standardised practice in both hospital and community settings. The ANTT® framework has been adopted by Public Health Wales and numerous NHS Trusts and primary care providers in England. See Supporting Evidence 1 for more information on this framework. You may also like to access the ANTT® website on www.antt.org. The ANTT® framework should not replace local policy where there is variation.

Supporting Evidence 1

Rowley, S. and Clare, S. (2011) ANTT ® : A standard approach to aseptic technique, *Nursing Times*, 107(36): 12–14

The authors of this article created the ANTT® framework highlighted in the NICE (2012) guidelines. The article presents the rationale and principles of the ANTT® framework and will develop your knowledge and understanding of this unique approach. The article can be accessed here:

https://www.nursingtimes.net/clinical-archive/infection-control/antt-a-standard-approach-to-aseptic-technique-09-09-2011/

Supporting Evidence

Loveday et al. (2014) epic3: National evidence-based guidelines for preventing healthcare-associated infections in NHS hospitals in England, *Journal of Hospital Infection*, 86(1): 1–70

You may be familiar with the national evidence-based guidelines for preventing infection from elsewhere in this textbook. The guidelines include direction on adoption of best practice for asepsis. The guidelines are produced by researchers and specialist clinicians following systematic review of the best available evidence on infection prevention and control and are designed to be adopted by approved healthcare providers. Section 2.6 of the guidelines focuses on asepsis and can be accessed here:

https://www.journalofhospitalinfection.com/article/S0195-6701(13)60012-2/fulltext#cesec1370

Touch Point **Standardised Practice is Safer Practice**

Evidence-based guidelines show that standardised practice is safer practice, reducing the risk of transmission of potentially harmful microorganisms (NICE 2012; Loveday et al. 2014). Standardised practice of aseptic non-touch technique is required within a healthcare organisation (Department of Health 2008), but no single approach has been shown in the evidence as more efficacious (Loveday et al. 2014), and there continues to be variation in how aseptic non-touch technique is undertaken between organisations. Nursing associate's awareness of and adherence to current local policy and procedure guidance is therefore vital.

Orange Flag

Infection prevention and control activities including aseptic non-touch techniques have the potential to cause adverse psychological effects. Non-touch techniques can lead to, for example, fear of contagion with either patients or nursing associates being fearful of the potential for spreading infection. Fear of contagion and the psychological impact of being physically isolated for reasons of infection control may be compounded for patients where isolation precautions are also required.

Applying the Principles: Preparing to Undertake an Aseptic Non-Touch Technique

Preparation for undertaking aseptic non-touch technique is key to a safe, effective procedure and varies according to the type of aseptic non-touch procedure required. An example of general preparation for undertaking aseptic non-touch techniques are provided in Box 44.1 that reflects the principles laid out in Table 44.1.

Guidance on undertaking specific procedures can be found in this textbook, for example, for venepuncture, see Chapter 11: Performing Venepuncture, or for wound care, see Chapter 29: Providing Wound Care.

Box 44.1 Applying the Principles of Aseptic Non-touch Technique: An Example of General Preparation for Undertaking a Procedure Requiring an Aseptic Non-touch Approach

1. Thoroughly wash and dry hands if using soap and water or use an alcohol-based hand rub if hands are visibly clean (see Chapter 47, on handwashing).
2. Clean the dressing trolley (start at top) or blue tray (if you are in a home setting) according to local policy using appropriate decontaminant and allow it to dry completely (see Chapter 48, on decontaminating equipment). Avoid areas of excessive air movement such as open windows or where beds are being made.
3. Place equipment on the bottom of the trolley or around blue tray.
4. Put on an apron (see Chapter 45, on the appropriate use of PPE).
5. Arrange the required equipment onto your sterile field or blue tray using a non-touch approach that protects key parts. Sterile packs are designed to be opened in specific ways. Open them carefully, following the instructions and without touching key parts of the contents. Never break/ tear open a sterile pack as this can lead to contamination. Note that flaps on sterile packs are designed to be peeled open, pointing the item away from the person opening the pack to avoid contamination. Drop the contents carefully onto your sterile/decontaminated field.
   Keep caps and covers in place to avoid contact with key parts. This is vital where using a blue tray to avoid key parts touching a non-sterile tray. Where it has been assessed that non-touch cannot be achieved during a procedure, select sterile gloves and/or sterile drapes and open packs maintaining the sterile field.
6. Decontaminate your hands and ensure that they are dry before immediately applying gloves (whichever type has been selected).
7. You are now ready to undertake the required procedure while continuing to observe the principles of aseptic non-touch technique.

Touch Point Applying the principles of aseptic non-touch technique

The nursing associate's scope of practice requires the undertaking of a range of clinical procedures that require aseptic non-touch technique, including wound care, injection administration and venepuncture. Application of the evidence-based principles of aseptic non-touch technique is required on every occasion that an aseptic non-touch procedure is required. Observing the principles are fundamental to ensure safe and effective technique, preventing the transfer of potentially infectious microorganisms to a key part or susceptible site.

Blue and Yellow Flags

Person-focused care is fundamental to any intervention (NMC 2018a, 2018b). Procedures requiring an aseptic non-touch technique require exposure of and contact with a patient's body, including parts of the body that may be considered 'private'. This may cause embarrassment or discomfort to varying degrees depending on the patient, the nursing associate or the environment (O'Lynn & Krautscheid 2011).

Nursing associates are required to balance the need for a safe aseptic non-touch technique with the requirement to demonstrate cultural awareness and consideration of a patient's needs and preferences (NMC 2018a, 2018b). Key to achieving this balance is communication that encourages patients to contribute to decisions made about how a procedure is undertaken. The nursing associate is required to make appropriate interventions that demonstrate sensitivity to the patient's experience of receiving care that requires exposure of their body parts. For more on demonstrating person-focused communication, see Chapters 2, 3 and 5.

Conclusion

Aseptic non-touch technique is the application of asepsis using a set of principles and practices applied to any procedure that breaches the body's natural defences. The aim of aseptic non-touch technique is to prevent the transmission of potentially infectious microorganisms via the nursing associate's hands or contaminated equipment. Nursing associates must use aseptic non-touch technique when undertaking procedures that breach the body's natural defences to prevent the transfer of potentially pathogenic microorganisms.

Nursing associate's scope of practice requires the undertaking of a range of clinical procedures that require aseptic non-touch techniques. The application of the principles of aseptic non-touch technique is required every time an aseptic non-touch procedure is undertaken, wherever it is undertaken, to ensure safe and effective practice. These principles help to ensure that the nursing associate does not transmit potentially infectious microorganisms to key parts of clinical equipment or to or between susceptible sites on a patient's body.

References

Department of Health. (2008) *The health & social care act*, London: Department of Health.

Loveday, H.P., Wilson, J.A., Pratt, R.J., Golsorkhi, M., Tingle, A., Bak, A., Browne, J., Prieto, J. and Wilcox, M. (2014) Epic3: National evidence-based guidelines for preventing healthcare-associated infections in NHS hospitals in England, *Journal of Hospital Infection*, 86(S1): 1–70.

NICE. (2012) *Infection control: prevention & control of healthcare-associated infection in primary & community care*, London: National Clinical Guidance Centre.

National Patient Safety Agency (*NPSA*). (2007) *Promoting safer use of injectable medicines*, NHS. [online] Available: https://www.sps.nhs.uk/wp-content/uploads/2016/12/2474_Inject_Multi-prof-1.pdf. Accessed September 2020.

Nursing & Midwifery Council (NMC). (2018a) *The standards of proficiency for nursing associates*. [online] Available: https://www.nmc.org.uk/globalassets/sitedocuments/nmc-publications/nmc-code.pdf. Accessed September 2020.

Nursing & Midwifery Council (NMC). (2018b) The code, *Professional standards of practice and behaviour for nurses, midwives and nursing associates*. [online] Available: https://www.nmc.org.uk/globalassets/sitedocuments/education-standards/nursing-associates-proficiency-standards.pdf. Accessed September 2020.

O'Lynn, C. and Krautscheid, L. (2011) How should I touch you?: a qualitative study of nurses attitudes to intimate touch in nursing care, *The American Journal of Nursing*, 111(3): 24–31. [online] Available: https://nursing.ceconnection.com/ovidfiles/00000446-201103000-00025.pdf. Accessed September 2020.

Royal College of Nursing (RCN). (2017) *Essential practice for infection prevention and control. Guidance for nursing staff*, London: RCN.

Rowley, S. and Clare, S. (2011) ANTT ™: a standard approach to aseptic technique, *Nursing Times*, 107(36): 12–14. [online] Available: https://www.nursingtimes.net/clinical-archive/infection-control/antt-a-standard-approach-to-aseptic-technique-09-09-2011/. Accessed September 2020.

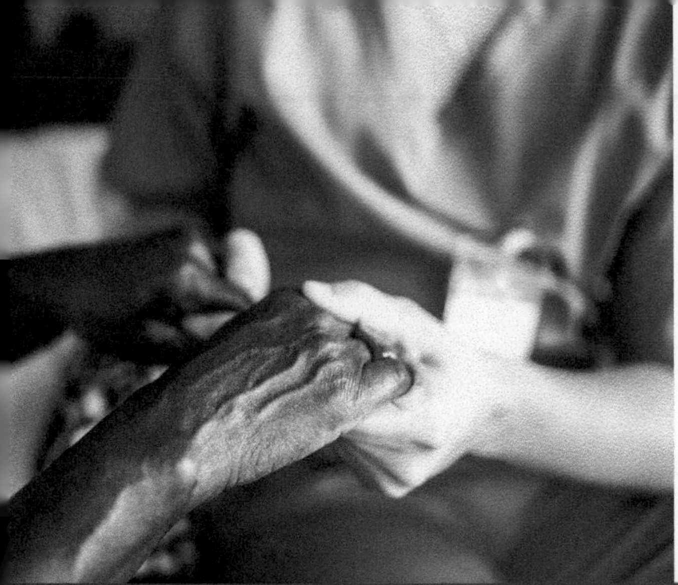

45

Using Appropriate Personal Protective Equipment

Nigel Davies

University of East London, UK

Chapter Aim

- This chapter discusses how the reader can adhere to standard precautions by using personal protective equipment (PPE) appropriately.

Learning Outcomes

- Discuss what PPE is and when it should be used.
- Describe some of the most common forms of PPE, including gloves, gowns and aprons.
- Outline issues faced by organisations related to the use of PPE and the accessibility and storage of equipment.

Test Yourself Multiple Choice Questions

1. Healthcare practitioners do not always comply with PPE guidelines. This may be due to a number of factors. Which of the following statement is FALSE?
   A) Individual knowledge of the patient and their risk factors can enable a nursing associate to judge what guidelines should be used or ignored
   B) Senior nurses on higher grades or bands with greater experience are more likely to comply
   C) Lack of availability of negative-pressure rooms can lead to a decision to not comply 100% with the policy
   D) Lack of training can mean staff are not aware of which guidelines to follow

The Nursing Associate's Handbook of Clinical Skills, First Edition. Edited by Ian Peate.

Companion website: www.wiley.com/nursingassociate

2. The following are equipment you *might* carry on your person in an acute care setting. Which item is part of your PPE?
   A) Pocket resuscitation mask
   B) Stethoscope
   C) Nurses fob-watch
   D) Mini alcohol gel dispenser

3. In which of these situations should clinical gloves NOT always be worn?
   A) When touching mucous membranes or breaks in the skin
   B) When performing or assisting with any invasive procedures, such as venepuncture or surgery
   C) When the healthcare practitioner has cuts, scratches, or other breaks in their own skin
   D) When assisting a patient to wash or giving a bed-bath
4. Wearing the correct sized gloves is important because:
   A) Gloves that are too small can limit hand dexterity and irritate your skin
   B) Incorrect sized gloves are more likely to rip or tear
   C) Gloves that are too large can be pulled off your hand
   D) All of the above
5. Disposable single-use plastic aprons are not required in which of the following cases?
   A) Performing or assisting in a procedure that might involve body fluids being splashed
   B) Performing or helping the patient with personal hygiene care
   C) Administering oral medications
   D) Carrying out cleaning tasks in the patient's bed area or living space, such as bed-making

Introduction

In Chapter 43, the principles of *Standard Precautions* were introduced. They aim to prevent the transmission of blood-borne and other infections in body substances where potentially infectious materials are present. The principal way this is achieved is through healthcare staff routinely using PPE as a protective barrier when anticipating contact with blood or body fluids (Loveday et al. 2014a). This chapter discusses the different types of PPE, circumstances when you should use PPE and some of the challenges you may face in complying with best practice guidelines for use of PPE.

Green Flag

The Health and Safety Executive (2013) considers that PPE is any equipment that protects the user against risks at work. In some industries, this might include items such as safety helmets and high visibility jackets. Within nursing, we mainly discuss its use in relation to specific infection control equipment (as in this chapter), but in fact other measures such as requirements to wear sturdy shoes or to wear lead aprons in the x-ray department are all part of your overall PPE. Employers have duties to provide adequate PPE for their workforce, but as a nursing associate, you have a responsibility to understand when and how to use it properly.

PPE must be provided and worn by staff in all instances where they will or may come into contact with blood, body fluids or repository secretions. This includes, but is not limited to, acute and community nursing care settings, dentistry, phlebotomy, processing of any bodily fluid specimen and post-mortem procedures. Different levels of PPE (see Figure 45.1) may be needed depending on either the setting or the individual. This will be determined following the completion of both work-place risk assessments and individual risk assessments.

- ***Work-place Risk Assessments***: At a hospital, team or ward level a risk assessment will be made by senior staff in association with infection control and health and safety professionals about the type of mask and other PPE required for different areas. For example, the use of masks, visors and fluid repellent full gown in critical care areas where patients with infectious diseases (like COVID-19) are being cared for.
- ***Individual Risk Assessments***: You will be asked to complete risk assessments relating to your own health and potential vulnerability to infection e.g. if you become pregnant it may not be advisable to care for patients with communicable diseases. Additionally, checks are also made at an individual level about whether equipment can safely protect you, for example, making sure a respirator type mask fits properly; this is often called "Fit Testing". This is particularly important for men with facial hair where a good 'fit' may be prevented by a beard.

Face Coverings, Surgical Masks and Respirator Masks

During the Covid-19 pandemic in 2020 the use of face covering by the public became widespread and for staff in hospitals and other health care facilities the wearing of masks became mandatory (Public Health England 2020). To distinguish between the different types of face protection a face mask generally refers to a mask which is designed and manufactured to conform to set standards (UK or previously European standards) to be used in a healthcare setting. Fluid-resistant surgical masks (FRSM) provide barrier protection against respiratory droplets reaching the mucosa of the mouth and nose. The protective effect of masks against severe acute respiratory syndrome (SARS) and other respiratory viral infections was well established prior to the Covid-19 pandemic. Level 2 PPE masks are commonly referred to as FFP3 (Filtering Face Piece) respirators. FFP3 masks should be used for any aerosol generating procedures, such as suctioning the respiratory tract, tracheostomy

PPE Level	What it is	When it should be worn
1	• Single pair of gloves • Disposable plastic apron • Fluid repellent surgical mask • Eye protection if you feel there is a risk of patient coughing, or splash or droplet exposure.	Any procedures when you may come into contact with blood or bodily fluids If airborne transmission of infection is likely e.g. when caring for individual patients with respiratory infection or in general if there is high prevalence of disease e.g. during the COVID-19 pandemic this level of PPE was advised for all face-to-face patient contacts within 2 metres
2	• Double pair of gloves to allow for changing top pair of gloves between patients or procedures. Bottom gloves should overlap the gown sleeves. • Long sleeved fluid repellent gown • FFP3 respirator mask • Eye protection (visor which can be disposable or reusable)	This level is required for all aerosol generating procedures, such as suctioning the respiratory tract, tracheostomy procedures, dental procedures like high-speed drilling, and induction of sputum. During the Covid-19 pandemic this level of PPE was standard in critical care settings at all times.

Figure 45.1 **Different levels of PPE.**

procedures, dental procedures like high-speed drilling, and induction of sputum. There is no evidence they add value over FRSMs for droplet protection when used with recommended wider PPE measures in clinical care.

The term face-covering is used for 'masks' that are (often home) made from general fabric or cloth to cover the mouth and nose. They offer some protection to the general public but are not appropriate in clinical settings.

Figure 45.2 provides further information about the use of gloves, masks, goggles, visors, gowns and disposable aprons.

Glove Use

Clinical gloves are disposable gloves used during nursing or medical procedures. Their use has become standard practice for surgical procedures and as part of standard precautions. There are two broad types of gloves:

1. Examination gloves (generally non-sterile)
2. Surgical gloves that have specific characteristics of thickness, elasticity and strength and are sterile

As a nursing associate, you should make sure that you know when and how to use gloves correctly. The correct technique for donning and removing gloves is shown in Figure 45.3.

Yellow Flag

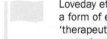

Loveday et al. (2014b) found that sometimes gloves are used inappropriately to give a sense of cleanliness and also to provide a form of emotional barrier against 'intimacy', for example, for washing a person's genitalia. Glove use can interfere with the 'therapeutic touch' associated with good nursing practice and could give patients the impression that they are somehow 'dirty' or contagious.

You should make sure you have access to the correct size gloves to ensure you maintain dexterity when performing tasks. Equally, you need to be aware of when to wear gloves and when their use is not appropriate. Recent studies (Loveday et al. 2014b; Wilson et al. 2017) suggest that the inappropriate use of gloves continues and that this is recognised by patients. Gloves are sometimes used for a wide range of care activities that do not involve direct contact with blood and body fluids and that in fact they are often put on too early, removed too late and their use may be linked to cross-contamination. The World Health Organisation (2009) has provided guidance on when gloves are required and when they are not indicated, including some common clinical examples (see Figure 45.4).

Take Note

Gloves are most commonly made from natural rubber latex due to its effectiveness (Wigglesworth 2019); however, latex can cause serious allergies or contact dermatitis. If you know you have an allergy or develop a sensitivity to latex, you should tell your employer so that alternative gloves can be supplied. Alternatives include neoprene and nitrile gloves, which may be readily available in large departments as several practitioners need them or you may need to obtain a personal supply. You may also need to adapt your glove use if a patient has an allergy and needs to avoid contact themselves with latex.

Gloves

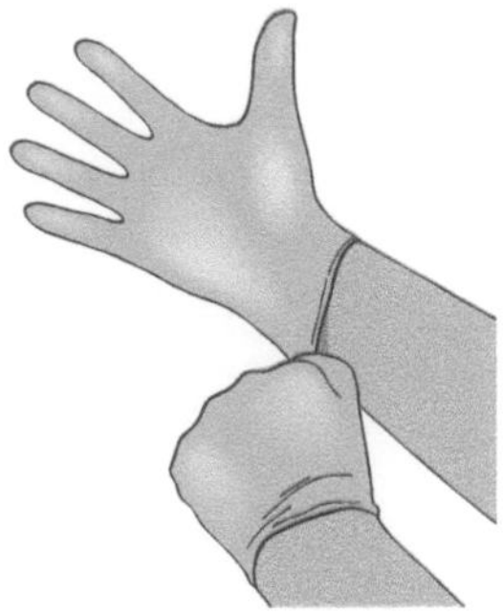

Latex gloves are recommended when dealing with blood or body fluids

- People with allergies to latex must be provided with other glove alternatives.
- Gloves must be changed after each client.
- Gloves should be worn:
  - When working with blood, blood products, semen, vaginal secretions and any other potentially contaminated body fluids such as cerebrospinal fluid, amniotic fluid and saliva
  - When touching mucous membranes or breaks in the skin
  - When performing or assisting with any invasive procedures, such as venepuncture or surgery
  - When working in situations where hand contamination may occur, such as with an uncooperative patient
  - When the healthcare practitioner has cuts, scratches or other breaks in their own skin

Masks, goggles and visors

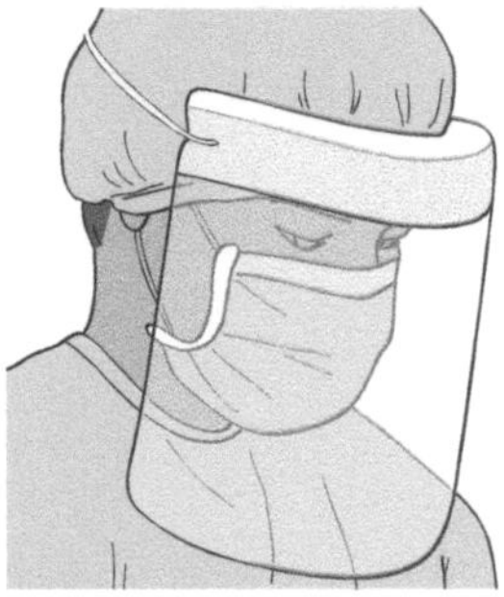

Masks, goggles or face shields should be worn

- During aerosol generating procedures
- During all invasive procedures and any procedure in which blood or body fluids may spatter or become airborne, e.g. during endoscopic procedures, during surgery
- During procedures in which heavy bleeding or other extensive fluid loss (such as peritoneal fluid) may occur

Gowns and plastic aprons

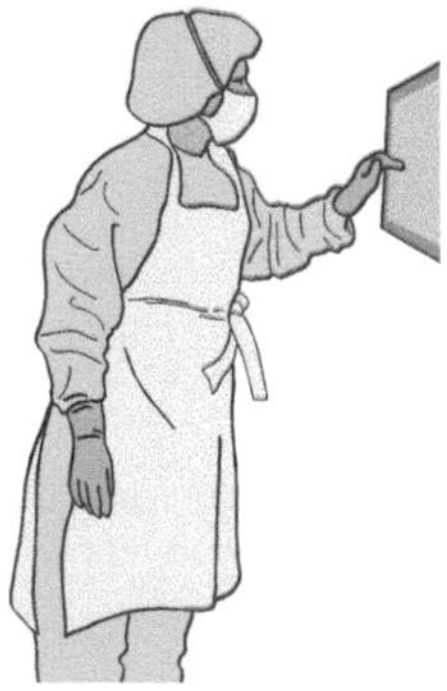

Gowns or aprons should be used when extensive fluid loss may occur

Reusable PPE must be cleaned and decontaminated or laundered by the employer. Lab coats and scrubs are generally considered to be worn as uniforms or personal clothing. When contamination is reasonably likely, protective gowns should be worn. If lab coats or scrubs are worn as PPE, they must be removed as soon as practical and laundered by the employer.

Disposal of equipment

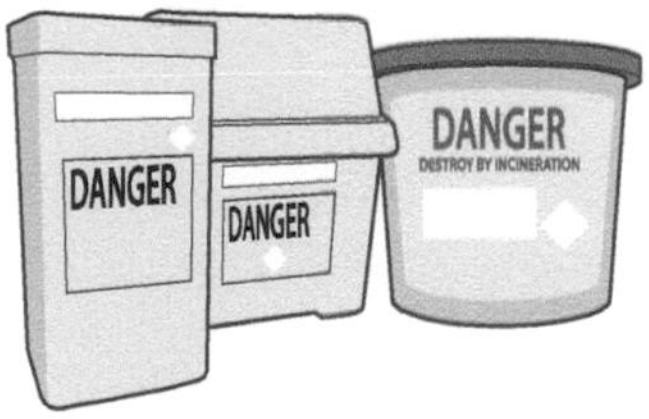

All equipment should be disposed of appropriately to prevent cross contamination

There is now a universal colour-coded system in use across the UK health service.

Needles must not be re-sheathed or re-capped after they are used. Syringes, needles and scalpel blades should be placed immediately in puncture-resistant containers ('sharps-bins'). Whenever possible, small sharps boxes should be taken to the bed side or point of care. (see Chapter 49)

Personal activities

Personal activities

- Eating (including sweets and chocolates), drinking, smoking, applying cosmetics or lip balm and handling contact lenses should be prohibited in work areas that carry the potential for occupational exposure
- Food and drink must not be stored in refrigerators, freezers or cabinets where blood or body fluids are stored or in other areas of possible contamination

Figure 45.2 **Protecting yourself and using Personal Protective Equipment (PPE).**

When the hand hygiene indication occurs before a contact requiring glove use, perform hand hygiene by rubbing with an alcohol-based handrub or by washing with soap and water.

I. HOW TO DON GLOVES:

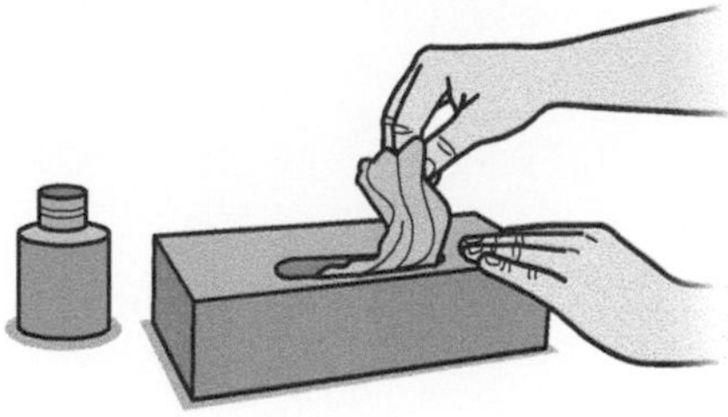

1. Take out a glove from its original box

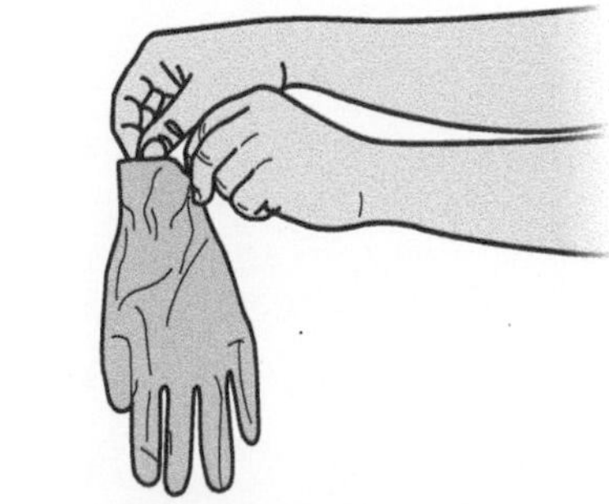

2. Touch only a restricted surface of the glove corresponding to the wrist (at the top edge of the cuff)

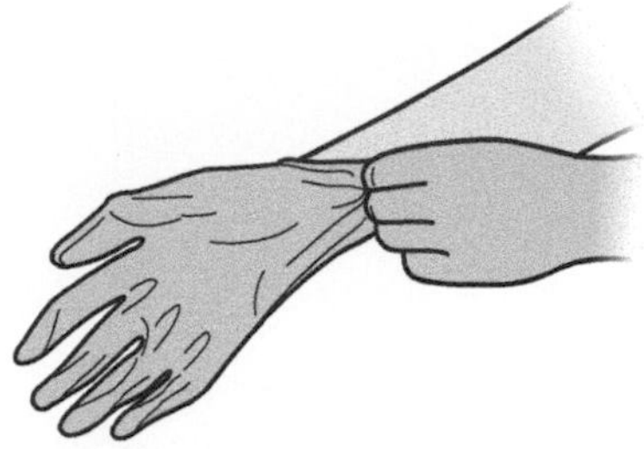

3. Don the first glove

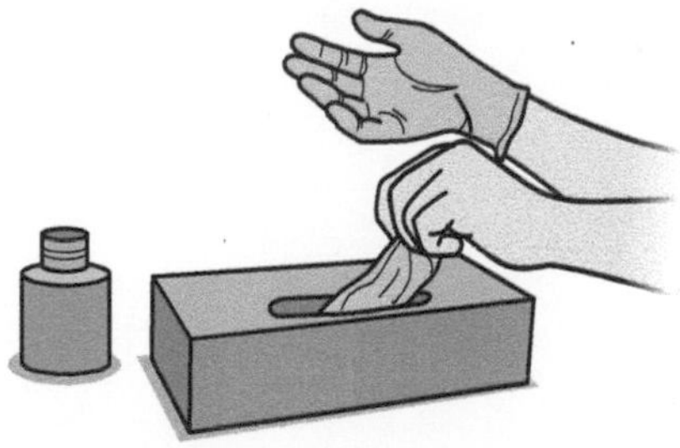

4. Take the second glove with the bare hand and touch only a restricted surface of glove corresponding to the wrist

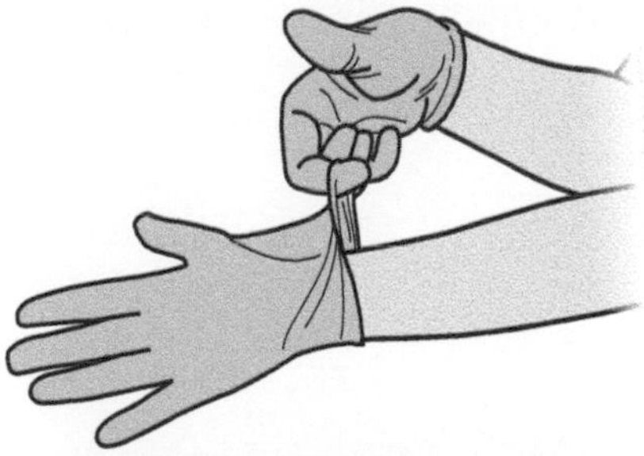

5. To avoid touching the skin of the forearm with the gloved hand, turn the external surface of the glove to be donned on the folded fingers of the gloved hand, thus permitting to glove the second hand

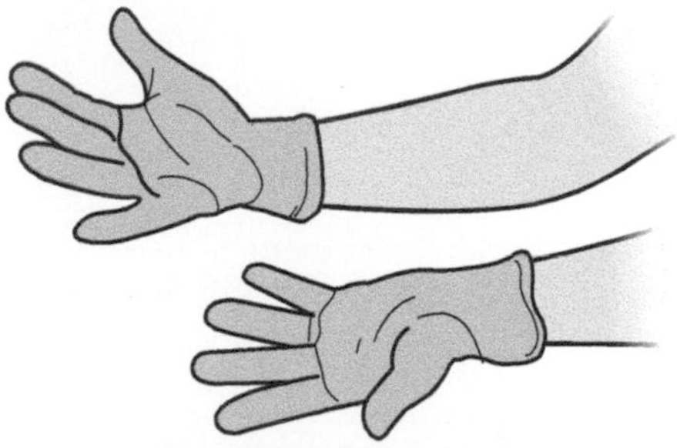

6. Once gloved, hands should not touch anything else that is not defined by indications and conditions for glove use

II. HOW TO REMOVE GLOVES:

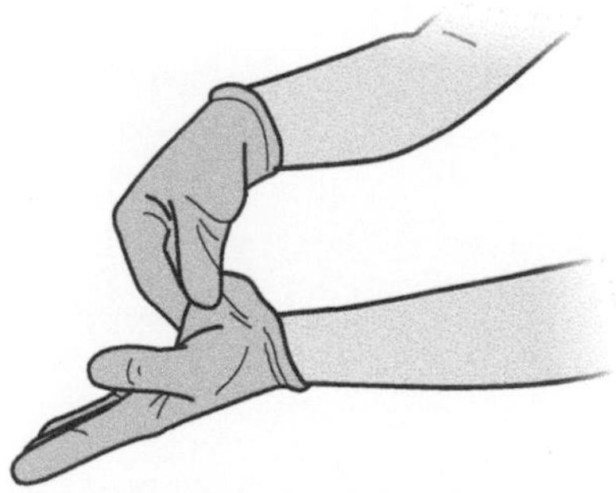

1. Pinch one glove at the wrist level to remove it, without touching the skin of the forearm, and peel away from the hand, thus allowing the glove to turn inside out

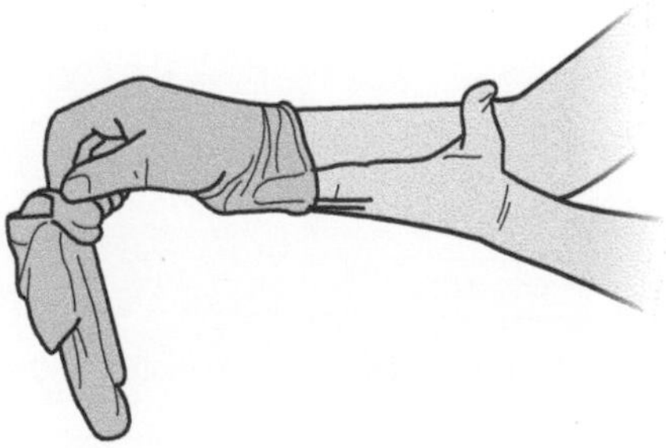

2. Hold the removed glove in the gloved hand and slide the fingers of the ungloved hand inside between the glove and the wrist. Remove the second glove by rolling it down the hand and fold into the first glove

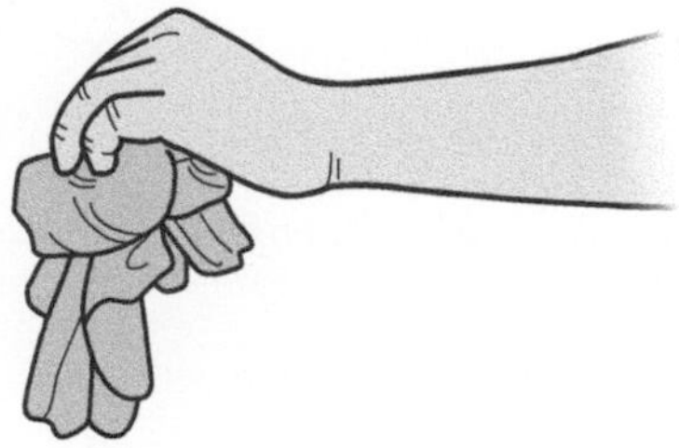

3. Discard the removed gloves

4. Then, perform hand hygiene by rubbing with an alcohol-based handrub or by washing with soap and water

Figure 45.3 Glove technique. *Source:* WHO (2009). © World Health Organization 2009.

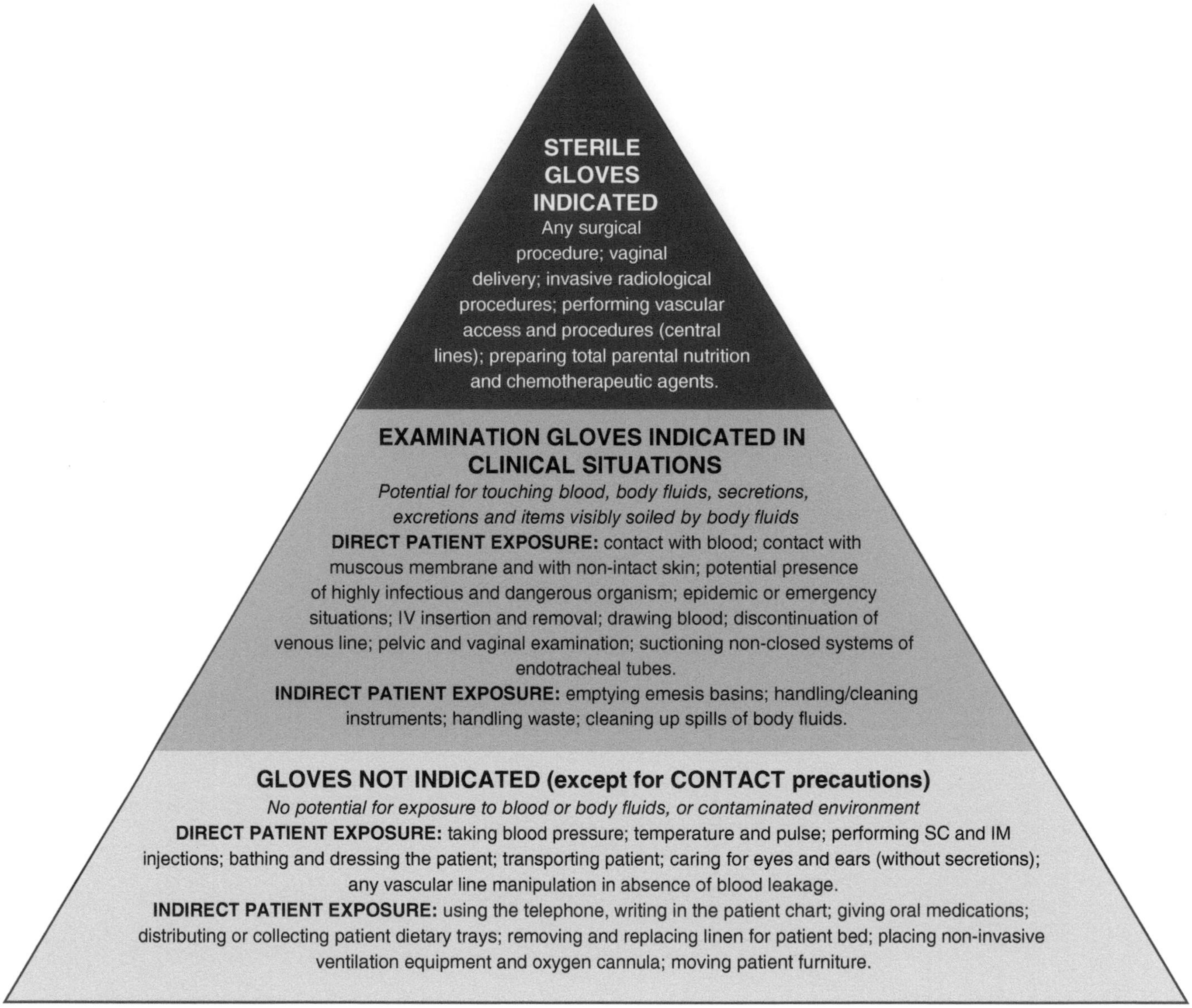
STERILE GLOVES INDICATED
Any surgical procedure; vaginal delivery; invasive radiological procedures; performing vascular access and procedures (central lines); preparing total parental nutrition and chemotherapeutic agents.
EXAMINATION GLOVES INDICATED IN CLINICAL SITUATIONS
Potential for touching blood, body fluids, secretions, excretions and items visibly soiled by body fluids
DIRECT PATIENT EXPOSURE: contact with blood; contact with muscous membrane and with non-intact skin; potential presence of highly infectious and dangerous organism; epidemic or emergency situations; IV insertion and removal; drawing blood; discontinuation of venous line; pelvic and vaginal examination; suctioning non-closed systems of endotracheal tubes.
INDIRECT PATIENT EXPOSURE: emptying emesis basins; handling/cleaning instruments; handling waste; cleaning up spills of body fluids.
GLOVES NOT INDICATED (except for CONTACT precautions)
No potential for exposure to blood or body fluids, or contaminated environment
DIRECT PATIENT EXPOSURE: taking blood pressure; temperature and pulse; performing SC and IM injections; bathing and dressing the patient; transporting patient; caring for eyes and ears (without secretions); any vascular line manipulation in absence of blood leakage.
INDIRECT PATIENT EXPOSURE: using the telephone, writing in the patient chart; giving oral medications; distributing or collecting patient dietary trays; removing and replacing linen for patient bed; placing non-invasive ventilation equipment and oxygen cannula; moving patient furniture.

Figure 45.4 **Glove Use Pyramid.**

Touch Point

- Gloves are used for a wide range of care activities.
- Clinical gloves come in two main categories: generally non-sterile examination gloves and surgical gloves, which are thicker, stronger and sterile.
- Gloves are sometimes used incorrectly, put on too early or removed too late, resulting in their use being linked to cross-contamination rather than preventing it.
- Patients often recognise when nursing staff use gloves inappropriately.

Gowns and Aprons

Disposable single-use plastic aprons are commonplace in many hospital and healthcare settings. They are not needed when undertaking most day-to-day activities with patients but are required for:

- performing or assisting in a procedure that might involve body fluids being splashed;
- performing or helping the patient with personal hygiene care;
- carrying out cleaning tasks in the patient's bed area or living space, such as bed-making.

Blue Flag

Some organisations use different-coloured aprons for different tasks, e.g. food/meal distribution and cleaning tasks, so you should check your local policy. This is done partly for infection control purposes to prevent cross-contamination but also to enhance public confidence so people can visibly see a separation of duties.

Take Note

When putting on, and after removing, a disposable apron, you should perform hand hygiene by either washing your hands with soap and water or using an alcohol gel sanitiser (see Chapter 47).

When you come to remove the apron, if gloves have also been worn, these should be removed first. The neck loop and waist straps should be broken and then the apron rolled downwards to fold the potentially contaminated surface inwards (Wigglesworth 2019). If you anticipate that there might be extensive splashing of blood or body fluids onto your skin or clothes, then a fluid-repellent full-body gown should be worn (Loveday et al. 2014a).

Using Personal Protective Equipment: Individual and Organisation Issues

While recognising the important infection prevention and control reasons for the use of PPE in practice for all healthcare practitioners, there are trade-offs between preventing exposure with the challenges of donning, wearing and removing PPE. This may tempt you and others to not always fully adhere to PPE and infection control protocols. The design of some items of PPE makes wearing them difficult. Over the last decade, manufactures have committed greater attention to the re-design of equipment so that compliance improves and to reflect the realities of the healthcare workplace (Institute of Medicine 2011).

Take Note

When you are using PPE, you need to consider the following factors related to the design of the equipment:

- maintaining good communications with patients, families and with your colleagues while wearing gowns and masks;
- being able to easily change PPE between different patients;
- making sure the PPE is as comfortable as possible over the duration of long shifts;
- being aware of how PPE might interfere with your dexterity to perform some intricate tasks, for example, removing sutures.

Supporting Evidence

The Institute of Medicine (2011) in the United States concluded that non-compliance with the use of PPE could be summarised into three categories:

1. individual factors, such as knowledge, beliefs, attitudes, perception of risk, history and sociodemographics
2. environmental factors, including availability of equipment and negative-pressure rooms
3. organisational factors, such as management's expectations and performance feedback, workplace policies and training and education programmes

Accessibility and Storage of Personal Protective Equipment

Equipment that is used frequently (e.g. gloves) needs to be readily available so staff can obtain the items quickly when needed. However, in some circumstances, this might be difficult because of safety issues for vulnerable patients or children.

Hughes et al. (2011) discuss some of the challenges to providing infection prevention and control measures within mental health settings, which are also relevant in other settings such as children's wards and emergency departments where there may be a need to adapt the approach taken and thought given to where equipment is stored to prevent items being used for self-harm or as potential weapons.

Conclusion

PPE is used to prevent the transmission of blood-borne and other infections in body substances where potentially infectious materials are present. The employer has a duty to provide PPE; however, as a nursing associate, you have a responsibility to understand when and how to use it properly.

Clinical gloves are used for a wide range of healthcare activities, and you must make sure you know how and when to wear them correctly. Likewise, if you need to wear masks, scrubs, gowns or use plastic aprons as PPE, then you must also be familiar with their correct use.

When using PPE, be aware of the unintended consequences the equipment might have, for example, how communication may be limited when wearing gowns and masks and how your dexterity to perform intricate tasks may be affected by wearing gloves which are not the correct size.

References

Health and Safety Executive. (2013) *Personal protective equipment (PPE) at work a brief guide.* [online] Available at: http://www.hse.gov.uk/pubns/indg174.pdf. Accessed 20 October 2019.

Hughes, J., Blackman, H., McDonald, E., Hull, S., Fitzpatrick, B. (2011) Involving service users in infection control practice. *Nursing Times*, 107(25): 18–19.

Institute of Medicine. (2011) *Preventing transmission of pandemic influenza and other viral respiratory diseases: personal protective equipment for healthcare personnel: update 2010*, Washington, DC: The National Academies Press.

Loveday, H., Wilson, J., Pratt, R., Golsorkhi, M., Tingle, A., Bak, A., Browne, J., Prieto, J.A. and Wilcox, M. (2014a) epic3: national evidence-based guidelines for preventing healthcare-associated infections in NHS hospitals in England, *Journal of Hospital Infection*, 86(Suppl. 1): S1–70.

Loveday, H., Lynam, S., Singleton, J. and Wilson, J. (2014b) Clinical glove use: healthcare workers actions and perceptions, *Journal of Hospital Infection*, 86 (2): 110–116.

Public Health England (2020) *COVID-19: infection prevention and control (IPC)*, [Online] Guidance on infection prevention and control for COVID-19. [online] Available at: https://www.gov.uk/government/publications/wuhan-novel-coronavirus-infection-prevention-and-control. Accessed 2 October 2020.

Wigglesworth, N. (2019) Infection control 3: use of disposable gloves and aprons, *Nursing Times*, 115(7): 34–36.

Wilson, J., Bak, A., Whitfield, A., Dunnett, A. and Loveday, H. (2017) Public perceptions of the use of gloves by healthcare workers and comparison with perceptions of student nurses, *Journal of Infection Prevention*, 18(3): 123–132. doi: 10.1177/1757177416680442.

World Health Organisation. (2009) *WHO guidelines on hand hygiene in health care: first global patient safety challenge. Clean care is safer care*, Geneva: WHO. [online] Available: http://whqlibdoc.who.int/publications/2009/9789241597906_eng.pdf. Accessed 20 October 2019.

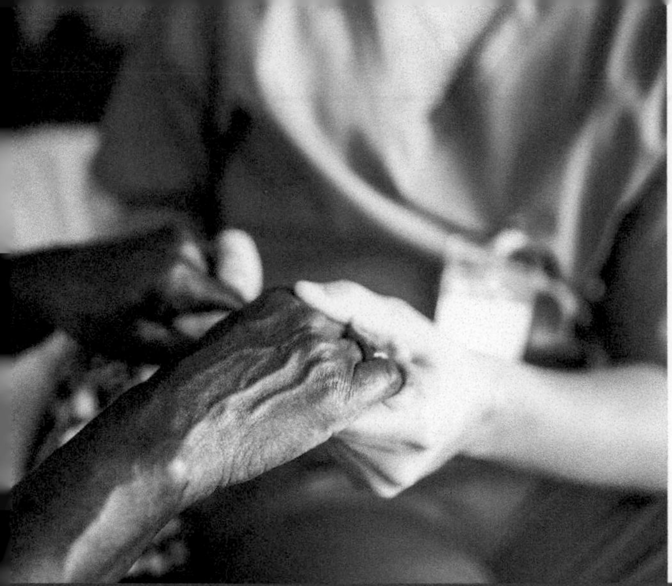

46

Implementing Isolation Procedures

Daniel Soto-Prieto

Former Lecturer at University of East London

Chapter Aim

- **This chapter aims to provide the reader with an overview of the principles required to implement effective isolation procedures.**

Learning Outcomes

- **To help the reader understand the rationale underpinning the need for isolation procedures**
- **To identify interventions required for specific clinical situations**
- **To ensure that care provision is patient-centred addressing all elements of care**
- **To convey the importance of the 6'Cs' associated with isolation procedures**

Test Yourself Multiple Choice Questions

1. **In what setting can the isolation precautions be implemented?**
   A) **Hospital**
   B) **Home**
   C) **Both**
2. **Which element is modified by the isolation procedures to reduce the spread of infection?**
   A) **Transmission**
   B) **Pathogen agent**
   C) **Reservoir**
3. **Which standard precaution can be excluded when a patient is under isolation precaution?**
   A) **Handwashing**
   B) **Decontamination**
   C) **None**

The Nursing Associate's Handbook of Clinical Skills, First Edition. Edited by Ian Peate.

Companion website: www.wiley.com/nursingassociate

4. **Can patients under isolation precautions be nursed in groups**
   A) Yes, always
   B) No, never
   C) Yes, if they are infected by the same agent
5. **How many patients in the United Kingdom acquire healthcare-associated Infections per year?**
   A) 100,000
   B) 200,000
   C) 300,000

Introduction

Isolation precautions are specific techniques aiming to prevent the spread of infection. Their main objective is to establish a barrier or physical obstacle that prevents the transmission of the infection from occurring. Isolation procedures extend beyond standard precautions, covered in Chapter 43. Standard precautions are designed to reduce the risk of transmission; however, in certain circumstances, some infectious agents might not be confined using standard precautions alone, therefore isolation procedures are required. Whereas standard precautions are always applicable to all patients regardless of their infectious condition, isolation procedures encompass explicit interventions applicable for specific clinical situations.

Violet Flag

Norovirus, an example of home isolation

During the winter of 2019, the National Health Service (NHS) closed more than 1,100 beds due to a norovirus outbreak (British Broadcasting Corporation 2019). Norovirus causes nausea, vomiting and diarrhoea for a short period of time (1–2 days). It is a highly contagious disease that spreads very easily through different routes. You can accidentally become infected by eating or drinking contaminated food, touching contaminated objects or having direct contact with someone who is infected.

Public Health England (PHE) recommended staying and treating the disease at home and not going to work or school until 48 hours after recovery from symptoms. PHE also recommended not to visit hospitals or general practitioner surgeries but to seek advice from NHS 111 for those with symptoms in order to avoid the spread of infection (Public Health England 2013).

According to the National Institute for Health and Care Excellence (2014), 300,000 patients a year acquired healthcare-associated infections as a result of care in the NHS. As first-line healthcare workers, in continuous contact with patients and relatives, nursing associates play a key role in implementing and maintaining appropriate and safe infection prevention and control measures as well as isolation procedures when needed. The proficiency of standards for nursing associates (Nursing and Midwifery Council (NMC) 2018) specifically identify the professional duty of 'implementing isolation procedures' in its section 8.5, and therefore, they are expected to demonstrate their proficiency while performing such techniques as well as providing a rationale underpinned by evidence-based practice. The NMC (2015) Code requires all registrants to ensure public safety, and this requirement applies when ensuring that the public and others are safe with regard to isolation prevention.

Source Isolation

This refers to the physical segregation of a patient with confirmed or suspected transmissible (contagious) disease to protect others from infection (Siegel et al. 2007). Its main objective is to restrain and confine the infectious pathogen to prevent infection from one person to another; it is also known as barrier nursing. These precautions are applicable for patients who are diagnosed or suspected to have an infectious disease or patients who are colonised or infected with a multi-resistant organism.

Orange Flag

Consider the physiological and social risk of being nursed in a single room under isolation conditions. There is evidence that anxiety, depression, mood disturbance, stigma or reduced contact might appear as a result of the partial or complete confinement (Barratt et al. 2011). Advocate for patients and put in place measures to prevent the adverse effects of isolation by providing social and emotional support, reassuring them, encouraging them to express their feelings, facilitating contact with family and friends in a safe environment.

Take Note

High-consequence infectious diseases (HCIDs) are contagious diseases which constitute a serious threat for human beings (Public Health England 2018). HCID transmission is normally by contact or airborne. Although HCID are rare in the United Kingdom, global mobility might produce an outbreak.

A detailed list of HCIDs, statistics, up-to-date guidance and advice can be found at https://www.gov.uk/guidance/high-consequence-infectious-diseases-hcid

There are three main categories of isolation precautions, classified according to the mechanisms of transmission: contact isolation, droplet isolation and airborne isolation. Sometimes, a disease may have more than one form of transmission which needs to be considered in order to implement isolation procedures.

Different isolation types will require specific procedures; nonetheless, they will also share some common principles as described in national and international manuals and guidelines.

Facilities: Isolation procedures will require, in most cases, a separate single-room or separated facility, including designated toilet. If single-rooms are in short supply, for instance during an outbreak, infected patients with the same infectious agent can be nursed in cohorts or groups (Fraise & Bradley 2009) under Infection and Prevention Control (IPC) team's supervision. In general terms, the room door must be kept closed, and warning signs will be displayed to notify that precautions and restrictions are applicable. Room surfaces must be cleaned and disinfected daily, specifically high-touched surfaces with designated cleaning equipment (Kundrapu et al. 2012).

Blue Flag

Healthcare Associated Infections (HAI) can be transmitted by healthcare workers. Each member of the team is responsible to adhere to infection prevention and control standards. Individuals inability to comply with policies and recommendations may breach infection control principles and risk patient´s health and safety.

Equipment: Use single-patient dedicated equipment to address the patient´s needs. If it is not possible ensure cleaning and disinfection is completed before using equipment with different patients. Information about decontamination process is covered in Chapter 48. Appliances will remain in the isolation room or cohort area. Evidence recommends using disposable non-critical items (in contact with intact skin) in the hospital settings (Siegel et al. 2007).

Visitors: Relatives and friends might be a source of infection; however, it is also important to facilitate patient contact with wider networking and socialising activities. This may require visitors to be screened before contacting with the patient, complying with standard infection control measures and in some cases to use PPE. Ensure that confidentiality is maintained at all times in line with your local policy and the NMC requirements (NMC 2015).

Patient transfers: As a general rule, patients under isolation precautions will be transferred only when necessary. It is crucial to inform the receiving service in advance so they can arrange the required precautions and activate protocols, for example, radiology, operating theatres or ambulance services for patients moving from care home to hospital settings (Nulens 2018). For unavoidable transfers of patients with airborne or droplet transmission diseases, patients will wear masks (Scotland NHS 2012).

Transmission: Some infectious agents might have more than one route of transmission (i.e. severe acute respiratory syndrome-associated coronavirus (SARS-CoV-1) is transmitted by droplets and contact), and therefore simultaneous transmission-based precautions may be used in addition to the standard precautions in order to ensure protection (Siege et al. 2007).

Red Flag

The meticillin-resistant *Staphylococcus aureus* (MRSA) is a common bacterium that lives harmlessly on the skin, nose, throat and groin; it is present in 1 in 30 people without causing disease. Meticillin-resistance refers to its capacity for being invulnerable to the antibiotics that are used to treat it.

MRSA can cause wound infections, endocarditis, urine infections, bacteraemia and sepsis if it penetrates the skin, and it contributes to high morbidity and mortality rates due to the challenges associated with treatment.

Nursing associates must read their local policy to find out when to start and discontinue isolation for patients infected with MRSA.

Watch the video 'Find out how MRSA is caught, what happens when you have it and how hospital staff and visitors can prevent infection' by Dr Brian Duerdan at https://www.nhs.uk/conditions/mrsa/.

Contact Precautions

Contact precautions aim to prevent and control infections that spread via direct contact (i.e. an open wound) or indirect contact (i.e. a contaminated object); this is the most common cause of cross-infection transmission. The pathologies listed in Box 46.1 require contact isolation.

Box 46.1 Indications for contact isolation

- Abscess, wound infection: major, draining
- Bronchiolitis
- Conjunctivitis: acute viral
- Gastroenteritis: *Clostridium difficile*, rotavirus, diapered (nappies) or incontinent persons for other infectious agents
- Diphtheria: cutaneous
- Hepatitis, type A and E virus: diapered or incontinent persons
- Herpes simplex virus: mucocutaneous, disseminated or primary, severe and neonatal
- Human metapneumovirus
- Impetigo
- Lice (pediculosis)
- Multidrug-resistant organisms: infection or colonisation
- Para-influenza virus
- Poliomyelitis
- Pressure ulcer: infected
- Respiratory infectious disease: acute, infants and young children
- Scabies
- Staphylococcal disease: furunculosis, scalded skin syndrome, burns

Source: Adapted from International Society for Infectious Diseases (Nulens 2018).

Take Note

Contact precautions aide-memoire

Hand Hygiene	Single-patient room	Gloves	Apron/Gown	Designated equipment	Eye protection	Patient transport
As in standard precautions	Recommended	Before entering	Before entering	Or ensure disinfection	Assess anticipated risk	Limited. Cover affected body areas

Contact precautions will require a single-patient room to nurse patients. If necessary, cohort (group) isolation is possible for patients with the same infection. In care home settings, patients will remain in their bedroom with the door closed. Avoid touching potential contaminated surfaces or objects. Use disposable or patient-designated medical devices and equipment (Scotland NHS 2012).

PPE recommendations: Wear non-sterile disposable gloves during the care episode which must be worn prior to entering the room and be removed before leaving the room. Also, wear a disposable apron or fluid-resistant gown according to anticipated contact and procedure. Remove gown and perform hand hygiene before leaving the room. Assess the anticipated risk of spraying or splashing, in which case surgical face mask and eye protection must be used (Siegel et al. 2007).

Limit patient transfers unless essential; in this case, before leaving the room, cover infected body areas. Notify in advance the receptor services so they will be able to make appropriate preparation. Linen and waste products will be considered as contaminated and disposed of accordingly. Conditions with specific risk for public health, i.e. haemorrhagic fever, will require special equipment such as an isolation suit (Siegel et al. 2007).

Droplet Precautions

Droplet precautions aim to prevent and control infections, spread by respiratory droplets larger than 5 micrometres (μm), which are discharged during coughing, sneezing, speaking or undergoing invasive procedures (oropharyngeal suction, laryngeal or endotracheal intubation and bronchoscopy). These droplets do not stay suspended on air for long periods, and they tend to settle quickly; therefore, transmission takes place in short distances (World Health Organisation 2014). The maximum distance for droplet transmission is still unclear; however, evidence has shown that highest transmission occurs within 1-metre (Bing-Yuan et al. 2018). 2-meters distance has been agreed as safe. The pathologies listed in Box 46.2 require droplet isolation.

Due to the nature of the transmission process, spatial separation of more than 1 metre has been demonstrated to be effective to protect people, although some infectious agents (i.e. smallpox), in certain conditions (i.e. environmental factors) may alter the transmission mechanism;

Box 46.2 Droplet isolation precautions

- Diphtheria: pharyngeal
- Influenza virus: seasonal
- Invasive disease: *Haemophilus influenzae* type B, *Neisseria meningitidis*, *Streptococcus* group A
- Mumps
- Parvovirus B19: erythema infectiosum
- Pertussis (whooping cough)
- Plague: pneumonic
- Pneumonia: adenovirus, *H. influenzae* type b (infants and children), *Mycoplasma*, rhinovirus
- Rubella
- *Streptococcus* group A disease: pharyngitis and scarlet fever (infants and young children)
- Viral haemorrhagic fevers due to Lassa, Ebola, Marburg and Crimean-Congo fever viruses

Source: Adapted from International Society for Infectious Diseases (Nulens 2018).

Take Note

Droplet precautions aide-memoire.

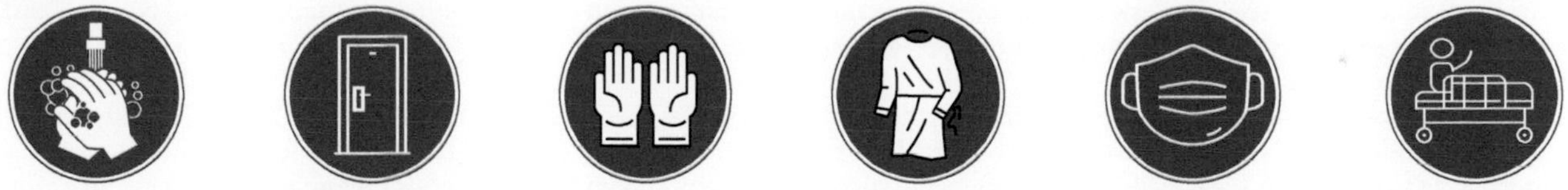

Hand Hygiene	Single-patient room	Gloves	Apron/Gown	Mask	Patient Transport
As in standard precautions	Recommended Maintain 1 to 2 meters distance	Before entering.	Before entering		Limited. Patient mask if unaviodable

therefore, masks will be used, at least, within 2meters from the patient. No special ventilation is required, and the door may remain open if mask precautions are maintained; which has been proved as the most effective element to prevent droplet infections (Scotland NHS 2012).

PPE recommendations: Wear Fluid resistant surgical face mask when entering in the room or close contact. Surgical masks can filter up to 80% particles; however, this filtration capacity is reduced if the mask is not appropriately fixed to the face. Disposable gloves and apron are also recommended however, more research is needed on eye protection recommendations (Siegel et al. 2007).

Avoid patient transfers. However, if transport is necessary, instruct patients to wear a mask.

Red Flag

Self-Isolation on COVID-19 Context

In early 2020, the COVID-19 pandemic spread out worldwide due to SARS-CoV-2 virus. Evidence has shown that this coronavirus strain is transmitted with close physical contact and respiratory droplets, although in some specific circumstances may also produce airborne transmission (WHO 2020a).

COVID-19 symptoms vary, ranging from mild (fever, cough, nasal congestion, sore throat, anosmia [partial or total loss of the sense of smell], headache, muscle or joint pain, nausea, diarrhoea) to severe symptoms (shortness of breath, confusion, persistent pain, high fever) affecting patients in very different degrees.

To prevent the transmission of SARS-CoV-2, many countries adopted infection control and non-pharmacological interventions such as hand washing, wearing masks, physical distance, isolation and quarantine, which has proved effective (Bailey & Wenzel 2020).

Self-isolation has been widely recommended for asymptomatic, or patients with moderate symptoms. Clinical decision to implement self-isolation relies on the evolution of patient condition, home setting suitability and monitoring capacity (WHO 2020b).

Self-isolation in the context of COVID-19 will follow contact and droplets isolation precautions, as below:

- Patient will remain in a separate room with appropriate ventilation.
- Wearing a facial mask is recommended.
- Reduce the number of household members and maintain 1-metre physical distance when they are in the same room. Caregivers will wear when present in the room. Maintain 1-meter physical distance as much as possible.
- Patient will have designated eating utensils, linen and towels. Waste material will be discarded on closed and strong bags.
- Daily cleaning and disinfection are recommended, especially for all high-touched surfaces and items.
- Maintain respiratory hygiene and cough etiquette (cover mouth when coughing or sneezing, use of disposable tissues, handwashing after touching mouth or nose).
- Perform hand hygiene following the “WHO 5 moments” covered in Chapter 47.

Airborne Precautions

Take Note

Airborne precautions aide-memoire.

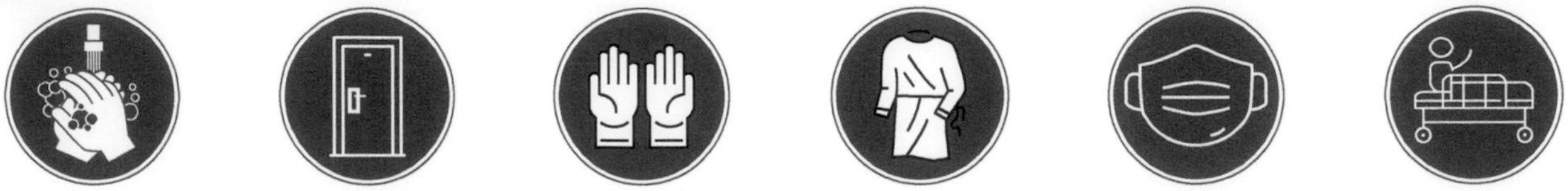

Hand Hygiene	Single-patient room	Gloves	Apron/Gown	Mask	Patient transport/ movement
As in standard precautions	Special ventilation. Door closed	Before entering.	Before entering	N95, FFP3 or higher	Limited to the special room. Patient mask if transported

Airborne precautions are specifically designed to prevent and control the transmission of infectious agents that are spread by small particles in the respirable size range (smaller than 5 μm) to patients and also healthcare and social care workers during the provision of care. Pathologies listed in Box 46.3 require airborne isolation.

Airborne precautions require rooms with special air ventilation systems as well as specific access arrangements to contain the infectious agent confined. These include neutral or negative air pressure systems (forced airflow from outside into the room to restrict contamination to adjacent areas), complete air renewal (6 to 12 changes every hour), high-efficiency filtration system for outgoing air (before air discharge) and a monitoring system to ensure appropriate functioning. If special rooms are not available, the patient should wear a surgical mask and should be kept aside until the appropriate facility becomes available. Seek for Infection Prevention and Control Team´s advice before cohorting patients, as antimicrobial study must be undertaken prior to grouping patients. Airborne isolation rooms often include an anteroom for airflow system purposes. It is also used for changing and hygiene purposes where PPE can be donned or removed (Nulens 2018).

Recommended PPE: Respiratory protection remains controversial, however there is agreement on wearing N95 or higher-level respirator masks when entering in the room. FFP3 respirators also offers protection for airborne particles. Their use requires to be fit-tested in advance to ensure they adjust to the contour of the user's face and they are properly sealed. All aerosol-generating procedures also require an FFP3 respirator mask and eye protection. They must be changed after each use, when damaged or contaminated. In contrast, surgical masks offer protection from splashes and droplets but do not protect from airborne particles (Siegel et al. 2007).

Use disposable gloves and disposable apron or fluid-resistant gown according to the procedure. Vulnerable or non-immune staff should restrict contact with patients known or suspected to be infected with airborne pathogens if other immune staff available (Siegel at el. 2007).

Limit patient transfers unless essential. If necessary, patients must wear masks. Waste products with respiratory secretions must be considered as contaminated and be disposed of accordingly (Scotland NHS 2012).

Box 46.3 Airborne isolation precautions

- Influenza A: avian H7N9, Asian H5NI
- Measles
- Middle East acute respiratory syndrome (MERS-coronavirus)
- *Mycobacterium tuberculosis*: laryngeal and pulmonary diseases, extra-pulmonary draining lesion
- Smallpox
- Varicella-zoster: disseminated disease, localised disease in immunocompromised patients

Source: Adapted from International Society for Infectious Diseases (Nulens 2018).

Protective Isolation

This refers to the physical isolation of patients who are especially susceptible to contracting contagious diseases and is designed to protect them from potentially harmful microorganisms. Patients are not infected but are at high risk. These procedures are applicable to patients with a compromised immune system (Dougherty & Lister. 2015).

Box 46.4 Protective isolation precautions

- Patients who have undergone transplantation
- Patients with leukaemia
- Those undergoing cancer treatment
- Patients with burns

Source: Adapted from International Society for Infectious Diseases (Nulens 2018).

The Centers for Disease Control and Prevention (CDC) removed this category from the isolation classification in 1983; however, over the years, it has specifically developed guidelines and recommendations regarding protective environment and immunocompromised patients as evidence develops, i.e. haematopoietic stem cell transplants. Pathologies listed in Box 46.4 require protective isolation.

Protective isolation facilities require specific and detailed design to ensure adequate functioning. Single rooms are recommended, including a single (unshared) toilet and bathroom. Also, anteroom with handwashing facilities and a double-door system, where at least one of the doors should be closed, at all times. Positive air pressure rooms are recommended for extreme immunocompromised patients, except if the infection agent could be airborne-transmitted. High-efficiency particulate air (HEPA) filters, effective-sealed rooms, low dust-production materials and air change system (12 air changes at least per hour) are also recommended (Department of Health, 2013).

Supporting Evidence

Do you want to learn more about isolation procedures and infection control? Do you want to gather information from an up-to-date source? Access the websites of the organisations below and their clinical recommendations for further information.

1. The International Society for Infection Diseases Guidelines accessible at https://isid.org/guide/infectionprevention/isolation-of-communicable-diseases/
2. Centers for Disease Control and Prevention. Guidelines accessible at https://www.cdc.gov/infectioncontrol/guidelines/isolation/precautions.html
3. The Northern Ireland Regional Infection prevention and Control Manual. Guidelines accessible at https://www.niinfectioncontrolmanual.net
4. National Institute for Health and care Excellence. Guidelines accessible at https://www.nice.org.uk/guidance/qs61

Staff and visitors with contagious diseases could be excluded from caring or accompanying these patients, as they could be a source of infection. Seek senior advice from IPC team.t is important to keep the room as clean as possible. Daily cleaning and disinfection are recommended. Cleaning equipment must be for exclusive use. Linen should be changed daily, and the mattress will be provided with special coating. Flowers are not allowed as they can act as reservoirs (Public Health Agency, 2015).

Follow standard precautions during each interaction. Staff must perform hand hygiene before and after patient contact. However, special procedures may need further precautions such as aseptic handwashing or sterile gloves according to local guidelines. Disposable aprons or gowns are recommended as a barrier clothing, but more evidence is required to appraise their role as a protective measure. Figure 46.1 demonstrates how to put on and remove PPE.

Conclusion

Isolation precautions should be used for those patients who are either known or suspected to have an infectious disease, are colonised or are infected with a multi-resistant organism or those who are particularly susceptible to infection.

There are a number of isolation procedures that contribute to effective infection prevention and control. Some of the procedures aim to prevent the transmission of infectious agents; however, they will only be effective if the nursing associate understands the rationale underpinning these procedures and the need to ensure that the patient's holistic needs are fully addressed.

Knowing the correct order to put on (donning) and remove (doffing) personal protective equipment is essential. Technique differs slightly depending on the type of the isolation precautions (contact, droplets or airborne) and equipment to be used. Public Health England released a quick guide in the context of COVID-19.

Donning:	Doffing:

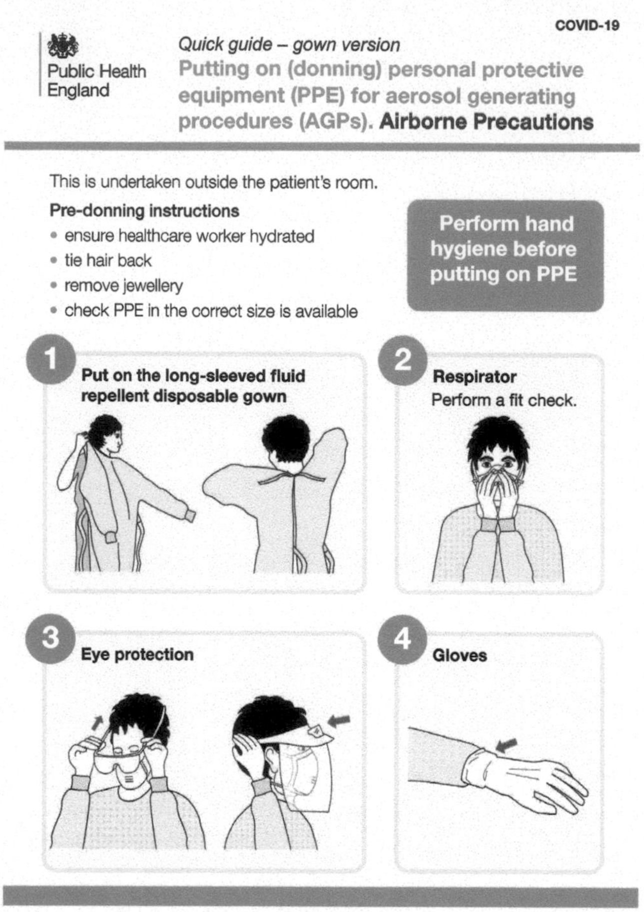

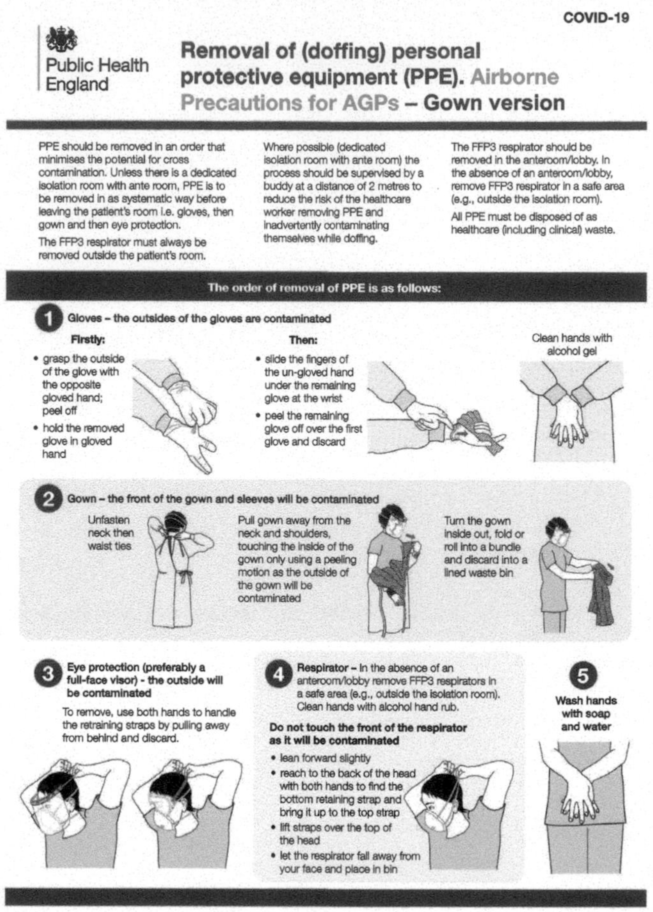

Figure 46.1 **Putting on and taking off PPE.**

References

Bailey, P., Wenzel, R.P. (2020) *The importance of non-pharmacological interventions for the prevention of COVID-19 Transmission. International Society for infectious Diseases. Guide to infection control in the healthcare settings.* [online] Available: https://isid.org/guide/pathogens/the-importance-of-non-pharmacologic-interventions-for-the-prevention-of-covid-19-transmission/. Accessed September 2020.

Barratt, R.L., Shaban, R., Moyle, W. (2011). Patient experience of source isolation: Lessons for clinical practice. *Contemporary Nurse: A Journal for the Australian Nursing Profession [Online].* 39(2): 180–193. Accessed November 2019.

Bing-Yuan, et al. (2018). Role of viral bioaerosols in nosocomial infections and measures for prevention and control. *Journal of Aerosol Science [Online]*, 117: 200–211.

British Broadcasting Corporation. (2019). *Norovirus closes 1100 hospital beds in England.* [online] Available: https://www.bbc.com/news/health-50673491. Accessed December 2019.

Department of Health. (2013) *Health building note 04-01 supplement 1: isolation facilities for infectious patients in acute settings*, London: Department of Health. [online] Available: www.gov.uk/government/uploads/system/uploads/attachment_data/file/148503/HBN_04-01_Supp_1_Final.pd.

Dougherty, L., Lister, S. (Eds.) (2015). *The Royal Marsden Manual of Clinical Nursing Procedures*. John Wiley & Sons.

Fraise, A., Bradley, C. (Eds.) (2009). *Ayliffe's Control of Healthcare-Associated Infection Fifth Edition: A Practical Handbook*. London, UK: CRC Press.

Kundrapu, S., Sunkesula, V., Jury, L.A., Sitzlar, B.M., Donskey, C.J. (2012). Daily disinfection of high-touch surfaces in isolation rooms to reduce contamination of healthcare workers' hands, *Infection Control & Hospital Epidemiology*, 33(10): 1039–1042.

National Institute for Health and Care Excellence. (2014). *Infection prevention and control, Quality Standard [QS61]*. [online] Available: https://www.nice.org.uk/guidance/qs61/chapter/About-this-quality-standard. Accessed November 2019.

Nulens, E. (2018). *Guide to infection control in the healthcare settings, Isolation of Communicable Diseases, International Society for Infectious Diseases.* [online] Available: http://isid.org/wp-content/uploads/2019/06/ISID_GUIDE_ISOLATION_OF_COMMUNICABLE_DISEASES.pdf. Accessed November 2019.

Nursing and Midwifery Council. (2015). *The Code.* [online] Available: https://www.nmc.org.uk/globalassets/sitedocuments/nmc-publications/nmc-code.pdf. Accessed November 2019.

Nursing and Midwifery Council. (2018). *Professional standards of practice and behaviour for nurses, midwives and nursing associates.* [online] Available: https://www.nmc.org.uk/globalassets/sitedocuments/education-standards/nursing-associates-proficiency-standards.pdf. Accessed November 2019.

Public Health Agency. (2015). *The northern Ireland regional infection prevention and control manual.* [online] Available: https://www.niinfectioncontrolmanual.net/isolation-patients. Accessed November 2019.

Public Health England. (2013). *Stop Norovirus spreading this winter.* [online] Available: https://assets.publishing.service.gov.uk/government/uploads/system/uploads/attachment_data/file/322947/Stop_norovirus_spreading_this_winter_leaflet.pdf. Accessed November 2019.

Public Health England. (2018). *High consequence infectious diseases (HCID)* [online] Available: https://www.gov.uk/guidance/high-consequence-infectious-diseases-hcid#definition-of-hcid. Accessed November 2019.

Scotland NHS. (2012) *National Infection Prevention and Control Manual (National Services Scotland).* [online] Available: http://www.nipcm.hps.scot.nhs.uk/ [Accessed November 2019]

Siegel, J.D., Rhinehart, E., Jackson, M., Chiarello, L., *The Healthcare Infection Control Practices Advisory Committee.* (2007 Last updated 2019). *Guideline for isolation precautions: preventing transmission of infectious agents in healthcare settings.* [online] Available: https://www.cdc.gov/infectioncontrol/guidelines/isolation/index.html. Accessed November 2019.

World Health Organization (WHO). (2014). *Infection prevention and control of epidemic-and pandemic prone acute respiratory infections in health care – WHO guidelines.* Geneva: World Health Organization. [online] Available at: http://www.who.int/csr/bioriskreduction/infection_control/publication/en/.

World Health Organization (WHO). (2020). *Cleaning and disinfection of environmental surfaces in the context of COVID-19: interim guidance, 15 May 2020* (No. WHO/2019-nCoV/Disinfection/2020.1). World Health Organization. [online] Available: https://apps.who.int/iris/bitstream/handle/10665/332096/WHO-2019-nCoV-Disinfection-2020.1-eng.pdf?sequence=1&isAllowed=y. Accessed September 2020.

World Health Organization (WHO). (2020). *Home care for patients with suspected or confirmed COVID-19 and management of their contacts.* Interim guidance, August 13, 2020. [online] Available: https://www.who.int/publications/i/item/home-care-for-patients-with-suspected-novel-coronavirus-(ncov)-infection-presenting-with-mild-symptoms-and-management-of-contacts. Accessed September 2020.

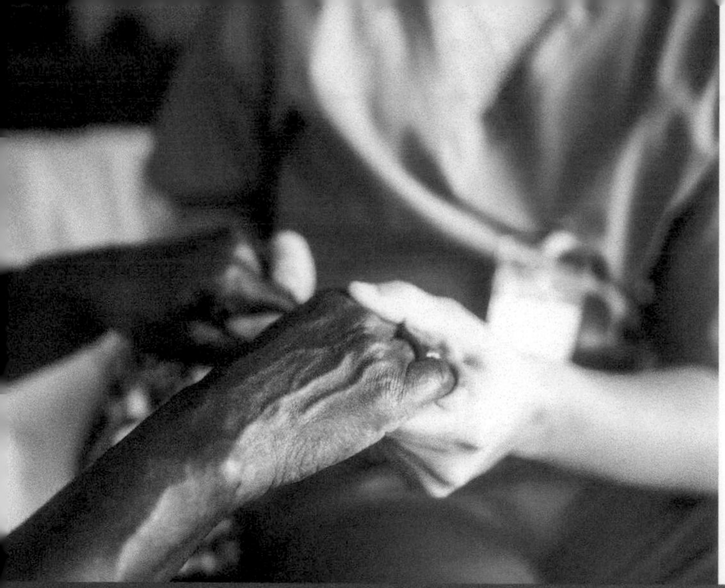

47

Using Hand Hygiene Techniques

Hazel Ridgers

Researcher and Lecturer in Nursing and Public Health

Chapter Aim

- **To provide clear guidance on what is expected regarding hand hygiene and present the evidence base for the use of hand hygiene across all healthcare settings.**
- **To explore the factors that influence decision-making regarding the choice of hand decontamination products.**
- **To establish how to safely, systematically and effectively use appropriate hand hygiene techniques.**

Learning Outcomes

By the end of this chapter, you should be able to:

- **Explain the evidence underpinning the need for appropriate, thorough hand hygiene techniques in healthcare settings.**
- **Describe the factors that should influence decisions regarding choice of hand decontamination products, including limitations to the use of alcohol-based hand-rubs.**
- **Demonstrate how to safely prepare for and then undertake systematic, step-by-step hand hygiene techniques using soap and water and alcohol-based hand- rub.**

Test Yourself Multiple Choice Questions

1. **Why is hand hygiene so important?**
   A) **To prevent the transfer of potentially pathogenic microorganisms on healthcare workers hands**
   B) **To prevent skin deterioration**
   C) **To adhere to local policy**
2. **How are pathogens like MRSA most commonly transmitted in healthcare settings?**
   A) **Through touch via healthcare workers hands**
   B) **Via body fluid spillage**
   C) **When patients cough**

The Nursing Associate's Handbook of Clinical Skills, First Edition. Edited by Ian Peate.

Companion website: www.wiley.com/nursingassociate

3. **When should nursing associates perform hand hygiene techniques?**
   A) At each of the '5 Moments for Hand Hygiene'
   B) At the start of their shift
   C) After contact with body fluids
4. **How should hand hygiene be performed?**
   A) Using a thorough, systematic step-by-step approach
   B) As long as you do it, the approach doesn't matter
   C) It depends on how much time is available
5. **Should alcohol-based hand-rubs be used for every episode of hand hygiene?**
   A) Yes
   B) Alcohol-based hand-rubs should be used for routine handwashing but there are evidence-based limitations to their use
   C) No, soap and water are always best

Introduction

The single most important factor in reducing healthcare-associated infections (HAIs) is the appropriate use of hand hygiene techniques. The hands are a major source of the transmission of potentially infectious microorganisms. Effective hand hygiene decreases microbe load and prevents onward transfer of potentially infectious organisms to patients.

Clean Hands Save Lives

HAI is critical to patient safety, and the impact of HAI on patient's morbidity and mortality cannot be overstated (National Institute of Health and Care Excellence (NICE) 2016; World Health Organisation (WHO) 2008).

Although using hand hygiene techniques may seem a simple intervention, the evidence shows that appropriate, effective hand hygiene techniques reduce the incidence of HAI (NHS 2019; Loveday et al. 2014), and as such, only clean hands are safe hands (WHO 2008). Therefore, hand hygiene must be used consistently wherever healthcare is delivered, including hospital, community and home settings.

In the United Kingdom, healthcare staff are required to undertake appropriate hand hygiene as part of standard infection control precautions. This means that appropriate hand hygiene techniques must be used by all staff, in all care settings, at all times, for all patients whether infection is known to be present or not (NHS 2019). For more discussion concerning SICP, see Chapter 43.

Green Flag **Professional Standards and Hand Hygiene**

As a nursing associate, you are required by the Nursing and Midwifery Council (NMC) (2018b) to demonstrate your commitment to preventing ill-health caused by HAI, to improving patient safety and the quality of care patients receive. Undertaking effective hand hygiene techniques are vital to demonstrate this commitment. National policy requires all healthcare staff to have the knowledge and skills to demonstrate competent hand hygiene practices (NHS 2019). The NMC expects trainee nursing associates to demonstrate the safe and effective use of hand hygiene techniques (NMC 2018a) and, once registered, to keep and promote these techniques (NMC 2018b).

How Healthcare Workers Spread Infections

Transient microorganisms are those found on the surface of skin. Hands easily become colonised by transient microorganisms, acquired by touching objects, equipment, patients and other people in the environment. Sources of further potentially infective microorganisms include blood and other body fluids, secretions or excretions, non-intact skin or mucous membranes and any equipment or items in the care environment that could have become contaminated (NHS 2019). Transient microorganisms may include pathogens such as MRSA or *Acinetobacter baumannii* which can be readily transferred onwards when healthcare professionals touch patients and equipment. If these microorganisms are transferred into susceptible sites such as in-dwelling devices or wounds, they can cause life-threatening infections. It is important to note that even transmission to non-vulnerable sites, such as a patient's intact skin, may still leave them colonised with a pathogen that may result in a HAI in the future (Loveday et al. 2014).

Touch Point **Why Hand Hygiene Techniques are Vital**

Hand hygiene techniques are used to prevent the nursing associate transferring microbes e.g. between patients or from the environment to a patient.

Effective hand hygiene techniques require a systematic approach, ensuring each step of the hand hygiene process is undertaken on each occasion that hand hygiene is performed.

The ability to apply consistent, effective hand hygiene is required to demonstrate fulfilment of the nursing associate proficiencies (NMC 2018a) and to comply with national policy on infection prevention and control (NHS 2019).

Preparing to Perform Hand Hygiene

Preparation for hand hygiene techniques is important to ensure all surfaces of the wrists and hands are accessible for cleansing. Remember that effective cleansing requires vigorous rubbing to create friction (Loveday et al. 2014) so anything that impedes this action should be removed in preparation:

- expose forearms (bare below the elbow)
- remove all hand and wrist jewellery (a single, plain metal finger ring is permitted but should be removed (or moved up)) during hand hygiene
- ensure fingernails are clean and short, and do not wear artificial nails or nail products
- cover all cuts or abrasions with a waterproof dressing

Supporting Evidence

There are national evidence-based guidelines for preventing infection which include guidance on the adoption of best practice for hand hygiene. The guidelines are produced by a nurse-led multi-professional team of researchers and specialist clinicians following systematic review of the available evidence on infection prevention and control. Section 2.3 of the guidelines focuses on hand hygiene. The guidelines are designed to be integrated into clinical practice and are updated periodically. You can access Section 2.3 on hand hygiene here:
https://www.journalofhospitalinfection.com/article/S0195-6701(13)60012-2/fulltext#cesec750

Source: Adapted from Loveday et al. (2014).

(NHS 2019)

Preventing Hai Requires Effective Hand Hygiene Techniques

The evidence shows that contaminated hands can directly transfer potentially pathogenic microorganisms, resulting in a patient acquiring a HAI. Effective hand hygiene techniques have been shown in research trials to prevent onward transfer of microorganisms and reduce incidences of HAI (Loveday et al. 2014).

Although hand hygiene may seem straightforward, to be effective, hand hygiene techniques require the correct preparation and a systematic and methodical approach to cleansing/washing. This ensures that all surfaces of the wrists and hands are decontaminated. Surfaces of the hands must be rubbed thoroughly during decontamination as it is the friction caused during rubbing that removes transient microorganisms.

Where hand washing is used, care must also be taken to dry hands thoroughly.

Where alcohol-based hand-rubs (ABHRs) are used, hands should be washed with liquid soap and water after several applications to prevent an excessive build-up of the ABHR product on the skin.

Safe Decision-Making: ABHRS or Liquid Soap and Water?

The National Policy on Hand Hygiene and Personal Protective Equipment (NHS 2019) states that ABHRs should be used for routine hand hygiene. ABHR dispensers should be available to healthcare staff as close to points of care as possible. Where this is not available, the policy advises that personal ABHR dispensers should be used. You should refer to local policy regarding the use and provision of ABHRs. All ABHRs used in healthcare settings must comply with current British Standards (Loveday et al. 2014).

Nursing associates must remember that there are evidence-based limitations to the use of ABHRs. Nursing associates must demonstrate an awareness of these limitations and apply this understanding to decisions made about which hand hygiene technique to use and when.

ABHRs do not remove dirt and organic matter (Loveday et al. 2014). Hands must be washed with liquid soap and water when they are visibly soiled.

Importantly, ABHRs must not be used when caring for patients with vomiting or diarrhoeal illnesses or if a gastrointestinal infection is suspected or confirmed. This is because evidence suggests ABHR is not effective against all microorganisms, e.g. norovirus or the spore-forming microorganism *Clostridium difficile* (Loveday et al. 2014). ABHRs may also be ineffective in some infection outbreak situations. If an outbreak occurs, local infection prevention and control teams should be asked for advice on hand hygiene methods.

To perform effective hand hygiene using ABHR, see 'How To Handrub' in Figure 47.1.

Touch Point When to Use and When Not to Use ABHR

Routine hand hygiene should be undertaken using ABHRs. However, nursing associates are expected to demonstrate sound evidence-based decision-making regarding the selection of an appropriate decontaminating agent (e.g. liquid soap and water or alcohol gel). Nursing associates are therefore required to demonstrate awareness that the evidence shows that there are limitations to the use of ABHRs, for example, ABHRs are not a safe method of hand decontamination when caring for a patient with diarrhoea or *C. difficile*.
http://www.nipcm.scot.nhs.uk/appendices/appendix-2-best-practice-how-to-hand-rub/

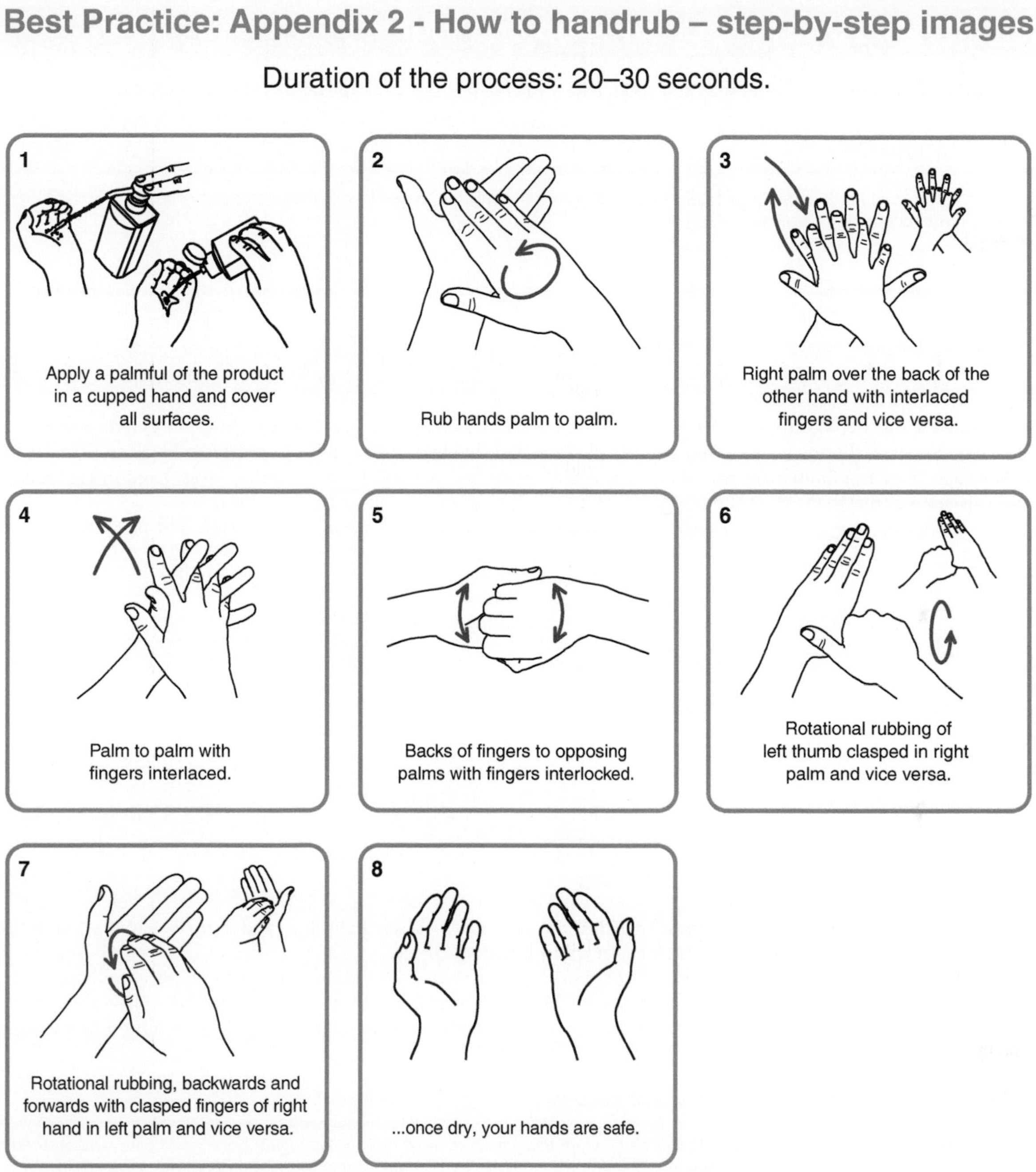
Best Practice: Appendix 2 - How to handrub – step-by-step images
Duration of the process: 20–30 seconds.
1
Apply a palmful of the product in a cupped hand and cover all surfaces.
2
Rub hands palm to palm.
3
Right palm over the back of the other hand with interlaced fingers and vice versa.
4
Palm to palm with fingers interlaced.
5
Backs of fingers to opposing palms with fingers interlocked.
6
Rotational rubbing of left thumb clasped in right palm and vice versa.
7
Rotational rubbing, backwards and forwards with clasped fingers of right hand in left palm and vice versa.
8
...once dry, your hands are safe.

Figure 47.1 Step-by-step guidance on how to effectively hand-rub with ABHR. *Source:* Health Protection Scotland (2019a). © 2019 Health Protection Scotland for the NHS National Services Scotland.

Undertaking Hand Washing Using Soap and Water

To perform effective hand hygiene using liquid soap and water, follow each step in the 'How To Hand Wash' in Figure 47.2.

Violet Flag – Turning Taps Off

In primary care or community settings where elbow taps are not available, paper towels may be used to turn off the tap to reduce the risk of contaminating clean hands.

Hand Drying and Skin Care

Drying is vital to remove moisture. Moisture can provide an environment favoured by pathogenic microorganisms. Good quality paper towels should be used to dry the hands thoroughly (Loveday et al. 2014). Attention should be paid to areas between the fingers and under a wedding band, if worn. Although there is a limited amount of research regarding the use of hand driers in clinical areas, hand driers are not recommended in healthcare settings due to the risks of microorganism movement and transfer (Loveday et al. 2014).

Alongside thorough drying, the NHS (2019) recommends using an emollient hand cream both at work and off duty to support skin integrity.

When to Perform Hand Hygiene Techniques

Knowing the critical moments to perform hand hygiene techniques before, during and after patient care is vital to prevent cross-transmission of microorganisms.

The following moments to perform hand hygiene have been identified:

1. Immediately before touching a patient
2. Immediately before clean or aseptic procedures
3. Immediately after body fluid exposure risk
4. Immediately after touching a patient
   Immediately after touching a patient's immediate surroundings
   (Loveday et al. 2014; NHS 2019; WHO 2008)

It is important to understand that hand hygiene must be performed immediately before putting on and immediately after removing gloves, as the moist, warm environment provided by gloves can be favoured by microorganisms.

The World Health Organisation (2008) has developed a pictogram of 'Your 5 Moments for Hand Hygiene' to support healthcare professional's awareness of when to perform hand hygiene techniques and why. The '5 Moments' approach has been adopted widely internationally, and '5 Moments' posters are commonly displayed in healthcare settings as an aide-memoire for staff. See Figure 47.3 'Your 5 Moments for Hand Hygiene' (WHO 2008).

Take Note When to Undertake Hand Hygiene Techniques

Nursing associates must demonstrate awareness of when to undertake hand hygiene during an episode of care. Understanding these key concepts enable nursing associates to keep patients safe and do the right thing for every patient, every time (NHS 2019). There are 5 key moments to undertake hand hygiene techniques (WHO 2008). These are shown in Figure. 47.3.

Take Note Hand Hygiene and Glove Use

Hand hygiene is required immediately before applying and immediately after removing gloves (NHS 2019). Wearing gloves is never an alternative to hand hygiene, and the decision to use gloves to complete a task should be based on a sound rationale and reflect personal protective equipment use policy (see Chapter 45).

Best Practice Where Hand Hygiene Facilities are Limited

National infection control policy (NHS 2019) recognises that healthcare may occur where running water is unavailable or hand hygiene facilities are lacking. If liquid soap and water hand hygiene is indicated but not available, staff may use hand wipes followed by ABHR and should wash their hands at the first opportunity.

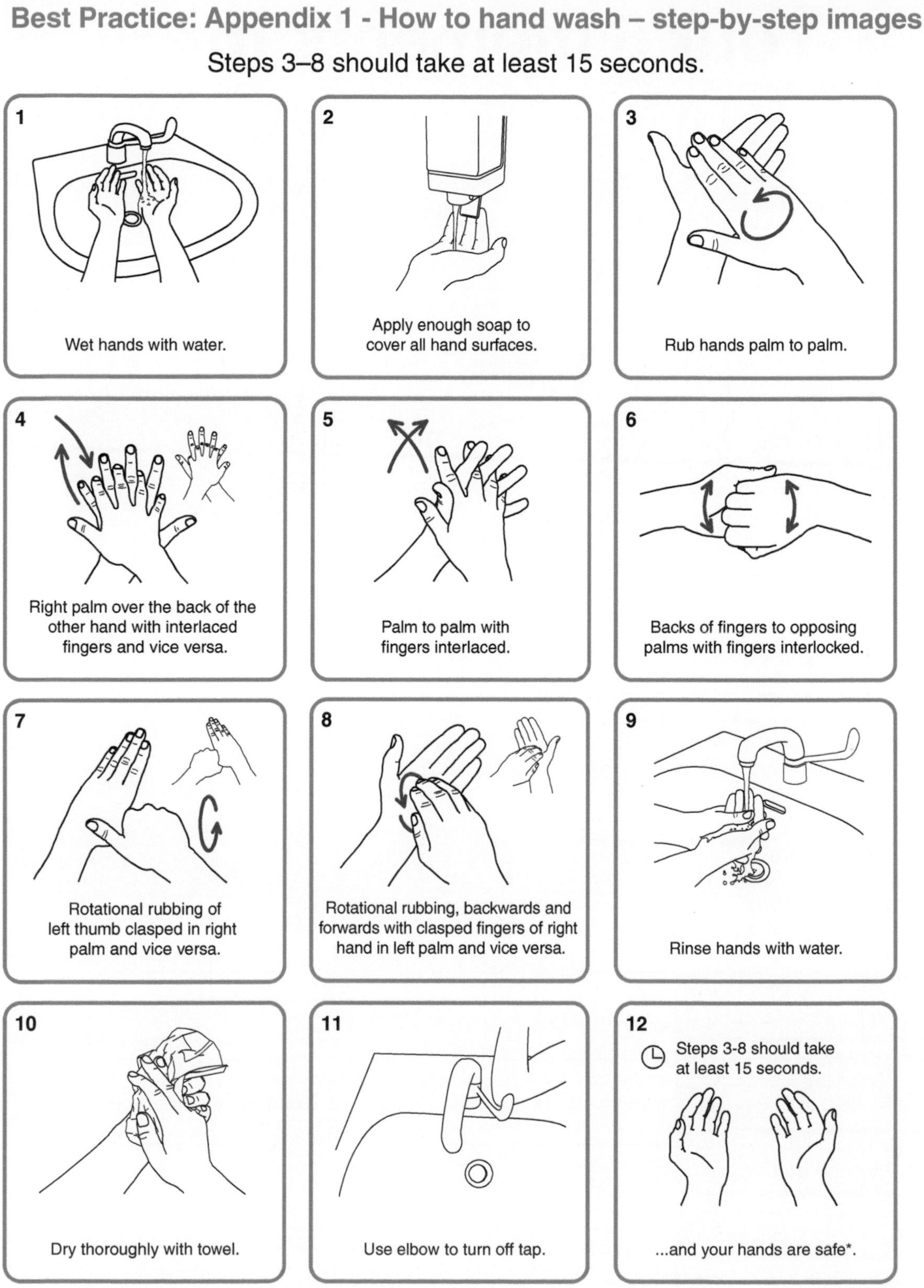
Best Practice: Appendix 1 - How to hand wash – step-by-step images
Steps 3–8 should take at least 15 seconds.
1
Wet hands with water.
2
Apply enough soap to cover all hand surfaces.
3
Rub hands palm to palm.
4
Right palm over the back of the other hand with interlaced fingers and vice versa.
5
Palm to palm with fingers interlaced.
6
Backs of fingers to opposing palms with fingers interlocked.
7
Rotational rubbing of left thumb clasped in right palm and vice versa.
8
Rotational rubbing, backwards and forwards with clasped fingers of right hand in left palm and vice versa.
9
Rinse hands with water.
10
Dry thoroughly with towel.
11
Use elbow to turn off tap.
12
Steps 3-8 should take at least 15 seconds.
...and your hands are safe*.

Figure 47.2 Step-by-step guidance on how to effectively wash hands with soap and water. *Source:* Health Protection Scotland (2019a). © 2019 Health Protection Scotland for the NHS National Services Scotland.

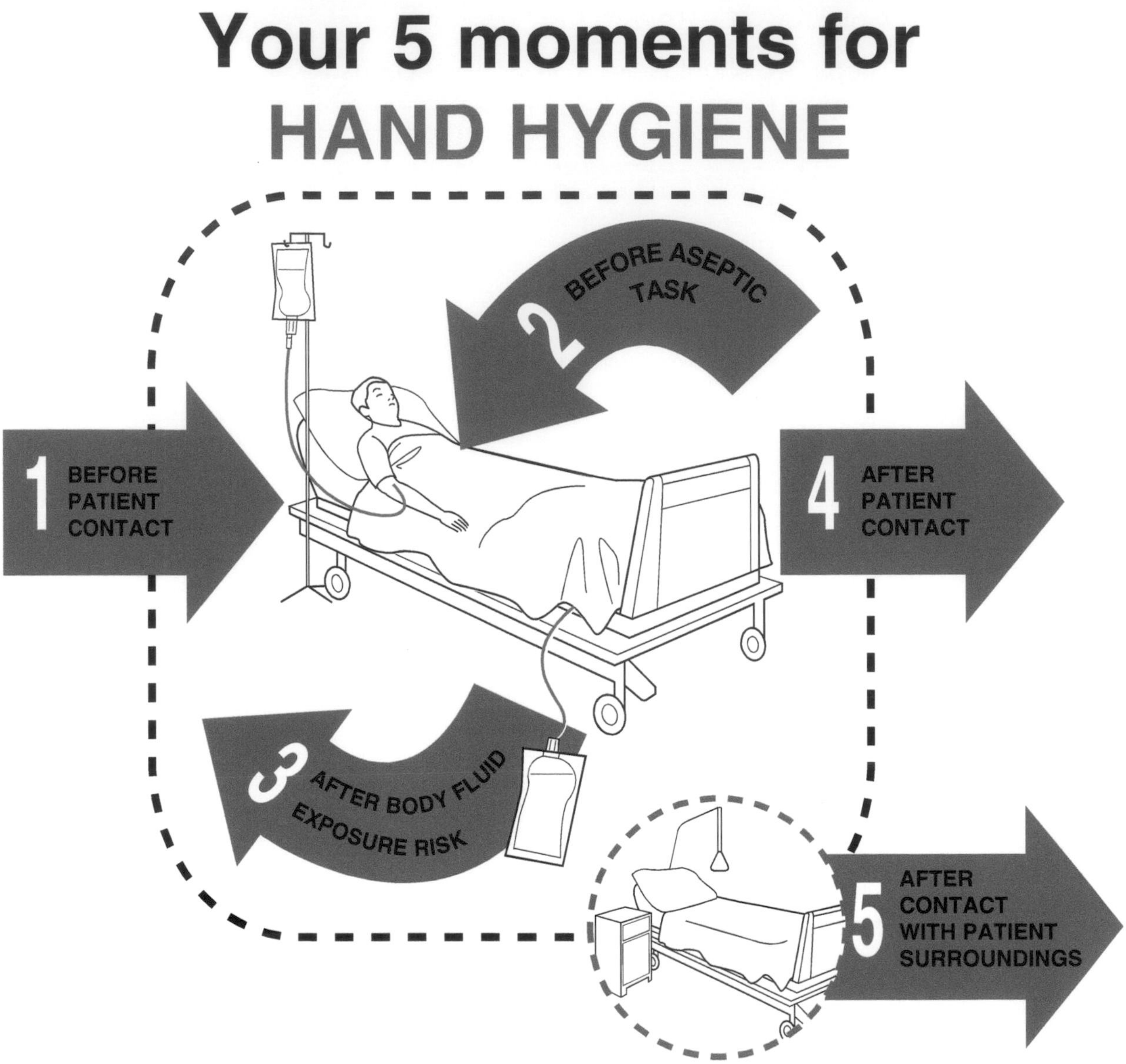

1 BEFORE PATIENT CONTACT	WHEN? Clean your hands before touching a patient when approaching them WHY? To protect the patient against harmful germs carried on your hands
2 BEFORE AN ASEPTIC TASK	WHEN? Clean your hands immediately before any aseptic task WHY? To protect the patient against harmful germs, including the patient's own germs, entering their body
3 AFTER BODY FLUID EXPOSURE RISK	WHEN? Clean your hands immediately after an exposure risk to body fluids (and after glove removal) WHY? To protect yourself and the health-care environment from harmful patient germs
4 AFTER PATIENT CONTACT	WHEN? Clean your hands after touching a patient and their immediate surroundings when leaving WHY? To protect yourself and the health-care environment from harmful patient germs
5 AFTER CONTACT WITH PATIENT SURROUNDINGS	WHEN? Clean your hands after touching any object or furniture in the patient's immediate surroundings, when leaving - even without touching the patient WHY? To protect yourself and the health-care environment from harmful patient germs

Figure 47.3 **The 5 moments when hand hygiene techniques must be performed to prevent onward transmission of potentially infectious pathogens.** *Source:* WHO Guidelines on Hand Hygiene in Health Care, WHO. © World Health Organization 2009.

Green Flag National Policy on Hand Hygiene in Healthcare

A recently published national policy document embeds evidence-based hand hygiene in practice. The Standard Infection Control Precautions for Hand Hygiene and Personal Protective Equipment Policy (NHS 2019) lays out the responsibilities of organisations, managers and staff regarding hand hygiene and personal protective equipment use:
https://improvement.nhs.uk/documents/4957/National_policy_on_hand_hygiene_and_PPE_2.pdf.

How Hand Hygiene Embedded in Policy and Practice

As noted throughout this chapter, the expectation upon employers and healthcare staff to comply with infection prevention and control measures that include hand hygiene is laid out in national policies (Department of Health 2008, NHS 2019). These policies include a requirement for employers to monitor and record healthcare staff compliance with hand hygiene techniques. This can take the form of a weekly hand hygiene audit, and nursing associates may be involved in completing these.

Supporting Evidence

Mody, et al. (2019) Multi-drug resistant organisms in hospitals: what is on patient hands and in their rooms?' Clinical Infectious Diseases.

Patient hand hygiene is often overlooked, but recent research from the United States suggests that supporting patients to decontaminate their hands is vital to the prevention and control of infection, particularly to prevent transfer of multi-drug resistant microorganisms such as MRSA. Researchers found that 29% of 'high touch areas' such as call-buttons and bedside trays were contaminated with MRSA (Mody et al. 2019). A summary of the article and a link to the article in full can be accessed here:
https://rcni.com/nursing-standard/newsroom/news/hand-hygiene-vital-patients-it-nurses-study-finds-148056

Conclusion

Hand hygiene techniques are vital to prevent nursing associates transferring potentially infectious microorganisms between patients or from the environment to a patient or between sites on patient's body. Effective hand hygiene techniques are systematic, and the nursing associates must ensure that each step of the hand hygiene process is undertaken on each occasion that hand hygiene is performed.

The ability to undertake consistent, effective hand hygiene techniques are key to fulfilling the requirements of the nursing associate proficiencies (NMC 2018a) and also to demonstrate compliance with national policy on infection prevention and control (NHS 2019). Routine hand hygiene should be undertaken using ABHRs. However, nursing associates are expected to demonstrate an evidence-based rationale regarding their choice of decontaminating agent (e.g. liquid soap and water or alcohol gel), for example, that ABHRs are not a safe method of hand decontamination when caring for a patient with diarrhoea or *C. difficile*.

References

Department of Health. (2008) *The health & social care act*, London: Department of Health.

Health Protection Scotland. (2019a) Appendix 2, Best practice: how to hand-rub, *National infection prevention and control manual*, NHS: National Services Scotland. [online] Available: http://www.nipcm.scot.nhs.uk/appendices/appendix-2-best-practice-how-to-hand-rub/ [accessed September 2020].

Health Protection Scotland. (2019b) Appendix 1, Best practice: how to hand wash, *National infection prevention and control manual*, NHS: National Services Scotland. [online] Available: http://www.nipcm.scot.nhs.uk/appendices/appendix-1-best-practice-how-to-hand-wash/ [accessed September 2020].

Loveday, H.P., Wilson, J.A., Pratt, R.J., Golsorkhi, M., Tingle, A., Bak, A., Browne, J., Prieto, J. and Wilcox, M. (2014) epic3: national evidence-based guidelines for preventing healthcare-associated infections in *NHS hospitals in England, Journal of Hospital Infection*, 86(S1): 1–70.

Mody, L., Washer, L.L., Kaye, K.S., Gibson, K., Saint, S., Reyes, K., Cassone, M., Mantey, J., Cao, J., Altamimi, S. and Perri, M. (2019) *Multi-drug resistant organisms in hospitals: what is on patient hands & in their rooms? Clinical Infectious Diseases*. [online] Available: https://doi.org/10.1093/cid/ciz092 [accessed September 2020].

NICE. (2016) *Healthcare-associated infections: quality standard QS113*, London: NICE. [online] Available: https://www.nice.org.uk/guidance/qs113 [accessed September 2020].

NHS. (2019) *Standard infection control precautions: national hand hygiene & personal protective equipment policy*, London: NHSE & NHSI.

Nursing & Midwifery Council (NMC). (2018a) *The standards of proficiency for nursing associates*, London: NMC

Nursing & Midwifery Council (NMC). (2018b) *The code: professional standards of practice and behaviour for nurses, midwives and nurse associates*, London: NMC.

World Health Organisation (WHO). (2008) *Your 5 moments for hand hygiene*, WHO. [online] Available: https://www.who.int/infection-prevention/campaigns/clean-hands/5moments/en/. Accessed September 2020.

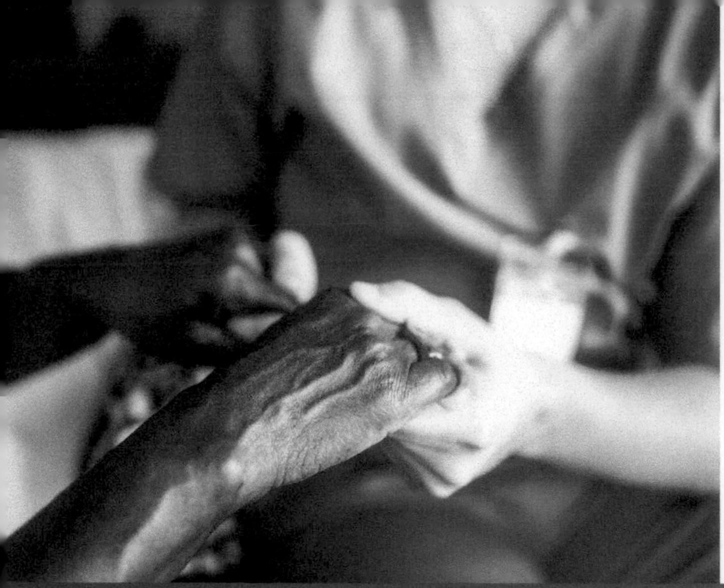

48

Decontaminating Equipment and the Environment

Daniel Soto-Prieto

Former Lecturer at University of East London, UK

Chapter Aim

- The aim of this chapter is to introduce the reader to the safe decontamination of equipment and the environment.

Learning Outcomes

By the end of this chapter, you should be able to:
- Explain the different levels of decontamination
- Describe the different methods and products for cleaning, disinfection, and sterilisation
- Identify the hazard pictograms, warning sentences, and information symbols in the product labels
- Describe the steps to undertake in case of blood or bodily fluids spillage

Test Yourself Multiple Choice Questions

1. What does antisepsis mean?
   A) The destruction or inhibition of pathogen microorganisms
   B) State of being free from bacteria and other living microorganisms
   C) Clinical approach to handle equipment avoiding touching key parts
2. What is the difference between antiseptics and disinfectants?
   A) Disinfectants destroy the majority of microorganisms and antiseptics destroy all microorganisms.
   B) Disinfectants are used to sanitise non-living objects or surfaces, and antiseptics are used to sanitise living tissues.
   C) Antiseptics are used to clean, and disinfectants are used to sterilise.

The Nursing Associate's Handbook of Clinical Skills, First Edition. Edited by Ian Peate.

Companion website: www.wiley.com/nursingassociate

3. How does hot water affect bleach action?
  - **A) Increase bleach action**
  - **B) Decrease bleach action**
  - **C) Does not affect bleach action**

4. This symbol can be found on some medical devices' packages. What does it mean? 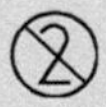
  - **A) Can be used twice only**
  - **B) Can be used once only**
  - **C) Can be used on a single patient, multiple times**

5. What does biocide mean?
  - **A) Destroy bacteria**
  - **B) Inhibit bacteria growth**
  - **C) Destroy only spores**

Introduction

A hygienic environment is vital for patient safety (Adams et al. 2008), a legal requirement (Department of Health 2015) and an ethical duty (Nursing and Midwifery Council (NMC) 2015). Nursing associates play a crucial role in protecting health and promoting hygiene through the decontamination of the spaces and equipment in contact with patients. Decontamination is the process of reducing the contamination to non-harmful levels and making objects and surfaces safe to use, which can be achieved by cleaning, disinfecting or sterilisation. Cleaning refers to the removal of dirt and consequently partial removal of microorganisms, disinfecting relates to the destruction of the majority of microorganisms or inhibition of their growth and sterilisation pertains to the destruction and elimination of all organisms, including resistant microbial forms such as spores (Parija 2012).

As a nursing associate, you are required to protect health and implement the principles of infection prevention and control. The Nursing and Midwifery Council (NMC) (2018) nursing associates proficiency standards specifically mention the duty of 'safely decontaminate equipment and environment' in its Section 8.7. Therefore, nursing associates are expected to demonstrate their proficiency in the decontamination of spaces and equipment as well as provide a rationale underpinned by evidence-based practice. The NMC (2015) Code requires all registrants to ensure public safety, and this requirement applies when ensuring that the public and others are safe with regard to the decontamination of equipment and the environment.

Take Note Glossary

Asepsis: Absence of microorganisms. Free of infection
Antisepsis: Destruction or inhibition of microorganisms using chemical agents
Bactericide: Destroy bacteria
Bacteriostatic: Inhibit or retard bacterial growth
Colonization: Presence, growth, and multiplication of microorganisms without clinical expression or immune response from the host
Contamination: Presence of potentially infectious agents before growth takes place
Infection: Presence, growth, and multiplication of potentially infectious microorganisms which causes immune response on the host

Supporting Evidence

Earl Spaulding (1957) classified medical equipment in relation to the risk of infection and established the levels of disinfection and sterilisation required prior to reutilisation in 1957. Over the years, this classification has been adapted to clinical practice in order to develop a methodological approach for decontamination purposes (World Health Organization (WHO) 2016).

The decontamination method chosen should be related to the risk of infection associated with a particular surface or equipment and in line with the local policies.

Table 48.1 Decontamination of reusable equipment.

RISK CATEGORY	RECOMMENDED LEVEL OF DECONTAMINATION	EXAMPLES
HIGH (critical items) Items that are involved with a break in the skin or mucous membrane or entering a sterile body cavity	Sterilisation	Surgical instruments, implants/prosthesis, rigid endoscopes, syringes, and needles
INTERMEDIATE (semi-critical items) Items in contact with mucous membranes or body fluids	Disinfection (high level)	Respiratory equipment, non-invasive flexible endoscopes, bedpans, and urine bottles
LOW (non-critical items) Items in contact with intact skin	Cleaning (visibly clean)	Blood pressure cuffs, stethoscopes, bedside table, and bed linen

Source: WHO (2016).

Table 48.2 Risk categories related to functional areas and required service levels.

RISK CATEGORY	FUNCTIONAL AREAS
Very high-risk functional areas	Such as operating theatres, intensive care units, emergency departments, departments where invasive procedures take place or immunosuppressed patients are cared for.
High-risk functional areas	Such as general wards, sterile services, and public toilets
Significant risks functional areas	Such as outpatient units, laboratory, and mortuary
Low-risk functional areas	Administrative areas, record stores, archives, and non-sterile supply areas

Source: Adapted from NPSA (2007).

Cleaning

Cleaning procedures aims to remove dirt and detritus and subsequentially microorganisms, decreasing the level of contaminants using mechanical (i.e. rubbing), physical (i.e. heat) or chemical (i.e. detergents) means.

The primary purpose of cleaning is to reduce the biological contamination for safe use, lessening the number of microorganisms present and preventing infection. Cleaning should be always conducted before disinfection and sterilisation, as these procedures cannot be effective on unclean objects.

The National Health Service (NHS) published the National Specifications for Cleanliness (National Patient Safety Agency (NPSA) 2007) which identify four risk categories which relate to the functional areas (see Table 48.2).

Cleaning Levels

In clinical practice, cleaning is often operationalised in three levels (Centers for Disease Control and Prevention (CDC) 2020) and normally undertaken in conjunction with domestic services as per local protocols:

- Routine cleaning: Comprise the daily basic cleaning and spot-cleaning using basic techniques.
- Terminal or discharge cleaning: Following the discharge of a patient who has been identified/suspected of being infected/colonised and in preparation for a new user.
- Deep cleaning: Thorough cleaning including all horizontal and vertical surfaces if required (walls, curtains, bed frame, and patient entertainment screens).

Cleaning Products

The equipment and materials used for cleaning include water, soap, detergents, enzymatic cleaners, brush, wipes, tissues, and scrubs scouring pads in combination with mechanical actions (friction or scrubbing).

Water

The chemical properties of water make it an excellent solvent where to dissolve many different substances.

Physical characteristics also influence its cleaning ability, such as temperature. For instance, lukewarm or warm water maximises the detergent enzyme's actions, while cold water is used with chloride-based products to prevent inactivation.

Enzymatic (Proteolytic) Cleaners

These substances contain enzymes (lipases, amylases or proteases) which break down different types of contamination. Enzymes facilitate cleaning process by accelerating chemical reactions, for example, protein stains. Enzymatic cleaners will degrade with latex gloves, so nitrile gloves are recommended instead (CDC 2020)

Detergents

Detergents are substances capable of dissolving dirt due to the following chemical properties:

- Dispersion: Breaks down the compact and solid dirt into smaller particles which can be easily eliminated
- Humectation: Reduces the attraction of water molecules so they can reach further areas
- Suspension: Wraps up and separates dirt particles which are removed away during washing out

There are different products for body hygiene, multi-surface cleaning, and dump dusting as well as detergents specially formulated for clinical equipment. Products intended for specific use cannot be utilised for a different purpose. Always select the detergent according to the use and technical specifications, and ensure that you are adhering to local policy and procedure. Also, detergents should not be mixed unless it is indicated.

Supporting Evidence

Poor or inadequate cleaning conditions might lead to contamination and transmission. Do you know how long microorganisms can remind viable on unclean surfaces? (Table 48.3)

Table 48.3 Microorganisms' survival time.

ORGANISM	SURVIVAL TIME
Meticillin-resistant *Staphylococcus aureus*	Up to 7 months
Acinetobacter	Up to 5 months
Clostridium difficile	Up to 5 months
Vancomycin-resistant *Enterococcus*	Up to 4 months
Escherichia coli	Up to 16 months
Klebsiella	Up to 30 months
Norovirus	Up to 7 days
SARS-CoV-2	Up to 4 days

Source: Dancer (2014) and Chin (2020).

General Principles of Cleaning

The list below gathers some of the most important and evidence-based (NPSA 2007; Provincial Infectious Diseases Advisory Committee 2018; CDC 2020) principles for effective and safe cleaning. This is not an exclusive list, as each case needs to be assessed in its own context and clinical environment.

- Clean daily or when visibly soiled.
- Clean from cleanest to dirtiest areas and from higher to lower, to prevent microorganisms contaminate areas already cleaned.
- Clean in a systematic and methodical manner to avoid missing areas.
- Use only designated equipment and follow local protocols.
- Use warm water (helps soften dirt) if it is compatible with manufacturer instructions, detergents, and surfaces to clean.
- Use fresh and disposable cloths and discard after use to avoid transmission.
- Follow manufacturer instructions regarding chemicals preparation, concentration, and contact time.
- Water or cleaning solutions may become contaminated or ineffective during cleaning procedures (organic material). Use fresh solutions for each use when it is visibly soiled or saturated.
- Clean heights within reach while standing on the floor. For higher surfaces or objects, contact domestic services or follow local protocol.
- Wear protective clothing: gloves, apron, gown, face masks, respirators, or eye protection if necessary.
- Rinse thoroughly with water to remove residues, if indicated.
- Dry thoroughly after cleaning using disposable towels.
- Decontaminate cleaning equipment after use.
- Where possible, use automated cleaning methods.

Cleaning Methods

Selecting a cleaning method for the environment (surfaces) or fomites (objects capable of carrying microorganisms) will be subject to the type of material or items to clean, and will follow the following principles (WHO 2016).

- *Manual cleaning* includes elements such as friction (i.e. rubbing, scrubbing) and fluidics (i.e. immersion or fluids under pressure) as well as other hand-operated methods (i.e. dry cleaning) to manually remove soil.
- *Mechanical cleaning* refers to the use of automatic devices such as washer-decontaminators which use pressure water, low intensity heat, etc., in combination with detergents or ultrasound cleaners (high-frequency ultrasonic waves transmitted in aqueous solutions to collide and break down dirt).

Disinfection

Disinfection is the action of sanitising surfaces, objects or tissues, destroying the majority of pathogenic microorganisms. It eradicates many microorganisms, but not all of them. Do not use disinfection as a substitute for cleaning. To be effective, cleaning must be performed before disinfection.

Box 48.1 Cleaning and Disinfecting Mattresses

Touch Point Cleaning and disinfecting mattresses

Although mattresses are considered as low-risk item, they might represent a substantial risk, given the close contact with patient skin and body fluids for long periods (Creamer & Humpreys 2008). Therefore, thorough cleaning and disinfection is required.

- Use hypochlorite solutions if approved by manufacturer to decontaminate mattress.
- Use chlorine 1000 ppm solution for regular decontamination or chlorine 10,000 ppm for blood-born microorganisms.
- Ensure mattress dries before storage to prevent moisture retention.

Table 48.4 Disinfection levels.

DISINFECTION	MICROORGANISMS ERADICATED			
	BACTERIA		VIRUS	FUNGI
	VEGETATIVE FORMS	SPORES		
Low intensity	Majority	–	Some	Some
Medium intensity	All	–	Majority	Majority
High intensity	All	Some	All	All

Source: Adapted from Parija (2012) and Rogers (2013).

Disinfection Levels

Disinfectants have different strength and effectiveness according to the capacity of eliminating microorganisms, which is classified in the Table 48.4.

Disinfection Methods

Disinfection can be carried out by physical (e.g. ultraviolet radiation or heat) or chemical means (e.g. disinfectants or antiseptics). Although the terms 'disinfectants' and 'antiseptics' are used interchangeably, disinfectants generally refer to the products used on inanimate objects (e.g. surfaces, equipment or machinery), whereas antiseptics usually relate to the products used on living organisms (e.g. skin or membranes).

Physical Methods

- Heat
  - Boiling: Objects are immersed in boiling water (Over 100°C) for a period of time. This inactivates the majority of pathogenic microorganisms; however, spores and some viruses can persist. Although it is an effective and affordable method, it is not recommended for thermolabile materials (subject to destruction by heat).
  - Moist-heat: This process takes place in an autoclave machine, which generates special conditions of temperature, steam and pressure up to 140°C breaking the microorganisms' membranes and denaturalising the protein structure. It is widely utilised in healthcare settings due to its process and control simplicity, extensive penetration and range, affordability, and absence of toxicity.
  - There are other forms of heat disinfection such as water steam (bedpan washers) and dry heat (ironing).
- Ultrasound: Produces high-speed vibrations (sound waves) which tear down bacteria's wall. It requires a designated device.
- Ultraviolet radiation: Requires a 'germicide lamp' that produces radiation (violet-coloured light). It can disinfect objects and air within short distances and superficially. This approach is commonly used in operating theatres and microbiology laboratories. The lamp requires periodic controls as efficacy decrease over time.

Chemical Methods

Disinfectants and antiseptic agents destroy or inactivate pathogenic microorganisms through denaturalisation of proteins and enzymes. This modifies the cytoplasmatic membrane (cell wall) which causes cellular oxidation and cell death. Table 48.5 provides an overview of agents used and their actions.

The chemical industry offers compounds for clinical practice which increase the sanitising effect without accruing disadvantages. Do not mix the product unless it is indicated otherwise, and always follow the manufacturer's specifications.

Table 48.5 Chemical agents and actions.

AGENT	ACTION	CHARACTERISTICS	SAMPLE
Alcohols	Disinfectant and antiseptic Bactericide	Water-soluble Medium intensity For surfaces and equipment disinfection	Ethyl and isopropyl alcohol
Aldehydes	Disinfectants	High intensity Very toxic Irritate skin and membranes Carcinogenic	Formaldehyde, glutaraldehyde
Oxidising agents	Disinfectants and antiseptics Biocide	Inactivate with organic substances, light or air Limited toxicity Short effect	Peroxide (used as liquid or gas)
Chlorine based	Disinfectants Wide biocide spectrum	Corrosive and irritating Use always diluted and with cold water	Sodium hypochlorite (bleach), chloramines
Chlorhexidine	Disinfectant and antiseptic Bactericide and fungicide	Safe and cost-effective. Ototoxic	Chlorhexidine, chlorhexidine gluconate
Iodine based	Disinfectant and antiseptic Effective germicide	Dilute with water, soap or alcohol solutions Do not mix with mercury, peroxide, and silver solutions	Povidone-iodine Alcohol-iodine
Mercury derivates	Antiseptic Bacteriostatic Effective against bacteria and some fungi	Very toxic Do not mix with iodine solutions	Thiomersal, merbromin
Cationic derivative forms quaternary ammonium	Disinfectants Bactericide and fungicide	Low activity against virus and spores Ineffective to tuberculosis bacillus	Cetrimide, benzalkonium chloride

Source: Adapted from WHO (2016) and Parija (2012).

Box 48.2 Managing Blood and Bodily Fluids Spillages

Touch Point

Any spillage of blood or body fluids is a potential infection hazard and must be dealt with promptly, safely, and appropriately to avoid contamination and infection. Priority must be given to the safe removal of the spillage rather than chemical inactivation.

In terms of infection control, body fluids are defined as 'any fluid found in, produced by or excreted from the human body which includes blood, urine, faeces, saliva, tears, breast milk cerebrospinal fluid (CSF), semen, vaginal fluid, amniotic fluid, pleural fluid, peritoneal fluid, bile, digestive juices, vomit, and pus, as they may contain infectious microorganisms' (Peate 2008)

Basic principles when dealing with blood or body fluids spillage

1. Wear appropriate personal protective equipment (PPE)
2. Identify (hazard sign) and contain the spillage (absorbent towels, cloths, granules) so it will solidify and not spread
3. Disinfect using biohazard designated kit or chlorine-based disinfectants, according to local protocol. Do not use chlorine-based disinfectants on urine spillages as it may release hazardous gases.
4. Clean thoroughly with detergent and lukewarm water
5. Safely collect and dispose all materials in adequate container (i.e. biohazard box, yellow bag)

The NHS Education for Scotland has produced an animation which explains the national policy and algorithm for the safe management of clinical spillages here, https://youtu.be/zec7CvWB7Us

Source: Adapted from National Patient Safety Agency (2009) and CDC (2020).

Red Flag

Cleaning and disinfecting in COVID-19 context

The Severe Acute Respiratory Syndrome Coronavirus-2 (SARS-CoV-2) is a strain of coronavirus responsible for the COVID-19 global pandemic (WHO 2020).

To date, the COVID-19 disease is transmitted with physical contact of respiratory droplets or some specific aerosol-generating medical procedures. COVID-19 transmission due to contact with environmental surfaces is still under investigation, although there is evidence of surface transmission with other coronavirus strains (Cheng et al. 2020). Studies have also suggested that SARS-CoV-2 can remain viable on surfaces such as cloth for 1 day, glass for 2 days, and metals/plastics for 3–4 days (Chin et al. 2020; van Doremalen 2020).

Although more research is needed to clarify the mechanisms of surface transmission, cleaning, and disinfecting are essential to maintain infection prevention and control standards and therefore reduce the spread of the virus. This is especially important since the SARS-CoV-2's, enveloped structure, is more vulnerable to disinfectants than other non-enveloped viruses such a rotavirus or norovirus (WHO 2020).

Cleaning: Follow the general cleaning principles as described in the cleaning section. Ensure that local policies are always followed and use PPE. It is important to use exclusive and designated equipment for COVID isolation areas which will be discarded according to local procedure.

Disinfecting: Disinfecting must take place after cleaning. Use disinfectants that have been proved effective against the coronavirus and other healthcare-associated pathogens

- Chlorine-based products at 0.1% (1000 ppm) for general purposes or minimum of 0.5% (5000 ppm) in case of body fluids or blood spills.
- Ethanol 70–90%
- Hydrogen peroxide ≥0.5%

Box 48.3 Decontamination further reading

Supporting Evidence

Decontamination (further reading)

- 2020: CDC and ICAN. Best practices for environmental cleaning in healthcare facilities in resource-limited settings. Atlanta, GA: US Department of Health and Human Services CDC, Cape Town, South Africa: Infection Control Africa Network; 2019. Available at https://www.cdc.gov/hai/prevent/resource-limited/index.html
- 2016 Decontamination of surgical instruments https://www.gov.uk/government/publications/management-and-decontamination-of-surgical-instruments-used-in-acute-care
- 2016 Decontamination of flexibles endoscopes https://www.gov.uk/government/publications/management-and-decontamination-of-flexible-endoscopes
- 2013 Decontamination in primary care dental practices https://www.gov.uk/government/publications/decontamination-in-primary-care-dental-practices

Sterilisation

Sterilisation is the process that destroys all living forms from an object. It represents the highest-level of sanitation as it eradicates both pathogen and non-pathogen microorganisms, including resistant forms or spores. Due to the nature of this process, sterilisation can only be applied to inanimate objects and not to living tissues. According to the WHO (2016), any medical device in contact with body tissues, fluids, or cavities (critical items) should be completely free of microorganisms, and therefore sterilised to avoid infection.

Sterilisation Methods

Sterilisation can be achieved by physical, chemical, or a combination of both means.

Physical Methods

These methods deliver some form of physical energy (i.e. radiant, thermal) to interrupt the normal development of microorganisms, causing their destruction (Parija 2012) (WHO 2016).

- *Dry heat*: Provided by high-temperature (160°C and above) ovens such as Pasteur's or Poupinel's ovens. Used to sterilise thermoresistant material such as glass, ceramic, or metallic objects. Also useful to sterilise powder and oleic substances. Dry heat does nor rust metal equipment.
- *Direct heat*
  - *Incineration*: Complete combustion to ashes using furnaces. Commonly used to destroy biohazard waste materials.
  - *Flaming*: Direct contact with flames. Very common in laboratories to sterilise equipment on-the-spot.
- *Steam*: Takes place in autoclave machines. Objects are packaged or wrapped with an auto-seal material activated when the temperature increases, preserving sterile conditions inside. Commonly used in clinical practice; affordable, quick, and safe.
- *Filters*: Use microporous materials to retain and remove small particles. Filters do not destroy microorganisms, only separate them. Its capacity will depend on the size of the porous materials. Very common to sterilise gaseous or liquid substances.

- *Radiation*
  - *Gamma radiation*: Achieves complete sterilisation under cold conditions. Commonly used to sterilise medical equipment in industrial facilities. Expensive.
  - *Ultraviolet* (UV): Commonly used to sterilise air in enclosed areas. Low efficacy.
  - *Ultrasound*: Produces high-speed vibrations (sound waves) in water or decontamination solutions, which damages and kill microorganisms.

Take Note Autoclave

The autoclave is an airtight, controlled chamber which regulates both high temperatures and high pressures. It is widely used in clinical settings to sterilise equipment due to its simplicity and cost-effectiveness. The autoclave heats distilled water, which increases pressure and temperature to boiling point. Sterilising action takes place when water steam reaches 121–144°C. The autoclave can be used for rubber, cloth, glass, and metal. Objects must be spread out, so that steam can circulate among them. Equipment must be adequately prepacked before sterilisation to protect and preserve the content once sterilised.

Chemical Methods

These methods are based on the chemical action of some elements on microorganisms. Chemical methods are appropriate for objects that cannot withstand high temperatures.

- *Ethylene oxide*: High antimicrobial activity and penetration. Commonly used for thermolabile. Ethylene oxide is toxic and flammable. The objects sterilised using this substance require ventilation to remove the excess.
- *Plasma gas*: Uses hydrogen peroxide vapour, which transforms into plasma at low temperatures. Appropriate for low-temperature sterilisation. It cannot be used with cloth, cellulose, powder, or liquids, which limits its application. Require polypropylene packaging. Quick procedure. Does not require ventilation.
- Ozone only or hydrogen peroxide and ozone gas: Great antimicrobial action. Uses oxygen chemical properties to decontaminate a wide range of materials used in clinical practice. No emission, and low operating temperature.
- *Formaldehyde gas*: Low operating temperature; however, toxic and probably cardiogenetic. Commonly used for haemodialysis equipment.

Take Note Medical Devices Package Symbols

As a healthcare worker, you will use medical equipment and devices whose package could be marked with some of the following symbols. Knowing the symbols is key to understanding how to safely use equipment, and to protect patients and yourself (Table 48.6).

Sterilisation Control Tests

Control tests are elements that verify the appropriate and effective sterilisation process.

- Physical tests: Verify sterilisation parameters and confirm the correct functioning order to the sterilisation – for instance, thermometers or timers.
- Chemical tests are substances which react and verify sterile conditions during the procedure. For instance, striped tapes (which demonstrate whether a specific temperature has been reached), Bowie–Dick test (vacuum pump control).
- Biological tests: Safest indicators to verify that an object has been sterilised. For instance, a vial with a sterilisation-resistant agent which is cultivated after sterilisation to confirm whether there is some abnormal growth.

Take Note COSHH Products

Many chemicals used to clean, disinfect, or sterilise are categorized under the Control of Substances Hazardous to Health (COSHH) Regulations. COSHH products are labelled with pictograms or warning sentences to provide information about the dangers or hazardous effects they may cause and preventing measures (European Chemical Agency 2008). In 2015, the Classification, Labelling and Packaging (CLP) Regulation (European Chemical Agency 2015) modified the old orange symbols for the new square red and black, unifying globally the identification system (Table 48.7).

Table 48.6 Medical devices and package symbols.

SYMBOL	MEANING
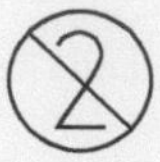	Do not reuse To be used on an individual patient, on a single procedure, and then discarded. Use only once
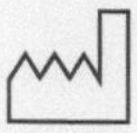	Date of manufacture Date a product has been manufactured. It will include a date
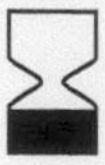	Use-by date Date the product is no longer safe to use. It will include a date
	Caution Special attention or awareness needed to avoid damage. See instructions for use
	Biological risks Biological hazard substance
SN	Serial number Indicates manufacturer's serial number identification. It will include alphanumeric characters
LOT	Batch code Indicates manufacturer's batch code identification. It will include alphanumeric characters
STERILE	Sterile Indicates sterile condition. Additional letters or symbols will indicate the method used to sterilise (i.e. radiation, heat, or ethylene oxide)
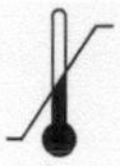	Temperature limit. It will include temperature values

Source: International Organization for Standardization (ISO) (2016).

Table 48.7 Warnings and Pictograms adapted from Health and Safety Executive.

WARNINGS		
	Hazard statements	That is, toxic if swallowed; causes severe eye damage
	Precautionary statements	That is, wear eye protection; avoid release to the environment
	Signal words	That is, warning; danger
PICTOGRAMS	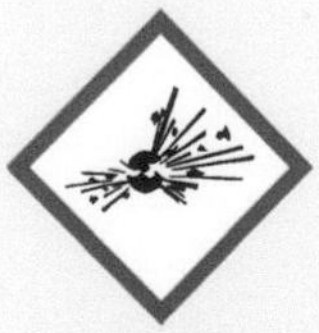	Explosive (symbol: exploding bomb)
		Flammable (symbol: flame)
		Oxidising (symbol: flame over circle)

(Continued)

Table 48.7 (Continued)

 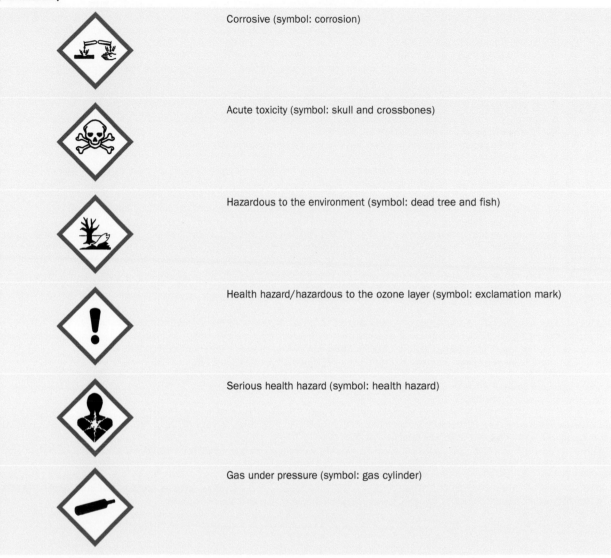	Corrosive (symbol: corrosion)
	Acute toxicity (symbol: skull and crossbones)
	Hazardous to the environment (symbol: dead tree and fish)
	Health hazard/hazardous to the ozone layer (symbol: exclamation mark)
	Serious health hazard (symbol: health hazard)
	Gas under pressure (symbol: gas cylinder)

Source: Health and Safety Executive (no date).

Conclusion

This chapter has introduced the reader to the principles of equipment and environment decontamination. This will provide nursing associates with the basic knowledge necessary to underpin clinical practice. Decontamination techniques are in constant evolution, so you might refer to a specialist for further information.

The decontamination method should be selected according to the risk of infection associated with a particular surface or equipment and in line with local policies. Special situations (accidental spillage or mattress sanitation) may require a higher level of decontamination.

Chemical substances might react in the presence of other substances. Use them only for the intended use, and do not mix them unless stated otherwise in the manufacturer specifications.

Medical equipment is marked with symbols which provide important information about usage requirements. COSHH products are marked with pictograms and warning sentences which provide information about the associated risks and preventing measures necessary when dealing with them.

References

Adams, J., Bartram, J., Chartier, Y. (Eds.). (2008) *Essential Environmental Health Standards in Health Care*. World Health Organization. [online] Available: https://apps.who.int/iris/bitstream/handle/10665/43767/9789241547239_eng.pdf?sequence=1. Accessed November 2019.

Centers for Disease Control and Prevention. (2020) *Best Practices for Environmental Cleaning in Healthcare Facilities in Resource-Limited Settings.* [online] Available: https://www.cdc.gov/hai/pdfs/resource-limited/environmental-cleaning-RLS-H.pdf. Accessed September 2020.

Cheng, V.C.C., Wong, S.-C., Chen, J.H.K., Yip, C.C.Y., Chuang, V.W.M., Tsang, O.T.Y., et al. (2020) Escalating infection control response to the rapidly evolving epidemiology of the coronavirus disease 2019 (COVID-19) due to SARS-CoV-2 in Hong Kong. *Infection Control & Hospital Epidemiology*, 41: 493–498.

Chin, A.W.H., Chu, J.T.S., Perera, M.R.A., Hui, K.P.Y., Yen, H.-L., Chan, M.C.W., et al. (2020) Stability of SARS-CoV-2 in different environmental conditions. *The Lancet Microbe.* [Accessed September 2020].

Creamer, E., Humphreys, H. (2008) The contribution of beds to healthcare-associated infection: the importance of adequate decontamination. *Journal of Hospital Infection*, 69(1): 8–23.

European Chemical Agency. (2008) Guidance on the application of the CLP criteria. Guidance to Regulation (EC) No. 1272/2008 on classification, labelling and packaging (CLP) of substances and mixtures.

European Chemical Agency. (2015) Guidance on the application of the CLP criteria. Guidance to Regulation (EC) No 1272/2008 on classification, labelling and packaging (CLP) of substances and mixtures. *Version* 4.1, June 2015.

Dancer, S.J. (2014). Controlling hospital-acquired infection: focus on the role of the environment and new technologies for decontamination. *Clinical Microbiology Reviews*, 27(4): 665–690.

Department of Health. (2015) *The Health and Social Care Act 2008: Code of Practice on the prevention and control of infections*, London. [online] Available: https://assets.publishing.service.gov.uk/government/uploads/system/uploads/attachment_data/file/449049/Code_of_practice_280715_acc.pdf. Accessed November 2019.

Health and Safety Executive [no date] [online] Available: https://www.hse.gov.uk/chemical-classification/labelling-packaging/index.html. Accessed November 2019.

International Organization for Standardization. Standard ISO 15223-1:2016(en) Medical devices - Symbols to be used with medical device labels, labelling and information to be supplied - Part 1: General requirements. Available from https://www.iso.org/standard/69081.html. Accessed November 2019.

National Patient Safety Agency. (2007) *The National Specifications for Cleanliness in the NHS: A Framework for Setting and Measuring Performance Outcomes.*

National Patient Safety Agency. (2009) *The Revised Healthcare Leaning Manual.* [online] Available: https://www.ahcp.co.uk/wp-content/uploads/NRLS-0949-Healthcare-clea-ng-manual-2009-06-v1.pdf. Accessed September 2020.

Nursing and Midwifery Council. (2015) *The Code.* [online] Available: https://www.nmc.org.uk/globalassets/sitedocuments/nmc-publications/nmc-code.pdf. Accessed November 2019.

Nursing and Midwifery Council. (2018). *Professional Standards of Practice and Behaviour for Nurses, Midwives and Nursing Associates.* [online] Available: https://www.nmc.org.uk/globalassets/sitedocuments/education-standards/nursing-associates-proficiency-standards.pdf. Accessed November 2019.

Parija, S.C. (2012). *Textbook of Microbiology and Immunology.* Elsevier (A division of Reed Elsevier India Private Limited).

Peate, I. (2008) Body fluids part 1: infection control. *British Journal of Healthcare Assistants*, 2: 6–10.

Rogers, W.J. (2013) *Healthcare Sterilisation: Introduction & Standard Practices* (Vol. 1). Smithers Rapra.

Provincial Infectious Diseases Advisory Committee. (2018) *Best Practices for Environmental Cleaning for Prevention and Control of Infections in All Health Care Settings*, 3rd Edition. Public Health Ontario.

Spaulding, E.H. (1957) Chemical disinfection and antisepsis in the hospital. *Journal of Hospital Research*, 9: 5–31.

van Doremalen, N., Bushmaker, T., Morris, D.H., Holbrook, M.G., Gamble, A., Williamson, B.N., et al. (2020) Aerosol and surface stability of SARS-CoV-2 as compared with SARS-CoV-1. *The New England Journal of Medicine*, 382: 1564–1567.

World Health Organization. (2016) *Decontamination and Reprocessing of Medical Devices for Health-care Facilities.* [online] Available: https://apps.who.int/iris/bitstream/handle/10665/250232/9789241549851-eng.pdf. Accessed November 2019.

World Health Organization. (2020). *Cleaning and disinfection of environmental surfaces in the context of COVID-19: interim guidance, 15 May 2020* (No. WHO/2019-nCoV/Disinfection/2020.1). World Health Organization. [online] Available: https://apps.who.int/iris/bitstream/handle/10665/332096/WHO-2019-nCoV-Disinfection-2020.1-eng.pdf?sequence=1&isAllowed=y. Accessed September 2020.

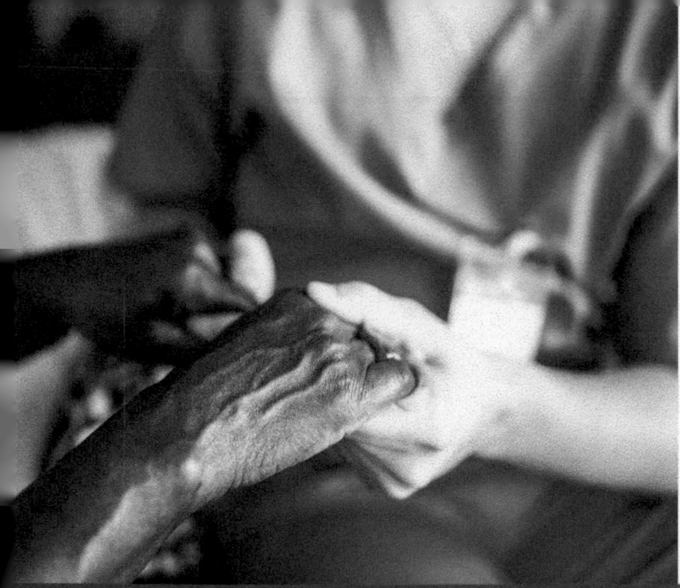

49

Safely Handling Waste, Laundry and Sharps

Nigel Davies

University of East London, UK

Chapter Aim

- This chapter discusses how to handle waste, laundry and sharps to ensure there is no infection risk for patients, yourself or your colleagues.

Learning Outcomes

- Outline the universal colour-code system used in healthcare environments to separate different types of waste
- Discuss how sharps should be handled and disposed of safely
- Describe how patients' linen and clothing should be handled and how your own uniform should be washed

Test Yourself Multiple Choice Questions

1. Which of the following is NOT one of the three broad categories which define clinical waste?
   A) Healthcare waste which poses a risk of infection
   B) Healthcare waste with a chemical hazard
   C) Medicines and medicinally contaminated waste
   D) General waste from a general practice surgery
2. What colour lid should a sharps box have in which you dispose of needles and empty syringes?
   A) Orange lid
   B) Blue lid
   C) Purple lid
   D) Red lid

The Nursing Associate's Handbook of Clinical Skills, First Edition. Edited by Ian Peate.

Companion website: www.wiley.com/nursingassociate

3. **Which colour bag would you dispose of paper hand towels in?**
   A) Yellow
   B) Blue
   C) Clear
   D) Black
4. **An oxygen mask should be considered a:**
   A) Single-use item
   B) Single-patient use item
   C) Reusable item
   D) Disposable item
5. **COSHH is the abbreviation for regulations which are concerned with safe handling of materials and waste. What does COSHH stand for?**
   A) Committee on Safety and Health Hazards
   B) Control of Secure Health Hazards
   C) Control of Substances Hazardous to Health
   D) Community of Safety for Human Health

Introduction

As a nursing associate, you have a key responsibility to ensure the correct management of waste to ensure that healthcare activities do not pose a risk or potential risk of infection to the public. There are systems in place in all healthcare environments which you must learn and follow to protect yourself, your colleagues and your patients. It is also important to recognise that this duty of care goes beyond your immediate environment, as other support workers and the public could come into contact with waste at a later stage. This responsibility is recognised in the proficiencies for nursing associates laid out by the Nursing and Midwifery Council (NMC 2018).

Green Flag

There are legal requirements concerning how waste is disposed. There has also been increased emphasis recently to consider best practice to minimise and segregate different types of waste to achieve more effective disposal by reducing the environmental and carbon impact by cutting back on incineration, landfill (Department of Health 2013) and plastic usage.

The legal requirements around healthcare waste are complex and derived from national and European laws. An important aspect of this is the Control of Substances Hazardous to Health (COSHH) regulations (Health and Safety Executive no date) which in different forms have existed for some time to safeguard staff and the public. You are likely to see posters and guidelines which reference COSHH regulations.

Clinical waste is defined as:

. . . any waste which consists wholly or partly of human or animal tissue, blood or other body fluids, excretions, drugs or other pharmaceutical products, swabs or dressings, syringes, needles or other sharp instruments . . . and any other waste arising from medical, nursing or similar practice being waste which may cause infection to any person coming into contact with it (Department of Health 2013, p. 22).

Colour-Code System

There is now a universal colour-code system in use across UK healthcare services for the segregation and disposal of waste (Department of Health 2013). This means different types of waste are allocated different colours to make management of different waste items easier and more efficient. The colour code is applied from the point waste is generated, for example, the bins and containers used at the bedside or in a clinic room, then during storage, transportation and disposal. Figure 49.1 provides an overview of the main categories you will see in general healthcare settings.

Touch Point

Clinical waste can be divided into three broad groups of materials:

a. Healthcare waste which poses a risk of infection
b. Healthcare waste which poses a chemical hazard
c. Medicines and medicinally contaminated waste

You need to be familiar with the colour-code system for waste disposal to ensure all waste is handled safety. This is to protect yourself and others.

Waste type	Classification	Colour coding	Description & disposal method
Infectious	Hazardous	YELLOW	Infectious waste for disposal by incineration
Infectious	Hazardous	ORANGE	Infectious waste for disposal by treatment or incineration
Cytotoxic/ Cytostatic	Hazardous	PURPLE	Containing cytotoxic waste for disposal by incineration
Offensive	Non-hazardous	YELLOW & BLACK	Offensive/hygiene waste for disposal by deep landfill
Anatomical	Hazardous	RED	Anatomical waste for disposal by incineration
Medicinal	Non-hazardous	BLUE	Medicinal waste for disposal by incineration
Dental	Hazardous	WHITE	Dental amalgam for recovery or recycling
Domestic	Non-hazardous	BLACK	General domestic for landfill
		CLEAR	Domestic recycling

Figure 49.1 Colour-code system for healthcare waste disposal.

Single-Use Devices

One approach to control infection is the single use of some devices. This refers to a medical device that is intended to be used on an individual patient during a single procedure and then disposed of. Medical devices that are for single use are labelled with the words 'do not reuse' or display the symbol shown in Figure 49.2. Other items may be for single-patient use; in contrast, this refers to a device that may be used more than once but only on one patient, for example, a nebuliser. In some cases where infection is known or anticipated, items such as blood pressure monitoring devices, which can usually be used between patients need to be deemed single-patient use to prevent cross-contamination.

Red Flag

Single-use devices must not be decontaminated and reused as this can affect their safety and effectiveness which may expose patients and staff to unnecessary risks.

Single-use medical devices

MHRA
Regulating Medicines and Medical Devices

How do I know if a device is for single-use?

It will have this symbol on the packaging or the device:

What does single-use mean?

Do not reuse. A single-use device is used on an individual patient during a single procedure and then discarded. It is not intended to be reprocessed and used again, even on the same patient.

Is single-patient use the same as single-use?

No. Single-patient use means the medical device may be used for more than one episode of use on **one patient only**; the device may undergo some form of **reprocessing** between each use.

Why shouldn't they be reused?

The MHRA is aware of serious incidents relating to reuse of single-use devices.

Reuse can be unsafe because of risk of:

- cross-infection — inability to clean and decontaminate due to design.
- endotoxin reaction — excessive bacterial breakdown products, which cannot be adequately removed by cleaning.
- patient injury — device failure from reprocessing or reuse because of fatigue, material alteration and embrittlement.
- chemical burns or sensitisation — residues from chemical decontamination agents on materials that can absorb/adsorb chemicals.

Also, if you reuse a single-use device, you may be legallyliable for the safe performance of the device.

Can I sterilise a single-use device?

A few single-use devices are marketed as non-sterile. These may require processing, in line with the manufacturer's instructions, to make them sterile and ready for use. You must not resterilise them.

Figure 49.2 Single-use medical devices. *Source*: MHRA (2013). © Crown copyright, except single-use symbol, reproduced with permission from: BSI www.bsigroup.com.

Supporting Evidence

The Medicines and Healthcare Products Regulatory Agency (MHRA) explains the consequences of using items more than once including an example of where a single-use bladder pressure transducer cover was not changed between patients, resulting in a *Pseudomonas* cross-infection where one patient developed septicaemia and died from a sub-arachnoid haemorrhage (MHRA 2013).

In another example, the MHRA points out that mechanical failure can also occur. In this case, a lithotripter kidney stone retrieval basket was incorrectly reused with the effects of re-decontamination thought to have caused a cable to snap leaving a device inside a patient who then required further surgery to retrieve it.

Take Note

Sometimes, healthcare practitioners break single-use only rules unwittingly. Care and attention should be applied in the following circumstances to ensure items intended for single-use are not re-used.

- Reusing a needle or especially a syringe to give medicine to more than one patient, e.g. when multiple immunisations like the 'flu vaccination' are given in general practice settings.
- Reusing a needle or syringe to withdraw medicine from a vial that is used for more than one patient, e.g. psychiatric medication, vaccines or local anaesthetic.
- Using multiple-dose vials for the same patient for longer than the manufacturer recommends once the seal is broken.
- Using fluid infusion and administration sets (i.e. tubing and connectors) for multiple infusions.
- Using blood glucose monitoring devices for more than one patient. Finger-stick retractable lancet devices are single-patient use items.
- Earpieces on auroscope or digital thermometers.
- Ensuring gloves and plastic aprons are used as single-use items.

Handling and Disposal of Sharps

Sharps refer to items such as needles, syringes, scalpel blades and stitch cutters, which if mishandled have a risk of causing blood-borne infection. Needles must not be re-sheathed or re-capped after use, and all sharps should be placed immediately in puncture-resistant containers ('sharps-bins') by the original person using the 'sharp' not left for others to clear away (National Clinical Guideline Group 2012).

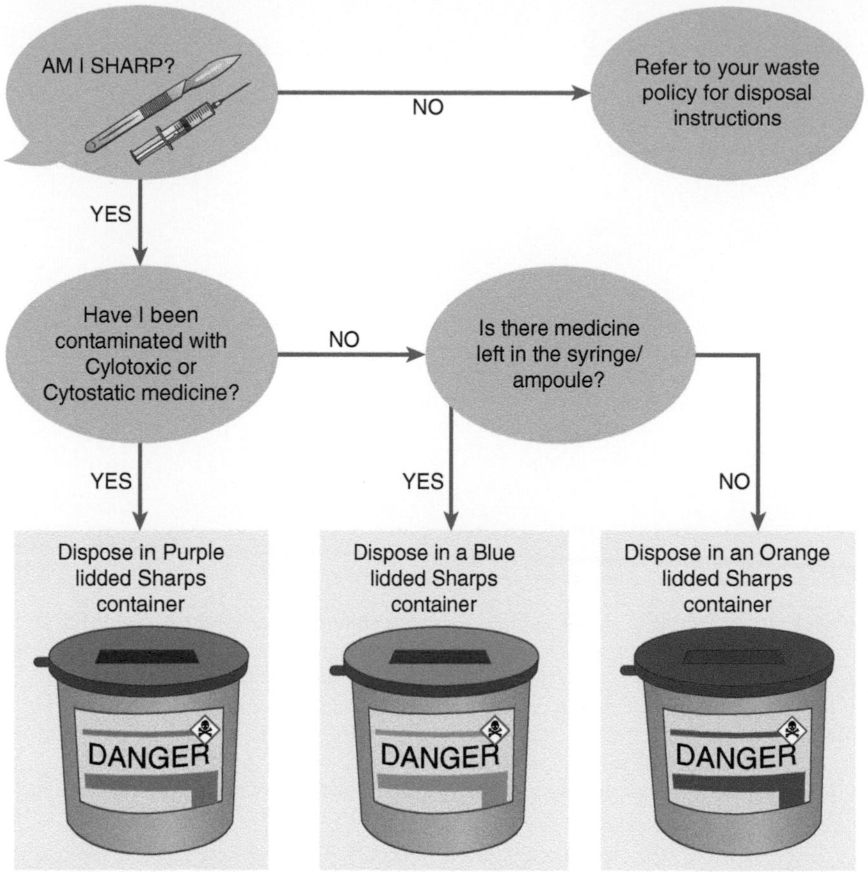

Figure 49.3 **Sharps disposal.**

The right size sharps containers should be selected depending on the anticipated use, and whenever possible, small sharps boxes should be taken to the bedside or point of care. They should be stored away from public areas and out of the reach of children or other vulnerable patients. They should not be overfilled and should be sent for disposal when the 'fill-line' is reached. The container must be labelled to conform with your organisation's traceability policy, and lids should be put on securely (National Clinical Guideline Group 2012). Boxes are generally yellow, but they follow the colour-code system depending on their content (see Figure 49.3).

Avoid unnecessary use of sharps by only using sharps when needed and use needle-free equipment if available. Manufacturers have attempted in recent years to devise new equipment which can help reduce the risk, for example, shields that slide to cover the needed after use. Where traditional-style needles are used, you should avoid recapping the needle after use. In some cases, a risk assessment may have been made that re-capping is preferable, but in these cases, a devise such as a needle-block to remove and hold the needle cap and allow safe one-handled recapping should be used (CQC 2019).

Some people may self-handle sharps, for example, people with diabetes who monitor their own blood glucose levels or administer their own insulin. In these cases, you should ensure they have the correct advice for disposal at home (via their local authority) with sharps boxes provided on prescription through their local pharmacy. If patients who self-administer are admitted to a care setting, you should ensure a risk assessment is completed including the use, safe storage and disposal of their sharps. This will need to take account of other patients in the vicinity, e.g. adjacent beds, as well as the individual patient's needs.

Touch Point

Handling sharps is an 'every-day' occurrence for many healthcare professionals. You should endeavour to follow the guidelines and make these as routine as possible as this will reduce the likelihood of receiving a 'needle-stick injury'. Having sharps boxes which you can take as close to the place where care is being delivered, and the sharp device used is recommended.

Avoiding the use of sharps, when at all possible, is advised especially if needle-free equipment is available. Consideration should also be given to the safety issues of storage, use and disposal of sharps if patients self-handle sharps.

Laundry

As with other waste, there are infection prevention and control implications of dealing with patients' laundry including bed linen and clothing. In hospitals, patients frequently wear hospital gowns or nightwear, and, therefore, any soiled items can be handled alongside bed linen. Linen bags also follow the colour-code system ensuring that soiled and infected linen is handled separately to standard or socially unclean linen and sent to an industrial laundry.

Yellow Flag

Promoting patients' dignity and self-respect by encouraging and enabling people to wear their own clothing has for many years been standard in long-term care but is also increasingly being seen in hospitals (see the "End PJ Paralysis" campaign: https://endpjparalysis.org/). This increases complexity with regard to laundry arrangements, especially if patients are incontinent and clothes are soiled. Family members will often be involved in the laundry arrangements, and this may provide an important involvement for them in the patient's care (Armstrong & Day 2017). Care and sensitivity need to be shown to families in the way soiled items are exchanged and information given if necessary to prevent cross-contamination.

Washing Your Own Uniform

You should be aware of the infection control implications of washing your own uniforms to ensure that you do not cross-contaminate other items of your clothing and that uniforms are clean for future use. It is recommended that uniforms are washed with a detergent at a temperature of 60˚C for at least 10 minutes (Department of Health 2010; Royal College of Nursing 2013) and that uniforms are subsequently ironed as a further infection minimisation measure. If you are not required to wear a uniform, for example, on mental health placements or in many sexual health clinics, then you should check local guidance about the suitability of the clothes you wear for clinical work and consider whether you are able to wash clothes at the correct temperature. As with standard precautions (see chapter 43), the answer lies in a multifaceted approach to minimise infection transmission, which includes clean uniforms/suitable clothes together with the use of PPE (Chapter 44) and good hand hygiene (Chapter 47).

Supporting Evidence

Riley et al. (2017) showed that most microorganisms are removed at 40°C, whereas all were at 60˚C, and therefore recommended that nurses launder their uniforms at 60°C to ensure safe removal of microorganisms. Riley et al. (2015, 2017) also determined that between a third and a half of staff questioned said they launder their uniforms below the recommended temperature which could potentially result in transmission of hospital-acquired infections. However, Loveday et al. (2007) consider that guidelines often differ and concluded that there is no good evidence to suggest uniforms are a significant risk of cross infection, that home laundering is inferior to commercial processing of uniforms or that it presents a hazard in terms of cross-contamination of other items in the wash-load. Furthermore, regardless of how or where uniforms are washed, bacterial recontamination can occur within hours of being re-worn.

Conclusion

Any waste containing human tissue, blood, other body fluids or excretions is considered clinical waste. Clinical waste can either pose a risk of infection, a chemical hazard or be medicines or items that are medically contaminated.

As a nursing associate, you should be familiar with the colour-code system for waste disposal to ensure all waste is handled safety. Consideration must also be given to the safety issues of storage, use and disposal of sharps for both your own practice and for patients who self-administer medicines.

Sharps guidelines should always be followed to prevent needle-stick injuries and where possible avoiding the use of sharps is recommended. The nursing associate must familiarise themselves with local policy and procedure regarding sharps injuries.

Handling bed linen and patients clothing has infection prevention and control implications. Sensitivity is needed when returning soiled clothing to relatives of patients for laundry.

The clothes that the nursing associate wears in clinical environments (whether uniform or your own clothes) should always be laundered in accordance with best practice guidance. It is recommended that nurses launder their uniforms at 60°C to ensure safe removal of microorganisms.

References

Armstrong, P. and Day, S. (2017) *Wash, wear and care: clothing and laundry in long term residential care*, Montreal: McGill-Queen's University Press.

Care Quality Commission (CQC). (2019) *Handling sharps in adult social care.* [Online] Available: https://www.cqc.org.uk/guidance-providers/adult-social-care/handling-sharps-adult-social-care [accessed December 2019].

Department of Health. (2010) *Uniforms and workwear: guidance on uniform and workwear policies for NHS employers*, London: The Stationery Office.

Department of Health. (2013) *Health technical memorandum 07-01: safe management of healthcare waste*, London: Department of Health. [online] Available: https://assets.publishing.service.gov.uk/government/uploads/system/uploads/attachment_data/file/167976/HTM_07-01_Final.pdf [accessed 19 October 2019].

Health and Safety Executive. (no date) *COSHH basics HSE*. [online] Available: http://www.hse.gov.uk/coshh/basics/index.htm [accessed 19 October 2019].

Loveday, H.P., Wilson, J.A., Hoffman, P.N. and Pratt, R.J. (2007) Public perception and the social and microbiological significance of uniforms in the prevention and control of healthcare-associated infections: an evidence review, *Journal of Infection Prevention*, 8(4): 10–21. doi: 10.1177/1469044607082078.

MHRA. (2013) *Single-use medical devices: implications and consequences of reuse*, London: Medicines and Healthcare Products Regulatory Agency. [online] Available: https://www.gov.uk/government/publications/single-use-medical-devices-implications-and-consequences-of-re-use [accessed 19 October 2019].

National Clinical Guideline Centre. (2012) *Partial update of NICE clinical guideline 2 infection: prevention and control of healthcare-associated infections in primary and community care*, London: National Clinical Guidelines Centre. [online] Available: https://www.nice.org.uk/guidance/cg139/evidence/control-full-guideline-pdf-185186701 [accessed 19 October 2019].

NMC. (2018) *Standards of proficiency for nursing associates*, London: Nursing and Midwifery Council.

Riley, K., Laird, K. and Williams J. (2015) Washing uniforms at home: adherence to hospital policy, *Nursing Standard*, 29(25): 37–43.

Riley, K., Williams, J., Owen, L., Shen, J., Davies, A. and Laird, K. (2017) The effect of low-temperature laundering and detergents on the survival of Escherichia coli and Staphylococcus aureus on textiles used in healthcare uniforms, *Journal of Applied Microbiology*, 123(1): 280–286.

Royal College of Nursing. (2013) *Guidance on uniforms and work wear*, London: Royal College of Nursing.

Unit 9

Meeting Needs for Care and Support at the End of Life

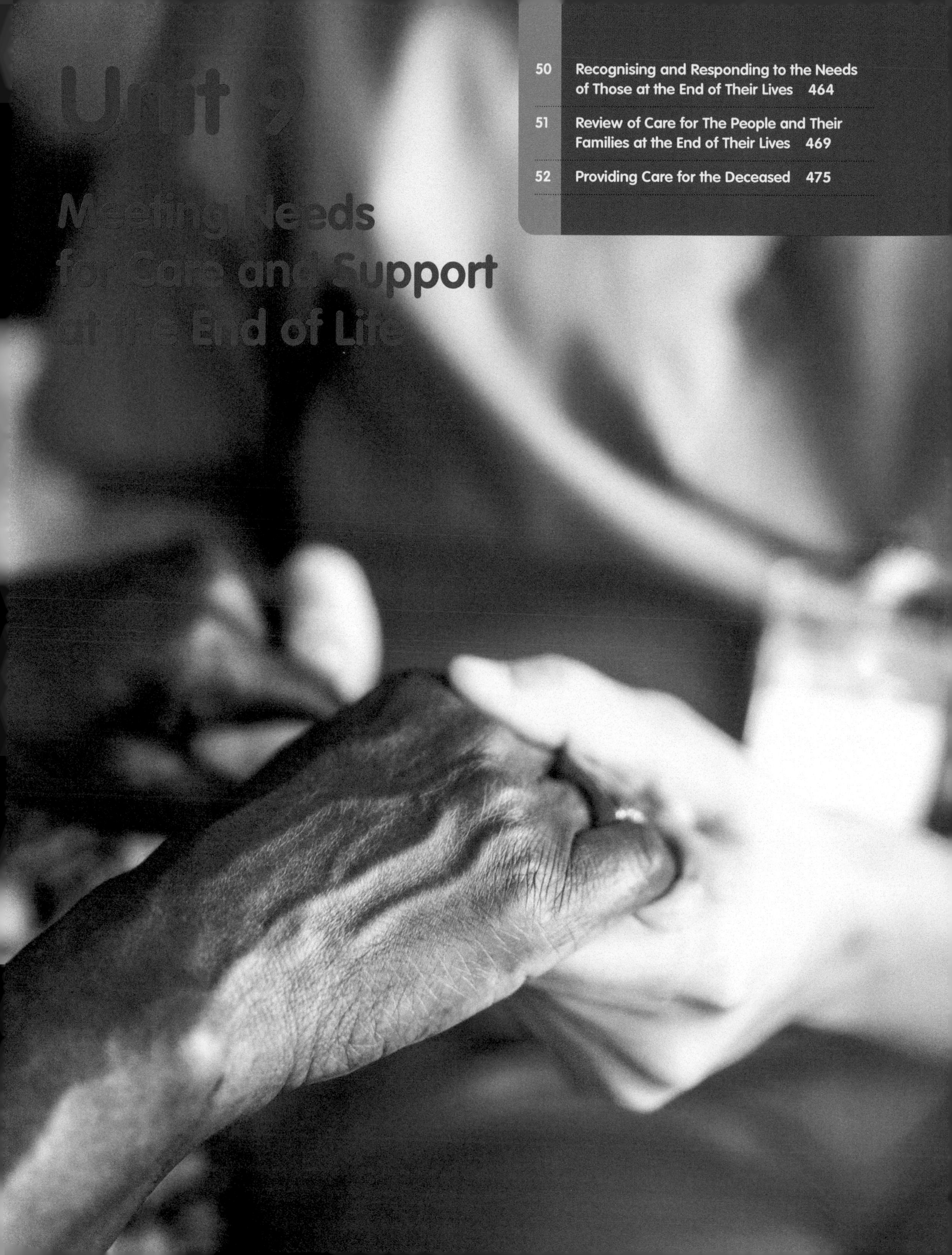

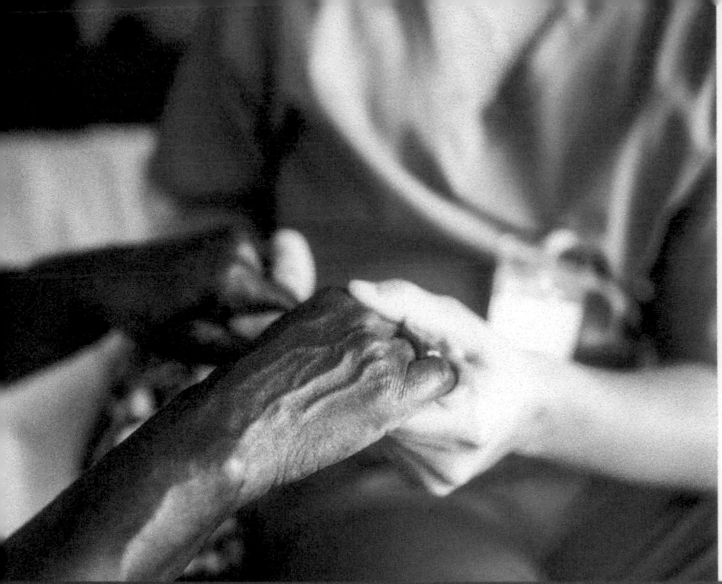

50

Recognising and Responding to the Needs of Those at the End of Their Lives

Karen Sumpter

University of Hertfordshire, UK

Chapter Aim

- **The aim of this chapter is for the reader to be able to recognise deterioration in a patient whose death is expected.**

Learning Outcomes

The reader will:

- **Be able to recognise when a patient is reaching the final phase of life.**
- **Understand the physiological changes that occur as end of life approaches.**
- **Be able to support the patient and family at the end of life.**

Test Yourself Multiple Choice Questions

1. ***Palliative care* is a term generally used:**
   A) **By the specialist palliative care team**
   B) **To describe the phase of illness whereby curative treatment is no longer available**
   C) **To describe when someone is dying.**
   D) **To diagnose dying**

The Nursing Associate's Handbook of Clinical Skills, First Edition. Edited by Ian Peate.

Companion website: www.wiley.com/nursingassociate

2. *Advance care planning* is a term used:
   A) To describe a care plan that the nurse writes before meeting a patient
   B) To describe a high-level care plan written by a consultant
   C) To describe care given to any patient
   D) To describe a structured discussion about an individual's wishes and thoughts in relation to their care at the end of life
3. A patient is sleeping more than usual; this may indicate:
   A) They are approaching the final stages of life
   B) They are tired
   C) They are anaemic
   D) They are approaching the final stages of life or they may be anaemic
4. A multi-professional approach to end-of-life care:
   A) Ensures all aspects of the patient's care are met and well co-ordinated
   B) Makes communication difficult
   C) Is confusing for patients as they don't know who is caring for them
   D) Is repetitious
5. If a patient asks, 'am I dying', it is best to:
   A) Reassure the patient that they will be OK
   B) Get the doctor to come and speak with the patient
   C) Answer honestly, showing empathy and compassion
   D) Change the subject

Introduction

Palliative care is an approach that improves the quality of life of patients and their families facing the problems associated with life-threatening illness, through the prevention and relief of suffering by means of early identification and impeccable assessment and treatment of pain and other problems–physical, psychosocial and spiritual (World Health Organisation 2016).

The chapter will support the nursing associate to be able to recognise changes to patients that have a palliative diagnosis, as they enter the last phase of life. This phase may be known as end-of-life care (Leadership Alliance for the Care of Dying People 2014), sometimes referred to as 'terminal care'. The length of the end-of-life phase can differ and can be difficult to determine. It can depend on the patient's condition, age and rate of disease progression (Boyd & Murray 2010).

This chapter will also consider advance care planning, including preparation for death, patient choice and funeral arrangements.

The NMC proficiencies and standards for nursing associates (Nursing and Midwifery Council 2018) related to this chapter require the nursing associate to demonstrate an understanding of human development to be able to recognise the dying phase. The nursing associate should be able to demonstrate knowledge in relation to changes to the functions of the body as patients enter the dying phase. The nursing associate should also demonstrate knowledge and communication skills to meet the needs of both the patient and their family during this final phase of life.

Diagnosing Dying

End-of-life care is a term that is usually used to describe the last weeks of life, generally when the patient's condition has deteriorated and no further treatments are available to prolong life (National Institute for Health and Care Excellence (NICE) 2011). During this phase, the patient is likely to tire quickly, sleep more, have a significantly reduced appetite and wish to stay in bed for long periods. Individuals may recognise themselves that they are getting weaker and may wish to talk about what is happening to them, or ask questions such as 'am I dying'? It is important to try and answer honestly to patients who ask such questions; these questions usually indicate that the patient wishes to talk about what is happening to them. They may be frightened and need reassurance–see section on communication.

The patient will decline further as they get nearer to death–the speed of this phase is often difficult to determine and can be different for every individual. Therefore, when caring for a patient in the last weeks of life, it is important to be able to recognise that the patient is entering the terminal phase of their illness. Regular patient review is important to check for deterioration; this is dependent on the care setting of the patient and may occur frequently throughout a shift if a patient is an in-patient (hospital, hospice or nursing home setting); or less frequently if the patient is at home. If you think the patient is becoming more unwell and showing signs that they might be entering the final phase of life, it is important to report this to the medical team, patient's GP or the palliative care team, depending on the care setting. Psychological support for both the patient and their family at this time is extremely important too. Box 50.1 provides an overview of the clinical indicators of dying.

Red Flag Potential reversible causes to exclude:

Some of the signs indicated in Box 50.1 could indicate other conditions that could be treated. For example, the patient may have an infection, which could be treated with antibiotics; they may be dehydrated and improve with the administration of intravenous fluids; blood tests may indicate other reversible causes such as anaemia or hypercalcaemia, which could be effectively treated with blood transfusions or intravenous medications (Noble 2019; Boyd & Murray 2010).

Remember, discussion with the patient and family as to whether treatment is appropriate or wanted should always be considered.

Box 50.1 Clinical Indicators of Dying: reaching the last days of life

Clinical indicators of dying may include:

- Confined to bed or chair and unable to care for self
- Having difficulty in taking oral fluids or not tolerating artificial feeding/hydration
- No longer able to take oral medication
- Increasingly drowsy, sleeping for long periods

Source: Based on Clinical Indicators for terminal care: Boyd & Murray (2010).

Communication

It can be a challenge for the nursing associate to initiate conversations with patients and family members about end-of-life wishes. Over recent years, much has been written about the benefits of doing this, and evidence has shown that often patients welcome the conversation and feel pleased if the health professional initiates the discussion (Travers & Taylor 2016). Take opportunities and be guided by cues from the patient– you may be talking to them whilst giving personal care or doing a dressing and they might mention that they have been feeling less well or have received bad news about their condition. They may broach the subject of dying directly. If this happens, try not to shy away from the subject. If you are busy at that time, think about when a good time might be to come back and talk. It can often feel uncomfortable, and nurses sometimes worry that they will not know what to say (Gillet et al. 2016; see Box 50.2). If possible, take opportunities to learn from other members of the team who may be more experienced in these conversations.

Multi-Professional Approach to End-of-Life Care

Whether you are caring for a patient at home, in a nursing home, in a hospice or in an acute hospital setting, there will be a multi-professional approach to the management of the patient and their family at this time. A co-ordinated approach to end-of-life care is paramount to ensure that care is holistic and all patient needs are met (NHS England 2016; NICE 2018). The nursing associate will form a part of the multi-professional team and participate in patient ward rounds, multi-disciplinary team meetings and patient care planning discussions (Figure 50.1).

Advance Care Planning

Advance care planning is a generic term used to describe a structured discussion about an individual's wishes and thoughts in relation to their care at the end of life (National Council for Palliative Care 2008). All patients should be offered a choice in how they are cared for at the end of life (Gov.UK 2015). Some patients choose to document their wishes formally many years in advance, whilst for others, the discussions are had once a palliative diagnosis had been made, or they are told they are approaching the end the life. Advance care planning is important; it ensures patient's wishes at the end of life are clearly documented (Sumpter 2017). Advance care planning is often initiated by a member of the Specialist Palliative Care team, or the patient may have discussed their wishes with their GP. A copy of an Advance Statement or Lasting Power of Attorney for Health may be present in the patient's records–in any patient setting: home, hospital, hospice or nursing home.

Box 50.2 Challenges to starting difficult conversations with patients about end-of-life care:

1. Fear and own preferences
2. Lack of experience and confidence
3. Patient and family factors
4. Lack of time and resources/choosing the right time to have the conversation
5. Insufficient communication within the healthcare team
6. Inaccurate or incomplete documentation
7. Institutional factors

Source: Adapted from Travers & Taylor (2016).

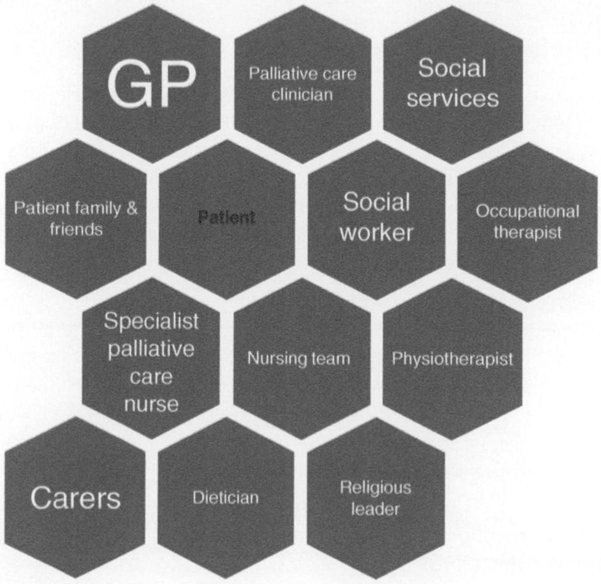

Figure 50.1 Multi-Disciplinary Team Members.

Supporting Evidence Advance Care Planning

An advance statement usually documents an individual's wishes of how they would like to be looked after at the end of life. This may include wishes in relation to care and treatment, but can also include beliefs, cultural wishes and other likes and dislikes. By preparing this in advance, it can support the family and the caregivers to ensure wishes are met should the individual lose capacity for decision-making or become very sleepy or unconscious as they reach the final stages of life. It is worth noting that any adult can make an advance decision – they do not have to have a life-limiting illness to do so.

An advance decision is a legally binding document that an individual makes to ensure their wishes are adhered to should they lose capacity to make decisions about their care (Compassion in Dying 2019). Advance decision documents are sometimes called living wills. An advance decision is focused on treatment and care wishes that may include, for example, whether the patient wishes to be resuscitated, whether they would wish to have antibiotics to treat an infection, or whether they would wish to have an acute hospital admission in the event of sudden deterioration. An advance decision requires a countersignature from a medical practitioner–this is often the patient's GP, unless completed in an acute care environment. Provided the individual has signed their advance decision, should they lack capacity to make decisions towards the end of life, the family and the multi-disciplinary team should support the wishes the patient has stated within their advance decision document.

A Lasting Power of Attorney for health and welfare is a legally binding document in which the patient passes over the responsibility for decision-making in relation to care and treatment to another (Compassion in Dying 2018). The individual must have mental capacity at the time of creating a lasting power of attorney, and it must be registered with the Office of Public Guardian (Gov.UK 2019). The lasting power of attorney only comes into effect when a patient no longer has capacity to make decisions about their own treatment and care. To make a lasting power of attorney for health and welfare, the document has to be registered with the office of public guardian. Further information about how to do this can be obtained from: https://www.lastingpowerofattorney.service.gov.uk/home

Preferred Place of Death

Allowing patient's choice on where they wish to die is a key element of the Department of Health's End of Life Care Strategy (DH 2012). Choosing where to die is commonly included in a patient's advance care plan and discussed with the patient by the Specialist Palliative Care team. Often patients indicate a wish to die at home; however, this is not always a practical option, depending on the patient's care needs, the family's ability to cope with the situation and availability of nursing or carer support (Pollock 2015). What is important is that the patient has the opportunity to discuss any wishes they might have and that a suitable place of death is agreed upon. If the patient is leaving an acute hospital setting with the plan to die at home, the nursing associate may be key in co-ordinating the complex patient discharge to ensure all care equipment and support are available to the patient and family after discharge.

Yellow Flag Cultural/religious beliefs and values

As patients enter the last weeks of life, it may be important to them to observe specific religious or cultural practices. Patients may wish to be visited by a faith leader to receive prayers or have time for reflection. Some patients may wish to seek spiritual guidance or discuss previous life events in order to find peace or acceptance prior to death (Costello 2019).

Discussing Plans After Death

As part of advance care planning, patients may wish to plan for their own funeral. This is a very individual thing: some patients may have discussed wishes already with their family or have documented wishes with a solicitor, whilst others may leave the arrangement with their family. Some may have specific religious requests for funeral arrangements; for example, there may be a specific time period between death and burial or cremation that is to be observed (Dickenson et al. 2000)–see chapter 52 for further information.

If you have developed a therapeutic relationship with the patient over a period of time, they may feel comfortable in discussing these arrangements with you. Patients may wish to prepare letters or put together a box of significant objects for family members they are leaving behind.

Violet Flag Funerals for patients with no relatives/next of kin

If the patient has no next of kin, no fixed residence and no finances, they are likely to be entitled to a 'pauper's funeral' (Funeral Guide 2019). This means the local authorities are obliged to pay for and arrange the funeral. For further information in relation to local authority funerals, please see https://www.funeralguide.co.uk/help-resources/arranging-a-funeral/what-is-a-paupers-funeral-public-health-funerals-explained.

Conclusion

Diagnosing death and supporting the patient to plan for end-of-life care can be emotionally challenging but extremely rewarding. The nursing associate should be able to recognise a deteriorating patient and provide support to the patient and family as they plan for the final stage of life.

References

Boyd, K. and Murray, S.A. (2010) Recognising and managing key transitions in end of life care, *BMJ*, 341(7774): 649–652. doi:10.1136/bmj.c4863.

Compassion in Dying. (2019) *Advance decisions (Living wills).* [online] Available: https://compassionindying.org.uk/wp-content/uploads/2016/05/AD04-v5.pdf. Accessed 11 December 2019.

Costello, J. (2019) *Adult palliative care for nursing, health and social care*, Los Angeles: SAGE.

Department of Health (DH). (2012) *End of life care strategy, Fourth annual report.* [online] Available: https://www.gov.uk/government/publications/end-of-life-care-strategy-fourth-annual-report. Accessed 11 December 2019.

Dickenson, D., Johnson, M., Katz, J. and Open University. (2000) *Death, dying and bereavement* (2nd edn), London: SAGE.

Funeral Guide. (2019) *What is a Paupers funeral?, Public health funerals explained.* [online] Available: https://www.funeralguide.co.uk/help-resources/arranging-a-funeral/what-is-a-paupers-funeral-public-health-funerals-explained. Accessed 11 December 2019.

Gillet, K., O'Neill, B. and Bloomfield, J.G. (2016) Factors influencing the development of end-of-life communication skills: a focus group study of nursing and medical students, *Nurse Education Today*, 36: 395–400. doi:10.1016/j.nedt.2015.10.015

Gov.UK. (2015) What's important to me, *A review of choice in end of life care.* [online] Available: https://assets.publishing.service.gov.uk/government/uploads/system/uploads/attachment_data/file/407244/CHOICE_REVIEW_FINAL_for_web.pdf. Accessed 11 December 2019.

Gov.UK. (2019) *Lasting power of attorney for health & welfare.* [online] Available: https://www.gov.uk/lasting-power-attorney-duties/health-welfare. Accessed 10 December 2019.

Leadership Alliance for the Care of Dying People (2014) *One chance to get it right.* [online] Available: https://assets.publishing.service.gov.uk/government/uploads/system/uploads/attachment_data/file/323188/One_chance_to_get_it_right.pdf. Accessed on 12 September 2020.

National Institute for Health and Care Excellence. (2011) *End of life care for adults.* [online] Available: https://www.nice.org.uk/guidance/qs13/resources/end-of-life-care-for-adults-pdf-2098483631557. Accessed 11 December 2019.

National Institute for Health and Care Excellence. (2018) *Multidisciplinary team meetings.* [online] Available: https://www.nice.org.uk/guidance/ng94/evidence/29.multidisciplinary-team-meetings-pdf-172397464668. Accessed 1 December 2019.

NHS England. (2016) *Specialist level palliative care: information for commissioners.* [online] Available: https://www.england.nhs.uk/wp-content/uploads/2016/04/speclst-palliatv-care-comms-guid.pdf. Accessed 1 December 2019.

Noble, S. (2019) Emergencies in palliative care, *Medicine*, 16(5): 514–520. doi:10.1016/j.mpmed.2019.10.011.

Nursing & Midwifery Council. (2018) *Standards of proficiency for nursing associates.* [online] Available: https://www.nmc.org.uk/globalassets/sitedocuments/education-standards/nursing-associates-proficiency-standards.pdf. Accessed 12 December 2019.

Pollock, K. (2015) Is home always the best and preferred place of death? *BMJ: British Medical Journal*, 351: h4855. doi:10.1136/bmj.h4855.

Sumpter, K. (2017) A happy ending, *Primary Health Care*, 27(8): 18–19. doi:10.7748/phc.27.8.18.s23.

Travers, A. and Taylor, V. (2016) What are the barriers to initiating end-of-life conversations with patients in the last year of life?, *International Journal of Palliative Nursing*, 22(9): 454–462.

World Health Organisation. (2018) *Definition of palliative care.* [online] Available: http://www.who.int/cancer/palliative/definition/en/. Accessed 2 December 2019.

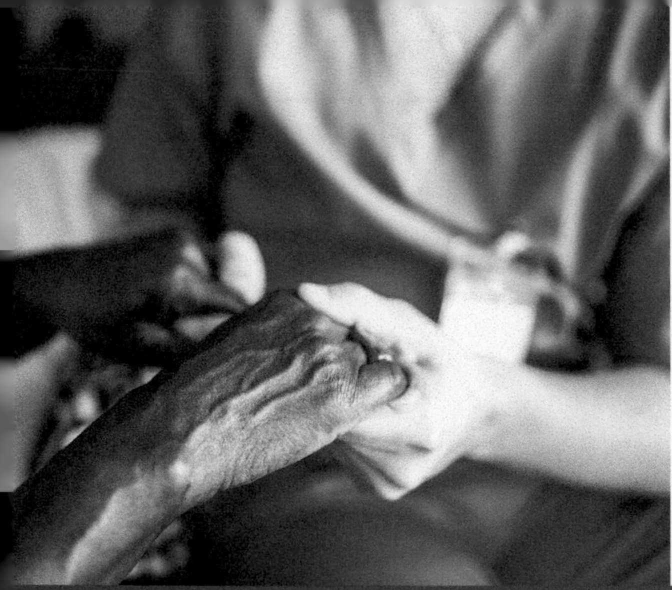

51

Review of Care for People and Their Families at the End of Their Lives

Karen Sumpter

University of Hertfordshire, UK

Chapter Aim

- This chapter aims to guide the reader in caring for patients and their families in the last days or hours of life.

Learning Outcomes

The nursing associate will:

- Gain an understanding of the common symptoms at the end of life and how to manage them.
- Gain knowledge in some of the common medications used to control symptoms at the end of life.
- Consider ethical issues that might influence care at the end of life.
- Be able to support the patient and family as they approach death.

Test Yourself Multiple Choice Questions

1. Care in the last days of life focuses on:
   A) Physical care of the patient
   B) Controlling patient pain
   C) Holistic care of the patient and their family
   D) Psychological care
2. Restlessness and agitation can be:
   A) Common symptoms in the last days of life
   B) Caused by stopping medication
   C) A sign of infection
   D) Caused by high doses of pain killers

The Nursing Associate's Handbook of Clinical Skills, First Edition. Edited by Ian Peate.

Companion website: www.wiley.com/nursingassociate

3. DNAR stands for:
 A) Do not assess respiration
 B) Do nothing at all
 C) Do not attempt resuscitation
 D) Do not attempt reasoning

4. The Mental Capacity Act was published in:
 A) 2019
 B) 1999
 C) 2013
 D) 2005

5. Medication to relieve symptoms at the end of life is most commonly given:
 A) Intravenously
 B) By mouth
 C) Not given–patients who are dying no longer need medication
 D) Subcutaneously via a syringe driver

Introduction

Caring for a patient in the last few days of life can be very rewarding and an opportunity for the nursing associate to provide holistic patient care. This chapter follows the principles discussed in Chapter 50 and will help the nursing associate to provide effective care to patients at the end of life.

When providing care in the last hours or days of life, priorities change. This phase may occur over a period of weeks, or happen quite quickly, seeing a fast deterioration at the end of life. This phase may occur within an acute hospital setting (including the Emergency Department), the home environment, a nursing home or a hospice. At this stage, there is no longer a need for curative treatment; the focus moves to control any physical symptoms the patient might have, as well as providing psychological and spiritual support to the patient and family (Chapman & Ellershaw 2015). A multi-disciplinary approach to care during this final phase of life is always encouraged.

The Nursing and Midwifery Council (NMC) proficiencies and standards for nursing associates (NMC 2018a) related to this chapter include the nursing associate being able to communicate effectively with patients and family members as the patient reaches the end of life. The nursing associate may need to act as an advocate for a patient, particularly if the patient has specific wishes for their end-of-life care.

The nursing associate will also demonstrate knowledge and skills to support patients with symptoms encountered at the end of life, including pain, discomfort and anxiety.

Stopping Treatment

As patients are identified as reaching the dying phase (Chapter 50), the multi-professional team will review the patient's treatment plan and prescribed medication. If not already in place, it may be necessary to complete a DNAR (do not attempt resuscitation) order. In the home or nursing home setting, this will be undertaken by the GP responsible for the patient; in hospital or hospice, the medical team will complete this. Medical teams should endeavour to include the patient in this decision unless it would cause the patient extreme psychological distress to do so (Resuscitation Council 2019). Providing the patient has capacity to be included in this discussion, family members' views, if different to the patient's would not need to be considered. The patient may already have an advance directive in place, which would aid decision making (Chapter 50).

Take Note

If a person is being cared for at home or in a care home, the GP has overall responsibility for that person's care. Community nurses will often visit the person at home, and family and friends may be closely involved in caring.

Violet Flag

From a human rights perspective, the right to freedom from torture, cruelty and punishment is a fundamental human right along, and this applies to prisoners or detainees who are also entitled to receive an appropriate level of health care. These rights have to be guaranteed irrespective of the nature of their crime or whether they are in a prison placement.

Most people do not think about dying in prison, but for some people in prison and places of detention, dying is more than a possibility or passing thought. For some, given their sentences, age and, often, their health status, specific consideration must be given to the possibility of dying in a place of detention. The Dying Well in Custody Charter (2018) sets out a framework to facilitate supportive end-of-life care in the prison setting. Further information can be found at http://endoflifecareambitions.org.uk/wp-content/uploads/2018/06/Dying-Well-in-Custody-Self-Assessment-Tool-June-2018.pdf

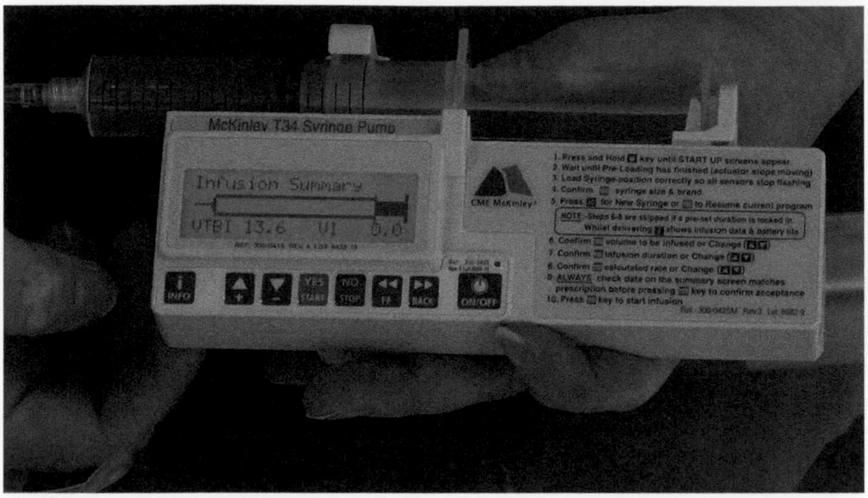

Figure 51.1 **McKinley T34 Syringe Pump.** ***Source:*** **CME Medical.**

Any unnecessary medications will be discontinued, for example, medications for high blood pressure or high cholesterol. Patients are usually eating very little by this stage and as they further deteriorate may only take sips of water (Chapman & Ellershaw 2015). At this time, family members may ask the multi-disciplinary team if they will administer artificial fluids to the patient. This may be supported by the team for comfort measures only (Dougherty & Lister 2015)–see section on Ethical Issues.

Touch Point

It is essential that support measures are put in place for the person who is at the end of life. Working with the multi-disciplinary team can help provide care that is holistic and person-centred.

Patients often require medication to help manage symptoms at the end of life. These are most commonly administered via continuous subcutaneous infusion using a syringe driver. See Figure 51.1.

Supporting Evidence DNAR & Mental Capacity

The Resuscitation Council provide clear guidelines on completion of DNAR forms, including helpful information for patients and family members. This can be sourced from https://www.resus.org.uk/dnacpr/

The Mental Capacity Act (2005) came into force to protect individuals to make their own decisions about how they are cared for (Gov. UK 2005). It is a useful document that guides health professionals to ensure that patients with capacity for decision making about their care are listened to; or to determine when patients are no longer able to make such decisions. Further information can be sourced from https://www.gov.uk/government/publications/mental-capacity-act-code-of-practice

Symptom Management

In the last days of life, patients may experience a number of physical and psychological symptoms. There are many different symptoms that patients may describe, and these will largely depend on the underlying illness or disease that the patient is dying from. For example, a patient dying from cancer is likely to experience pain at the end of life, whereas a patient in the final stages of chronic obstructive pulmonary disease (COPD) is likely to experience extreme breathlessness (Costello 2019). For this reason, it is important that the nursing associate be able to undertake a holistic review of the patient to ensure that all symptoms are managed as effectively as possible. It should be noted that in the final stages of life, a patient may be very drowsy or semi-conscious, and therefore, unable to communicate any symptoms they may have, which is why regular checks are important (Dougherty & Lister 2015).

Red Flag

Too many patients die an undignified death with uncontrolled symptoms, and this can lead to a distressing and undignified death. Resources should be made available to enable patients to die with dignity in a setting of their choice.

Common Symptoms and How to Manage Them

It is impossible to mention every symptom that a patient may experience as they are approaching death, as different conditions may bring about different symptoms. In order to guide the nursing associate in supporting patients at the end of life, Box 51.1 contains a list of the most common symptoms patients may experience and how they might be managed.

Take Note

There are seven standards associated with the provision of palliative care, these are referred to as the seven C's, developed by the Gold Standards Framework:

- Communication
- Co-ordination of care
- Control of symptoms
- Continuity including 'out of hours'
- Continued learning for the multi-professional team
- Career support
- Care in the dying phase

Source: Strickland (2019)

Spiritual Care

Spiritual needs in end-of-life care can be described as finding peace; and may or may not be linked to religion. Spiritual distress can be displayed by patients in the final phase of life, particularly if they are anxious or afraid of death (Marie Curie 2019). Spiritual distress is often displayed by either physical or psychological symptoms at the end of life, which may include pain, anxiety, restlessness or agitation (Costello 2019). In addition to providing symptom relief for these symptoms (Box 51.1), if the patient is conscious, talking therapies are often helpful. The nursing associate could spend time with the patient, listening to any worries the patient may share. However, if the distress is persistent or severe, the nursing associate may refer the patient to other members of the multi-professional team such as counsellors, psychologists, chaplains (or faith/religious leaders), spiritual care co-ordinators or palliative care social workers (NHS England 2013).

Yellow Flag

Spirituality means different things to different people; a part of a person's spirituality can include their religion and faith; however, spirituality is not always religious. We all have spiritual needs throughout our lives regardless of whether we follow a religion or not. Spiritual needs can include the need:

- for meaning and purpose in our lives
- for love and to feel loved
- to feel that you belong
- to experience hope, peace and gratitude

Box 51.1 Management of common symptoms at the end of life

Pain
Good pain assessment is key (Chapter 19)–talk to the patient if you are able. If the patient is very drowsy or semi-conscious, look for non-verbal signs of pain such as facial grimacing or change in position. Towards the end of life, analgesia is usually administered continuously via a subcutaneous syringe driver. The most common analgesia administered via this route is morphine.

Nausea and Vomiting
Nausea and vomiting can be attributed to the patient's disease or can be caused by medications the patient is receiving. Anti-emetic medications such as cyclizine or metoclopramide are often given subcutaneously in the syringe driver with the analgesia.

Respiratory Secretions
Excessive respiratory secretions are common in the final days of life. Medications to dry up the secretions are helpful in the management of this symptom–hyoscine butylbromide or glycopyrronium are commonly used. These medications are often included in the subcutaneous syringe driver prescription.

Breathlessness
Patients may become breathless in the last days of life; or if suffering from a respiratory condition, breathlessness may increase as the patient's condition deteriorates. Oxygen may be prescribed and administered, even though it is unlikely to have a therapeutic effect–patients often find it comforting. Fan therapy may be of benefit. Low doses of opioid medication or anxiolytics can also be of benefit.

Some patients will request to see a specific person in the last days of life – for example, a Catholic patient may ask for the priest to receive the sacrament of the last rights (or the anointing of the sick) (Ellershaw & Wilkinson 2003), or an individual may wish to make peace with another individual before death, for example, an estranged family member.

Blue Flag

The last stage of life brings with it opportunities for individuals and their families to address important issues such as putting practical matters in order, making amends with alienated loved ones and with their loved ones moving towards closure.

Spiritual care is a key aspect of holistic nursing care and is particularly relevant when supporting patients at the end of life (Elcock et al. 2019). Further information on religious or cultural beliefs at the end of life can be found in Chapter 52.

Orange Flag **Terminal Restlessness and Agitation**

Restlessness and agitation in the last days of life can indicate patient distress. Patients are often unaware of this symptom; however, for family members this can be very distressing to witness. Patients are usually semi-conscious, sometimes appear confused whilst awake. They may call out or be seen to be 'plucking at the bed sheets' (Hosker & Bennett 2016). Review and recognition of this symptom is key. Try to eliminate any obvious causes such as urinary retention, medication reactions or hypoxia. Good communication skills are important in this situation, providing reassurance to the patient and to the family. Sometimes the use of touch or a very gentle massage will help the patient to become more settled. The use of sedating medication may be of benefit in this situation–usually midazolam. This would be discussed with the patient's family prior to administration and would be added to the subcutaneous syringe driver alongside other medication.

Source: Dougherty & Lister (2019); Chapman & Ellershaw (2015)

Ethical Issues: Nutrition and Hydration in the Last Days of Life

As patients reach the last days of life, they often lose the ability to swallow food or fluids by mouth (Boyd & Murray 2010). This would be seen as a key indicator that the patient in entering the final phase of life (see Chapter 50 for more information). At this time, the multi-disciplinary team can be faced with difficult decisions in relation to providing artificial nutrition (via a nasogastric feeding tube) or artificial hydration (via administration of intravenous or subcutaneous fluids). Sometimes there can be conflicting views amongst the team, often dependant on knowledge in relation to this subject (Heuberger & Wong 2019). The insertion of either a nasogastric tube or an intravenous cannula to an individual who is dying can be a painful procedure and one that is unlikely to be of benefit to the patient; however, if the patient and family are willing for artificial nutrition or hydration and it provides comfort at the end of life, then it may be considered (General Medical Council 2019). If a patient has signs of dehydration and is showing distress, then administering subcutaneous fluids very slowly may help (Dougherty & Lister 2015; NICE 2015); however, the evidence to suggest whether this is of actual benefit to the patient is still inconclusive (Raijmakers et al. 2011).

It is worth noting that patients may have already considered this and have an advance decision to refuse treatment in place, clearly stating their wishes in relation to artificial nutrition and hydration, should they lack capacity to be involved in the decision at the time. In this situation, the medical team would manage the patient's care in accordance with their wishes, as an advance decision to refuse treatment is a legally binding document (British Medical Association 2018).

The nursing associate should be aware of the ethical discussions that commonly occur in end-of-life care and use the biomedical ethical framework in Supporting Evidence box to guide practice; alongside the NMC's Code of Conduct, which states that 'nurses should act in the best interests of people at all times' (NMC 2018b).

Supporting Evidence **Principles of Biomedical Ethics**

AUTONOMY	Patients' rights to make their own decisions.
BENEFICENCE	To act in patients' interest and do good.
NON-MALEFICENCE	To do no harm
JUSTICE	To treat all patients in a similar manner

Source: Modified from Beauchamp & Childress (2001)

Conclusion

Caring for a patient in the last days of life can be challenging when faced with multiple symptoms that the person may be experiencing. This chapter has given the nursing associate knowledge in relation to common symptoms and how to manage them, including some commonly administered medications. It has also considered some of the ethical dilemmas at the end of life in relation to artificial nutrition and hydration.

References

Ambitions for Palliative and End of Life Care Partnership. (2018) *Dying well in custody charter.* [online] Available: http://endoflifecareambitions.org.uk/wp-content/uploads/2018/06/Dying-Well-in-Custody-Self-Assessment-Tool-June-2018.pdf. Accessed 13 December 2019.

Beauchamp, T.L. and Childress, J.F. (2001) *Principles of biomedical ethics* (5th edn), Oxford: Oxford University Press.

Boyd, K. and Murray, S.A. (2010) Recognising and managing key transitions in end of life care. *BMJ*, 341(7774): 649–652. doi:10.1136/bmj.c4863.

British Medical Association. (2018) *Advance decisions.* [online] Available: https://www.bma.org.uk/advice/employment/ethics/consent/consent-tool-kit/9-advance-decisions. Accessed 10 December 2019.

Chapman, L. and Ellershaw, J. (2015) Care in the last hours and days of life, *Medicine*, 43(12): 736–739.

CME Medical. (2019) *McKinley T34 syringe driver.* [online] Available: https://www.cmemedical.co.uk/product/t34tm-ambulatory-syringe-pump/. Accessed 12 December 2019.

Costello, J. (2019) *Adult palliative care for nursing, health and social care*, Los Angeles: Sage.

Dougherty, L. and Lister, S. (2015) *The royal Marsden manual of clinical nursing procedures: professional edition* (9th edn), Hoboken: Wiley.

Elcock, K., Wright, W., Newcombe, P. and Everett, F. (2019) *Essentials of nursing adults*, London: SAGE.

Ellershaw, J. and Wilkinson, S. (2003) *Care of the dying: a pathway to excellence*, Oxford: Oxford University Press.

General Medical Council. (2019) *Ethical guidance: clinically assisted nutrition and hydration.* [online] Available: https://www.gmc-uk.org/ethical-guidance/ethical-guidance-for-doctors/treatment-and-care-towards-the-end-of-life/clinically-assisted-nutrition-and-hydration. Accessed 12 December 2019.

Gov.UK. (2005) *The mental capacity act.* [online] Available: https://www.gov.uk/government/publications/mental-capacity-act-code-of-practice. Accessed 13 December 2019.

Heuberger, R. and Wong, H. (2019, 2018) Knowledge, attitudes, and beliefs of physicians and other health care providers regarding artificial nutrition and hydration at the end of life. *Journal of Aging and Health*, 31(7): 1121–1133. doi:10.1177/0898264318762850.

Hosker, C.M.G. and Bennett, M.I. (2016) Delirium and agitation at the end of life, *BMJ (Online)*, 353: i3085. doi:10.1136/bmj.i3085.

Marie Curie. (2019) *Providing spiritual care.* [online] Available: https://www.mariecurie.org.uk/professionals/palliative-care-knowledge-zone/individual-needs/spirituality-end-life#needs. Accessed 10 December 2019.

National Institute for Health and Care Excellence. (2015) *Care of dying adults in the last days of life.* [online] Available: https://www.nice.org.uk/guidance/ng31/chapter/Recommendations#maintaining-hydration. Accessed 10 December 2019.

NHS England. (2013) *Leadership alliance for the care of dying people.* [online] Available: https://www.engage.england.nhs.uk/consultation/care-dying-ppl-engage/supporting_documents/lacdpengage.pdf. Accessed 10 December 2019.

Nursing & Midwifery Council. (2018a) *Standards of proficiency for nursing associates.* [online] Available: https://www.nmc.org.uk/globalassets/sitedocuments/education-standards/nursing-associates-proficiency-standards.pdf. Accessed 10 December 2019.

Nursing & Midwifery Council. (2018b) *The code: professional standards of practice and behaviour for nurses and midwives.* [online] Available: https://www.nmc.org.uk/globalassets/sitedocuments/nmc-publications/nmc-code.pdf. Accessed 10 December 2019.

Peteet, J.R. and Balboni, M.J. (2013) Spirituality and religion in oncology, *CA: A Cancer Journal for Clinicians*, 63(4): 280–289. doi:10.3322/caac.21187.

Raijmakers, N.J.H., van Zuylen, L., Costantini, M., Caraceni, A., Clark, J., Lundquist, G., Voltz, R., Ellershaw, J.E. and van der Heide, A. on behalf of OPCARE9. (2011) Artificial nutrition and hydration in the last week of life in cancer patients. A systematic literature review of practices and effects, *Annals of Oncology*, 22(7): 1478–1486. doi:10.1093/annonc/mdq620.

Resuscitation Council (UK). (2019) *Do not attempt CPR.* [online] Available: https://www.resus.org.uk/dnacpr/. Accessed 14 December 2019.

Strickland, K. (2019) Nursing patients who need palliative care, in Peate, I. (ed.) *Alexander's nursing practice hospital and home Ch 31* (5th edn), Oxford: Elsevier, 757–773.

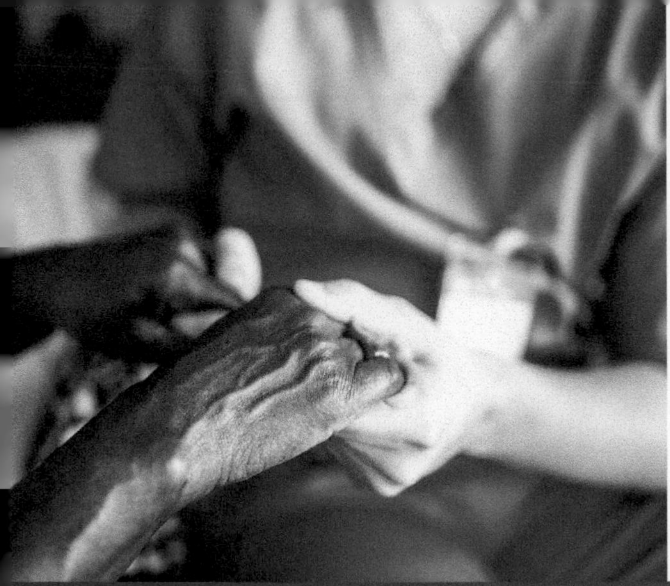

52

Providing Care for the Deceased

Karen Sumpter

University of Hertfordshire, UK

Chapter Aim

- This chapter aims to guide the reader in the care of the deceased patient and their family.

Learning Outcomes

The reader will:
- Be able to care for the body of a patient following death.
- Understand legal and religious/cultural implications for care after death.
- Be able to support the family/friends of a patient after death.

Multiple Choice Questions

1. Caring for person after death:
   A) Is a legal requirement
   B) Must be carried out within 48 hours of the person's death
   C) Has be undertaken in the presence of the family
   D) None of the above
2. Some people are uncomfortable talking about dying and death:
   A) Because of this, the nursing associate performs care activities according to their values and beliefs
   B) Meaning that when they come to the end of their lives friends and loved ones are not aware of their preference
   C) As result of this there is no requirement to adhere to local policy and procedure
   D) All of the above
3. Providing care for the deceased is also known as:
   A) Last offices
   B) Final duties
   C) Death rites
   D) Laying out obligations

The Nursing Associate's Handbook of Clinical Skills, First Edition. Edited by Ian Peate.

Companion website: www.wiley.com/nursingassociate

4. **Involving families in providing care for the deceased:**
   - A) May help to get the patient moved quicker
   - B) Should only be permitted if local policy and procedure permits
   - C) May help with grieving
   - D) Is an infection risk
5. **In sudden death:**
   - A) The nursing associate is required to inform the police
   - B) A coroner's input is likely to be required
   - C) There is no need to inform the coroner
   - D) You must only provide care to the deceased in the presence of the family

Introduction

Caring for someone after they have died should be a continuum from caring prior to death. Patients should be treated with dignity and respect at all times, ensuring privacy is maintained (Delves-Yates 2018; Merlane & Armstrong 2019).

This chapter will consider the care of a patient following death, both in preparation for the family to view; and in preparation for delivery to the mortuary or collection by funeral director (depending on the setting). It will also enable the nursing associate to consider care of family members or friends, communication skills required, religious or spiritual considerations and any legal implications.

Death can occur in a variety of healthcare settings – hospital, hospice, home, or nursing home. Elements of care after death may need to be adapted, depending on the environment in which death has occurred.

The NMC proficiencies and standards for nursing associates (Nursing and Midwifery Council 2018) related to this chapter and the provision of care to the deceased require the nursing associate to demonstrate an understanding of human development so as to enable delivery of person-centred care. The nursing associate is required to demonstrate knowledge, communication and relationship management skills that are needed to offer people, families and carers accurate information responding to their needs with a focus on people's dignity and privacy.

Delivering sensitive and compassionate end-of-life care and support to people to plan for their end of life means giving information and support to those who are dying, their families and the bereaved. The nursing associate has to act in line with any end-of-life decisions and orders, organ and tissue donation protocols, infection protocols, advanced planning decisions, living wills and lasting powers of attorney for health.

Meeting needs and offering support at the end of life requires the provision of care for the deceased person as well as the bereaved family.

Communication

Following the death of a patient, communication with family members or friends is of paramount importance. They may be present at the bedside at the time of death; or they may be called to come to the hospital/nursing home/hospice environment following a sudden death; or in the home setting, they may not live with the deceased person, or they may be contacting the nurse in the community to inform them of the expected death.

The nursing associate must consider the communication skills required to provide support in the most appropriate way, depending on the situation. Relatives/family/friends may be very upset (crying), angry, or silent after death has occurred, so adaptable responses are important here – see Box 52.1

Box 52.1 Breaking the Bad News – Communication Model

This model may help you when giving bad news to family members at the time of death or when discussing sensitive subjects such as referral to the coroner or choosing cremation or burial.

Preparation	Of self, recipient and environment
Communication	Delivery of the information
Planning	Agreeing what happens next
Follow-up	Documentation
	Provision of written information
	Liaison with other agencies

Source: Modified from Royal College of Nursing (2013).

Yellow Flag Religious or Cultural Awareness

Prior to expected death, there may be an opportunity to discuss any specific religious or cultural preferences following death. It may be possible to explore these with the patient or with family members. Although there is much written information available to guide staff on specific religious requirements after death, do not always assume that because an individual has stated their religion, they wish to observe the customs of this religion after death. There are a number of religions that determine the time of burial or cremation after death, so it is important to be aware of these.

Supporting Evidence Religion and Culture

Further information in relation to specific religious practices can be found at https://religionmediacentre.org.uk/factsheets/death-funeral-rituals-in-world-religions/ Many healthcare organisations have policies and guidelines related to specific religious practices at the end of life, so do access these to guide you. If the patient and/or family wishes are not known, follow the local guidelines in relation to any religious considerations after death, dependent on the religion recorded in the patient records.

Further reading: this easy to read guide for health professionals has been developed by Suffolk Inter-Faith Resource https://www.sifre.org.uk/SIFRE/downloadlib/EP_Faith_Card.pdf#zoom=75

Green Flag Legal Implications

Before washing the body after death, consideration should be given to any legal implications. If the death is unexpected, the patient may have to undergo a post-mortem examination (Dougherty & Lister 2015, p. 413). The coroner may need to be contacted. The medical staff should advise if there are specifics that need to be observed prior to or whilst preparing the body for transportation to the mortuary, for example, if wound drains or cannulas should remain in place. There is information available on the NHS website (NHS 2018) for families in relation to post-mortem, why it might need to happen and what to expect. It can often be distressing for families, so being able to direct them to clear information, if they would like it, can be of benefit. The government provides clear guidelines for medical staff as to when a patient death should be reported to the coroner. Local trust or organisation policies will be in place to guide staff also. Usually these will include a death within 24 hours of surgery or hospital admission; or when the cause of death is unknown (Dougherty & Lister 2015, p. 414; Gov. UK 2019; Merlane & Armstrong 2019) – See Box 52.2, Referral to the Coroner.

Organ and Tissue Donation

Patients' wishes in relation to organ or tissue donation should be documented prior to death (Chapter 51). This generally only happens if the patient has made their wishes known to the staff caring for them, or if the patient's family is aware of the patient's wishes at the time of death. If the patient has expressed this wish, advice should be sought from NHS Trusts Organ donation teams, or via the UK Organ Donation website (NHS Organ Donation 2019). From 2020, all adults in England will be automatically entered on to an organ donor national register. Individuals who do not wish to donate organs after death have to opt out. This means that if an individual has not opted out, their organs may be considered for donation without specific permission from the deceased's family (NHS Organ Donation 2019). This new law does not apply to individuals under the age of 18 years, those who lack mental capacity and those who have lived in the United Kingdom for less than 12 months.

Supporting Evidence Organ Donation

Further information and factsheets to enhance your knowledge are available from: https://www.organdonation.nhs.uk/

Such information may be of benefit to share with patients and/or relations either before death, or after death (relatives).

Box 52.2 Referral to the Coroner

- Cause of death is unknown
- Death was violent or unnatural (e.g. homicide or suicide)
- Death was sudden or unexplained
- Person who died was not seen by the medical practitioner who signed the medical certificate within 14 days before death or after they have died
- Death occurred during surgery or before the person came around from an anaesthetic
- Medical certificate suggests the death may have been caused by an industrial disease or industrial poisoning

Note: not all patients who are referred to the coroner require a post-mortem. The coroner will decide if one is required.

Source: Modified from Gov.UK (2019).

Care of the Deceased Body

Personal care is provided after death. This section will consider what equipment is required and the care after death procedure. The nursing associate may need to consider a number of factors, some of which may depend on the location of the deceased patient at the time of death. These may include whether or not to remove cannulas, drains or catheters; privacy and dignity of the deceased body, particularly in a ward environment when the patient is in a bay with other patients; and whether or not to include the patient's family in the process.

Yellow Flag Cultural Or Religious Considerations

In some cultures, or for some individuals, it is extremely important for family members to be involved in this care after death has occurred (Martin & Bristowe 2015; Urzell 2018).

Usually, two healthcare professionals will work together to provide personal care after death. Gather all the equipment required prior to starting the care to avoid having to leave the environment part way through. A comprehensive list of equipment can be seen in the Box 52.3. Talking to the patient as if you were providing care when they were alive is a way of showing compassion during this process (Martin & Bristowe 2015; Laurant et al. 2016).

Procedure

This procedure is to guide you in providing personal care of the deceased patient. Depending on the care setting, you should consider local policies or guidelines, together with any previously stated patient wishes or those of the patient's family.

- Gather all equipment as per list in Box 52.2 and put on gloves and aprons.
- Position the patient as flat as possible, lying on the back, with legs straight and arms by the sides. Gently rest your hands on the eyelids and close them (try to do this part of the procedure as soon as possible after death).
- Remove any electronic devices attached to the patient – for example – subcutaneous syringe driver, monitoring equipment. Remove any cannulas and apply gauze and dressing in the usual way.
- Remove any drains and apply gauze and dressing. Spigot urinary catheters to prevent leakage. Any leaking wounds should have gauze and dressings applied. Cover stomas with a clean stoma bag.
- Wash the patient's body with soap and warm water and dry thoroughly. Note: in some religions washing by health professionals after death is not permitted, so be guided by the patient's family and observe these practices if requested to do so.
- Bodily fluids may continue to leak from the body after death. Ensure pads or incontinence sheets are used if this happens.
- Usually, in a care setting, the patient will be dressed in a plain white shroud after death – this is usually made of disposable material, and covers the patient from neck to toe, with long sleeves and fastens at the back – see Box 52.3. If the patient is at home, a clean nightdress or pyjamas may be used. Consider any religious or cultural preferences as requested by the family.

Box 52.3 Equipment

- Disposable personal protective equipment (PPE) – gloves and aprons (further PPE may be worn if patient infectious)
- Bowl of warm water
- Patients own toiletries
- Towels x 2
- Patient's own razor/disposable razor
- Comb or hairbrush; nail brush
- Equipment for mouth care, including care of dentures as appropriate
- Plastic bags for disposal of clinical and domestic waste (as per policy)
- Bed pan or other contain to collect expressed urine (not required if patient is catheterised)
- Clean bed linen
- Patient documentation as required by law or local policy
- Shroud or patient clothing as requested by the family – this is usually clean nightwear but could also be religious or culturally specific (Figure 52.1)

If the patient is in hospital/hospice/care home:

- Linen skip for soiled linen
- Patient ID bands × 2
- Valuables/property register and bags for patient's belongings

If required:

- Gauze, dressings, tape to cover any wounds, or IV/cannula sites
- Caps, spigots for urinary catheters, drains or cannulas if they are to be kept in situ

Source: Dougherty & Lister (2015)

- Remove all jewellery – ensure two nurses are present for this so that all removed items are checked and recorded (as per local policy). If requested, a wedding band or any religious jewellery may be kept in place; however, this must be clearly documented. Rings may be kept in place using surgical tape.
- Organisational patient labels should be attached to the patient – follow local policy. Generally, patient identity labels are placed on the wrist and the opposite ankle.

Red Flag Infectious Patients After Death

- If the patient is not infectious, they may then be wrapped in a sheet. If there is severe leakage of bodily fluids, consider the use of a body bag. Any patients with known infections will be placed in a body bag. An identification label is placed on the sheet or the body bag. If the patient is infectious, this must be clearly documented to advise mortuary and/or funeral director staff.
- Finally, ensure the patient is transferred from the care setting with privacy and dignity.

Source: (Dougherty & Lister 2015; Merlane & Armstrong 2019).

Removal of the Body

What happens to the deceased patient after performing personal care is very dependent on the setting in which the death has occurred. If an individual dies in a hospital setting, most commonly they will be transported from the clinical environment to a hospital mortuary. It may be possible for family members to view the body in a hospital chapel of rest sometime after death, whilst the body is in the mortuary. The deceased patient is usually collected from the ward by the portering team. It is important to prepare staff and other patients/visitors for this happening by ensuring privacy is maintained.

If a patient has died in a nursing home, place of detention (i.e. a prison), hospice or at home, the usual practice would be to transfer the patient to a funeral director. The choice of funeral director is usually determined by the next of kin. The exception to this would be if there were to be a post-mortem; in this situation, the patient would be transferred to the nearest hospital mortuary prior to the post-mortem procedure.

Often family members may be unclear what to do after someone has died. They may ask for information in relation to funeral directors, cremation or burials or how to register a death. Information given by nursing staff may depend on the setting and local policies. Some organisations have bereavement support teams who will provide family with this information, whereas in other settings it may be part of the nursing role. Family will need to collect a certification of death, which is completed by a doctor. This certificate is then needed for family to be able to

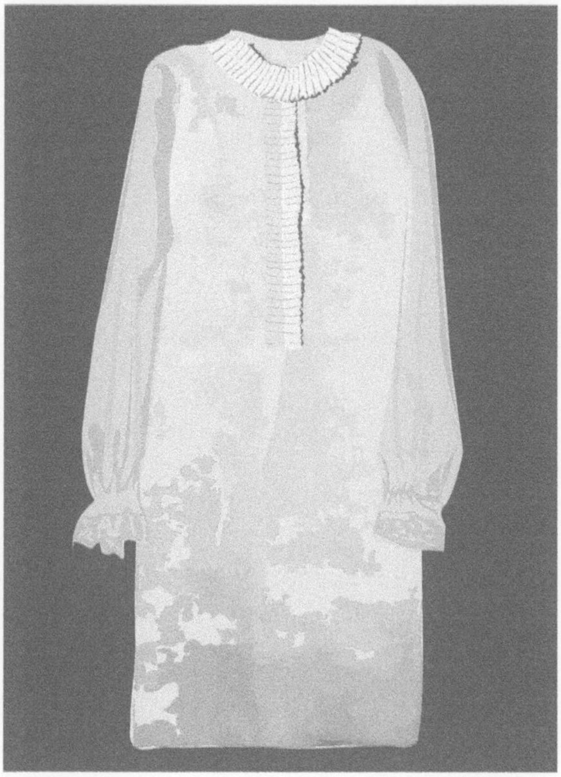

Figure 52.1 A hospital shroud. *Source:* Lindsay et al. (2018).

formally register the death. Deaths should be registered within 5 days, unless the death is reported to the coroner (Gov. UK 2019). Most organisations have written information to give to family members when they collect the death certificate, or information can be found online from https://www.gov.uk/after-a-death. This website can also advise on how to organise a funeral and provide other information related to finances.

Bereavement Support for Family/Close Friends

At the time of death, the nursing associate should ensure there is time made for family members to see the deceased patient if they wish – this is particularly important in a care setting outside of the patient's home (hospital, nursing home, hospice). Family may or may not wish to do this. However, it can be beneficial for many; having the opportunity to say a final goodbye can help longer term in relation to bereavement. Sometimes families may wish to take photographs of loved one after death, particularly when the deceased person is a baby, child, or young person (Laurent et al. 2016).

Organisations may offer bereavement support for family members – check whether this is available where you work and how to make a referral. Cruse bereavement care is a charity that offers bereavement support for individuals that might not wish to have bereavement support through a healthcare organisation or if there is no other support available. Individuals can self-refer to Cruse via the telephone or online through https://www.cruse.org.uk/.

Individuals react to death in many different ways and there is no one way in which you might expect someone to respond. The most well-known model of grief was developed by Kubler-Ross (1969) in the 1960s. This model suggests that individuals work through five stages from denial to acceptance (Kubler-Ross & Kessler 2005); Worden (2009) provides an alternative model that is much more active and often used by an individual in conjunction with a counsellor (see Box 52.4). However, Klass et al. (1996) suggest that grieving is a continuous process and that although individuals may learn to come to term with their loss, they use memories to continue to remember the person who has died, thus maintaining spiritual links with the dead person.

Looking after Yourself

Whilst it has been written that providing personal care after death is a privilege and an opportunity for nurses to show kindness and empathy (Henoch et al. 2017); for some, it can be quite overwhelming or indeed quite frightening. Ensure that you speak with the nurse you are working with if you are worried about performing this task; discuss any worries you have. Set some time aside after the procedure to reflect on your experiences (Porritt 2017).

Conclusion

Caring for a patient who has died is the final act that a nurse will carry out for a patient. When preformed with compassion, respect and dignity, this act can lead to closure for the nurse and the family. The nursing associate must have understanding of families' needs and offer ensuing support. This chapter has provided some of the practical considerations and reactions to death that the nursing associate may encounter. Relevant information that families might need to know about the death of their loved one and care provision for different groups of patients have been outlined.

Box 52.4 Stages of Grief

Kubler–Ross model

- Denial
- Anger
- Bargaining
- Depression
- Acceptance

The time span associated with each stage may be different in each individual.

Source: Kubler–Ross & Kessler (2005)

Tasks model:

Task 1: Accept the reality of the loss
Task 2: Manage/process the pain of loss/grief
Task 3: Adjust to life without the deceased
Task 4: Emotional relocation (moving on).

Source: modified from Worden (2008, 2009)

References

Delves-Yates, C. (2018) *Essentials of nursing practice* (2nd edn), Los Angeles: SAGE.

Dougherty, L. and Lister, S. (2015) *The Royal Marsden manual of clinical nursing procedures: professional edition* (9th edn), Hoboken: Wiley.

Gov.UK. (2019) *When to report a death to the Coroner.* [online] Available: https://www.gov.uk/after-a-death/when-a-death-is-reported-to-a-coroner. Accessed 25 October 2019.

Henoch, I., Melin-Johansson, C., Bergh, I., Strang, S., Ek, K., Hammarlund, K. and Browall, M. (2017) Undergraduate nursing students' attitudes and preparedness toward caring for dying persons - a longitudinal study, *Nurse Education in Practice*, 26: 12.

Laurent, S., Samuel, J. and Dowling, T. (2016) Fifteen-minute consultation: Supporting bereaved parents at the time of a child's death, *Archives of Disease in Childhood* - Education & Practice Edition, 101(6): 292–294. doi:10.1136/archdischild-2015-309960.

Klass, D., Silverman, P.R. and Nickman, S.L. (eds.). (1996) *Continuing bonds: new understandings of grief*, Washington, DC: Taylor & Francis.

Kübler-Ross, E. (1969) *On death and dying*, Routledge.

Kübler-Ross, E. and Kessler, D. (2005) *On grief and grieving: finding the meaning of grief through the five stages of loss*, London: Simon & Schuster.

Lindsay, P., Bagness, C. and Peate, I. (2018) *Midwifery skills at a glance: 9781119233985* (1st ed.), Great Britten: Wiley-Blackwell.

Martin, S. and Bristowe, K. (2015) Last offices: nurses' experiences of the process and their views about involving significant others, *International Journal of Palliative Nursing*, 21(4): 173–178. doi:10.12968/ijpn.2015.21.4.173.

Merlane, H. and Armstrong, L. (2019) Care after death, *British Journal of Nursing*, 28(6): 342–343. doi:10.12968/bjon.2019.28.6.342.

National Health Service (NHS). (2018) Post-Mortem. [online] Available: https://www.nhs.uk/conditions/post-mortem/. Accessed 25 October 2019.

NHS Organ Donation. (2019) *Organ donation.* [online] Available: https://www.organdonation.nhs.uk/. Accessed 25 October 2019.

Nursing & Midwifery Council. (2018) *Standards of proficiency for nursing associates.* [online] Available: https://www.nmc.org.uk/globalassets/sitedocuments/education-standards/nursing-associates-proficiency-standards.pdf. Accessed 18 December 2019.

Porritt, R. (2017) Maintaining dignity in death: performing last offices for the first time was an emotional but ultimately rewarding experience, *Nursing Standard*, 31(51): 36–36. doi:10.7748/ns.31.51.36.s41.

Royal College of Nursing. (2013) *Breaking bad news: supporting parents when they are told of their child's diagnosis*, RCN guidance for nurses, midwives & health visitors. [online] Available: https://www.rcn.org.uk/professional-development/publications/pub-004471. Accessed 2 July 2019.

Urzell, J. (2018) *Death/funeral rituals in world religions.* [online] Available: https://religionmediacentre.org.uk/factsheets/death-funeral-rituals-in-world-religions/. Accessed 10 November 2019.

Worden, J.W. (2008, 2009) *Grief counseling and grief therapy: a handbook for the mental health practitioner* (4th edn), New York, NY: Springer Publishing Company.

Unit 10

Procedural Competencies for Administering Medicine Safely

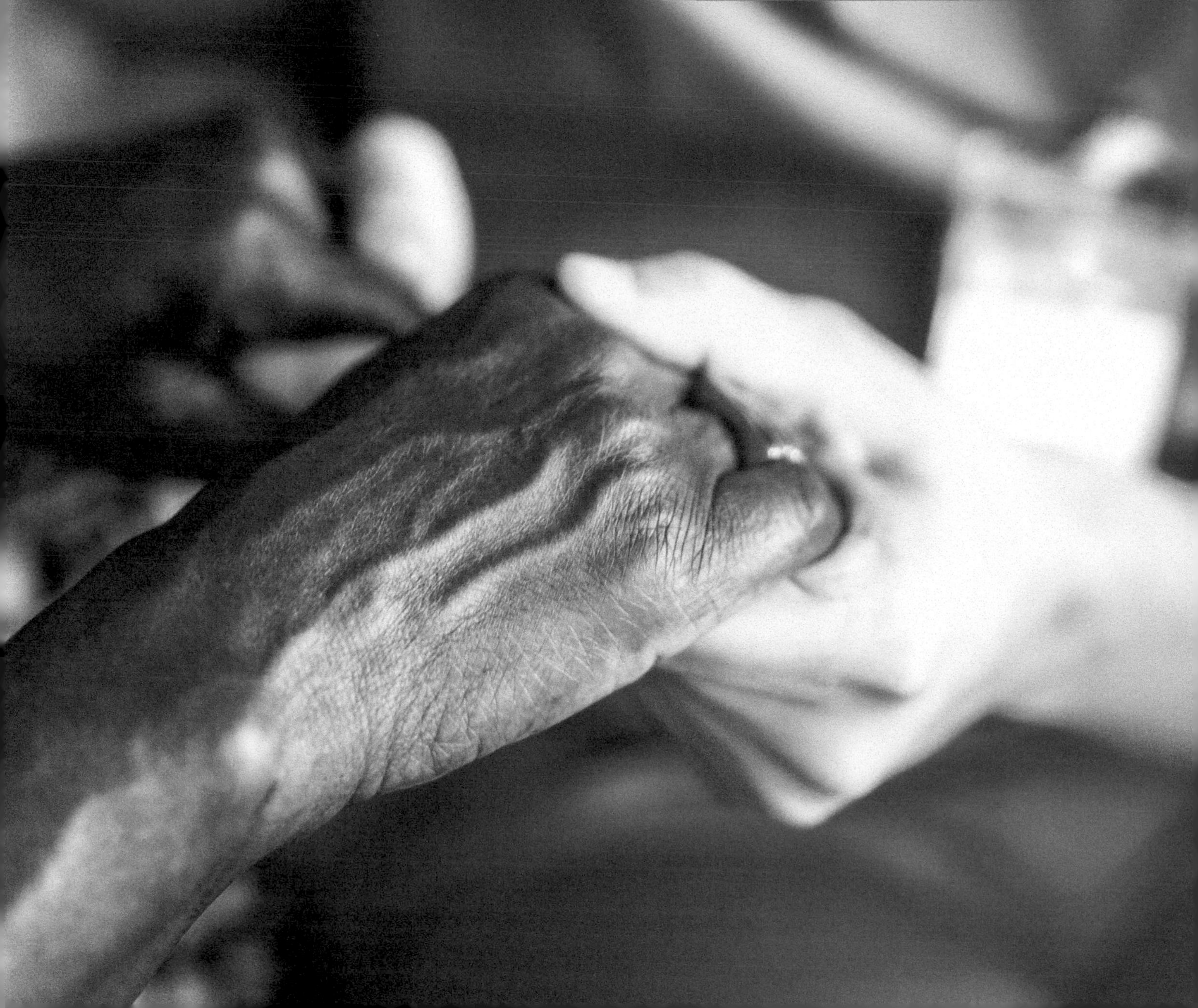

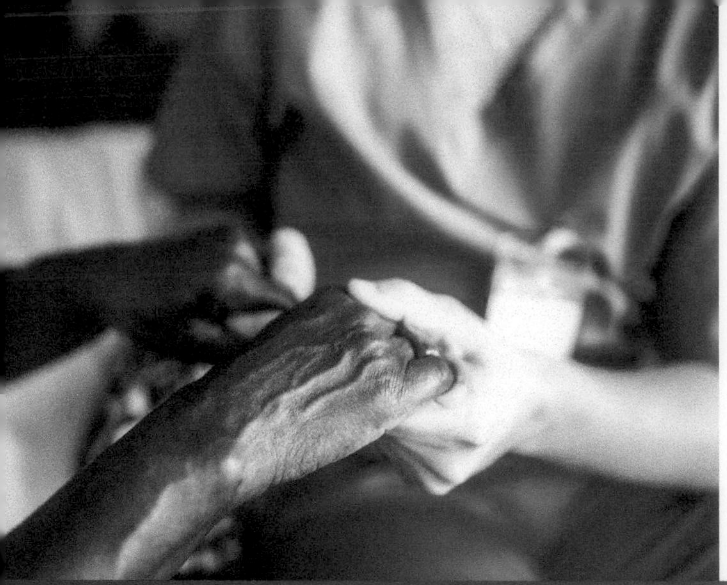

53

Reviewing a Person's Ability to Administer Their Own Medicines

Ian Peate

School of Health Studies, Gibraltar

Chapter Aim

- **This chapter aims to provide the reader with insight into the review of a patient's ability to self-administer their own medicines.**

Learning Outcomes

- **To demonstrate an awareness of how important it is to review a patient's ability to self-administer their own medicines.**
- **To discuss the key issues associated with medication self-administration.**
- **Outline the key components for successful implementation of self-administration.**

Test Yourself Multiple Choice Questions

1. **Self-administration is:**
   A) **When a person can look after and take their own medicines**
   B) **When a person can look after and take only two types of their own medicines**
   C) **When a person can look after their own medicines and does this in the presence of a nursing associate**
2. **People should:**
   A) **Never be supported to self-administer their medicines as this would risk the safety of others**
   B) **Be supported to self-administer their medicines if they wish to and it does not put them or others at risk**
   C) **Be supported to self-administer their medicines only if they have a carer with them 24 hours a day**

The Nursing Associate's Handbook of Clinical Skills, First Edition. Edited by Ian Peate.

Companion website: www.wiley.com/nursingassociate

3. **The effect of inpatient self-administration of medication is:**
   A) **Underused**
   B) **Under researched and unclear**
   C) **Both of the above**
4. **The person responsible for the self-administration of medicines after risk assessment has taken place and is said to be level 3 is:**
   A) **The nursing associate**
   B) **The manager**
   C) **The patient**
5. **The opportunity for self-administration of medicines should be:**
   A) **Offered only to patients aged between 18 and 55 years of age**
   B) **Offered to all competent patients**
   C) **Offered only to patients in residential care homes**

Introduction

There are a number of chapters in this text that are associated with medicines management. Medicines management according to the Royal Pharmaceutical Society of Great Britain (RPSGB) (ND) aims to maximise health gain through the best use of medicines. It includes all aspects of medicines used, from the prescribing of medicines to the ways in which medicines are taken or not taken by patients.

This chapter provides insight into the review of a person's ability to administer their own medication. Because a person has been prescribed medication, it should not be expected that they will be able to administer their medication themselves. Chapter 59 of this text provides a discussion of the safe storage of medicinal products.

Green Flag

The Nursing and Midwifery Council (NMC) has laid down a number of requirements that at the point of registration the nursing associate has to demonstrate, for example, how to continually assess and monitor people receiving care and their on-going ability to administer their own medications (NMC 2018a). The NMC Code also places demands on the nursing associate, who is required to ensure the safety of the patient including the administration of medicines (NMC 2018b).

A trainee nursing associate has to demonstrate knowledge and competence in relation to the safe administration of medications under the direct supervision of a registered nurse. There is a need to:

- Apply knowledge of pharmacology, how medicines act and interact in the systems of the body and their therapeutic action
- Prepare and administer medications safely in a timely manner and maintain accurate records at all times
- Correctly and safely undertake all medicines calculations
- Demonstrate appropriate professional behaviours and expected attitudes during the administration of medicines
- Maintain safety and safeguard the patient/service user from harm
- Know when a person is able (or not) to administer their own medicines

Self-Administration of Medicines

The Care Quality Commission (CQC) (2019) suggest that 'self-administration' is when a person can look after and take their own medicines; they add that people have the right to choose to manage their own medicines and staff should consider a person's choice and determine if there is a risk to them or others. Self-administration of medication can be seen as a 'transfer of responsibility' that is dependent on a patient's ability to manage the tasks involved as well as giving their consent to do so (RPSGB 2005).

The National Institute for Health and Care Excellence (NICE) (2014) note that staff should assume a person can self-administer (unless after undertaking a risk assessment this indicates otherwise). When people are receiving short-term respite, or intermediate care, they need to maintain their skills, and this includes keeping skills they need to take their own medicines when they return home.

Red Flag

Risk assessments are key to determining what support a person requires to help them to self-administer different medicines, allowing care providers to ensure that necessary support is available. Risk assessment must be reviewed periodically and whenever circumstances change, so as to address the need to make adjustments to support that may be needed.

The RPSGB (ND) recommend that within social care settings, whenever possible, children and adults should take responsibility for their own medicine. This, they comment, preserves independence regardless of the social care environment, and it is a significant feature of intermediate care as it prepares people to look after their own medicines when they return home. The nursing associate and others must not make the assumption that medicines can automatically be removed from people when in a care setting.

Self-administration is a philosophy of patient care that considers patients should be as independent as possible; they should participate in their own care, make decisions about their treatment in partnership with nursing, medical and pharmacy staff and as such; they should, therefore, be able to make informed choices. The opportunity for self-administration should be offered to all competent patients, particularly those who wish to self-administer and where the timing of the medications is crucial, for example, diabetes, Parkinson's disease and asthma.

The key components for successful implementation of self-administration must work in conjunction with national (e.g. NICE and CQC) and local policies of medicine storage and how this is organised. The principle of self-administration applies to all patient groups; this chapter offers a generic discussion for the nursing associate in order to aid successful implementation; the content includes the residential care home setting and the facilitation of patients having the custody of and administering their own medicines, while in hospital. Traditionally, in hospital, patients have had their medicines administered to them, and this should continue especially where medication regimens are complex or for those for whom self-administration of medicines has been assessed as inappropriate.

Supporting Evidence

NICE (2015) Medicines Management in Care Homes www.nice.org.uk/guidance/qs85

This quality standard addresses the prescribing, handling and administering of medicines for all people (including adults, children and young people) living in care homes and the provision of care or services relating to medicines to those people.

The principles discussed in this document can be applied to other care areas.

The chapter focuses on those who are deemed suitable for self-administration of their medicines. With regard to children and young people, the majority of parents/carers are encouraged to participate in medicine administration. There are some children and young people who are able to self-administer if they have been deemed to have an appropriate level of understanding of their treatment. This is particularly common in those children undergoing long-term treatment or those with long-term conditions (Macqueen et al. 2012).

Touch Point

It should be assumed that all people can self-administer medication unless after undertaking a risk assessment that indicates otherwise. Not all people are suitable for self-administration of medications. Guidance has been produced to assist with safe and appropriate administration.

Self-Administration: Maintaining Safety

While nursing associates will contribute to most aspects of care, including the delivery and monitoring of care, it is the registered nurses who take the lead on assessment, planning and evaluation. Registered nurses will also lead on managing and coordinating care with full input from the nursing associate within the integrated care team, and this includes the delivery of medicines. Table 53.1 sets out the differences between the role of the nursing associate and the registered nurse.

The nursing associate must ensure that when making the assessment to ascertain if the person is able to self-administer their own medications that local policy and procedure is adhered to at all times. There are some medications, administered via a particular route, for example, the intramuscular, intravenous or intrathecal route and one-off doses of medication that may fall outside of policy.

Table 53.1 The platforms.

NURSING ASSOCIATE	REGISTERED NURSE
An accountable practitioner	An accountable practitioner
Promoting health and preventing ill health	Promoting health and preventing ill health
Provide and **monitor** care	Provide and **evaluate** care
Working in teams	**Leading and managing nursing care and** working in teams
Improving safety and quality of care	Improving safety and quality of care
Contributing to integrated care	**Co-ordinating care**
	Assessing needs and planning care

Source: NMC (2018a, 2018c).

Policies and procedures are there to support the nursing associate and to ensure that where appropriate, patients are enabled to self-administer their medication having been adequately assessed, provided with appropriate information and supported to self-administer their medicines.

The self-administration of medicines occurs through safe medicines management. This includes ensuring that the patient is safe, the assessment is documented and the process has been assessed and agreed with the patient. The aim is to establish a routine for medication administration, which can enable the patient to continue a regimen they were following prior to admission or to help establish a routine that can be continued on discharge from hospital.

Usually, medicines are stored in a locked cabinet at the patient's bedside or in the patient's room. When the patient and the nurse agree that the patient is able to self-medicate, they are given a key to the medicine cabinet. The key is to be kept on the person at all times, and the medicine cabinet is locked whenever it is not being used. Responsibility lies with the patient. The nursing associate asks, at agreed time frames, if the medication has been taken, helping with any problems that occur. It should be noted that at any time the patient can withdraw from the programme.

Self-administration involves teaching and offering advice to patients concerning medicines, where this is needed. This applies to patients who will self-administer as well as for those patients administering medicines under supervision. This permits patients to:

- Improve their understanding about their medicines
- Practise the administration of their medicines
- Identify medication problems with health care staff at an early stage
- Enjoy more independence and empowerment

Touch Point

Local (and national) policies and guidance are available to help support the nursing associate to ensure that where appropriate patients are empowered to self-administer their medication once assessed, provided with appropriate information and encouraged to self-administer their medicines.

Blue Flag

Self-administration of medicines has the potential to develop trust, and as a result of this, relationships with the nursing associate and other health care staff. It can also increase knowledge and understanding of treatment and improve patient concordance with medication.

Violet Flag

There are several areas in the health and social care field where specific requirements are in place regarding medicines management. These requirements can be associated with the law (legislation) and the specific organisation's own regulations (standard operating procedures and policies) that apply. These can include:

- An adult placement
- Boarding schools, school care accommodation, special residential schools
- Schools
- Care at home, domiciliary care
- Childcare, early education
- Children's home, secure accommodation, short break and respite services
- Day care
- Drug and alcohol rehabilitation
- Foster care
- Housing support, supported living
- Palliative care
- Residential care for adults, residential care for older people, short break and respite services
- Residential family centre
- Places of detention (including prisons and detention centres)
- Hospitals and hospices

The nursing associate must determine the standard to which they are required to work, and this will include how people in various care areas are assessed regarding their ability to administer their own medication.

Risk Assessment

The self-medication process is not without its risks. A risk assessment can indicate if a person has the ability to self-administer their own medication. An individual risk assessment can help ascertain how much support a person needs to carry on with self-administration. Determine if any previously unidentified support is needed to enable the person to continue administering and looking after their medicines themselves. NICE (2014) recommend risk assessment should consider:

- The person's choice
- If self-administration may be a risk to the person or to others
- If the person can take the correct dose of their own medicines at the right time and in the right way (e.g. do they have the mental capacity and manual dexterity for self-administration?)
- How often to repeat the assessment based upon individual needs
- How medicines will be stored
- The responsibilities of staff, which should be written in the person's care plan

Orange Flag

The traditional methods that are used within some mental health inpatient environments to administer medication are very often paternalistic and closely aligned to the medical approach to care. There is a need to develop further innovative methods in the management of medicines for people with mental health problems so as to redress the power imbalance for patients.

Table 53.2 provides an example of a risk assessment tool.

The individual risk assessment should use a coordinated approach determining who should be involved. It should involve the patient and their family members or carers if appropriate, other health and social care practitioners, for example, the practice nurse, GP, doctor and pharmacist. The aim is to help identify whether the medicine regimen could be adjusted so as to enable safe self-administration.

Yellow Flag

Patients who administer their own medicines while in hospital are more likely to report their overall care as excellent and are more satisfied with the discharge process than those patients who had not. The traditional drug round can encourage patient dependency, ignoring the lifestyle of each individual, restricting patients to a passive role, demanding that everyone takes their medication at the same time.

Table 53.2 Example of the content of a risk assessment tool.

	YES	NO	ACTION TO BE TAKEN
1. The person can verbalise that they wish to self-medicate (consent)			
2. The person is able to explain what each drug is for (not in medical terms), that is, Atenolol–my blood pressure tablet, Simvastatin–my cholesterol tablet			
3. The person is able to read the instructions on their medications and can verbalise these: a. The dose required b. How many times to be taken c. Any special instructions such as after food d. Date the medication expires			
4. The person is unable to undertake the requirements above, have they marked their drug containers with their own symbols so as to differentiate between each drug, or do have they a checklist designed by themselves?			
5. The person demonstrates an awareness that their medicine can cause side effects and any concerns they may have should be reported to the person in charge			
6. The person will inform the person in charge when their medication is 'running out'			
7. The person has the right aids to assist them in self-medication			
8. The person agrees and understands that they have to store the medication in the secure storage provided in their room at all times			
9. The person agrees that they must only take drugs as prescribed for themselves and if any other remedies or over the counter products are used the person in charge is informed in case of any drug interactions			

Take Note

Documentation used in conjunction with self-administration must adhere to robust systems, ensuring any information is accurate and kept up to date when and if changes occur. Regular monitoring of patients' progress whilst on self-medication is essential, with the multidisciplinary team reviewing information and taking appropriate action where required.

Self-Medication–Levels

When self-medication is being considered, the following factors need to be taken into account:

- The skills and ability of the patient to take the correct medication at the correct time. This needs to include the ability to remove the medication from the dispensed container and to take the prescribed number of dose units for each medication, using the labelled instructions as required.
- The level of prompting and observation required by nursing staff to ensure that the patient is taking their medication correctly.
- The security of medication, which can either be fully with nursing staff or devolved to the patient, where the quantity kept by the patient will be closely monitored and risk assessed.

Self-administration levels are related to patient assessment (risk assessment) and indicate the level of self-administration and/or supervision required; different health and social care providers may have different levels; see Table 53.3 for an example.

The aim of the assessment is to ascertain the patient's ability to self-administer safely, to ensure there are no unacceptable risks and to identify and if possible, resolve any potential difficulties. The level of support and subsequent responsibility of the nursing associate should be written in the care plan for each person, including how to monitor whether the person is still able to self-administer medicines. The assessment is an on-going process. Monitoring how the person manages to take their medicines and regular reviews are integral elements of the person's care.

Take Note

A risk assessment using a risk assessment tool must be undertaken to determine if a patient is suitable for self-administration of medications. Some medications may be excluded from self-administration, for example, controlled drugs or medication that is classified as schedule 3, medication to be given as a one-off dose (stat dose medication), medication to be given as and when required (PRN medication).

Table 53.3 Levels of self-administration and supervision.

LEVEL	DESCRIPTOR
Level 1	The nursing associate or a registered nurse will administer medicines to the patient from either a trolley or a bay medication locker. The patient is asked to put any medication in the bedside medication lockers on admission. The key for the locker is held securely by the ward staff and is not available to the patient.
Level 2	The patient is encouraged to dispense and administer their own medication personally from their individual bottles/containers. This process is supervised and checked throughout by the nursing associate or a registered nurse. The key for the locker is stored securely on the ward and is not accessible to the patient.
Level 3	The patient administers their own medication and has responsibility for the key to the bedside locker. The patient needs to be able to understand that for the safety of others their medicines must be kept locked within the bedside locker whilst they are on or off the ward.

Conclusion

The overarching aim of the self-administration of medicines is to improve health outcomes for people and is a key theme in empowering patients to take an active role in the management of their conditions. Self-administration of medications by patients has the potential to improve adherence and comfort and empowers patients as they are actively involved in their care.

All appropriate patients should be assessed to determine if they are eligible for self-administration, especially on admission. Patients are deemed eligible if they are assessed as suitable for self-administration following completion of a self-administration pre-assessment form and the self-administration assessment form to self-administer.

References

Care Quality Commission (CCQ). (2019) *Self-administered medicines in care homes*. [online] Available: https://www.cqc.org.uk/guidance-providers/adult-social-care/self-administered-medicines-care-homes. Accessed December 2019.

Macqueen, S., Bruce, E.A. and Gibson, F. (2012) *The great Ormond street hospital manual of children's nursing practices*, Oxford: Wiley.

National Institute for Health and Care Excellence. (2014) *Managing medicines in care homes*. [online] Available: https://www.nice.org.uk/guidance/sc1/resources/managing-medicines-in-care-homes-pdf-61677133765. Accessed December 2019.

Nursing and Midwifery Council (NMC). (2018a) *Standards for pre-registration nursing associate programmes*. [online] Available: https://www.nmc.org.uk/standards/standards-for-nursing-associates/standards-for-pre-registration-nursing-associate-programmes/. Accessed December 2019.

Nursing and Midwifery Council (NMC). (2018b) *Future nurse: standards of proficiency for registered nurses*. [online] Available: https://www.nmc.org.uk/globalassets/sitedocuments/education-standards/future-nurse-proficiencies.pdf. Accessed December 2019.

Nursing and Midwifery Council (NMC). (2018c) The code, *Professional standards of practice and behaviour for nurses, midwives and nursing associates*. [online] Available: https://www.nmc.org.uk/globalassets/sitedocuments/nmc-publications/nmc-code.pdf. Accessed December 2019.

Royal Pharmaceutical Society of Great Britain (RPSGB). (2005) *The safe and secure handling of medicines: a team approach*. [online] Available: https://www.health-ni.gov.uk/sites/default/files/publications/dhssps/the-safe-and-secure-handling-of-medicines.pdf. Accessed December 2019.

Royal Pharmaceutical Society of Great Britain (RPSGB). (ND) *The handling of medicines in social care*. [online] Available: https://www.rpharms.com/Portals/0/RPS%20document%20library/Open%20access/Support/toolkit/handling-medicines-socialcare-guidance.pdf. Accessed December 2019.

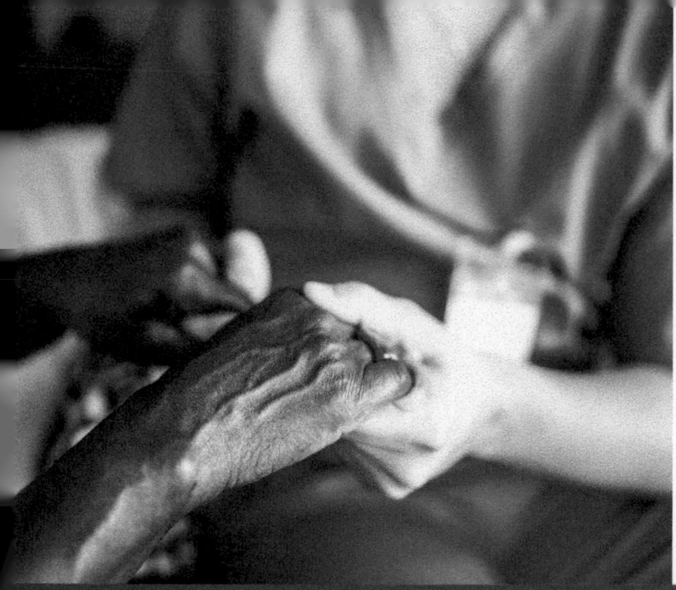

54

Undertaking Accurate Drug Calculations

Matthew van Loo

South Tees Hospitals NHS Foundation Trust, UK

Chapter Aim

- **The aim of this chapter is to provide the reader with the knowledge to accurately undertake drug calculations for a variety of common routes and methods of administration.**

Learning Outcomes

By the end of this chapter you will:

- **Have an understanding of the metric system, SI systems and units of measurement.**
- **Be able to accurately calculate doses by converting between units of measurement and using weight.**
- **Have the confidence to undertake accurate calculations of solid medications, liquid medication and infusion rates.**

Test Yourself Multiple Choice Questions

1. **Convert 735 milligrams to grams.**
   A) **0.735 grams**
   B) **7.35 grams**
   C) **735 grams**
   D) **73.5 grams**
2. **Convert 1.3 litres to millilitres.**
   A) **130 millilitres**
   B) **1.3 millilitres**
   C) **1,300 millilitres**
   D) **13 millilitres**

The Nursing Associate's Handbook of Clinical Skills, First Edition. Edited by Ian Peate.

Companion website: www.wiley.com/nursingassociate

3. **A patient is prescribed 80 milligrams of atorvastatin. 40 milligram tablets are available. How many tablets should you administer?**
   A) 5 tablets
   B) 1 tablet
   C) 2.5 tables
   D) 2 tablets
4. **A patient is prescribed mirtazapine 45 milligrams; you have a liquid preparation of 15 mg/mL. How many millilitres should be administered?**
   A) 1 millilitre
   B) 3 millilitres
   C) 5 millilitres
   D) 7.5 millilitres
5. **A 40-kilogram patient requires paracetamol 15 mg/kg. Paracetamol 250 mg/5 mL is in stock. How many millilitres should the child receive?**
   A) 0.12 millilitres
   B) 1.2 millilitres
   C) 12 millilitres
   D) 22 millilitres

Introduction

A key feature of the nursing associate's role is the safe administration of medicines. To enable the safe administration of medication, a nursing associate will need to accurately perform drug calculations. Undertaking this function requires a competent ability in basic mathematics.

The Nursing and Midwifery Council (NMC) (2018a) standards of proficiency require the nursing associate to be able to accurately calculate in a number of areas. This chapter will explore the mathematical functions that any nursing associate must be proficient in. The nursing associate has to, for example, measure weight and height, calculate body mass index and recognise healthy ranges and clinically significant low/high readings. The chapter will further explore the clinical application of mathematics to enable the safe and accurate calculation of medicines.

Mathematical Concepts

To safely undertake accurate drug calculations for the administration of medications, an understanding of arithmetic is needed. Arithmetic and mathematics are based around the rules of numbers and how numbers are used and manipulated. Understanding these rules is essential for accurate medication administration.

Green Flag

The four key themes within the Code (NMC 2018b) are:
1. Prioritise people
2. Practice effectively
3. Preserve safety
4. Promote professionalism and trust

When the nursing associate demonstrates proficiency in undertaking accurate drug calculations, they are adhering to the four themes that underpin practice and patient safety.

Whole Numbers and Fractions

The calculations involved in accurate medication administration will primarily use whole numbers and fractions. A whole number is any number that does not have a fraction, for example 1, 5, 18, 460. A fraction is any number that is not a whole number, for example, $\frac{1}{2}$, $\frac{7}{8}$ and $\frac{28}{9}$. The top number in a fraction is called a numerator and the bottom number is called the denominator.

Proper, Improper and Mixed Fractions

There are three types of fractions:
- A proper fraction is where the numerator is less than the denominator $\frac{1}{2}$, $\frac{3}{8}$ and $\frac{6}{11}$
- An improper fraction is where the numerator is greater than the denominator $\frac{17}{4}$, $\frac{31}{16}$ and $\frac{118}{7}$

- A mixed fraction contains a whole number and a proper fraction $2\frac{1}{3}$, $9\frac{7}{8}$ and $45\frac{2}{5}$

An improper fraction can be converted to a mixed fraction. This is particularly helpful in accurate medication administration. Imagine you have undertaken a medicine calculation to work out the correct number of tablets to administer, and you get the answer $\frac{9}{2}$. This answer is not helpful in its current form and needs to be simplified. Convert it to a mixed fraction $\frac{9}{2}=4\frac{1}{2}$ tablets, which is a form that can now be applied to medicines administration.

Converting improper fractions to a mixed fraction requires a couple of steps.

Example

What is $\frac{9}{2}$ as a mixed number?

Step one is to divide the numerator (9) by the denominator (2). 9 ÷ 2 = 4 *remainder* 1.

Step two is to rewrite the new fraction. The answer (4) is the whole number and the remainder (1) becomes the numerator of the fractions, so the answer is $4\frac{1}{2}$.

Note that the denominator remains unchanged.

Decimals

A number between two whole numbers is a decimal, for example 1.6, 6.33 and 0.245. Decimal places are the numbers to the right of the decimal point.

- 1.6 has 1 decimal place
- 6.33 has 2 decimal places
- 0.245 has 3 decimal places

When you have an answer with decimal points, there are two rules to remember.

Rule one. If the answer is greater than 1, give the answer correct to 1 decimal point

- 2.331 litres = 2.3 litres
- 96.24 milligrams = 96.2 milligrams

Rule two. If the answer is less than 1, give the answer correct to 2 decimal points

- 0.923 grams = 0.92 grams
- 0.544 millilitres = 0.54 millilitre

Mathematical Operations

In the accurate calculation of medications, there are four commonly used operations.

- Addition: when two or more numbers are added together their sum is found.
- Subtraction: a second number is subtracted from the first number to find the difference between the two numbers.
- Multiplication: two numbers are multiplied together to find the product of the two numbers.
- Division: the first number is divided by the second number to find the quotient of the two numbers.

Metric System

Touch Point

The SI system is core to accurate medicines calculations. Understanding how this system works provides the nursing associate with confidence to apply the theory to practice.

Introduced in France in the late seventeenth century, the *International System of Units* is the international decimal weight system. This is commonly known as the SI system, from the French *Le Système International d'unités*. This system provides a standardised measurement of weight (gram), volume (litre) and length (metre); the terms in brackets represent the base unit–the building blocks of the system. Through this system, the approach to calculations is then based on a standardised decimal framework that provides the nursing associate with familiarity and consistency.

The fundamental reason for consistency in the SI system is the fact that it is constructed around the use of the decimal system.

Multiplication By 10, 100 and 1000

To multiply by 10, move the decimal point 1 place to the right, for example 0.36 × 10 = 3.6

To multiply by 100, move the decimal point 2 places to the right, for example 0.36 × 100 = 36.0 *or* 36. Where the answer is a whole number, the decimal point may be omitted.

To multiply by 1000, move the decimal point 3 places to the right, for example 0.36 × 1000 = 360.0 *or* 360. Use zero to make up the places, to complete the whole number.

Division By 10, 100, and 1000

To divide by 10, move the decimal point 1 place to the left, for example 81.2 ÷ 10 = 8.12.

To divide by 100, move the decimal point 2 places to the left, for example 81.2 ÷ 100 = 0.812. For numbers less than one, write a zero before the decimal point.

To divide by 1000, move the decimal point 3 places to the left, for example 81.2 ÷ 1000 = 0.0812.Use zeros to make up places, where necessary.

In medicine calculations, there are five commonly used prefixes, which you will use (Table 54.1).

Combining these prefixes with the base units below allows the nursing associate the ability to express the measurement accurately.

Expression of Weight

The base unit for weight is gram. The gram is a common unit of measurement in medicine calculations. The measurement is used in two situations. First, the measurement of a medicine. This will be seen in the prescription, for example furosemide 40 mg. In this description the drug is furosemide; the expression of weight is 40 mg (milligrams). This is making reference to 40 mg of furosemide in each tablet. The second use of weight in medicines calculation is the patient weight. Typically, this will be measured in kilograms (kg), although grams (g) will be used in the neonatal and infant populations. The scale of difference in weight between a newborn child and a fully grown adult necessitates the need to adjust medication to the size of the patient. In expressions of weight, the following should be remembered.

- 1 kilogram (kg) = 1000 grams (g)
- 1 gram = 1000 milligrams (mg)
- 1 milligram = 1000 micrograms*
- 1 microgram = 1000 nanograms (ng)

*To avoid confusion between milligram and microgram the abbreviation of micrograms should not be used in clinical practice. Microgram should always be written in full.

Expression of Volume

The base unit for volume is a litre, and a litre is used to define a volume of liquid or solid that could be poured, for example a powder. Two expressions of litre are used in medicines administration: litre (L) and millilitre (mL).

In expressions of volume, the following should be remembered.

1 litre (L) = 1000 millilitres (mL)

Table 54.1 Commonly used prefixes.

PREFIX	DECIMAL	ENGLISH WORD
Nano	0.000 000 001	One billionth
Micro	0.000 001	One millionth
Milli	0.001	One thousandth
Centi	0.01	One hundredth
Kilo	1,000	One thousand

Expression of Length

The base unit for length is a metre. The metre is used to measure the height of a patient.

In the expression of length, the following could be remembered.

- 1 metre = 1000 millimetres (mm) or 100 centimetres (cm)
- 1 centimetre = 10 millimetres (mm) or 0.01 metre (m)
- 1 millimetres = 0.1 centimetre (cm) or 0.001 metre (m)

By itself, the measurement of height is not particularly important in medicines administration, but when used with weight, it can support the administration of medicine. This can be achieved by measuring the body surface area, which is the total surface area of the body. It is essential to know the body surface area for the administration of some creams and lotions.

Conversion of Large Units to Smaller Units

Conversion of a larger unit to a smaller unit requires multiplication, for example kilograms to grams, litres to millilitres, metres to centimetres.

Example

Change 0.7 kilograms to grams.

This is a large unit (kilograms) to a smaller unit (grams); therefore, multiplication is needed. 1 kilogram = 1000 grams, so to multiply by 1000, the decimal point is moved 3 places to the right. 0.7 × 1000 = 700.0, *which is written as* 700 *grams.*

Example

Change 2.55 litres to millilitres.

This is also a large unit (litres) to a smaller unit (millilitres); therefore, multiplication is needed. 1 litre = 1000 millilitres, so to multiply by 1000, the decimal point is moved 3 places to the right. 2.55 × 1000 = 2550 *millilitres*. Remember to add the extra zero to fill the space after 255.

Conversion of Small Units to Larger Units

Conversion of a smaller unit to a larger unit requires division, for example milligrams to grams, millilitres to litres, centimetres to metres.

Example

Change 1635 micrograms to milligrams

This is a small unit (micrograms) to a larger unit (milligrams); therefore, division is needed. 1000 micrograms = 1 milligram, so to divide by 1000, the decimal point will be moved 3 places to the left. 1635 *micrograms* = 1.635 *milligrams.*

Example

Change 3490 millilitres to litres

This is also a small unit (millilitres) to a large unit (litres); therefore, division is needed. 1000 millilitres = 1 litre, so to divide by 1000, move the decimal point 3 places to the left. 3490 *millilitres* = 3.490 *which is written as* 3.49 *litres.*

Take Note

Using the prefixes nano, micro, milli, centi and kilo with the expressions of weight, volume and length accurately describes the measurements used in drug calculations.

Clinical Calculations

Touch Point

There are a small number of medicines calculations a nursing associate needs to know to safely administer medicines. These calculations will apply to solid medicines, liquid medicines and infusion rates.

The term *enteral* describes medicines that are administered directly to the gastrointestinal tract. Enteral medications are typically available in solid and liquid forms. The prescription will indicate the amount to be administered. The nursing associate will then need to calculate the correct number of tablets or capsules, or volume of liquid, to administer. This calculation should be done on each administration to avoid error. There will be common medications in the clinical area, with which the nursing associate becomes very familiar; however, it is safe and prudent to confirm the calculation at the time of administration. There will be occasions when the pharmacy supplies a medication, from a different manufacturer, or the strength of the medication changes.

Red Flag

Each one of us has an essential role to play in checking the dose of a drug given to a patient; any of us has the potential to discover an accidental error, which might otherwise lead to the wrong dose.

A drug error has the potential to impact negatively on a patient's health and well-being.

Supporting Evidence **Human factors and medication errors: a case study**

Human beings are error prone. A significant component of human error is flaws inherent in human cognitive processes; these are exacerbated by situations in which the person who made the error was distracted, stressed or overloaded, or the person does not have satisfactory level of knowledge to carry out an action correctly. The scientific discipline of human factors deals with environmental, organisational and job factors, as well as human and individual characteristics, which influence behaviour at work in a way that potentially gives rise to human error. Gluyas & Morrison (2014) discusses how cognitive processing is related to medication errors.

Solid Medications, that is Tablets, Capsules and Suppositories

The most common form of medication is the solid form. Calculations as to the volume to administer are normally straight forward. From the medicine prescription, you need to identify the amount of medication you need. This will be in grams, milligrams or micrograms. Next, you need to refer to the medication available, or the stock strength, and identify the amount of medication in each tablet or capsule. Using the following formula, you will then be able to calculate the correct number of tablets or capsule.

$$\frac{medicine\ prescribed}{stock\ strength} = volume\ required$$

Example

A patient is prescribed Glicazide 160 mg, 40 mg tablets are in stock.

$$\frac{medicine\ prescribed}{stock\ strength} = \frac{160}{40} = 4\ tablets\ to\ be\ administered$$

Example

A patient is prescribed rifampicin 450 mg; 150 mg capsules are in stock.

$$\frac{medicine\ prescribed}{stock\ strength} = \frac{450}{150} = 3\ capsules$$

Example

A patient is prescribed paracetamol 1 gram, 500 milligram tablets are in stock. In this example, the prescribed dose and the stock strength are in different units. It is essential that the prescription and the stock are in the same units.

- Step 1. Convert to the same units 1 *gram* = 1000 *milligrams*; therefore, the prescription shall be reconsidered as paracetamol 1000 milligrams is prescribed; 500 milligram tablets are available.
- Step 2. Calculate the number of tablets required.

$$\frac{medicine\ prescribed}{stock\ strength} = \frac{1000}{500} = 2\ tablets$$

Take Note

You need to identify, from the medicine prescription, the amount of medication that is needed–grams, milligrams or micrograms. Next, refer to the medication available, or the stock strength and identify the amount of medication that is in each tablet or capsule

Compound Medications

Medications that contain two or more active ingredients are called compound medications or compound preparations. The strength of a compound medication is expressed as follows: co-codamol 8 mg/500 mg. In this example each tablet contains 8 milligrams of codeine phosphate and 500 milligrams of paracetamol. To approach calculations with compound medications, treat each active ingredient separately. Calculate how many tablets are to be administered using one active ingredient, then repeat the calculation with the other active ingredient. Both calculations should give the same answer. There must be an element of caution with compound medications, due to medications of the same name being available in different strengths. Co-codamol, is available in 8 mg/500 mg, but is also available in 30 mg/500 mg.

Example

A patient is prescribed co-amilofruse 5 mg/40 mg; 2.5 mg/20 mg tablets are available in stock. Co-amilofruse is a combination of amiloride and furosemide. How many tablets should be administered? As this is a compound medication, each active ingredient should be calculated separately.

Amiloride component

$$\frac{\textit{medicine prescribed}}{\textit{stock strength}} = \frac{5}{2.5} = 2$$

Furosemide component

$$\frac{\textit{medicine prescribed}}{\textit{stock strength}} = \frac{40}{20} = 2$$

Both calculations confirm that 2 tablets should be administered.

Liquid Medications, that is Syrups and Injections

The calculation of liquid medication takes a similar initial approach, but with the addition of a further step. With liquid calculations, the volume of the solution needs to be considered. Stock solution will be written in the following for 250 mg/5 mL. This means that there are 250 milligrams of medication in every 5 millilitres of solution. So, if a patient is given 5 millilitres, they will receive 250 milligrams of medicine. If the dose is doubled and the patient receives 10 millilitres of the same medicine, they will now receive 500 milligrams of medicine.

$$\frac{\textit{medicine prescribed}}{\textit{stock strength}} \times \textit{volume of stock solution} = \textit{volume required}$$

The same approach is used for liquid oral medications and injections.

Example

A patient is prescribed amoxicillin 500 mg; 125 mg/5 mL solution is in stock. How many millilitres should be administered?

$$\frac{\textit{medicine prescribed}}{\textit{stock strength}} \times \textit{volume of stock solution} = \frac{500}{125} \times 5 = 4 \times 5$$
$$= 20\ \textit{millilitres}$$

Example

A patient is prescribed tinzaparin 3500 units; 10,000 units/mL is in stock. How many millilitres should be administered?

$$\frac{\textit{medicine prescribed}}{\textit{stock strength}} \times \textit{volume of stock solution} = \frac{3500}{10000} \times 1 = 0.35 \times 1$$
$$= 0.35\textit{millilitre}$$

Note where the stock solution is written without a number before the mL, this means 1 mL. For example, 10 mg/mL = 10 mg/1 mL.

Infusion Rates

The administration of infusions is likely to be limited to subcutaneous infusions; intravenous infusions are not in the nursing associate's scope of practice. Accurate calculations of infusion rates are related to the volume of the infusion and the time over which the infusion is to be administered. The prescription will state the volume, in millilitres or litres, and time will be in minutes or hours.

The calculation of a flow rate will inform the nursing associate the speed at which the infusion should be administered, which will be expressed as millilitres per an hour (mL/hr).

$$Rate = \frac{volume\,(mL)}{time\,(hr)}$$

Example

A patient is prescribed 500 mL of sodium chloride to be administered over 4 hours. At how many millilitres per hour should the pump be set?

$$\frac{volume\,(ml)}{time\,(hr)} = \frac{500}{4} = 125\,mL\ per\ hour$$

Example

A patient is prescribed 1 litre of sodium chloride to be administered over 12 hours. At how many millilitres per hour should the pump be set? The prescription is 1 litre, and the pump is programmed in millilitres; therefore, the first step is to convert to the same unit.

Step one–conversion to millilitres

$$1\ litre = 1000\ millilitres$$

The prescription should now be reconsidered as a patient is prescribed 1000 mL of sodium chloride to be administered over 12 hours. At how many millilitres per hour should the pump be set?

Step two–calculate the infusion rate

$$\frac{volume\,(ml)}{time\,(hr)} = \frac{1000}{12} = 83.3\,mL\ per\ hour$$

Weight-Related Calculations

There are situations where the weight of the patient needs to be factored into the medicine calculation. This is especially common in the field of child nursing, where the calculation of correct medication doses will normally involve the child's weight. Recognition of the patients' weight will allow the precise dosing of a medication. The weight-related calculation will be in one of the following forms and will use a multiplication calculation.

- Milligram per a kilogram
- Microgram per a kilogram
- Nanograms per a kilogram
- Units per a kilogram
- Millilitres per a kilogram

Example

A patient is prescribed furosemide 2 mg/kg; 20 mg/5 mL solution is in stock. The child weighs 12 kilograms.

Step one is to calculate the dose required.

$$milligrams\ required \times patient\ weight\ (kg) = 2\ milligrams \times 12\ kilograms = 24\ milligrams$$

The prescription should now be reconsidered as a patient is prescribed furosemide 24 milligrams; 20 mg/5 mL solution is in stock. How many millilitres should be administered?

Step two is the liquid medication calculation.

$$\frac{medicine\ prescribed}{stock\ strength} \times volume\ of\ stock\ solution = \frac{24}{20} \times 5 = 1.2 \times 5 = 6\ millilitres$$

Example

A patient is prescribed dexamethasone 150 micrograms/kg; 2 mg/5 mL solution is in stock. The child weighs 20 kilograms. Note the dose required is in micrograms and the solution available is in milligrams. A three-step approach will be needed.

Step one is to calculate the dose required.

$$milligrams\ required \times patient\ weight\ (kg) = 150\ micrograms \times 20\ kilograms = 3000\ micrograms$$

Step two is to convert the dose required from micrograms to milligrams. 3000 *micrograms* = 3 *milligrams*

The prescription should now be reconsidered as a patient is prescribed dexamethasone 3 milligrams; 2 mg/5 mL solution is in stock. How many millilitres should be administered?

Step three is the liquid medication calculation.

$$\frac{medicine\ prescribed}{stock\ strength} \times volume\ of\ stock\ solution = \frac{3}{2} \times 5 = 1.5 \times 5 = 7.5\ millilitres$$

Take Note

Medicines calculations, at first glance, can seem daunting. Using a stepped approach will provide structure to the calculation.

1. Calculate the dose (in a weight-related prescription).
2. Ensure that the prescription and stock supply are in the same units.
3. Calculate the amount to be administered or the speed of infusion.

Conclusion

Safe medication administration is a fundamental role of the nursing associate, and the ability to make accurate calculations is essential to delivering professional, high-quality care. A broad understanding of a range of mathematical principles is required. Knowledge and understanding of the SI system and its application to the expression of weight, volume and length provides the foundations of safe and accurate medicines administration. These mathematical principles can then be applied to the prescribed medicines, enabling the correct amount to be administered to every patient, on every administration.

References

Gluyas, H. and Morrison, P. (2014) Human factors and medication errors: a case study, *Nursing Standard*, 29(15): 37–42. doi: 10.7748/ns.29.15.37.e9520.

Nursing and Midwifery Council (NMC). (2018a) *Standards of proficiency for nursing associates.* [online] Available: https://www.nmc.org.uk/globalassets/sitedocuments/education-standards/nursing-associates-proficiency-standards.pdf. Accessed November 2019.

Nursing and Midwifery Council (NMC). (2018b) The code, *Professional standards of practice and behaviour for nurses, midwives and nursing associates.* [online] Available: https://www.nmc.org.uk/globalassets/sitedocuments/nmc-publications/nmc-code.pdf. Accessed November 2019.

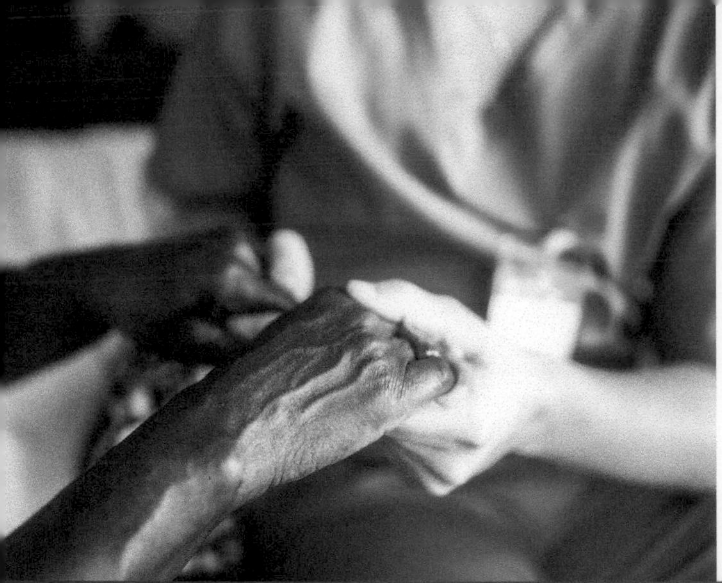

55

Accountability in Ensuring the Safe Administration of Medicines

Claire Pryor

Northumbria University, UK

Chapter Aim

- This chapter highlights the importance of accountability and how this is demonstrated when administering medicines.

Learning Outcomes

By the end of this chapter the reader will be able to:

- Demonstrate an understanding of professional accountability in relation to medication administration.
- Describe how patient factors may influence medicines administration decisions.
- Recognise the routes of administration permitted of the nursing associate and what influences adverse reactions or effects of medicines administration.

Multiple Choice Questions

1. Enteral administration of medicine:
   A) Avoids the gastrointestinal tract
   B) Takes place using the gastrointestinal tract
2. A PSD is:
   A) A form of medication administration chart
   B) A route of administration
3. Select two features of covert medication administration:
   A) The patient is unaware of the administration of medicines
   B) Can be undertaken at any time
   C) Can be done following a best interest decision having been made
   D) Is only undertaken once

The Nursing Associate's Handbook of Clinical Skills, First Edition. Edited by Ian Peate.

Companion website: www.wiley.com/nursingassociate

4. **Select one adverse effect of sublingual GTN:**
   A) **Pain**
   B) **Headache**
   C) **Hypertension**
5. **Nursing associates may administer medication via all routes available to registered nurses:**
   A) **True**
   B) **False**

Introduction

As a registered healthcare professional with the Nursing and Midwifery Council (NMC), nursing associates are responsible and accountable for maintaining safe and effective practice. Nursing associates may administer medicines and as such are responsible and accountable for not only their own professional practice but also ensuring standards of practice of others and maintaining safety. This accountability is seen not only in the NMC Code of Conduct and other codes of practice (Health Education England 2017a; NMC 2018a), but also in line with the proficiencies set out by the NMC for nursing associates specifically (NMC 2018b). Incorporated into both of these governing frameworks is practice relating to the safe administration of medication. The nursing associate must be able to work to both.

Annex B, section 10 of the standards of proficiency for nursing associates (NMC 2018b) details procedural competencies required for administering medication safely. Particular attention is paid in this chapter to 10.3 (accountability in safe administration (NMC 2018b) as the nursing associate applies their knowledge of accountability in ensuring safe administration of medication, providing and monitoring care, improving patient safety and quality of care. The process and procedure of medication administration using a variety of routes is detailed in chapter 56, with adverse effects of medication discussed in detail in chapter 58.

Accountability

Nursing associates are professionally registered healthcare professionals and as such are accountable for their actions and omissions in practice. Health Education England (HEE) clarifies the term accountability, in line with responsibility, discussing that:

'Accountability is to be responsible for the decisions you make and be answerable for your actions' (Health Education England 2017b).

Part of this accountability is to understand how to administer medicines safely, appropriately and have an understanding of the complex nature of issue pertaining to medicines administration and adverse reactions to medicines.

Whilst nursing associates may administer medicines, strict parameters are set on what can be administered, and how (i.e. route of administrations). Part of accountability is the understanding of permitted actions and those that are not permitted. Nursing associates are able to administer medicines using a variety of routes. These are shown in Box 55.1, and nursing associates are expected to administer medicines in a timely manner but must ensure that they only administer medications using routes they have been educated and assessed as competent in specific settings where such routes are appropriate and must ensure that they act in accordance with local policy (Health Education England 2017b).

Alongside permitted actions, some actions related to medicines are not permitted to be undertaken by nursing associates. The understanding of both what is and what is not within the scope of nursing associate practice will ensure accountability is demonstrated at all times.

Red Flag Actions not permitted relating to medicines

- Decisions to change the prescribed plan of care
- Supply or administer medicines under a patient group directive
- Prescribing medicines

Source: Adapted from Health Education England (2017b)

Box 55.1 Routes of administration

- Oral
- Topical
- Inhalation
- Subcutaneous injection
- Intramuscular injection
- Enteral
- Rectal (noted as enema and suppositories only)

Touch Point

Accountability relates to taking responsibility for your actions and being answerable for them.Nursing associates must ensure that they use both national and local guidance to ensure they work within the scope of practice. This relates to the wider role of the nursing associate, the local environment in which they are working, but also their own level of education, skill and competency base.

Whilst some components of care are not permitted for nursing associates, it is expected that they demonstrate a level of autonomy: this must be under the direction of a registered nurse and they must ensure that professional judgement is used to ensure they work within their scope of professional practice (Health Education England 2017b). In addition to administration, accountability for safe medication practice includes the reporting or raising of concerns or errors relating to medicines administrations and keeping accurate documentations and records.

Classification of Medications

The people nursing associates provide care to may come to the clinical setting (or the nursing associate into theirs if they are being nursed at home or in residential care). It is important that the nursing associate has an awareness of the different legal classifications of medicines that may be prescribed for patients or those that they may have purchased without any healthcare intervention or advice. All medicines or medicinal products are legally classified as general sales list (GSL), pharmacy medicines (p), or prescription-only medicine (POM) (as seen in Table 55.1). This classification system is detailed in the Medicines Act (1968) and as such is part of UK law.

Whilst patients (especially in their own homes) may self-administer medicines, the nursing associate must ensure that they only administer medicines specifically identified on the patient's medicines administration chart, following all the associated instructions. This includes medication that the patient may have purchased previously themselves (GSL medication).

Green Flag

Some medicines may be POM, P or GSL depending on quantity sold or quantity dispensed. Paracetamol comes in 500 mg tablets. People can buy this without any supervision in packs of no more than 16 tablets. This means a box of 16 paracetamol 500 mg tablets is classed as GSL.

If the person requires more than 16 tablets, it must be discussed with and sold by a pharmacist. Pharmacists may sell packets of up to 32 tablets of paracetamol 500 mg. More than 32 tablets of paracetamol 500 mg require a prescription and as such, paracetamol 500 mg tablets now are a POM.

As seen above, whilst the medicine does not change (paracetamol 500 mg tablets), the quantity impacts on the legal classification (Medicines and Healthcare Products Regulatory Agency 2009; Joint Formulary Committee 2019).

Source: Adapted from Pryor & Hand (in press).

Controlled drugs (or medicines) are prescription-only medicines that are subject to extra controls set out in the Misuse of Drugs Act (1971) and have specific 'schedules' of medicines depending on the specific controls and regulations in place for them. As a distinct classification of prescription-only medicines, nursing associates must (as with any drug administration) be fully competent and confident to administer, observe effect and report appropriately any concerns or effects to the registrant. Nursing associates may legally administer schedule, 2, 3 or 4 controlled drugs (CDs) providing that they are following the directions of a regulated prescriber (e.g. doctor or non-medical prescriber). In addition, employers should identify in policy the scope of CD administration for nursing associates (Health Education England 2017a). This will include any CDs allowed for administration and guidance on permitted routes of administration. This may be located in a medicines management policy or safety critical medicines documentation. Safety critical medicines are those that carry potentially a higher risk of harm to patient (e.g. warfarin, insulin or opioids) (Health Education England 2017a). As such, the nursing associate needs to fully understand the medication to be

Table 55.1 Legal classifications of medicines.

CATEGORY	DESCRIPTION
POM–prescription-only medicine	A product that may only be sold or supplied to the public on a practitioner's prescription, for example, levothyroxine
P–pharmacy-only medicine	A product that may only be sold in a registered pharmacy under the supervision of a registered pharmacist
GSL–general sales list (also known as over the counter (OTC))	A product that may be sold from a retail outlet without the supervision of a registered pharmacist
ACBS–Advisory Committee on Borderline Substances	A product that may be prescribed for the treatment of certain conditions. Prescriptions for these products must be endorsed

Source: Adapted from Pryor & Hand (in press).

administered, permitted route of administration and any additional safety considerations or policy actions or follow-up requirements prior to administration.

Touch Point

Nursing associates may administer specific schedules of CDs under direction of a prescriber and in line with a documented medicines administration chart.

Local policy regarding administration of CDs must be understood prior to administration as this may vary between employers or clinical settings.

Capacity and Consent

As with any care procedure, the nursing associate must consider the patient's capacity to consent to treatment prior to delivering care (including medication administration). A person's mental capacity is their ability to make a specific decision at a specific time. It is not an overall statement or a singular concept. As such, the nursing associate is responsible for ensuring that they consider a person's capacity at every interaction as capacity can fluctuate. Often capacity and the assessment of capacity is thought of as a medical assessment, and it may well be for complex decisions. However, the person responsible for providing care needs to be confident in the patient's capacity and the decisions and actions surrounding it. Considerations of capacity, the need for capacity assessment and consent is not limited to complex decisions or medical actions. It applies to everyday decisions such as food or clothing choice, through the total spectrum of decisions and includes life-sustaining treatments. This is embedded in law in the *Mental Capacity Act* (MCA) and indicates that everyone working with or caring for an adult who may lack capacity to make specific decisions must comply with the Act when making decisions or acting for that person, when the person lacks capacity to make a particular decision for themselves (Mental Capacity Act 2005).

Touch Point

- Everyone over the age of 16 should be presumed to have capacity unless it can be demonstrated otherwise.
- Capacity is both decision and time specific.
- Capacity can fluctuate.

As a healthcare professional responsible for delivering care, you need to ensure that you consider the patient's capacity and that consent is needed to perform your care role.

Crucially, the MCA stipulates that everyone over the age of 16 years should be presumed to have full, legal capacity unless it is demonstrated otherwise. Judgements should not be made about a person's capacity based on past medical history or diagnosed conditions (such as dementia or learning disability as well as age). Key here is to remember that capacity is not an overarching term; it is decision and time specific. Prior to carrying out care, the nursing associate is accountable and responsible for ensuring that they obtain informed consent for the care to be given.

Capacity is assessed using a two-stage approach which considers:

1. If the person has an impairment of the mind or brain, or is there some sort of disturbance affecting the way their mind works?
2. If that impairment or disturbance means that the person is unable to make the decision in question at the time it needs to be made?
   (Mental Capacity Act 2005)

Patients are said to have capacity and be able to consent to treatment (including taking medicines) when they have been provided with all the appropriate information they need in a manner suitable for them, they understand that information, can retain the information, weigh up the information as part of their decision making process and communicate their decision (in a manner that is suitable to them) (Mental Capacity Act 2005; National Institute for Health and Care Excellence (NICE) 2018). Consent can be verbal, written or demonstrated, but it is paramount that the nursing associate documents the consent given.

Yellow Flag

A person may have capacity but make a decision that is seen as unwise (by the healthcare professionals or family, e.g.) or refuse treatment. If the person has capacity, the nursing associate must respect this decision, document it clearly and discuss it with the appropriate professional in a timely manner.

People may make decisions based on their religion, culture, previous experiences and values (to name a few). The nursing associate must respect these decisions and support the patient in their choices. Alternatives or mediating factors may be discussed; however ultimately a person with capacity has the right to make decisions others may see as unwise.

A person is said to lack capacity when they are unable to make a specific decision at a specific time due to an impairment of, or disturbance of function of the mind or brain (Mental Capacity Act 2005).This is demonstrated in an inability to either understand the information relating to the decision, an inability to retain the information for an appropriate time, inability to use the information to make a decision or an inability to communicate their decision. It is paramount, therefore, that the nursing associate considers each patient individually, at each care episode to ensure the principles and process of consent is maintained.

If a person lacks capacity, the healthcare team will make specific decisions about what, when and how care will be provided following the legal process of 'best interest' decisions.

Take Note

Capacity, consent, unwise decisions and decisions made in a person's 'best interest' (also known as best interest decisions) are specific terms defined by the Mental Capacity Act and should be used in line with this legislation.

It is inappropriate to use 'best interest' as a care premise without following the MCA principles.

If a medicine is expected to be administered by a nursing associate (or nurse) as part of their healthcare role, it needs to be documented as a Patient Specific Direction chart (PSD) (Royal College of Nursing (RCN) 2019). This is a form of medication administration chart that has been completed by the prescriber, following assessment of the individual patient. The nursing associate uses this chart to sign for medicines following administration. A PSD is often confusingly called a 'prescription' by people who use them for administration of medicines; They are administration charts and, should not to be confused with a prescription that is given to a patient in order to obtain a supply of medicines from a pharmacy or dispensary (RCN 2019). They are also not to be confused with Patient Group Directions (PGD), which give instructions for supply and administration of specific medicines to a specific group of patients rather than individuals. Nursing associates are not allowed to administer or supply medicines using PGDs (Health Education England 2017a).

Whilst administration charts (PSD charts) will vary from employer to employer, they will all be completed in a similar manner with similar information given. The writing of the prescriber should be clear and unambiguous. The name of the medicine and any additional information of special properties relating to its medicinal form (enteric coating, modified release, additional monitoring instructions or parameters) must be present. The route of administration, timing, special precautions or actions to take and information about dose intervals or maximum dose in 24 hours should be explicit. The instruction must be signed by the prescriber. The nursing associate needs to ensure that they are happy with all the information on the chart, that they feel comfortable and competent in the administration required, have an appropriate knowledge of the medicine to be given and any additional monitoring, precautions or safety instructions. A signature is required to indicate that the medicine has been given as instructed and that all appropriate instructions and actions have been followed (Jones 2019). Acting outside of this may compromise patient safety and professional responsibility.

Process of Administration

Whilst the individual routes of medicines administration are discussed in chapter 56 in more depth, it is paramount to understand accountability in relation to the process prior to and following administration.

Firstly, it is recommended that before any consideration of administration, allergy status is known. Being aware of your patient's allergies or sensitivities is vital before administering medicines irrespective of it being a first dose, or something that have been taking for a long time. The PSD should give clear indication of any allergies or sensitivities, and this must be checked on every administration. Ensure that both medicines and any other substances (food or latex for example) are considered. Coloured wristbands with specific details may be used in clinical practice; however, in a patient's own home, outpatient or other settings these may not be present. The nursing associate should always check the documentation available and ask the patient about any allergies or sensitivities. If a new allergy or sensitivity is reported, it is essential that all records are updates immediately and medicines are reviews prior to administration (Meechan-Rodgers & Paget 2019). The process of allergic reactions, treatment and documentation is discussed in chapter 58 in depth.

Violet Flag

In the community and residential setting, patients may not have patient identity and allergy wrist bands. It is essential that you can positively identify the correct patient and confirm allergy and sensitivity status prior to administering any medication using alternative methods of positive patient identification.

Following this, the nursing associate should apply the 5 rights (5 Rs) to medicines administration.

1. Right patient
   Positive patient identification is mandatory prior to administering any medicine or treatment. This should include asking the patient their name and date of birth (the patient should verbalise this when asked for their name and date of birth: verbalising their name and date of birth yourself and asking for confirmation may produce errors if the patient incorrectly identifies himself or herself). You should check their information against the PSD. Other form of identification may include electronic bar codes in some clinical areas or photographs.
2. Right drug
   You must identify the correct medicine for administration and be aware of its action, risks, interactions and potential side effects. If you are unsure about this, you must seek further information using reputable sources of information such as the British National Formulary (BNF) or the Electronic Medicines Compendium.

3. Right time
   Timing of medicines is carefully considered to ensure maximum therapeutic effect and to moderate any interactions or side effects. It is paramount that all medicines are given at their specified times according to the PSD. If you are concerned about the timing of medicines, you must seek guidance prior to administration, filling in any documentation (or the PSD) required in line with the advice given. This is to ensure that the required time between doses is clearly maintained.
4. Right dose
   The correct dose of medicine is essential. There may be requirement to select a dose from an indicated range depending on specified clinical features or undertake dose calculations. Being aware of the units of measurement and any calculations required is paramount to ensure safe and accurate medication doses are administered.
5. Right route
   Route of administration affects the action of medicines within the body. Errors in administration routes may pose significant risk to the patient. You must ensure that you are familiar with the routes of administration and that they are clear on the PSD (Routes of administration are discussed in depth in chapter 56).

The 5 Rs above represent a sound base for safe and accountable medicines administration; however, additional Rs have been suggested to further increase safety and promote accountability in practice. These include, but are not limited to: right documentation, right history and assessment, right approach and the right to refuse, right drug-drug interaction and evaluation, right education and information, right reason (for administration) and right response. Careful consideration of all of these will increase patient safety and ensure accountable and responsible practice: specific focus should be paid to the core 5 Rs and should not be substituted out, but possibly added to.

Chapter 56 of this text provides further detail concerning the administration of medicines.

Touch Point

Nursing associates must only administer medicines following the PSD or medicines administration chart; this includes GSL, P and POM medicines.

Some medication may require additional actions to be taken either pre- or post-administration. This may include, for example, ensuring vital signs (blood pressure, pulse, oxygen saturation) are within a specified range prior to administration or post administration actions are required (e.g. specific monitoring post administration or body positioning).

Professional accountability extends past the actual physical process of administration, to the wider knowledge and clinical decision making both pre- and post-administration. Patient education may be required in relation to what the medicine is for, what its desired effects are, or what side effect it may have. Discussion of how the patient may manage or report these should be considered and what follow-up actions are required.

It is essential that all documentation and any required reports to an appropriate health professional are both timely and accurate.

Covert Medication

Covert medication administration is when medicines are given in a disguised format without the knowledge or consent of the patient (Care Quality Commission 2019). This is not a process that is to be undertaken without careful and thorough consideration of the wider healthcare team. In order for medication to be given covertly, the patient needs to have been deemed as lacking capacity to make decisions pertaining to that medication and that the medication is essential to their health. It is not a 'quick fix' or undertaken without strict guidance. Employers should have specific policies in place relating to covert medicines administration, and it is essential that you seek guidance around the nursing associate's role in this process and if you are allowed to give medicines covertly in your organisation as well as specific clinical setting. Any consideration of covert administration of medicines should be carefully care planned for the individual patient and medicines in accordance with the MCA (2005). These plans should include: who is involved and responsible for the decisions, advice and guidance from the prescriber about the medication (e.g. consideration of discontinuation), details of the best interest decision meeting in which covert medication administration was agreed, which medicines can be given covertly and specific instructions of how the medicines will be given (following pharmacist advice) (NICE 2017, 2019).

It is paramount that nursing associates receive clearly documented authorisation, specific training and instructions regarding their role in covert administration of medicines. If permitted to administer medicines covertly, the nursing associate must always follow the care plans and administration instructions for each medicine, as disguising medicines in food or drinks (for example) may change their mode of action in the body. As such, pharmacy guidance is paramount to maintain safety and therapeutic action of the medicines involved.

Orange Flag

Covert medicines should only be administered following the formal assessment of capacity and a best interest decision meeting in accordance with the Mental Capacity Act (2005). The covert administration of medicines should follow a clearly documented process, which is patient and medicine specific. This plan should be made in partnership with the care provider, prescriber, pharmacist and consider who can administer medicines covertly, which medicines should be administered covertly and how they are to be administered.

If you are involved in covert administration, you are professionally accountable for having a sound knowledge of the patient's individual covert medicines care plan prior to administration, as with any other medicine administration.

Routes of Administration and Adverse Effects

With the range of routes of administration allowed by nursing associates, it is essential that consideration is given to how adverse reactions could present. The nursing associate is accountable for their knowledge base and clinical competence and as such should understand that both the mechanism of administration and the pharmaceutical properties of the medicine itself may cause adverse reactions. The mechanisms and processes associated with each mode of administration are discussed further in chapter 56.

Take Note

Adverse reactions may occur due to

1. The action of the medication
2. The route of administration

The nursing associate must have an awareness of both of these to administer medication safely and effectively.

Adverse reactions may present in a number of different ways: local presentations such as inflammation or irritation of the site of administration, systemic reactions due to the action of the medication, or more unspecified presentations that may not be easily identified as being due to the medication such delirium (a new change in awareness or attention: often called acute confusion) in an acutely unwell person and following the commencement of a new medication.

Enteral Administration

Enteral routes of administration include all routes of administration that involved the gastrointestinal tract (most commonly oral, buccal, sublingual, rectal and through specially placed tubes such as nasogastric or jejunostomy tubes). The PSD/medication administration chart must make explicit which route is to be used and any special considerations regarding medication preparation, feed discontinuation or flushing requirements pre- and post-medication administration if it is via enteral tube access.

Commonly, enteral administration refers to administration via a specific administration tube into the gastrointestinal tract.

Oral

The oral route of administration may be most familiar to the nursing associate and involved the patient swallowing medicine in a variety of forms (e.g. tablets, capsules or liquids). The importance here is to note the medicine is swallowed and as such, absorption does not occur in the mouth (this is different in sublingual or buccal administration in which the sites of administration are specific regions within the mouth itself). The nursing associate must ensure prior to administration that the oral form of medicine is suitable for the patient (e.g. ensuring swallow is not impaired or checking patient confidence in taking tablets) and that the correct form of medicine is administered. Many oral medicines have special preparation coatings, which will be indicated on the PSD/administration chart. Such coatings alter the site of absorption (e.g. enteric coating is used to prevent absorption in the stomach–this may be abbreviated to EC). In addition, medicines may be coated or formulated to delay absorption in relation to time (modified release or continuous release analgesics). Any preparation considerations should be clearly documented on the prescription chart; any abbreviations should be standardised and clearly understood and indicated on the medication packet. If there is any uncertainty regarding medication preparation, the nursing associate should seek further advice from a registrant or the prescriber.

Oral medications are systemically absorbed, but vary greatly in their desired and undesired effects. As such the nursing associate must know (as with any medicine) the medicine's common side effects or potential adverse effects prior to administration and the appropriate actions to take if an effect is seen.

Red Flag

The nursing associate must differentiate between **oral**, **sublingual** and **buccal** routes of administration. Whilst all commence with the oral cavity (mouth), the routes of administration are different due to the location of absorption.

The nursing associate must ensure that they are permitted to give medicines via the sublingual or buccal route and have received appropriate training and acquired competence prior to administration. This may be an extended role, or outside the scope of the nursing associate role and practice.

Sublingual and Buccal

Sublingual (under the tongue) and buccal (against the cheek) administration is used for rapid absorption into the systemic circulation due to the readily available supply of blood and lymphatic vessels in the mouth (oral cavity). Whilst rapid absorption may be beneficial, local effects may be felt, such as tingling with glyceryl trinitrate (GTN), and patients may find it uncomfortable to keep a tablet in place whilst it is being absorbed (Aronson 2009). It would be prudent to visualise the oral cavity prior to buccal or sublingual administration to check for ulcers or broken skin and discuss any concerns with positioning or administration of medicines if present. In addition, loose fitting dentures could cause potential complications such as a risk of medication becoming trapped in or under the denture. Drug-related adverse effects or side effects may present due to the pharmacodynamics of the medicine, such as headache, dizziness or nausea caused by the action of GTN.

Rectal

The rectal route may be used when the oral route is not available, due to the medicine itself (such as wanting to bypass the effect on the stomach or small intestine) or when the desired effect is localised to the rectum. As with sublingual and buccal routes, absorption is into the systemic circulation (Aronson 2009). Local adverse effects may be seen following administration including discomfort, itching or expulsion of the medication prior to absorption or desired effect. Adverse effects may be medication specific: rectal GTN administration may cause the same adverse effects as sublingual GTN due to the nature of the medicine.

The rectal route of administration may cause additional distress or concern for the patient due to the personal nature of the route. The nursing associate must employ respectful, clear and empathetic communication to ensure patient comfort, privacy and dignity is maintained. This is particularly pertinent when gathering information on the medication effect and supporting the patient through the required absorption time (such as with enema administration). The nursing associate is responsible for documenting and escalating any failure of treatment (such as with early expulsion of enemas or suppositories) or reporting local adverse effects (e.g. pain, itching or bleeding at the rectum) as well as completion of administration and the desired effects.

Blue Flag

Nursing associates must foster a therapeutic and trusting professional relationship with the patient to ensure that medication administration via the rectal route is conducted in a sensitive manner and appropriate support is given when discussing any adverse events or side effects associated with this route.

Parenteral Administration

Parenteral administration takes place via any route that does not use the gastrointestinal system. For nursing associates, this includes topical, inhalation, subcutaneous and intramuscular injections. Registered nurses and other suitably trained healthcare professionals may use intravenous methods of parental administration.

Commonly, the term 'parental administration' is used to signify intravenous administration via specially placed access lines and is outside the normal scope of the nursing associate.

Subcutaneous Injection

Subcutaneous injections are used when the oral route is not appropriate (e.g. the patient is unable to swallow or has nausea or vomiting) or due to the nature of the medication and desired effect. The subcutaneous route allows slower absorption into the systemic circulation through injection, infusion or implantation of medicines. Adverse effects may be localised to the injection site such as pain, bruising or haematoma around heparin injection sites, or lipodystrophies (a disorder of the adipose tissue caused by insulin). This may present locally as visible changes in fat distribution around injection sites (either fat loss, or fatty swellings (Tsadik et al. 2018)) or can sometimes be identified by fluctuations in blood glucose readings due to altered absorption rates caused by the changes in tissue. Changes in insulin have reduced the incidence of lipodystrophy but the nursing associate may still be aware of them and may consider their presence when choosing an injection site.

Supporting Evidence

The British National Formulary: Online resource of medicines information (also available in print version) https://bnf.nice.org.uk/

The Mental Capacity Act: A brief summary provided by the NHS https://www.nhs.uk/conditions/social-care-and-support-guide/making-decisions-for-someone-else/mental-capacity-act/

Conclusion

The NMC provides standards that must be met by any nurse, midwife or nursing associate who wishes their name to be entered on to the professional register that are known as proficiencies. This chapter has addressed the key issues associated with accountability in ensuring that medicines are administered safely. The nursing associate is responsible and accountable for maintaining safe and effective practice. This accountability is highlighted in the NMC's Code of Conduct (NMC 2018a).

References

Aronson, J. (2009) Routes of drug administration: uses and adverse effects. Part 2: sublingual, buccal, rectal and some other routes, *Adverse Drug Reaction Bulletin*, 254: 975-978.

Care Quality Commission. (2019) *Administering medicines covertly.* [online] Available: https://www.cqc.org.uk/guidance-providers/adult-social-care/administering-medicines-covertly. Accessed 26 October 2019.

Health Education England. (2017) *Advisory guidance: administration of medicines by nursing associates* [Online], Health Education England. [online] Available: https://www.hee.nhs.uk/sites/default/files/documents/Advisory%20guidance%20-%20administration%20of%20medicines%20by%20nursing%20associates.pdf. Accessed 9 October 2019.

Health Education England. (2017) *Nursing associate curricula framework*, England: Health Education England.

Joint Formulary Committee. (2019) *British national formulary: how to use BNF publications online [Online]*, London: Joint Formulary Committee. [online] Available: https://bnf.nice.org.uk/about/how-to-use-bnf-publications-online.html. Accessed 2019.

Jones, N. (2019) Documentation, in Peate, I. (ed.) *Learning to care: the nursing associate*, London: Elsevier.

Medicines And Healthcare Products Regulatory Agency. (2009) *Paracetamol 500mg tablets (paracetamol) PL31308/0007-9 UK public assessment report [Online]*, Medications and Healthcare products Regulatory Agency. [online] Available: http://www.mhra.gov.uk/home/groups/par/documents/websiteresources/con071056.pdf. Accessed 17 September 2019.

Meechan-Rodgers, R. and Paget, K. (2019) Medicines management and administration, in Elcock, K., Wright, W., Newcombe, P. & Everett, F. (eds.) *Essentials of nursing adults*, London: Sage.

Mental Capacity Act, C. (2005) *Mental capacity act.* [online] Available: http://www.legislation.gov.uk/ukpga/2005/9/part/1/data.pdf. Accessed 26 October 2019.

Misuse Of Drugs Act. (1971) *C38.* [online] Available: http://www.legislation.gov.uk/ukpga/1971/38/data.pdf. Accessed 26 October 2019.

National Institute For Health And Care Excellence (NICE). (2017) *Managing medicines for adults receiving social care in the community [Online], National institute for health and care excellence.* [online] Available: https://www.nice.org.uk/guidance/NG67/chapter/Recommendations#giving-medicines-to-people-without-their-knowledge-covert-administration. Accessed 29 October 2019.

National Institute for Health and Care Excellence (NICE). (2018) *Decision-making and mental capacity NG 108.* [online] Available: https://www.nice.org.uk/guidance/NG108. Accessed 14 September 2020.

National Institute for Health and Care Excellence (NICE). (2019) *Giving medicines covertly: A quick guide for care home managers and home care managers providing medicines support.* [online] Available: https://www.nice.org.uk/about/nice-communities/social-care/quick-guides/giving-medicines-covertly. Accessed 14 September 2020.

Nursing and Midwifery Council (NMC). (2018a) *The code: professional standards of practice and behaviour for nurses, midwives and nursing associates [Online]*, The Nursing and Midwifery Council. [online] Available: https://www.nmc.org.uk/standards/code/. Accessed 20 September 2019.

Nursing and Midwifery Council (NMC). (2018b) *Standards of proficiency for nursing associates [Online]*, Nursing and Midwifery Council. [online] Available: https://www.nmc.org.uk/standards/code/. Accessed 20 September 2019.

Royal College of Nursing. (2019) *Patient specific directions (PSDs) and patient group directions (PGDs).* [Online] Available: https://www.rcn.org.uk/clinical-topics/medicines-management/patient-specific-directions-and-patient-group-directions. Accessed 26 October 2019.

The Medicines Act. (1968) [online] Available: http://www.legislation.gov.uk/ukpga/1968/67/contents. Accessed 26 October 2019.

Tsadik, A.G., Atey, T.M., Nedi, T., Fantahun, B. and Feyissa, M. (2018) Effect of insulin-induced lipodystrophy on glycemic control among children and adolescents with diabetes in Tikur Anbessa specialized hospital, Addis Ababa, Ethiopia, *Journal of Diabetes Research, para* 2.

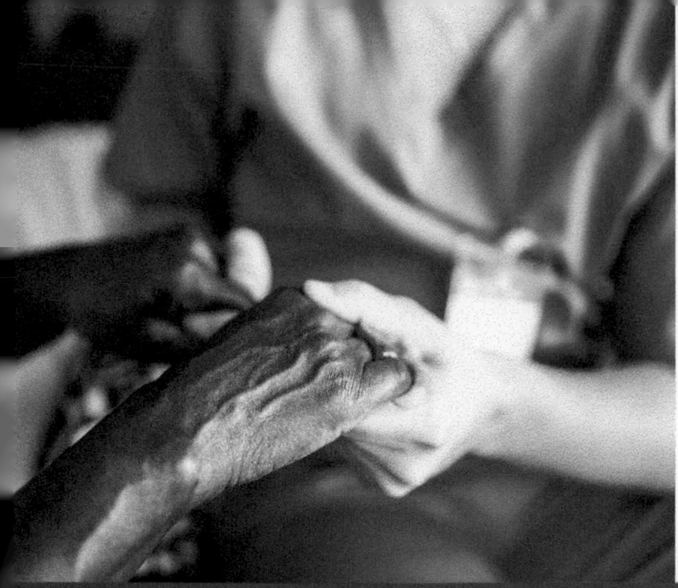

56

Administering Medicines

Tom Walvin

University of Plymouth, UK

Chapter Aim

- This chapter aims to provide the reader with an overview of the safe administration of medicine.

Learning Outcomes

- Understand the principles underpinning the administration of medicines.
- Discuss the five rights of medication administration.
- Maintain medication safety practices.
- Understand the nursing associate's scope of practice.

Test Yourself Multiple Choice Questions

1. Who is accountable for the administration of a drug which has been prescribed?
   A) The prescribing doctor
   B) The person administering the medication
   C) The patient's consultant
   D) The ward manager
2. What are the minimum number of 'rights' or checks should be considered before administering a medication?
   A) 2
   B) 3
   C) 5
   D) 10

The Nursing Associate's Handbook of Clinical Skills, First Edition. Edited by Ian Peate.

Companion website: www.wiley.com/nursingassociate

3. **If a medication is prescribed to be given 'PO', what does this mean?**
   A) **In the rectum**
   B) **In the morning**
   C) **Before bed**
   D) **In the mouth**
4. **Decontamination of the skin should be performed before giving any injection?**
   A) **Yes**
   B) **No**
   C) **Follow the employer's policy**
   D) **Make your own choice**
5. **Does using a spacer with an inhaler make the inhaler more effective?**
   A) **Yes, but only in children**
   B) **Yes, for all ages**
   C) **No, not at all**
   D) **It depends on the type of inhaler**

Introduction

Medicines administration historically is a key procedure that registered nurses have always performed and certainly within the hospital ward environment is a procedure that registered nurses undertake regularly throughout the shift. The extent and role the nursing associate plays in administering medications is determined by the employer; however, the nursing associate curriculum requires trainee nursing associates to be trained, educated and to demonstrate competence in safe and timely drug administration, medicines management and drug calculations, so that they can be delegated to perform these roles (Health Education England 2017).

One of the key drivers for nursing associates to become registrants with the Nursing and Midwifery Council (NMC) was in regard to their role in medicines administration (Health Education England 2017). Although administration of medicines may be viewed as a 'task to be completed' by healthcare workers, the reason registration is so important to a role in administering medications is its link to patient safety.

To safely administer medications, the registrant needs to be accountable for their actions, demonstrate a working knowledge of the drug's action on the body, therapeutic doses and side effects (Baillie 2014). The NMC (2018a) requires the nursing associate to demonstrate proficiency in relation to the procedural competencies that are required for administering medicines safely. This needs to combined with knowledge of the patient, disease process and ongoing assessment of the patient – remember, a drug prescription is written for the patient at the time they required the drug, but the patient's condition or situation may change; it is the role of registered nurses and nursing associates administering drugs to identify if the drug remains safe and suitable to administer.

Administering medicines is an important element of professional practice and must never seem solely a mechanistic task to be undertaken in strict deference with the written prescription. It requires thought and the use of professional judgement. There are a number of other chapters within the text that refer to, or are closely related to, the administration of medicines. Chapter 42, for example, discusses the management of inhalation, humidification and nebuliser devices.

Take Note

Drug administration is not the simple task of giving out medication following a prescription. You need to understand the medication and appropriate dose being given, within the context of the patient's health and other medications and treatments being given. The person administering the drug is accountable for its safe administration, regardless of the prescription.

Green Flag

The NMC Code of Conduct (NMC 2018b) Section 18 is specifically related to drug administration:

Section 18: Advise on, prescribe, supply, dispense or administer medicines within the limits of your training and competence, the law, our guidance and other relevant policies, guidance and regulations.

18.1 – You must prescribe, advise on or provide medicines or treatment, including repeat prescriptions (only if you are suitably qualified), if you have enough knowledge of that person's health and are satisfied that the medicines or treatment serve that person's health need.

18.3 – You must make sure that the care or treatment you advise, prescribe, supply, dispense or administer for each person is compatible with any other care or treatment they are receiving, including (where possible), over-the-counter medicines.

Touch Point

In summary, the NMC Code of Conduct (NMC 2018b) holds nursing associates to account for their decisions to administer or withhold medications. You must ensure you have sufficient knowledge of the patient's current health and ensure medications administered are safe to administer in the context of other medications prescribed and administered.

Safe Drug Administration

Safe drug administration can be aided by utilising the 'five rights of drug administration' as check before administering a medication:

- The Right Patient
- The Right Medication
- The Right Dose
- The Right Route
- The Right Time

However, it is noted that whilst these steps may help improve patient safety, they do not offer a guarantee of safe drug administration as there may be other organisational or system failures that can contribute to drug errors (Jones & Treiber 2018).

The Right Patient

It is crucial that the prescribed medication is administered to the correct patient. The prescription (drug) chart (or any other form of direction to administer) must clearly indicate the patient's full name, hospital number and date of birth as a minimum. Prior to administering any medication, compare the patient's full name, hospital number and date of birth on the prescription (drug) chart against:

1. The patient's identity wristband
2. The patient's verbal confirmation of their name and date of birth
   (Hastings 2009)

Where a patient may not be able to communicate verbally, confirming the identity carefully against the wristband carries importance.

Violet Flag

Administration of medications may take place in community settings such as a patient's own home, nursing homes, care homes or sheltered care environments. Patients in these settings will not wear identity bands and the nursing associate administering medications will need to take additional care to identify patients when administering medications. Best practice is to always identify the patient by at least two forms of identification (e.g. full name and date of birth) against the prescription or other direction to administer. Services in such community settings will likely have a drug administration policy detailing exact procedures which the nursing associate must know. Examples include:

- Confirming the name and date of birth with the patient directly
- Confirming the name and date of birth with a relative if the patient's condition is such that they are unable to confirm or likely to agree if their name is suggested
- Use of patient photographs (which must be kept to date)
- Confirming the identity with care staff who may have been working long-term with the patient

Mortell (2019) recognises that the 'five rights' do not include a check of the patient's known allergies; and as part of a case study involving the administration of antibiotics to a patient who was known to be allergic, suggests that additional sixth right: 'right known allergy status'. This can again be confirmed by a visual check of the patient's drug chart where allergies should have been recorded on admission; and a verbal confirmation of allergies from the patient where possible.

Some health care providers may choose to use red wristbands to further identify patient allergies; however, Ismail et al. (2008) identified in their study that wristbands for identification of allergies were not always used effectively, and consequently, this cannot be used alone as a reliable method.

The Right Medication

Administration of incorrect medication is the cause of up to a third of medication errors (Elliot & Liu 2010). Consequently, when administering medication, the registrant must be absolutely sure the drug selected for administration matches the drug that has been prescribed. Drugs normally have a 'generic name' as well as a 'brand name', therefore, be cautious. The person administering must also be sure the medicine is appropriate for that patient (Dougherty et al. 2015) at the time of drug administration, and therefore knowledge and assessment of the patient's condition is necessary. If the medication does not appear appropriate for the patient's condition, or there is now a contraindication the drug should be withheld, the reason documented and the prescriber contacted immediately.

The Royal Pharmaceutical Council (2019) directs that the prescription should be also checked for any ambiguity and ensure it meets legal requirements; and in any case that it does not, the prescriber should be contacted without delay.

The Right Dose

Many drugs come in a range of doses depending on the extent of treatment that is required. Therefore, it is important that if the nursing associate is not familiar with the dose, it must be checked for accuracy.

This can be achieved by using the British National Formulary (BNF), which provides information regarding uses, cautions, contraindications, side-effects, doses and costs (Joint Formulary Committee 2019). The BNF, however, does not contain information about the pharmacology of the medication and as such, accessing appropriate resources regarding the pharmacokinetics and pharmacodynamics is important to help understand how the drugs work.

Table 56.1 Abbreviations for the most common medicine administration routes.

ABBREVIATION	MEANING
PO	By mouth
IM	Intramuscular
SC	Subcutaneous
IV	Intravenous
PR	Via the rectum
PV	Via the vagina
SL	Sublingual (under the tongue)
Neb.	Via nebuliser
Inh.	Inhaler
Top.	Topical (applied to skin)

Table 56.2 Some abbreviations used on prescription charts and their meanings.

ABBREVIATION	MEANING
OD	Once a day
BD	Twice a day
TDS	Three times a day
QDS	Four times a day
OM	In the morning
ON	At night

Take additional care where decimal places and/or abbreviations are used in a prescription as these can lead to errors in calculations and administration of drugs. It is now recommended that prescribers try not to use decimal places and write concentrations of drugs in full (e.g. milligrams instead of mg) (World Health Organization (WHO) N.D). Drugs which require a complex calculation to achieve the dose may need second checking by an appropriately qualified person (Baillie 2014). Chapter 54 of this text discusses drug calculations.

The Right Route

The rate of absorption of a drug, or the onset of action, varies between different routes (Elliot & Liu 2019), and consequently, it is important that the registrant administers the medication via the prescribed route to ensure accurate and safe administration of the medication.

Although it is recommended that abbreviations are not used in prescriptions, the most common abbreviations indicating different routes of administration can be found in Table 56.1.

The Right Time

Regularly prescribed medications will be indicated for administration at intervals throughout the day if more than one dose is administered. The nursing associate must ensure that the drug is administered at the correct times to ensure the intervals between the doses are appropriate. This is normally to ensure that the concentration of the medication remains at the appropriate therapeutic level for the patient, so it is important to ensure that timing is adhered to.

Prescription charts will normally specify the exact time for administration; however, common abbreviations exist regarding frequency of administration, see Table 56.2.

Touch Point

Use of the five rights of drug administration aid the safe administration of medications. The five rights of drug administration are:

1. The Right Patient
2. The Right Medication (Drug)
3. The Right Dose
4. The Right Route
5. The Right Time

The person administering the drug must have sufficient knowledge about the medication and the patient's health in order to make safe decisions about drug administration. It may be appropriate to withhold a drug if it is believed to be unsafe to administer, even if it has been prescribed.

Administration of Oral Medication

Medication administered orally may come in different forms which can be seen in Table 56.3.

Oral medications offer the advantage that they are easy and practical for patients to take and therefore more convenient. No additional equipment or procedural knowledge is required as may be the case with other routes (e.g. injectable mediations) and as such it is more economical (Ruiz & Montoto 2018).

Table 56.3 Types of oral medications.

TYPE	EXPLANATION
Tablets	Tablets come in various shapes, sizes and coatings. Many will be a simple white compressed powder. Some tablets having a sugar coating, providing a more appealing colour. 'Enteric coated' medications are used for drugs which may cause gastric irritation; 'modified-release' or other such terms mean the medication will gradually break down and release the medication.
Capsules	Capsules are made of a hard gelatine, broken down by gastric acid to release the medication inside.
Elixir, syrups and linctus	These are liquid preparations, containing the active ingredient (the drug) mixed with sugars or alcohols. They are often sweetened or flavoured.
Suspensions and emulsions	These are two chemicals or liquids combined together to ensure thorough distribution of the active ingredient through the mixture. These medications need to be mixed well by shaking the bottle before administration, ensuring an even mix throughout the drug to be sure the correct dose by volume is achieved.
Sublingual and buccal medication	Sublingual medications are tablets or sprays placed under the tongue for absorption. Buccal medications are normally dissolving tablets placed between the gum and lips. These medications are normally rapidly acting (see Figure 56.1)

Source: Baillie (2014); Dougherty et al. (2015); Aschenbenner & Venebal (2009).

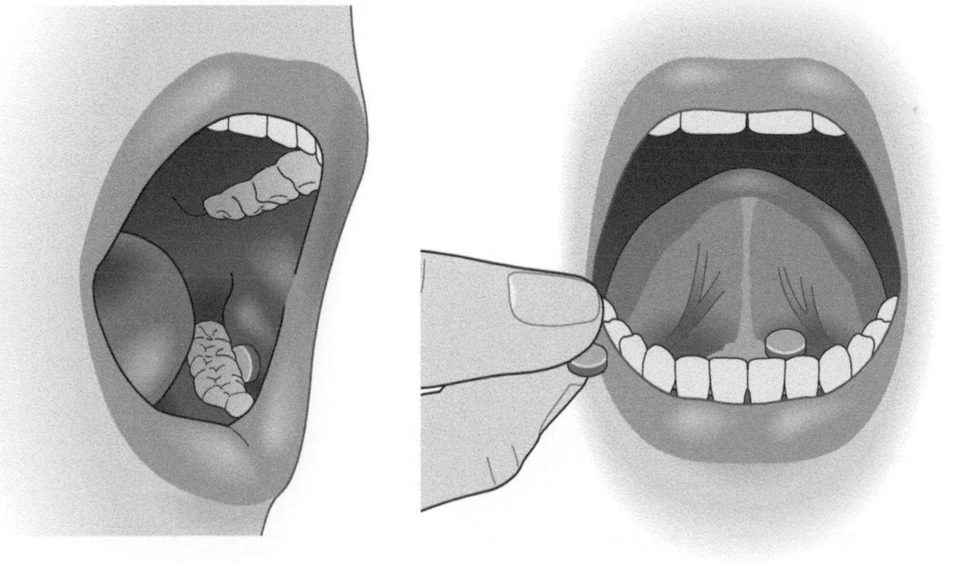

Figure 56.1 Sublingual and buccal routes. ***Source:*** **Peate & Wild (2017), figures 19.8 and 19.9, p. 389.**

Oral routes are slower acting as they must first pass through the digestive system before being broken down into smaller components that can be absorbed into the blood via the intestines and therefore, not useful for medications, which need to be quick acting. Tablets must not be crushed, and capsules must not be opened, as this could change the action and absorption of the medication, as well as altering any protective covering or slow-release formula.

Take Note

Whole tablets and capsules are designed for drug administration via the human digestive system and may be adapted to break down or absorb in a specific part or gradually over time. Altering tablets by cutting or crushing may make the medication ineffective or work too rapidly or produce intended side effects.

Green Flag

Administering a medication that has been altered or crushed means that the medication is being administered differently to its licence. The person administering the medication then becomes legally responsible for that medication's effects. Always seek the written authorisation of the prescriber and/or pharmacist prior to altering or crushing medication.

Preparing for Oral Drug Administration

Oral medications will normally be the most common form of drug. It is, therefore, important to take care when administering these drugs, especially in cases where you might be familiar with the common medications administered and with the patients you have administered medication to before. Lapses in concentration are the most common reported unsafe acts in drug administration (Keers et al. 2013).

Medications required may be found in a common place such as a store cupboard or drug trolley; increasingly hospital pharmacies dispense 'patient's own' medications to increase safety and monitoring of medications. The patient's prescription (drug) chart should be consulted and the appropriate medication taken out for administration. The details on the medication box or bottle label should be checked against the prescription; and the expiry date also checked. You should also check any foils inside medication boxes to make sure the foil pack matches the medication box and prescribed medication.

Hand hygiene must be performed prior to dispensing any medication. Gloves are not required for oral drug administration (WHO 2009).

If administering tablets or capsules, use a 'non-touch technique' to remove the required number of tablets/capsules from a bottle, into a medicine pot. Tablets/capsules in a foil blister pack can be pushed through the foil from the underside of the packaging directly into the medicine pot.

If administering liquids with a syringe, a specially coloured and labelled oral medication syringe must be used as a visual aid to prevent inadvertent intravenous (IV) administration (National Patient Safety Agency 2006). Measuring pots may also be available; however, the Joint Formulary Committee (2012) suggests that syringes should be used to measure quantities other than 5 mL in order to ensure accuracy.

Supporting Evidence

National Patient Safety Agency – Patient Safety Alert 2017/19

This national alert required the introduction of coloured, labelled oral medication syringes following the IV administration of oral liquid medication resulting in multiple patient harm, deaths and near misses between 1997 and 2006.

Administration Considerations

Perform hand hygiene prior to administering any medications. Consider the patient's position; they should preferably be sitting upright to receive the oral medication. Complete a safe patient ID check against the drug chart as described earlier, even if you have administered medication to the patient previously. Check known allergies on the drug chart and verbally with the patient. Identify any medications on the chart that have a specific medication requirement (e.g. must be administered with food) and ensure these administration conditions are met.

Ensure the patient has a glass of water to swallow tablets with prior to administering the first tablet. Assess the patient's ability to administer the medications themselves directly from the medicines pot; otherwise use a spoon to administer the medication to the patient (Baillie 2014) (Chapter 53 of this text considers the patient's ability to administer their own medicines). The patient has a right to informed consent; therefore, check the patient's knowledge of the medication and provide education if needed.

After Administration

Remain with the patient to ensure that all oral medications administered have been taken. The prescription (drug) chart should only be signed once the patient has been observed to take the medication to prevent inaccurate recording of medications administered. The patient should be assessed to ensure the medication has been effective and to observe any self-effects (Baillie 2014).

Administration of Topical Medication

Topical medications are medications that are applied to the skin. There a vast range of different topical medications, some of the most common types are explained in Table 56.4.

Table 56.4 Types of topical medications.

TYPE	EXPLANATION
Creams	Creams are a preparation of medication with oil (such as petrolatum) with a water base; allowing the medication to be applied and spread over the required skin area.
Ointments	Ointments are very similar to creams; except the preparation of the medicine is mixed with water with an oil base. Consequently, ointments tend to be oilier and greasier when applied.
Lotions	Lotions are similar to creams and ointments, with droplets of oil mixed in water; but are much less thicker than creams and ointments allowing it to absorb into the skin more quickly.
Powder	Powders can be the pure form of the medication itself; or the medication mixed with another substance such as corn starch.
Transdermal patch	Transdermal patches are stuck to the skin in a similar way to a plaster or sticky dressing. They contain medication within the patch and normally release the medication gradually, absorbed through the skin. Transdermal patches normally have a 'time' which they are effective for and therefore need replacing at the end of this time period.

Topical medications are absorbed through the skin into the small capillaries; and then enter the systemic circulation via these capillaries. For many patients, it may well be likely that they are able to administer their own topical medications. However, if the medication is being administered by somebody else, it is important that gloves are worn to prevent inadvertent contact with the skin of the person administering; or in the case of powders, care should be taken not to inhale (Doyle & McCutcheon 2012). Doughety et al. (2015) suggest that topical creams and solutions should be applied to skin using a sterile topical swab. Transdermal patches should never be applied to broken or irritated skin as this can cause further irritation, nor should they be applied to scarred or hard skin as absorption may not be satisfactory (Hastings 2009).

Take Note

Topical medications are absorbed into the blood supply through the skin or mucous membranes. Care should be taken if administered to a patient to prevent inadvertent self-administration.

Administration of Injections

There are a number of different injection routes; this chapter will focus on subcutaneous and intramuscular injections. Medicines injected subcutaneously are injected into the hypodermis; the fatty layer of the skin constructed of adipose and connective tissues. Intramuscular injections are much deeper; given directly into a suitable muscle in the body.

Injections offer some advantages over administration by other routes. Injected medications are generally faster in their action because they reach the systemic circulation faster than in oral medications. Similarly, medications that can be rendered ineffective due to the action of the digestive system can be injected. Injectable routes are also useful for patients who are unable to swallow or who are nil-by-mouth.

Subcutaneous (SC) Injections

Subcutaneous injections are administered into the more 'fatty' areas of the body commonly:

- The abdomen
- Upper hips
- Upper back
- Outer upper arms
- Thighs

(Hastings 2009).

See Figure 56.2 highlights various sites that may be used for subcutaneous injections.

Because subcutaneous tissue does not have a rich blood supply, absorption of medication by this route is slower than intramuscular injection. Subcutaneous injections are limited to a volume of 0.5 mL–1 mL (Rushing 2004). Some sources, however, indicate up to 2 mL is acceptable.

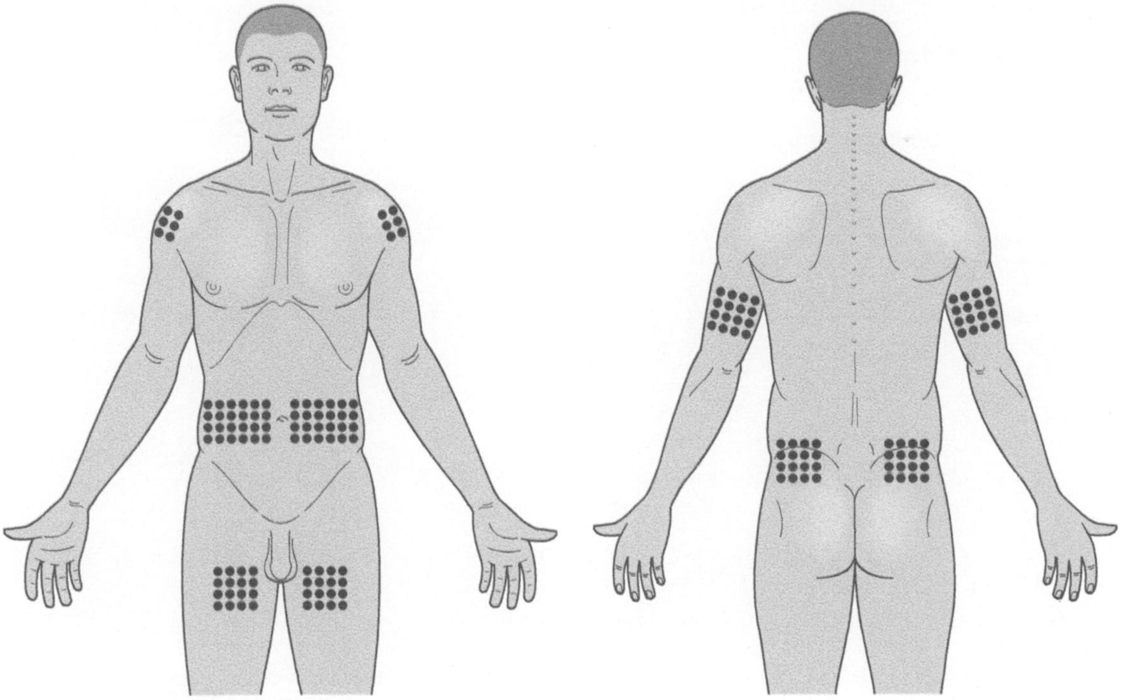

Figure 56.2 Subcutaneous injection sites. ***Source:*** **Peate & Wild (2017), figure 19.14, p. 392.**

Due to lack of rich blood supply in the subcutaneous tissue, routine 'drawing back' of the syringe plunger whilst the needle is in place (aspiration) to check for inadvertent administration into a blood vessel is not required for subcutaneous injections.

In order to ensure that the medication is administered correctly into the subcutaneous layer, the subcutaneous tissue is lifted away from the muscle by use of a gentle 'pinching' action between forefinger and thumb and lifting the subcutaneous tissue upwards. This is often easily achieved using skin folds.

Injectable medications that require drawing up and the use of a separate needle and syringe are inserted into the subcutaneous tissue at a 45-degree angle to the skin. The needle used for subcutaneous injection is normally the 25-gauge 'orange' needle (Shepherd 2018b). However, many regularly used subcutaneous injections, often coming in a pre-filled syringe (examples including insulin pens, or low-molecular-weight heparins such enoxaparin or deltaparin), have an extremely fine small needle requiring the injection to be administered at a 90-degree angle to the skin. Local policy and procedure must be adhered to at all times.

It is also possible to use the subcutaneous route to administer infusions of fluids; commonly used in palliative care or for the elderly, rather than for emergency fluid resuscitation (Doughety et al. 2015). A butterfly needle is inserted subcutaneously at 45 degrees and covered with a transparent dressing (Bowen et al. 2014).

Intramuscular (IM) Injections

Muscles are highly vascular tissues with an excellent blood supply; therefore, intramuscular injections offer a much faster response to the medication being absorbed into the systemic circulation quickly; although slower than with intravenous (IV) administration directly into the bloodstream. The acceptable volumes for administration in intramuscular injections vary depending on the type of muscle used. The most common sites used for intramuscular injections and the maximum volumes are in Table 56.5. See Figures 56.3, 56.4 and 56.5 depicting key issues related to intramuscular injections.

It has been previously taught that once the needle has been inserted into the muscle, before the medication is administered, the person administering should aspirate (pull the syringe plunger back with the needle in place) to check for the presence of blood indicating risk of injection into a vein resulting in accidental intravenous administration. Hettinger and Jurokevic (ND) described that there is no reported evidence

Table 56.5 Intramuscular injection sites.

SITE	LOCATION	MAXIMUM VOLUME
Deltoid	Upper arm	1–2 mL
Ventrogluteal	Hip	3 mL
Dorsogluteal	Upper outer buttock	4 mL
Vastus lateralis	Outer thigh	5 mL
Rectus femoris	Upper thigh	5 mL

Source: modified from Chadwick & Withnell (2015).

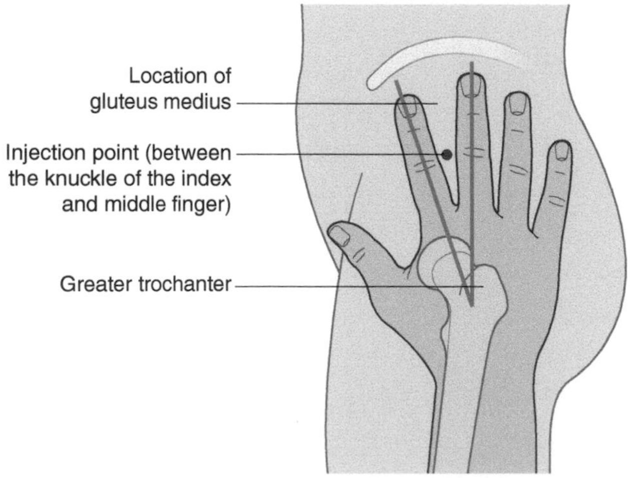

Figure 56.3 Location of the gluteus medius muscle. ***Source:*** **Peate & Wild (2017), figure 19.11, p. 390.**

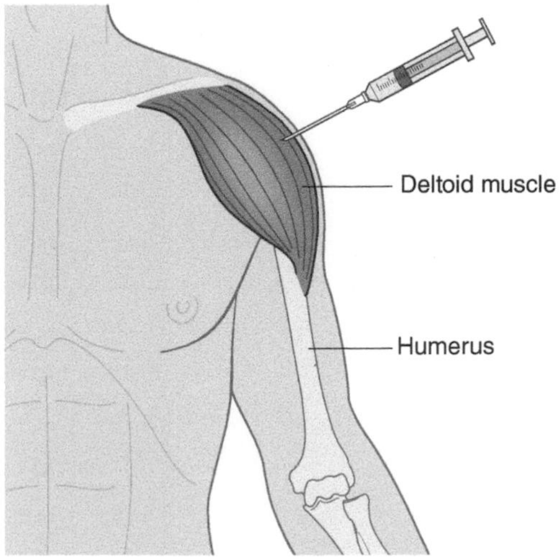

Figure 56.4 Location of the deltoid muscle. ***Source:*** **Peate & Wild (2017), figure 19.12, p. 391.**

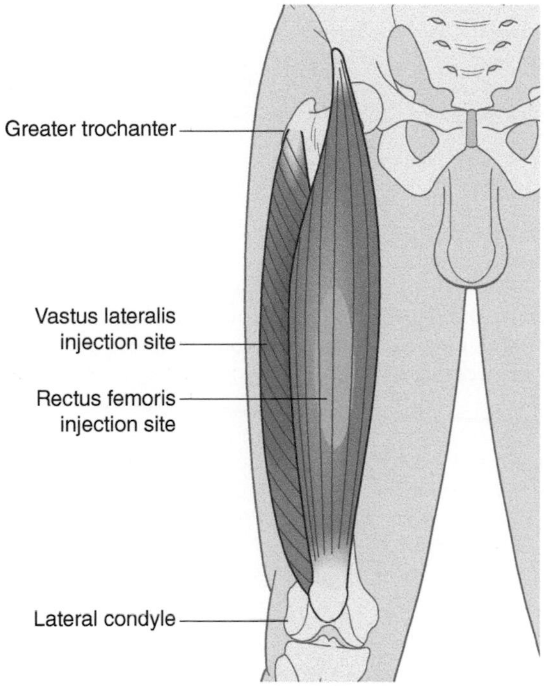

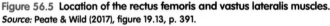

Figure 56.5 Location of the rectus femoris and vastus lateralis muscles. *Source:* Peate & Wild (2017), figure 19.13, p. 391.

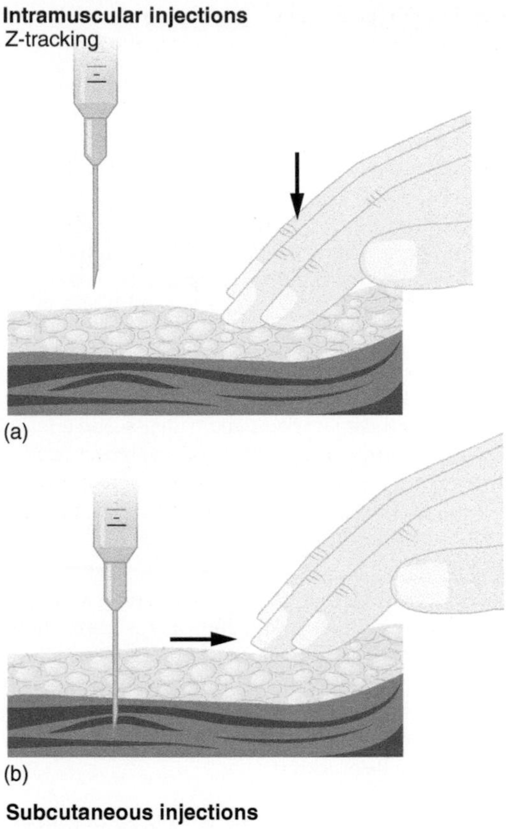

Figure 56.6 Z-track injection technique. *Source:* Lindsay et al. (2018), figures 73.1(a) and (b), p. 152.

that aspiration with or without blood return confirms correct needle placement and further suggests that eliminating aspiration reduces injection duration and injection pain. This is supported by Public Health England (2013) who detail that aspiration is not normally required, with the exception of the dorsogluteal site that is highly vascular and as such, believes there is a risk of accidental intravenous administration. Consequently, aspiration at the ventrogluteal, deltoid and vastus lateralis sites are not recommended as they are not in close proximity to blood vessel or nerves.

Muscles are much deeper than the subcutaneous layer; therefore, a larger needle size is required. The 21G 'green' needle is used for intramuscular injections in most patients; however, the person administering the injection must assess the size and musculature of the patient, in some cases, a smaller needle (often the 23G 'blue' needle) may be required if the person has smaller or atrophied muscle.

When administering the intramuscular injection, it should be administered at a 90-degree angle to the skin and a 'dart-like' movement using the dominant hand to insert the needle deeply into the muscle (Chadwick & Withnell 2015).

The skin should be 'stretched' between forefinger and thumb to reduce the layer of subcutaneous tissue with the injection inserted in the gap between them. However, the 'Z-track technique' is often recommended because it prevents the backflow of injected medication into the subcutaneous tissue by 'sealing in' the injected medication in the muscle by the production of a zig-zag path rather than a direct straight path into the muscle (Pullen 2005). The effect of backflow of medication into the subcutaneous tissue is irritation and discomfort.

The Z-track technique is achieved by the person administering the medication applying their thumb to the patient's skin and displacing the skin. This brings the subcutaneous skin out of alignment with the muscle and then the tension is released, the layers return to normal closing the needle track (Hastings 2009) (see Figure 56.6).

It is important to develop competence in intramuscular injection as poor technique can increase pain, bleeding, formation of abscesses, infection, muscle fibrosis and injuries to nerves or blood vessels (Shepherd 2018a).

Yellow Flag

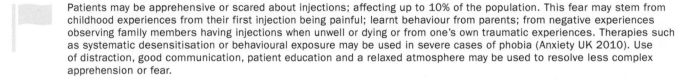

Patients may be apprehensive or scared about injections; affecting up to 10% of the population. This fear may stem from childhood experiences from their first injection being painful; learnt behaviour from parents; from negative experiences observing family members having injections when unwell or dying or from one's own traumatic experiences. Therapies such as systematic desensitisation or behavioural exposure may be used in severe cases of phobia (Anxiety UK 2010). Use of distraction, good communication, patient education and a relaxed atmosphere may be used to resolve less complex apprehension or fear.

Other Injection Considerations

Skin preparation

Research into the need to undertake alcohol-based decontamination of the skin has not reached a consensus. Studies performed by Dann (1969) on more than 5000 participants found that there was no case of local or systemic infection caused by intramuscular injections.

Recent publications appear to lean towards social cleanliness being sufficient to prevent infection, suggesting that dirty, soiled skin does require cleaning prior to an intramuscular injection, but this can be achieved using soap and water (Scottish Centre for Infection and Environmental Health 2015; Vaccine Administration Taskforce 2001). However, assessment of the patient's current health status is crucial; where a patient is recognised to be immunocompromised, skin decontamination is still recommended (Royal College of Paediatrics and Child Health (2002). The nursing associate, when administering injections, however, must follow workplace policy; many workplace policies indicate that alcohol-based decontamination is expected.

Use of gloves

There also remains debate around the use of wearing non-sterile gloves whilst administering injections. The World Health Organisation (WHO) (2010) states that gloves are not required to be worn when administering routine intradermal, subcutaneous and intramuscular injections, where both the healthcare worker's and patient's skin are healthy and intact. The WHO (2010) also states that wearing gloves does not reduce risk of transmission from a needlestick injury; however, Din & Tidley (2014) describe how gloves may have a 'wiping' effect on a used needle potentially reducing the risk of transmission. There is no consensus found in this area; subsequently, the practitioner should make an evidence-informed choice about wearing gloves for injections, in conjunction with local workplace policy.

Needlestick injury

It is essential that when administering an injection, a sharps box is taken to the patient so that the needle can be immediately disposed of once withdrawn from the patient: 'skin to bin'. Sharps boxes should be sealed once reaching the indicated fill line and never be allowed to overflow beyond that line. Many workplaces now use 'safety needles' in which a protective cover can be applied over the sharp end of the needle once removed from the patient, reducing the risk of a needlestick injury; this however, does not mean the risk is no longer present and should still be disposed of immediately. Even with protective measures and education in place, needlestick injuries will inevitably occur. If you do have a needlestick injury, follow these actions:

1. Remove the needle quickly
2. Encourage the wound to bleed
3. Place the wound under running water and clean with plenty of soap
4. Cover with a dressing or plaster
5. Contact your workplaces' occupational health department; or attend the nearest Emergency Department

Do not scrub or suck the wound site (National Health Service 2018).

> **Touch Point**
>
> Injections offer advantages and disadvantages over oral medication. The main routes of injection are subcutaneous and intramuscular. Subcutaneous routes are slower and more suitable for medicines needing a slow uptake; intramuscular injections absorb quicker and suit conditions where a faster onset of action is required. Always be careful when handling sharps; always take a sharps bin to the patient. Follow you employer's policy regarding skin decontamination and wearing gloves.

Administration of Inhaled Medications

Inhaled medications come in two forms – inhalers and nebulisers. Chapter 42 of this text discusses in more detail the use of inhalers and nebuliser devices.

The most commonly encountered inhaler will be 'metered dose' inhaler, a plastic device containing a pressurised canister that releases the dose of medication as an aerosol, which is inhaled by the patient. Inhalers may also be 'dry powder inhalers' where the dose is delivered as dry powder either stored in the inhaler device or obtained via the insertion of a capsule that is pierced by the inhaler before use and then the contents inhaled. A spacer should be used for child and adults wherever possible as this increases the effectiveness of the inhaled medication.

Nebulisers use the flow of air or oxygen from its source to break up medication liquid into minute droplets suspended within the air or oxygen, which is then inhaled into the lungs. This occurs in the specialised 'nebuliser chamber' device attached to an oxygen mask or mouth piece.

Inhaled medications are used primarily for the treatment of respiratory conditions. The advantage with this route is that medications can be absorbed directly in the respiratory system where they are required to work (Baillie 2014).

Take Note

Inhaled medications such as inhalers and nebulisers are suitable for treatment of respiratory disease as the medication can directly reach the respiratory system. Patients need good education and ongoing supervision to make sure they are effectively receiving the medication.

Administration of Rectal Medications

Suppositories and enemas are the most common forms of medication given rectally. In both cases, the medication can be used to manage a local issue/condition in the rectum itself (such as constipation); or as medication is easily absorbed into the bloodstream in the rectum, systemically acting medications can be given effectively this way too (such as analgesia). A suppository is medicine in a solid form, normally in a 'bullet' shape with a waxy texture, which dissolves rapidly at body temperature promoting the local affect or absorbing quickly into the bloodstream for a systemic affect. An enema, however, is a liquid form of medication, which is introduced into the rectum and similarly can have a local or systemic affect.

Yellow Flag

Patients often are fearful and embarrassed about medicines delivered via the rectum. It is important to assess the suitability of the rectal route before administration; and if required, educating the patients about the benefit of the route is helpful. The patient will need to expose their buttocks and anus for this route, therefore, maintaining privacy and dignity is absolutely essential – provide blankets, draw curtains, ensure a commode is available next to the bed, minimise the number of people nearby.

Suppositories

Suppositories are commonly used for the management of constipation either by softening the stool by encouraging more water into the bowel and providing lubrication or by stimulating bowel movement. Suppositories in other forms of medication such as steroids and analgesia can be administered for their systemic effect taking advantage of rapid absorption into the blood supply.

Before administering a suppository, informed consent must be obtained. There are few risks in suppository administration, however; assessing the risk and maintaining caution is advised in patients who have had rectal or lower colon surgery, gynaecological surgery or radiotherapy, or any known or observed abnormality of the perianal region (Higgins 2007). Note that the patient may prefer to self-administer their suppository, in which case they will need to be offered advice regarding the procedure before they perform it.

The patient should lie down on their left side with knees flexed upwards towards the chest with buttocks near the edge of the bed (the nursing associate may be required to assist the patient in order to assume this position), allowing ease of administration of the suppository into the rectum as the normal anatomy of the colon can be followed; this will ultimately reduce discomfort as the suppository is pushed through the anal sphincter (Dougherty et al. 2015).

To prepare the suppository, the end of the suppository should be lubricated with an appropriate lubricating gel. There is some disagreement as to what 'end' of the suppository should be lubricated with some suggesting that the blunt end should be lubricated and inserted first to reduce anal irritation and increase retention of the suppository (Mitchell 2019). The other option is to first lubricate and then insert rounded, pointed end of the suppository. Baillie (2014) recommends following the manufacturer's advice or adhering to the employer's policy.

An incontinence sheet should be placed underneath the patient. Prior to administration, a digital rectal examination (DRE) should be performed (Royal College of Nursing 2019). This confirms that the patient has constipation and the location of stool. Where stool is present, the suppository should be moved around the side of the stool as to be in contact with the mucosa rather than embedded in the stool which would be ineffective (Baillie 2014). If the suppository is for constipation and no stool is found, the suppository should not be administered (Peate 2015).

When the suppository is administered, a lubricated index finger is used to gently push the suppository past the anus and into the rectum. The full length of the index finger is required to achieve this (Mitchell 2019). Following insertion, the process should be repeated if a second suppository is prescribed; otherwise, ensure the patient is left clean in anal and buttock areas. Ensure the patient is left with a bedpan, commode or call-bell as appropriate. Hand hygiene should be performed both prior to administration and after administration.

Enema

Enemas are administered for the same reasons described for a suppository, although the effect of an enema is often more immediate, especially in regard to the management of constipation. Some enemas are designed to be retained by the patient for longer, ensuring full evacuation of the bowel prior to procedures or investigations of the bowel. Some enemas also deliver medication, for example, the delivery of steroids to reduce inflammation in the mucosa of the colon.

Many of the same contraindications and cautions for suppositories are the same, for example recent bowel or gynaecological surgery. Additionally, enemas should be not administered to patients with a paralytic ileus, where the normal peristaltic movement of the bowel is lost (Higgins 2006).

Preparation of the procedure is also similar. Hand hygiene should be performed prior to administration; inform the patient about the procedure and obtain informed consent; place an incontinence sheet under the patient; complete a DRE if not already done so. Administration of cold enema liquid into the bowel causes cramping; therefore, the solution should be warmed. Higgins (2007) suggests a temperature of 40.5–43.3 degrees Celsius.

The enema will come with a long nozzle-like structure above the liquid, which should be inserted into the patient's anus. The cap should be removed, and the tip and sides of the nozzle lubricated prior to insertion. Gently lift the patient's uppermost buttock in order to visualise the anus. The nozzle should penetrate the anus slowly and smoothly towards the direction of the umbilicus whilst the patient is instructed to breathe deeply through the mouth, relaxing the anal sphincter (Rushing 2003). The nozzle should be inserted to approximately 10 centimetres in adults (Higgins 2007). The enema liquid should then be squeezed from the base of the enema container upwards preventing backflow. Once complete, slowly remove from the patient. Ensure that a commode or bedpan is immediately available to the patient; or they are positioned near to a toilet.

Take Note

Suppositories and enemas contain medications administered rectally. They are commonly used to provide treatment for constipation; although they may also contain medications such as steroids or analgesia. Rectal administration can be uncomfortable and embarrassing for patients; care needs to be taken to ensure privacy and dignity. Patients should always be near a toilet, commode or use a bedpan and given a call bell as the effects of rectal medications can occur quickly. Procedures to administer are similar, but there are some major differences in administration techniques and onset of action.

Conclusion

There are a wide range of different routes of medicine administration available; all routes offer advantages and disadvantages. The processes of ensuring safe patient identity checks and drug administration remain the same; however, the nursing associate when administering medication, must be able to demonstrate proficiency when administering medication by any route.

References

Anxiety UK. (2010) *Injection phobia and needle phobia: a brief guide*, Manchester: Anxiety UK.

Aschenbenner, D. and Venable, S. (2009) *Drug therapy in nursing* (3rd edn), London: Wolters Kluwer.

Baillie, L. (ed.). (2014) *Developing practical nursing skills* (4th edn), Oxon: CRC Press.

Lindsay, P., Bagness, C. and Peate. I. (eds) (2018) *Midwifery skills at a glance*, UK: Wiley-Blackwell.

Bowen, P., Mansfield, A. and King, H. (2014) Using subcutaneous fluids in end-of-life care, *Nursing Times*, 110(40): 12–14.

Chadwick, A. and Withnell, N. (2015) How to administer intramuscular injections, *Nursing Standard*, 30(8): 36–39

Dann, T. (1969) Routine skin preparation before an injection: an unnecessary procedure, *The Lancet*, 2: 96–97.

Din, S. and Tidley, M. (2014) Needlestick fluid transmission through surgical gloves of the same thickness, *Occupational Medicine*, 64(1): 39–44.

Dougherty, L., Lister, S. and West-oram, A. (2006) *The royal Marsden manual of clinical procedures* (9th edn), Chichester: Wiley-Blackwell.

Doyle, G. and McCutcheon, J. (2012) *Clinical procedures for safer patient care*. [online] Available: https://opentextbc.ca/clinicalskills/. Accessed 25 November 2019.

Elliot, M. and Liu, Y. (2010) The nine rights of medication administration: an overview, *British Journal of Nursing*, 19(5): 300–305.

Hastings, M. (ed.). (2009) *Clinical skills made incredibly easy*, London: Wolters Kluwer.

Health Education England. (2017) *Advisory guidance: administration of medication by nursing associates*, Leeds: Health Education England.

Hettinger and Jurokevic. (ND) *Evidence based injection technique: to aspirate or not to aspirate*, Sanford Health.

Higgins, D. (2006) How to administer an enema, *Nursing Times*, 102(20): 24.

Higgins, D. (2007) Bowel care part 6 – Administration of a suppository, *Nursing Times*, 103(47): 26–27.

Ismail, Z., Ismail, T. and Wilson, A. (2008) Improving safety for patients with allergies: an intervention for improving allergy documentation, *Clinical Governance: An International Journal*, 13(2): 86–94.

Joint Formulary Committee. (2019) *British national formulary* (78th edn), London: BMJ Group and Pharmaceutical Press.

Jones, J. and Treiber, L. (2018) Nurse's rights of medication administration: including authority with accountability and responsibility, *Nurse Forum*, 2018(53): 299–303.

Keers, R., Williams, S., Cooke, J. and Ashcroft, D. (2018) Causes of medication administration errors in hospitals: a systematic review of quantitative and qualitative evidence, *Drug Safety*, 36(11): 1045–1067.

Mitchell, A. (2019) *Administering suppositories: how to, care of, monitoring, reporting: at a glance*. [online] Available: https://repository.uwl.ac.uk/id/eprint/6049/1/Mitchell_BJON_2019_Administering_a_suppository_types%2C_considerations_and_procedure.docx. Accessed 6 December 2019.

Mortell, M. (2019) Should known allergy status be included as a medication administration 'right'? *British Journal of Nursing*, 28(20): 1292–1298.

National Health Service. (2018) *What should I do if I hurt myself with a used needle?* [online] Available: https://www.nhs.uk/common-health-questions/accidents-first-aid-and-treatments/what-should-i-do-if-i-injure-myself-with-a-used-needle/. Accessed 5 December 2019.

National Patient Safety Agency. (2007) *Patient safety alert: promoting safer measurement and administration of liquid medicines via oral or other enteral routes*, National Patient Safety Agency: London

Nursing and Midwifery Council (NMC). (2018a) The code, *Professional standards of practice and behaviour for nurses, midwives and nursing associates*. [online] Available: https://www.nmc.org.uk/globalassets/sitedocuments/nmc-publications/nmc-code.pdf. Accessed December 2019.

Nursing and Midwifery Council (NMC). (2018b) *Standards for pre-registration nursing associate programmes*. [online] Available: https://www.nmc.org.uk/standards/standards-for-nursing-associates/standards-for-pre-registration-nursing-associate-programmes/. Accessed December 2019.

Peate, I. (2015) How to administer suppositories, *Nursing Standard*, (30)1. 34–36.

Peate, I. and Wild, K. (2017) *Nursing practice. knowledge and care* (2nd edn), UK: Wiley Blackwell.

Public Health England. (2013) *Immunisation procedures: the green book*, London: Public Health England.

Pullen, R. (2005) Administer medication using the Z-Track method, *Nursing*, (35)7: 24.

Royal College of Nursing. (2019) *Bowel care: management of lower bowel dysfunction, including digital rectal examination and digital removal of faeces*, London: Royal College of Nursing.

Royal College of Paediatrics and Child Health. (2002) *Position on statement of injection technique*, London: Royal College of Paediatrics and Child Health.

Royal Pharmaceutical Society. (2019) *Professional guidance on administration of medicines in healthcare settings*, Royal Pharmaceutical Society: London.

Ruiz, M. and Montoto, S. (2018) Routes of drug administration: dosage, design and pharmacotherapy success, in Talevi, A. and Quiroga, P. (eds.) *ADME processes in pharmaceutical sciences*, Switzerland: Springer, 97–113.

Rushing, J. (2003) Administering an enema to an adult, *Nursing*, (33)11: 28.

Rushing, J. (2004) How to administer a subcutaneous injection, *Nursing*, (34)6: 32.

Scottish Centre for Infection and Environmental Health. (2015) *Skin disinfection: a review of the literature.* [online] Available: https://www.documents.hps.scot.nhs.uk/hai/infection-control/publications/skin-disinfection-review.pdf. Accessed 5 December 2019.
Shepherd, E. (2018a) Injection technique 1: administering drugs via the intramuscular route, *Nursing Times*, 114(8): 23–25.
Shepherd, E. (2018b) Injection technique 2: administering drugs via the subcutaneous route, *Nursing Times,* 114(9): 55–57.
Vaccine Administration Taskforce. (2001) *UK Guidance on best practice in vaccine administration,* London: Sherwell Publications.
World Health Organization. (2009) *Glove use information leaflet*, Geneva: World Health Organisation.
World Health Organization. (2010) *WHO best practices for injections and related procedures toolkit*, Geneva: World Health Organization.
World Health Organization. (ND) *Guide to good prescribing: a practical manual*, Geneva: World Health Organization.

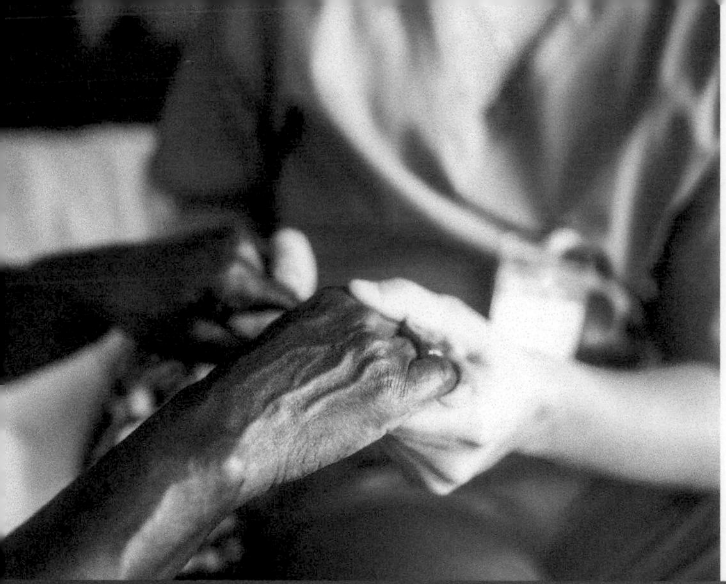

57

Managing the Effectiveness of Symptom Relief Medications

Dominic Simpson

Northumbria University, UK

Chapter Aim

- **This chapter aims to introduce the reader to the importance of measuring the effectiveness of symptom relief medications.**

Learning Outcomes

- **Recognise the importance of understanding symptom relief.**
- **Understand the difference between a symptom and a sign.**
- **Interpret why managing the effectiveness of medication is important to the role of a nursing associate.**

Test Yourself Multiple Choice Questions

1. **When is a symptom considered to be chronic?**
   A) **A symptom lasting longer than a week**
   B) **A symptom lasting longer than a month**
   C) **A symptom lasting longer than six months**
   D) **A symptom that is related to a chronic condition**
2. **When patients describe their symptoms this should be considered as what?**
   A) **Objective data**
   B) **Subjective data**
3. **Select the correct definition of; the therapeutic window of drug administration:**
   A) **The specific time frame in which a drug should be given**
   B) **The range of drug dosages which can treat symptoms/disease effectively without becoming toxic**
   C) **An evidence-based guideline for safe drug administration**
   D) **A mindfulness activity to reduce pharmaceutical burden within acute care**

The Nursing Associate's Handbook of Clinical Skills, First Edition. Edited by Ian Peate.

Companion website: www.wiley.com/nursingassociate

4. **Which of the following would not form part of your questioning when trying to understand a patient's symptom?**
   A) **Site**
   B) **Severity**
   C) **Relieving factors**
   D) **Past medical history**
5. **The systematic problem-solving approach towards providing individualised care is known as:**
   A) **The nursing care plan**
   B) **The Health and Social Care Act**
   C) **The nursing process**
   D) **Nurses Practice Act**

Introduction

Symptom relief and symptom control can mean many things. This chapter provides an overall discussion concerning the ways in which the nursing associate can contribute to managing the effectiveness of symptom relief. In this chapter pain is discussed as a symptom and the measures taken to review and reassess efficacy of interventions. The Nursing and Midwifery Council (2018a, 2018b) require nursing associates to manage and monitor effectiveness of symptom relief medication as well as ensuring that they evaluate the quality of their work and also that of the team.

Difference Between a Sign and a Symptom

Before understanding the management of symptom relief, it is important to understand what a symptom is. Often the terms 'sign' and 'symptom' are used interchangeably; however, it is important to note that the two are different. A sign of illness is something which is objective; for example hypotension could be a sign of illness; this is something that can be observed, measured and quantified. Patients suffering with hypotension may be nauseous; therefore, nausea is a symptom of hypotension. In contrast to this a symptom is something that is subjective as it can only be perceived by the patient experiencing the symptom. Examples of symptoms of illness include pain, fatigue and anxiety (Peate 2019). A symptom should be regarded as a physical or mental feature, which is indicating a condition or disease (Knapp 2018). This chapter will focus on understanding the effectiveness of symptom relief only.

Three main types of symptoms are outlined in Table 57.1.

Some conditions show no symptoms at all. For example, a person could have hypertension for years without knowing. Some cancers have no symptoms until the later, more aggressive stages. These are known as *asymptomatic conditions*, and even though the idea of symptoms is often linked to discomfort or abnormal function, a condition without symptoms can be deadly.

As a nursing associate, it is important that you consider the presenting complaint of the patient. You will need to ask some questions to understand your patient's symptom(s) further; this is known as the history of the presenting complaint; an example of this is shown in Table 57.2.

Table 57.1 Types of symptoms.

TYPE OF SYMPTOMS	DESCRIPTION
Remitting symptoms	When symptoms improve or resolve completely, they are known as *remitting symptoms*. For example, symptoms of the common cold may occur for several days and then resolve without treatment.
Chronic symptoms	These are long-lasting or recurrent symptoms, typically lasting longer than six months. Chronic symptoms are often seen in ongoing conditions, such as diabetes mellitus, asthma or cancer.
Relapsing symptoms	These are symptoms that have occurred in the past, resolved and then returned. For instance, symptoms of depression may not occur for years at a time but can then return.

Table 57.2 Understanding a patient's presenting history of a symptom.

PRESENTING COMPLAINT	SHORTNESS OF BREATH.
Further details of complaint	Duration: ½ hour. Onset: Patient was walking up the stairs at the time. Site: Central chest. Severity of pain: 4 out of 10 Character: Tightness in chest. Precipitating factors: Came on with exertion. Relieving factors: Improved with use of an inhaler and rest. Previous similar symptoms: Has happened several times before.
Effects of the symptom on the patient's life	Impacts on the patients' ability to carry out usual activities of living, unable to walk long distances/upstairs.

As a nursing associate, it is your responsibility to find out about a patient's symptom(s) to ensure you can properly treat them; to do this you should ask about:

- The site – Where is the symptom originating.
- Duration – How long has the symptom been affecting the patient.
- Onset – When did it start, was the patient carrying out a particular task at the time.
- Severity – For example, you could ask patient to score pain on a scale of 1–10.
- Character – What are the features of the symptom, is it dull/sharp etc.
- Precipitating factors – What makes it worse.
- Relieving factors – What makes it better.

Red Flag

Whenever reviewing a patient's symptoms, it is important to consider what is the underlying pathology causing these symptoms, is this being caused by a potentially life-threatening condition. A tool to aid your decision-making in this is NEWS2 (Royal College of Physicians 2017); see, for example, Chapter 6 in this book. If unsure, refer to a senior colleague.

Take Note

As a nursing associate, using the appropriate approach, you will need to identify and support the management of a range of commonly encountered physical and non-physical symptoms, including:

- Pain, nausea and vomiting
- Dehydration
- Restlessness
- Agitation
- Mood swings
- Anxiety
- Breathlessness
- Pyrexia and hypothermia
- Skin rashes and itching
- Fatigue
- Insomnia
- Angina

The NMC standards of proficiency (NMC 2018a, 2018b) make it a requirement that you assist with monitoring the above symptoms, observing and reporting signs of improvement or deterioration and escalate any concerns.

Nursing Process

As a nursing associate when managing symptoms, it is recommended to utilise the nursing process (Barrett et al. 2019). Understanding what symptom(s) are affecting the patient you are caring for is the initial step in the nursing process. This involves the systematic and continuous collection of data; sorting, analysing and organising that data; and the documentation and communication of the data collected. Critical thinking skills applied during the nursing process, provide a decision-making framework to develop and guide a plan of care for the patient incorporating evidence-based practice concepts. This concept of precision education to tailor care based on an individual's unique cultural, spiritual and physical needs, rather than a trial-by-error, one-size-fits-all approach, results in a more favourable outcome (Allen et al. 2018; Dunham & MacInnes 2018).

Yellow Flag

The nursing associate (NMC 2018b) has a duty to ensure that the person's unique needs – physical, spiritual and cultural – are taken into account when determining if symptom control has been effective.

There are five steps associated with the nursing process:

- **Assessment:** Utilising some of the methods discussed earlier, you will use your clinical decision-making skills to identify the presenting complaint. You may need to use a number of different tools to accurately make a holistic assessment as well as utilising the skills of other practitioners. While nursing associates contribute to most aspects of care, including delivery and monitoring, registered nurses will take the lead on assessment, planning and evaluation, managing and coordinating care with full contribution from the nursing associate within the integrated care team.
- **Nursing diagnosis:** This is different from the medical diagnosis that focuses on disease; the nursing diagnosis aims to focus on the human need associated with illness/symptoms. You will utilise data and information collected in the assessment phase to understand how the symptoms of this complaint are impacting upon the patient.
- **Planning:** This phase is conducted in partnership with the patient (and if appropriate the family) and the multi-disciplinary team; as a nursing associate, you will help to prioritise identified needs, being mindful of keeping safety and patient comfort as top priorities. This stage involves setting realistic goals, such as the patient may want to be pain free. When setting goals, it is useful to ensure that these are S.M.A.R.T., meaning they are:
  - *Specific*, being direct, detailed and meaningful
  - *Measurable*, how is this quantifiable? How will you know that intended treatment has been effective?
  - *Attainable,* is it realistic and achievable?
  - *Relevant,* does the proposed outcome link with the patients wants/needs?
  - *Time-Based,* what is the time frame for achieving this goal?
- **Intervention:** This phase of the nursing process involves implementing the planned treatment. While being mindful that assessment is a continuous, ongoing part of the patient care. During the course of any prescribed interventions, as a nursing associate, you will need to seek advice about making clinical decisions regarding how to proceed based upon data collected. Medications such as anti-hypertensive or cardiac drugs may require specific assessments prior to intervention, for example, measuring blood pressure or recording a pulse rate.
- **Evaluation:** This final step of the nursing process is vital to a positive patient outcome. After any intervention or treatment you are required to reassess or evaluate. This is important in determining if the goal of the treatment has been achieved and if the patient feels that the desired outcome has been met. Reassessment may frequently be needed depending upon overall patient condition. The plan of care may be adapted based on new assessment data. Evaluation is key to ascertain if symptoms have been relieved.

Take Note

The nursing associate requires specific skills related to the review and re-assessment of symptoms and the use of medications/interventions as treatment plans. They include the following elements:

- Understanding and following the correct procedures, as guided by local and national policy, for checking if a medication is appropriate for the patient.
- Understanding and following correct procedures for the administration of medications.
- Understanding how to identify and minimise risks associated medication administration.

Therapeutic Effect

When administering medication with the intention of symptom relief, for example, the administration of analgesia to relieve pain, it is important to consider the therapeutic effect, or therapeutic window of that specific drug. Therapeutic window of drug administration is defined as the range of drug dosages that can treat symptoms/disease effectively without becoming toxic (Kim et al. 2018). When a drug is administered, there will be a lag period while the drug is absorbed. When the drug begins to relieve symptoms, this is the onset of the effect and the drug plasma concentration (Cp) is within the therapeutic window.

A drug will reach its peak effect when the maximum amount of that drug has been absorbed into the bloodstream; as the drug is metabolised, the Cp will reduce and eventually drop below the therapeutic range. When trying to relieve patients' symptoms, it may take multiple doses of a drug to maintain Cp within the therapeutic window. For this reason, it is important to continually and systematically reassess patients when managing their symptoms.

Figure 57.1 shows a bell graph demonstrating a typical drug administration; each drug will have a minimum effective concentration (MEC) to be effective at relieving symptoms or treating a condition. there will also be an MEC for adverse responses before a drug becomes toxic. Drug toxicity is when Cp becomes dangerously high.

Green Flag

When administering medication, it is important you are aware of and understand the MEC for effective treatment and the MEC for drug toxicity. In practice you can use the British National Formulary (Joint National Formulary 2019) to guide you in the safe administration of drug dosages.

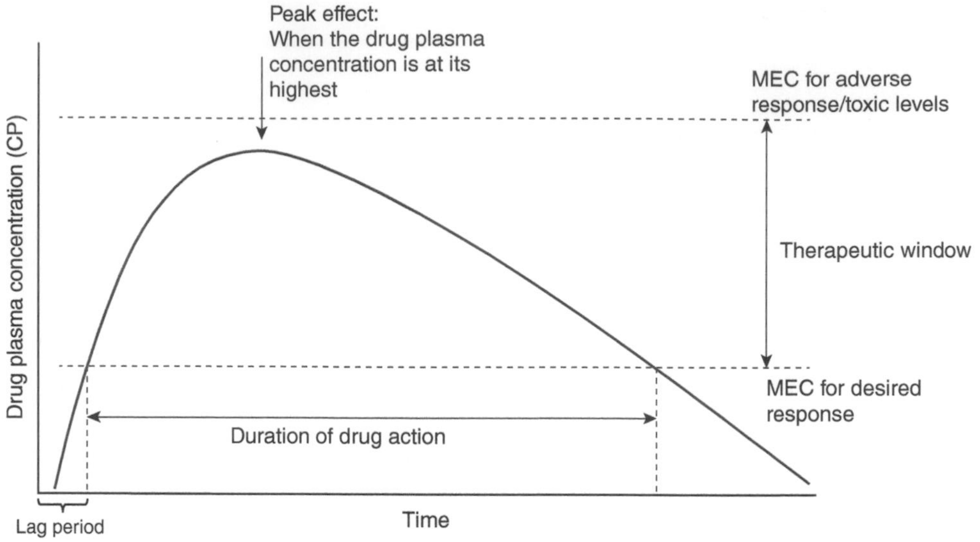

Cp = Drug plasma concentration.
MEC = Minimum effective concentration.

Figure 57.1 **Minimum Effective Concentration.**

The main factors that influence how quickly a drug reaches its therapeutic range are:

- The route of administration
- The rate of absorption
- How the drug is distributed

When administering medication, the overall aim is for the medication to exert its effect within a certain time frame, especially in the case of one-off doses of medication, such as analgesia. As a nursing associate, it is your responsibility monitor and report on its effect.

Duration of Effect

The duration of effect for a drug is the period of time from onset to the time at which sufficient drug has been removed from the body, to render it as therapeutically ineffective. This is largely controlled by hepatic (liver) metabolism and renal (kidney) excretion. It is important to know how long a drug will have optimum efficacy as this dictates the dosing schedules. Drugs need to be administered more than once to have a continued effect. There are some drugs that may need to be administered daily, but some need to be given more often to maintain effective drug action. This can be deduced from the duration of action of the drug.

This aspect of the chapter will now focus on the symptom of pain. The nursing process will be applied as an example of how you might understand and manage the effects of symptom relief for patients.

Green Flag

It is important to note that any treatment offered and care provided should always be underpinned by evidence-based practice and adherence to local policy and procedure within the organisation.

Pain

Many patients may present with pain as a symptom. Pain can be acute, starting suddenly and lasting a short time, or chronic, defined as pain lasting longer than six months, or pain continuing after the tissue has healed (Mankelow et al. 2019). Pain can also be referred, coming from one part of the patient's body but being felt in another (e.g. pain originating in the gall bladder causing the patient to experience shoulder tip pain), or phantom, being felt in a part of the body that has been removed (e.g. the amputation of a digit or a limb). Pain could also be described as total pain which includes emotional, social and spiritual factors that affect a person's experience of pain (Tierney & Gregory 2019). See Table 57.3 for an example of the nursing process as applied to pain.

Table 57.3 The nursing process as applied to pain.

NURSING PROCESS APPLIED TO PAIN		
Assessment	When assessing the patient's pain, it is important to understand the following: site, duration, onset, severity and character. As well as assessing what are the precipitating factors and relieving factors. Younger et al. (2009) provide an overview of evidence-based assessments and techniques for the measurement of pain. Some of them are multi-dimensional (such as the short-form McGill Pain Questionnaire or Brief Pain Inventory); these tools give you the opportunity to fully explore how the symptom of pain is impacting on the patient's life. In practice the most common assessment of pain is a unidimensional scale such as asking patients to score pain on a scale of 1–10. There are some objective measures that can be observed in a patient's assessment, such as a tachycardia. Patient's self-reported pain gives you subjective data; however, this should not be considered less valuable than the objective measure.	**Example:** Patient presents with complaint of pain following plastic surgery for removal of non-malignant melanoma. On assessment, the patient's NEWS2 score is 3 with tachycardia and tachypnoea. The patient scores pain 8 out of 10.
Nursing diagnosis	When formulating a nursing diagnosis for a patient, it is important to understand how this symptom is impacting upon their activities of living. Is this pain chronic or remitting?	Patient unable to properly mobilise due to pain. This is an acute onset of pain post-surgery.
Planning	When planning how to manage the patient's pain, you must set goals that are SMART. How will the patient's pain be managed? Who else needs to be involved in the management of the patient's pain?	S = Reduce pain to a level where the patient can mobilise. M = Measure using the 1–10 scale. A = Achievable with multi-disciplinary team involvement. R = It is relevant to the patient's goal. T = Within 6 hours. Plan to refer to specialist pain team for a prescription of morphine via a patient-controlled analgesia pump, set up and administered by a registered nurse according to local policy.
Intervention	The decided intervention in this instance was to administer morphine via a pump Patient could also be referred to physiotherapists to support mobility post-surgery.	Interventions: • Give break through pain relief (although this could not be opiate based due to Morphine PSA). • Communicate with specialist pain team. • Communicate with physiotherapy team.
Evaluation	This final essential step is required to check back and see if the interventions have been successful, if they have worked, what was it that worked, if it has not worked how can you further support the patient in achieving their goal to be able to mobilise again without pain.	Review pain score using the same tool that was used during the assessment phase, has the reported pain reduced? Have the patient's vital sign observations stabilised and returned to normal?

Conclusion

The aim of this chapter was to highlight important areas of knowledge required to be a registered nursing associate in relation to the management and monitoring of symptom relief medication for your patient(s). Having read this chapter, you will now have a good level of understanding about what a symptom is, how it can be effectively managed utilising the nursing process and how drugs are metabolised within the body to achieve a therapeutic effect.

This chapter has focused primarily on the assessment and measurement of symptoms, for example by using validated tools. It is important that you understand how to use these tools effectively, alongside your clinical decision-making to ensure treatment is effective. You should always seek clarification and further advice from other clinicians should this be needed. The essential step in understanding how effective treatment has been is the evaluation post treatment. It is essential as a nursing associate that you continuously assess patients presenting symptoms to understand if care and treatment have been effective.

References

Allen, E., Williams, A., Jennings, D., Stomski, N., Goucke, R., Toye, C., Slatyer, S., Clarke, T. and McCullough, K. (2018) Revisiting the pain resource nurse role in sustaining evidence-based practice changes for pain assessment and management, *Worldviews Evidence Based Nursing*, 15(5): 368–376.

Barrett, D., Wilson, B. and Woollands, A. (2019) *Care planning: a guide for nurses*, Oxfordshire: Routledge.

Dunham, M. and MacInnes, J. (2018) Relationship of multiple attempts on an admissions examination to early program performance, *Journals of Nurse Education*, 57(10): 578–583.

Joint Formulary Committee. (2019) *British national formulary (online)*, London: BMJ Group and Pharmaceutical Press. [online] Available: www.medicinescomplete.com https://doi.org/10.18578/BNF.525838558. Accessed September 2020.

Kim, P.K., Zhao, P. and Teperman, S. (2018) Evolving treatment strategies for severe *clostridium difficile* colitis: defining the therapeutic window, in Sartelli, M., Bassetti, M. and Martin-Loeches, I. (eds.) *Abdominal sepsis. Hot topics in acute care surgery and trauma*, Switzerland: Springer.

Knapp, T.R. (2018) Symptom: cause, effect, both, or neither? *Clinical Nursing Research*, 27(4): 391–394.

Mankelow, J., Ryan, C., Taylor, P., Simpson, D. and Martin, D. (2019) Effectiveness of pain education to improve pain related knowledge, attitudes and behaviours in health care students and professionals: a systematic review protocol, *International Journal of Therapy and Rehabilitation*, 26(8): 1–8.

Nursing and Midwifery Council (NMC). (2018a) *Standards for pre-registration nursing associate programmes.* [online] Available: https://www.nmc.org.uk/standards/standards-for-nursing-associates/standards-for-pre-registration-nursing-associate-programmes/. Accessed September 2020.

Nursing and Midwifery Council (NMC). (2018b) The code, *Professional standards of practice and behaviour for nurses, midwives and nursing associates.* [online] Available: https://www.nmc.org.uk/globalassets/sitedocuments/nmc-publications/nmc-code.pdf. Accessed September 2020.

Peate, I. (2019) *Learning to care the nursing associate*, Edinburgh: Elsevier.

Royal Colleges of Physicians. (2017) *National early warning score (NEWS) 2.* [online] Available: https://www.rcplondon.ac.uk/projects/outputs/national-early-warning-score-news-2. Accessed September 2020.

Tierney, P. and Gregory, J. (2019) Caring for the acutely ill adult, in Burns, D. (ed.) *Foundations of adult nursing.* London: Sage, pp. 313–360.

Younger, J., McCue, R. and Mackey, S. (2009) Pain outcomes: a brief review of instruments and techniques, *Current Pain and Headache Reports*, 13(1): 39–43. doi:10.1007/s11916-009-0009-x.

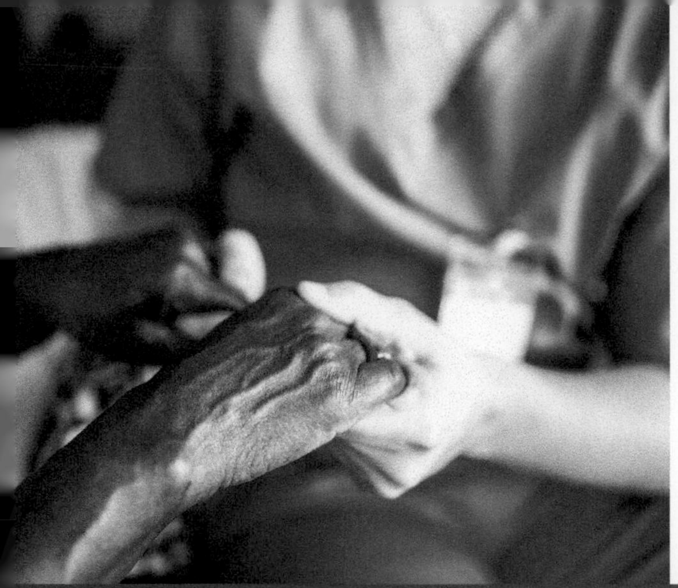

58

Recognising and Responding to Adverse Effects of Medications

Claire Pryor and Carol Wills

Northumbria University, UK

Chapter Aim

- This chapter will highlight the importance of recognising and responding to adverse reactions of medications.

Learning Outcomes

By the end of this chapter, the reader will be able to
- Demonstrate understanding of what an adverse drug reaction is.
- Describe how adverse drug reactions may present.
- Recognise and respond appropriately to adverse drug reactions.

Multiple Choice Questions

1. What is a *safety critical* medication?
   A) Medications that require extra storage considerations
   B) Medications that have time limited use
   C) Medications that carry a higher risk of harm
   D) Medications that need special handing
2. An adverse drug reaction (ADR) is also a type of adverse event.
   A) True
   B) False

The Nursing Associate's Handbook of Clinical Skills, First Edition. Edited by Ian Peate.

Companion website: www.wiley.com/nursingassociate

3. **Select two features of a type A ADR.**
   A) **Is a dose-related reaction**
   B) **Occurs on withdrawal of medication**
   C) **Can be an exaggeration of the drug's normal action**
   D) **Is unexpected**
4. **Select two features of a type B ADR.**
   A) **Is predictable**
   B) **Is related to drug accumulation**
   C) **Is uncommon**
   D) **Is not related to the usual action of the drug**
5. **What colour is the card system used to report adverse drug reactions?**
   A) **Blue**
   B) **Red**
   C) **Orange**
   D) **Yellow**

Introduction

Medications are given with the intention of having a beneficial effect on a persons' health; however, any medication has the potential to produce an adverse, unwanted or unexpected effect or reaction (National Institute for Health and Care Excellence 2019a). Reactions may range from minor side effects to extreme reactions, which may be difficult to predict. It is important, therefore, to understand how medicines work. This may support risk reduction and early recognition of the different types of adverse reactions, and how you should respond to these.

Annex B, section 10 of the Standards of proficiency for nursing associates (Nursing and Midwifery Council 2018b) details procedural competencies required for administering medication safely. Particular attention is paid in this chapter to section 10.9 (recognising and responding to adverse and abnormal reactions to medications including reporting and escalation of concerns) (Nursing and Midwifery Council 2018b). Accountability and safety in medicines administration has been discussed in chapter 55, followed by the process and procedures of medication administration using a variety of routes, detailed in chapter 56.

Platforms in the nursing associate proficiencies

In applying knowledge of recognising and responding to adverse effects of medications, you will practice within:

Platform 1 'Being an accountable professional'
Platform 3 'Provide and monitor care'
Platform 5 'Improving safety and quality of care'

And specifically

Annexe B 'Procedures to be undertaken by the nursing associate'

Adverse events related to medicines can include allergic reactions, drug sensitivities, contraindications and adverse drug reactions (ADRs). Side effects are secondary, often unwanted effects of medication that occur during drug therapy, but are usually predictable, and patients are often advised of them before commending a new medicine. Some medication may be chosen specifically for its side effect action (e.g. mirtazapine use in anorexia due to its known side effect of weight gain) (Leheny 2017).

An ADR may happen immediately or evolve over a long period of time (Ferner & McGettin 2018). It could simply be described as an unpleasant effect, or it could equally be life threatening and require an urgent response to save the person's life. Patients may not associate their symptoms with a medication (Ferner & McGettin 2018). As such, the nursing associate must have an understanding of not only the medication's desired effect, but also potential adverse effects and how to manage these within the scope of their practice. Side effects, contraindications and cautions for medicines can all be found using the British National Formulary (print or online), the Electronic Medicines Compendium (EMC online) as well as accessing both patient information leaflets (PILs) or the summary of product characteristics (SmPCs). PILs are the leaflets that are included in the medication packets for patient use. This information is written specifically to increase patients' understanding of the medication they are taking. SmPCs are written specifically for healthcare professionals and details how the medication acts and how it is to be used.

Touch Point

Make a note of the medicines that are commonly used in your area of practice. Find out the following for each medicine:

- What are the common or very common side effects listed?
- What are the rare or uncommon side effects listed?
- Which of these would require urgent medical attention or discontinuation/change of therapy?

The World Health Organization (WHO) defines an adverse reaction as:

> *'a response to a medicine which is noxious and unintended, and which occurs at doses normally used in man'*
>
> (World Health Organization 2000)

The definition expresses clear relationships between the medication and the unwanted reaction to that medication. In practice, this terminology can often be confused with adverse events. An adverse event is defined as:

> 'any untoward medical occurrence that may appear during treatment with a pharmaceutical product but which does not necessarily have a causal relationship with the treatment'
>
> (World Health Organization 2002)

Adverse reactions are commonly termed ADRs. The differentiation between the two terms is seen in the causal relationships, and the dose indication. ADRs are noted to be directly linked to and caused by a specific medication when used at the intended dose. Adverse events happen during a treatment period. However, they may or may not be caused by medication (just happen in the same timeframe as a medication is being used). In addition, they may be caused by inappropriate dose schedule or other factors that do not relate to the pharmacology of the drug being given. As such, ADRs are classed as a type of adverse event (Schatz & Weber 2015).

Touch Point

An adverse reaction is harmful, occurs with a normal therapeutic dose and is not the response which was intended- it is directly linked to a medicine being used.

ADRs can present with varied severity inclusive of minor, moderate, severe and fatal reactions. In addition, ADRs are categorised from A to D depending on both the nature of the reaction and the timescale. Table 58.1 details the full ADR classification system and gives examples using the guidance determined by the Medicines and Healthcare Products Regulatory Agency (MHRA 2018). Most commonly, ADRs are categorised as type A or type B. Type A reactions (augmented) are seen when a medication is given at the usual therapeutic dose, but the action of the drug is exaggerated. It is important to note that not only the desired action of the drug should be recognised, but also any known undesired actions. Augmented Reactions (Type A ADRs) are the most common type of reaction; in other words, they can be expected from what we know about the pharmacology of the drug and how it works. It is an exaggerated response, which occurs with the normal therapeutic dose of the product. An example of this would be a person taking anti-coagulants to treat or prevent blood clots. Blood clots can be life threatening and can cause a stroke so people susceptible to this may be prescribed an anticoagulant, for example, warfarin (warfarin sodium). These drugs work by making the blood take longer time to clot (some call this thinning the blood), so the person would have frequent blood tests to ensure that the time the blood takes to clot is within safe and therapeutic limits. Expected side effects may include bruising from a relatively minor knock or upset stomach. A Type A reaction, however, would be sudden or severe internal bleeding as a result of taking a normal dose of the drug, for example, vomiting blood or passing blood in faeces. The risk of a serious internal bleed is varied but is said to be around 2% (British Heart Foundation 2019) and requires urgent medical attention. Some Type A adverse reactions can be minimised by reducing the dose of the drug (National Institute for Health and Care Excellence 2017), so a referral back to the prescriber or health professional managing their care is indicated if this is suspected so that they may assess the nature and severity of the reaction and subsequent care.

Type B reactions ('bizarre') are reactions that are unexpected and not predicable in relation to the normal action of the drug ('novel'). These types of reactions are rare in comparison with Type A reactions, but they are life threatening and need fast responses to prevent death. A Type B reaction requires immediate recognition and treatment. These often present as allergic reactions such as skin rashes or anaphylaxis.

Recognising ADRs

Practicing in accordance with the NMC (2018b) Standards of proficiency for nursing associates section 3.15, nursing associates must be able to recognise the effects of medication as well as recognise allergies, drug sensitivity, side effects, contraindications and adverse reactions.

Violet Flag

ADRs can occur in any health or social care setting. In addition to hospital- or clinic-based care, you may be involved in caring for people in the wider community or social care setting: For example in patients' own homes following commencement of a new mediation by the General Practitioner, or reactions to vaccinations in clinic or in their own home.

Community nursing teams who administer specific medications in people's own homes or community settings may carry emergency medication to treat severe reactions (such as anaphylaxis).

No matter what area of care you are involved in, it is paramount that you consider this setting and are aware of the local policy and process for requesting support or emergency care.

Table 58.1 Classification of adverse drug reactions.

TYPE OF ADR	TITLE	FEATURES	EXAMPLE
A	Augmented	• Reaction occurs at normal therapeutic drug dose • Usually dose dependant • Can be an exaggeration of the drugs normal actions	Respiratory depression with opioids
B	Bizarre	• Unexpected/novel reactions • Not expected by the drug action • Often allergic • Medication induced disease	Rash with antibiotics Anaphylaxis
C	Continuing	• Sometimes named 'chronic' • Persists for a long duration	Osteonecrosis of the jaw due to bisphosphonates
D	Delayed	• Do not present initially • Occur sometime after medication use • Some are time critical	Leucopenia presenting up to six weeks post lomustine (a chemotherapy drug) administration
E	End-of-use	• Present after the drug has been stopped/withdrawn	Insomnia following benzodiazepine discontinuation

Source: Medicines and Healthcare Products Regulatory Agency (2018)

Recognising ADRs may appear complex; however, a good understanding of the patient's condition, history and the pharmacokinetic and pharmacodynamic properties of the medicines they take will support timely recognition and appropriate action. As shown in Table 58.1, ADRs may not always present on first administration of medication; subsequent administrations may produce an ADR, or they may present after a considerable amount of time taking the medication. Vigilance in recognising signs or symptoms of potential ADRs is vital. It could be a change in skin colour, shortness of breath, a new skin rash, confusion or a report from the patient feeling non-specifically unwell, or an exaggeration of the desired effect that gives the first cue that an ADR may be present. Whilst it is often the registered nurse or doctor who takes a medication history, patients may offer information to you during your interactions, and appropriate questioning and careful listening may glean important clues and details. The history of taking specific medications, first dose or long-term treatment may assist in categorisation of ADR; additional medications including herbal, supplements or over-the-counter medications is essential as these too may produce ADRs and contribute to potential medication interactions for example.

Previous drug reactions are documented in the patient's notes and medication charts. This should be matched by a patient wristband that clearly identifies what medication has caused the reaction. It is vital that this information is checked and updated when a new reaction is identified.

Touch Point

ADRs do not only occur in prescribed medication (prescription-only medicine or POM). They may be caused by medications bought from shops without any health professional guidance, for example at a garage (known as general sales list product or GSL) or following the guidance of a pharmacist (pharmacist-only medication or P). Additionally, recreational drugs may cause ADRs, and more recently special attention has been placed on vape devices and e-cigarettes.

A number of different factors may influence a person's susceptibility to ADRs including age, gender, pregnancy, ethnicity, the presence of specific diseases and the number of other medications being given (Kaufman 2016). Multiple medicines prescribed to one person is termed polypharmacy (Duerden et al. 2013). Polypharmacy can be both appropriate, if the medications are required and have been carefully optimised, but also problematic when inappropriate prescribing of multiple medications has occurred. The presence of polypharmacy increases the risk of medication interactions and ADRs (Duerden et al. 2013) and requires vigilance in identifying and reporting potential ADRs.

Touch Point

Oxygen is often given in emergency situations and for ongoing care needs. It should be considered as medication and prescribed accordingly (National Institute for Health and Care Excellence 2019b). Oxygen should be included in discussion and notes of prescribed medications (chapter 39, managing the administration of oxygen discusses this further).

Green Flag

Nursing associates must practice within the scope of the NMC Code (Nursing and Midwifery Council 2018a) and the NMC standards of proficiency for nursing associates (Nursing and Midwifery Council 2018b).

The NMC Code 15.1 stipulates that in an emergency you must act in line with your knowledge and competence and arrange for appropriate emergency care access and provision (15.2).

The NMC standards of proficiency for nursing associates stipulate in 10.9 that you must be able to recognise and respond to adverse and abnormal reactions to medications. This includes appropriate escalation of concerns.

Both of the above NMC standards must be adhered to in line with your specific organisational policies, procedures and role responsibilities. Different employers will allow nursing associates to take on different roles and responsibilities. It is paramount that you have a clear understanding of these to allow safe and appropriate practice.

Allergic Reactions

Allergic reactions have both patient- and drug-related risk factors. Having an awareness of medication sensitivities and allergic reactions is vital when providing patient care. Allergies or hypersensitivity occurs due to the body recognising a usually harmless antigen (such as a drug or pollen) and harmful. The immune system overproduces antibodies to the antigen in an attempt to protect the body (Carne & Owen 2019). A severe allergic reaction is caused by a person being exposed to a drug for a second time and which their body has already produced antibodies against. The second exposure triggers an immediate response by the antibodies and mast cells which flood a range of chemicals, including histamine, into the bloodstream and tissues (Carne & Owen 2019). This can occur with any medicine (or indeed non-medicine e.g. food allergy or bee-sting), and so it is extremely important to check for allergies and ensure that any allergies are recorded in the medical notes. There are some medicines, which we know are more likely to trigger allergic reactions; these include antimicrobials (antibiotics), non-steroidal anti-inflammatory drugs (NSAIDS e.g. ibuprofen) and anaesthetic medicines (Resuscitation Council 2008). Some patients may be at increased risk of allergic reactions due to a number of different factors. Some of these are shown in Box 58.1.

An allergic reaction may be immediate, or it may take hours. In an anaphylactic reaction, this can be within 5–60 minutes of the allergen being taken (depending on the route).

Anaphylaxis

Anaphylaxis is a type of allergic reaction. The Resuscitation Council defines anaphylaxis as:

'A severe, life threatening, generalised or systemic hypersensitivity reaction'

(Resuscitation Council UK 2008)

An anaphylactic reaction can result as a hypersensitivity or a severe allergic reaction and is a medical emergency. A review of the data by Turner et al (2015) relating to hospitalised patients in England and Wales over a 20-year period to 2012 with anaphylaxis advises that the incidence of anaphylaxis in the UK is increasing, but the estimated 20 deaths per year has stabilised.

Red Flag

Anaphylaxis is a serious and life threatening allergic reaction. It is rapid in onset and presents with compromise to airway, breathing and circulation. In addition, mucosal and skin changes are often present.

- All patients irrespective of clinical setting should expect:
- Recognition that they are severely unwell
- A prompt and early request for assistance
- Assessment and treatment following the ABCDE process
- Adrenaline therapy if indicated. (Adrenaline is also known as Epinephrine)
- Referral and follow up by an allergy specialist

Source: Resuscitation Council UK (2008).

Box 58.1 Allergic reactions: patient-related risk factors

- Immune status: Previous reaction to the same or related compound.
- Age: Younger adults are more likely to have an allergic reaction than infants or the elderly.
- Gender: Women are more likely than men to suffer skin reactions.
- Genetic: Atopy–a predisposition to developing some allergic reactions. Atopy may have a genetic component.
- Concomitant disease: Some viral infections such as HIV and herpes are associated with increased risk of allergic reactions. Cystic fibrosis is associated with increased risk of allergic reactions to antibiotics.

Source: Dougherty et al. (2015); Mirakian et al. (2008)

A diagnosis of anaphylactic reaction is 'likely if a patient who is exposed to a trigger (allergen) unexpectedly develops a sudden illness (usually within minutes of exposure) with rapidly progressing skin changes and life-threatening airway and/or breathing and/or circulation problems' (Resuscitation Council 2008). The patient will feel and look unwell and can become very anxious.

Rapid in onset, anaphylaxis presents with:

- airway compromise
- difficulty in breathing (bronchospasm with tachypnoea)
- skin and mucosal changes
- problems with the circulatory processes (hypotension and/or tachycardia)

(Resuscitation Council UK 2008; National Institute for Health and Care Excellence 2011).

The two most commonly noted medications in anaphylactic reactions are non-steroidal anti-inflammatory drugs (NSAIDs) and β-lactams (beta-lactams) (Takazawa et al. 2017) (β-lactams include some types of antibiotics such as penicillins, e.g. amoxicillin or flucloxacillin, and cephalosporins, e.g. cephalexin). Other common causes of anaphylactic reactions include environmental agents such as stings from insects, contact with latex or hair dye, food and nut allergies (Pumphreys 2004).

Blue Flag

The psychological impact of anaphylaxis is not limited to the patient. Family, friends and healthcare professionals may need additional support following involvement in (or prior to) an anaphylactic reaction.

Anaphylaxis Presentation and Actions to Take

To reiterate, anaphylactic reactions present suddenly and have a rapid progression over several minutes. The patient may visibly appear unwell or report feeling unwell and be anxious. Often patients report 'a sense of impending doom' (Ewan 1998; Kaplan 2007) and this vital clue should not be overlooked. The Resuscitation Council (UK) stipulate that three criteria indicate that an anaphylactic reaction is present:

1. sudden onset with rapid progression
2. life threatening compromise of airway, and/or breathing, and/ or circulation
3. finally, skin or mucosal changes

The Resuscitation Council advocate an ABCDE approach to recognition and management (Resuscitation Council UK 2008).

The airway, breathing and circulation (ABC) compromise may present as difficulty in breathing due to airway swelling (throat or tongue oedema) or stridor (a high-pitched noise heard on inspiration). Importantly, the patient may self-report feeling as if their throat is closing, or have a hoarse voice (Resuscitation Council UK 2008). Compromised breathing may be signalled by shortness of breath, wheeze or increased respiratory rate (tachypnoea). The shortness of breath and an increased respiratory rate may result in tiredness and ultimately lead to cyanosis and respiratory arrest.

Circulatory issues may present as pale clammy skin (indicating shock), hypotension (low blood pressure) and tachycardia (increased pulse rate). The patient may have a change in consciousness or lose consciousness due to circulatory compromise; and ultimately a slowing of the pulse leading to cardiac arrest.

As noted previously, both respiratory or cardiac arrest may occur (Resuscitation Council UK 2008) due to a compromised airway (A), breathing (B) and circulation (C). Disability (D) may relate to an altered neurological state (confusion, agitation, loss of consciousness and so on) due to decreased brain perfusion or gastrointestinal issues such as pain, vomiting or incontinence. Through exposure (E), skin and mucosal changes may be evident and often are the first indications of a reaction occurring.

Skin and mucosal changes can be subtle or dramatic such as flushing of the skin, itchy hives or welts (urticaria) or a deeper reaction causing swelling of the tissues, commonly eyelids, lips and mouth or throat (angioedema) and a patchy or red rash (erythema), which are important criteria to support the diagnosis. Such skin and mucosal signals are present in over 80% of anaphylactic reactions and often the first notable feature. It is important to remember, however, that skin reactions without the life-threatening ABC problems do not signify an anaphylactic reaction.

The Resuscitation Council (UK) anaphylaxis algorithm is presented in Figure 58.1. Offering a clear process for emergency management, the nursing associate must ensure that they work within their scope of practice, confidence and competence at all times. Depending on clinical setting and responsibilities, actions to be taken may include recognising a potential reaction, alerting the clinical team quickly, documentation, monitoring of vital signs, liaising with and supporting the patient, family members and clinical team. The scope of practice, actions and responsibilities must be undertaken in line with the local setting and role expectations.

Orange Flag

Anaphylaxis is a serious and life threatening allergic reaction. The person who has had an anaphylaxis reaction may experience anxiety as a result of fear of subsequent reactions. Important factors for supporting someone with a history of anaphylaxis include:

1. High-quality information on what anaphylaxis is
2. Clear information on what their trigger allergen is
3. Appropriate management strategy education for anaphylaxis
4. Appropriate referral to an allergy specialist
5. Follow up are provision

Support and guidance given should be tailored to the individual and always follow the advice of the medical or specialist clinical teams.

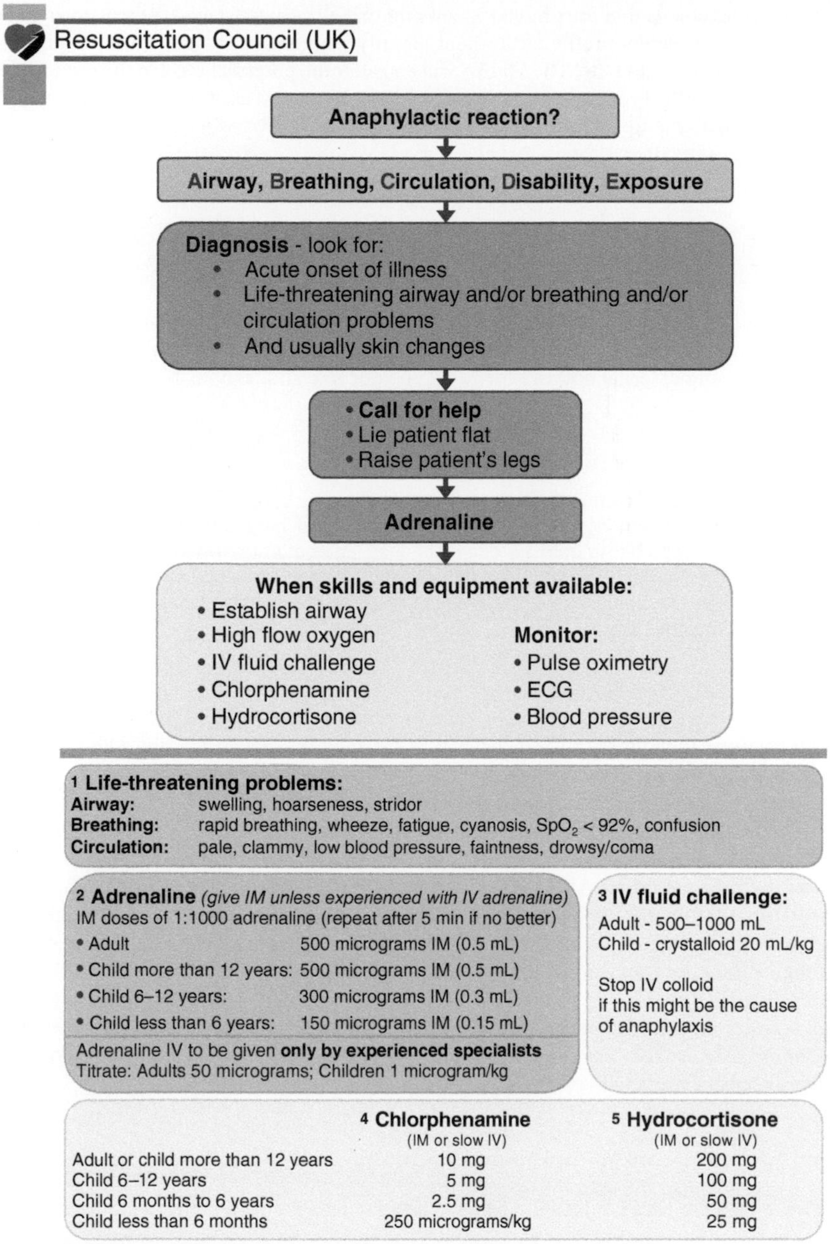

Figure 58.1 **Anaphylaxis algorithm.** *Source:* Resuscitation Council UK (2008). © Resuscitation Council UK 2008.

Background to Medicine Safety

In the early 1960s, a phenomenon was identified that babies across the world were being born without limbs. This was linked and later proven to be caused by the drug thalidomide, which was taken by pregnant women to combat their nausea. There was no central system at the time to collect this type of data and alert other prescribers and thus the Yellow Card Scheme was introduced as a monitoring system for the United Kingdom. This is integrated within the role of the Medicines and Healthcare products Regulatory Agency (MHRA). A worldwide monitoring system was later introduced in 1971 by the WHO.

The MHRA governs the licensing of medicines and medical devices in the United Kingdom. Prior to being authorised with a product licence (or marketing authorising), the product must have undergone clinical trials to demonstrate its effectiveness and safety profile. The safety profile will detail the types of reactions, contraindications and cautions identified within the clinical trial data. This offers practitioners information about what is to be expected from the product. A limitation of this, however, is that clinical trials are undertaken on a very select group of people, for example a specific age range or people with a specific condition. It is not until there is more widespread use of the product that we then begin to find out how some people may react to the product or how it may interact with other drugs or new reactions etc. that may not have been identified. These new products (or sometimes old products with a new use or ingredient) are assigned a black triangle (see the British National

Formulary (BNF)) to warn health professionals that the product is new and that all suspected adverse reactions must be reported to the MHRA. This information is then used to build the safety profile further and identify any risks associated with the product (pharmacovigilance) and consider whether they are common, rare or serious etc. The MHRA will consider the potential risks to the patient if not treated with the medication and the risk associated with the side effects of the medication. Health professionals are then alerted to any identified risks through safety alert systems and drug leaflets and medicine formularies such as the BNF. The MHRA work collaboratively with the European Medicines Agency and the WHO so that all drug safety data is monitored and shared.

Reporting ADRs

All healthcare professionals have a responsibility for reporting suspected ADRs; the NMC (2018b) states in section 10.9 that nursing associates must *recognise and respond to adverse or abnormal reactions to medications, and when and how to escalate any concerns*. This may include reporting ADRs through both organisational and external bodies depending on your role and responsibilities established by your employer.

Yellow Flag

It is important to build a therapeutic relationship with your patients so you can have an open and in-depth discussion regarding any potential ADRs and support the person in reporting to you their symptoms, concerns or worries.

Fear or a feeling of not wanting to be 'trouble' or 'complain' may limit patients' reports of what they perceive to be minor ADRs.

In addition, the nature of the medication or problem being treated may be sensitive in nature. Knowing your patient, their social and cultural background, diagnosis, being aware of the wider context of the medical issue being treated, the medication and route of administration are all important factors to consider.

Careful supportive communication and compassion will help facilitate effective discussions.

The MHRA is responsible for ensuring that quality and efficiency is maintained, and also providing education to healthcare professionals and the public on the safety of medicine and devices; the MHRA collects information and reports regarding ADRs to influence regulatory frameworks ensuring any risk associated with a medicine or device is proportionate and effective.

The MHRA accepts reports from all healthcare professionals and self-reports from patients or consumers of products. Information collected relates to side effects (or ADRs), medical device adverse incidents, defective medicines, counterfeit or fake medication or devices, and from 2016, the MHRA started collecting information on ADRs in relation to e-cigarettes (Medicines and Healthcare Products Regulatory Agency 2019). With the increased use of the internet and online technology, trade in fake or counterfeit drugs is increasing, with the WHO reporting that in 50% of cases, medicines bought online, using illegal sites with concealed physical addresses, were fake products (World Health Organization 2010). This highlights the importance of reviewing where a patient accesses their medication, but also questioning appropriately about non-prescribed, self-bought medicines.

Medical device information is collected as well as medicines information, and may include issues with wheelchairs, condoms, thermometers and instructions for use, for example. Medical devises should carry CE mark (Figure 58.2) to show it has reached the approved requirements of the Medicinal Devices Directive as outlined by the MHRA (2015a, 2015b).

Yellow Card System

Alongside local processes for reporting suspected ADRs, it is good practice for healthcare professionals to report any suspected ADRs or incidents to the MHRA using the yellow card scheme. This facilitates accurate reporting and recognition of ADRs both known and new in relation to medicines, interactions between medicines and medical devices. Reporting can take place using hard copies of the yellow cards found at the back of print version of the BNF, online via https://yellowcard.mhra.gov.uk/ or through the yellow card mobile app.

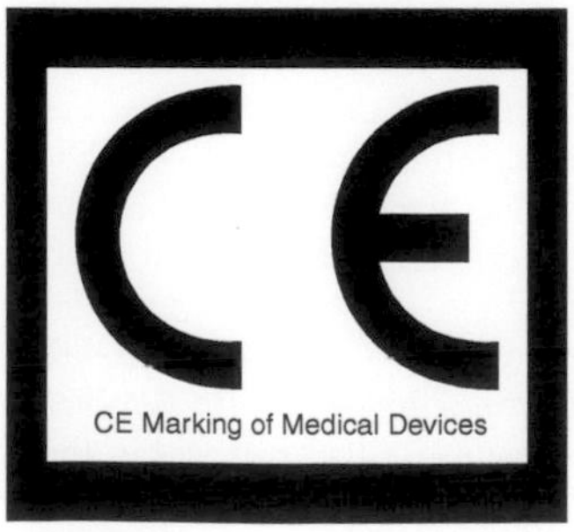

Figure 58.2 CE mark of approved devices.

The cards have four distinct sections which are critical for accurate reporting. It is asked that all as much information is provided. The MHRA request information (if known) in relation to:

1. The suspect drug
   - Administration route
   - Dose information, including frequency and daily dose
   - Date/dates of administration
   - Brand and batch number if the ADR relates to a vaccine
2. The suspect reaction
   - When the suspect reaction happened
   - The severity of reaction
   - Treatment administered
   - Reaction outcome
3. Patient information
   - Sex of patient
   - Age when reaction occurred
   - Weight
   - Patient initials and identification number.

The MHRA requests at least one piece of information from section 3 and the note that requesting the patient initials and identification number does not breach any confidentiality agreement between the patient and healthcare provider (Medicines and Healthcare Products Regulatory Agency 2015b).

4. Details of the reporting individual
   - Name and address should be provided for receipt of the report, future contact or follow-up

In addition to these four criteria, additional information may be provided including any medicines taken in the past three months including prescription medicines and those bought over the counter, medical history and known allergies, any pertinent test results, drugs taken during pregnancy (if applicable) and any congenital abnormalities and date of last menstrual period (if applicable) (Medicines and Healthcare Products Regulatory Agency 2015b) and any re-challenge of the medicine. A medicine de-challenge and re-challenge test (re-exposure test) is when a practitioner reintroduces a medicine that has previously caused a reaction in a patient (Meyboom 2013). Or it may be that medications are removed (de-challenge) and are not reintroduced. The aim of these tests is to establish causality (i.e. is it the drug causing the reaction (ADR) or that a reaction has occurred during treatment, but is not caused by the drug (ADE) (Marante 2018), or to obtain information knowledge that may benefit future patients or to establish patient tolerance at a lower dose (Meyboom 2013).

It is paramount to note here that such challenges may pose significant and life-threatening danger to patients and should only be conducted by appropriately trained practitioners under strict regulation and guidance.

In addition, if it is unclear if someone else has reported the ADR, it is advisable to send an additional yellow card, or if new information is available. The MHRA will collate the reports and omit any duplication of information (Medicines and Healthcare Products Regulatory Agency 2015b). It is recommended that a copy of the completed yellow card should be included in the patent's notes to ensure accurate documentation and future reference.

Touch Point **Reporting ADRs**

All healthcare professionals (including nursing associates) have a part to play in recognising, responding to, reporting ADRs, and any concerns relating to drugs or medical devices. This must be in line with the employer's policy, role and responsibilities.

The MHRA yellow card scheme supports reporting and investigation of concerns and suspected issues or incidents. These are inclusive of

- ADRs
- Incidents where a medical device was involved
- Medicines of poor quality (defective)
- Fake medication or devices
- Safety information or concern regarding e-cigarettes and refill devices

Modes of reporting can be through

1. Hard copy yellow cards as found in the print version of the BNF
2. Online via https://yellowcard.mhra.gov.uk/
3. Using the yellow card mobile app

Safety Critical Medications

Nursing associates may administer medicines in line with their role or according to their scope of practice and local policies. Some medicines carry and increase risk of harm to the patient and are often termed *Safety Critical Medicines*. These drugs may include (but are not limited to) warfarin, digoxin, insulin and opiates. Health Education England (2017) made recommendations to all employers of nursing associates. They requested that the employers name in policy or documentation all safety critical medications that their nursing associate may administer. This should be coupled with additional administration or safety guidance to reduce the associated risk related to the medication (Health Education England 2017) and to support the nursing associate in their practice.

Touch Points Revisited

- This chapter has addressed key features of ADRs including their categorisation as a unique form of adverse event.
- It is important that the nursing associate recognises and responds appropriately to ADRs.
- The nursing associate must always work within their scope of practice aligned to the NMC Code, the standards of proficiency for nursing associates and local policy and procedure.
- The nursing associate and other health care professionals have a responsibility for reporting suspected ADRs; this may include reporting ADRs through both organisational and external bodies depending on role and responsibilities determined by your employer.
- Systems for reporting ADRs have been discussed alongside the introduction of safety critical medicines.

Supporting Evidence and Useful Resources

Patient- and drug-related risk factors for ADRs

Dougherty, L., Lister, S. and West-Oram, A. (2015) Medicines management, *The royal Marsden manual of clinical nursing procedures* (9th edn), John Wiley and Sons Ltd.

Anaphylaxis guidance including treatment and management

Resuscitation Council UK. (2008) *Emergency treatment of anaphylactic reactions: Guidance for healthcare providers*, Resuscitation Council UK

The British National Formulary: Online resource of medicines, medicinal products and prescribing information https://bnf.nice.org.uk/

The Electronic Medicines Compendium: Online resource of medicines, medicinal products, patient and prescribing information https://www.medicines.org.uk/emc/

References

British Heart Foundation. (2019) *Warfarin; an experts view.* [online] Available: https://www.bhf.org.uk/informationsupport/heart-matters-magazine/medical/warfarin/expert. Accessed 16 September 2020.

Carne, E. and Owen, N. (2019) Care of the adult with an immunological condition, in Elcock, K., Wright, W., Newcombe, P. & Everett, F. (eds.) *Essentials of nursing adults*, London: Sage, p. 568.

Dougherty, L., Lister, S. and West-Oram, A. (2015) *Medicines management, The Royal Marsden manual of clinical nursing procedures* (9th edn), John Wiley and Sons Ltd.

Duerden, M., Avery, T. and Payne, R. (2013) *Polypharmacy and medicines optimisation: making it safe and sound*, London: The King's Fund.

Ewan, P. (1998) Anaphylaxis, *The British Medical Journal*, 316: 1442–1445.

Ferner, R. and Mcgettin, P. (2018) Adverse drug reactions, *The British Medical Journal*, 363(9237): 1255–1259.

Health Education England. (2017) *Advisory guidance: administration of medicines by nursing associates [Online]*, Health Education England. [online] Available: https://www.hee.nhs.uk/sites/default/files/documents/Advisory%20guidance%20-%20administration%20of%20medicines%20by%20nursing%20associates.pdf. Accessed 9 September 2019.

Kaplan, M. (2007) Anaphylaxis, *Permanente Journal*, 11: 53–56.

Kaufman, G. (2016) Adverse drug reactions: classification susceptibility and reporting, *Nursing Standard*, 30(50): 53–61.

Leheny, S. (2017) *'Adverse event', not the same as 'side effect'.* [online] Available: https://www.pharmacytimes.com/contributor/shelby-leheny-pharmd-candidate-2017/2017/02/adverse-event-not-the-same-as-side-effect. Accessed 18 September 2019.

Marante, K. (2018) The challenges or adverse drug reaction evaluation, *Journal of Pharmacovigilance*, 6:3. DOI: 10.4172/2329-6887.1000260

Medicines and Healthcare Products Regulatory Agency. (2019a) *Medicines and healthcare products regulatory agency: about us.* [Online] Available: https://www.gov.uk/government/organisations/medicines-and-healthcare-products-regulatory-agency/about#contents. Accessed 15 October 2019.

Medicines and Healthcare Products Regulatory Agency. (2015a) *Medical devices: conformity assessment and the CE mark, Medications and Healthcare products Regulatory Agency.*[Online] Available: https://www.gov.uk/guidance/medical-devices-conformity-assessment-and-the-ce-mark. Accessed 16 September 2020.

Medicines and Healthcare Products Regulatory Agency. (2015b) *What to include in your yellow card of an adverse drug reaction.* [Online] Available: https://assets.publishing.service.gov.uk/government/uploads/system/uploads/attachment_data/file/404416/What_to_include_in_your_Yellow_Card_of_an_adverse_drug_reaction.pdf. Accessed 12 October 2019.

Medicines and Healthcare Products Regulatory Agency. (2018) *Guidance on adverse drug reactions: classification of adverse drug reactions [Online], Medications and Healthcare products Regulatory Agency.* [online] Available: https://assets.publishing.service.gov.uk/government/uploads/system/uploads/attachment_data/file/752688/Guidance_on_adverse_drug_reactions.pdf. Accessed 12 October 2019.

Medicines and Healthcare Products Regulatory Agency. (2019b) *Yellow card: about yellow card.* [Online] Available: https://yellowcard.mhra.gov.uk/the-yellow-card-scheme/. Accessed 15 October 2019.

Meyboom, R. (2013) Intentional rechallenge and the clinical management of drug-related problems, *Drug Safety*, 36(3): 163–165.

Mirakian, R., Wewan, P., Durham, S., Youlten, L., Dugue, P., Friedmann, P., English, J., Huber, P. and Nasser, S. (2008) BSACI guidelines for the management of drug allergy, *Clinical and Experimental Allergy*, 39(1): 43–61.

National Institute for Health and Care Excellence. (2011) *Anaphylaxis: assessment and referral after emergency treatment*, London: National Institute for Health and Care Excellence.

National Institute for Health and Care Excellence. (2017) *Adverse drug reactions.* [Online] Available: https://cks.nice.org.uk/adverse-drug-reactions. Accessed 19 October 2019.

National Institute for Health and Care Excellence. (2019a) *British national formulary: adverse reactions to drugs, Yellow card scheme [Online], National Institute for Health and Care Excellence.* [online] Available: https://bnf.nice.org.uk/guidance/adverse-reactions-to-drugs.html. Accessed 12 October 2019.

National Institute for Health and Care Excellence. (2019b) *British national formulary: oxygen [Online], Joint Formulary Committee.* [online] Available: https://bnf.nice.org.uk/treatment-summary/oxygen.html. Accessed 16 October 2019.

Nursing and Midwifery Council (NMC). (2018a) *The code: professional standards of practice and behaviour for nurses, midwives and nursing associates [Online]*, The Nursing and Midwifery Council. [online] Available: https://www.nmc.org.uk/standards/code/. Accessed 20 September 2019.

Nursing and Midwifery Council (NMC). (2018b) *Standards of proficiency for nursing associates [Online]*, Nursing and Midwifery Council. [online] Available: https://www.nmc.org.uk/standards/code/. Accessed 20 September 2019.

Pumphreys, R. (2004) Fatal anaphylaxis in the UK. 1992-2001, in: Bock, G. and Goode, J. (eds) *Novartis Foundation Symposia*, 257: 116–128.

Resuscitation Council UK. (2008) *Emergency treatment of anaphylactic reactions: Guidance for healthcare providers*, UK: Resuscitation Council UK.

Schatz, S. and Weber, R. (2015) Adverse drug reactions, in: Lee, M. and Murphy, J. (eds) *Pharmacology Self-Assessment Program (PSAP), book 2, CAN and pharmacy practice*. American collage of clinical pharmacology, pp. 5–26.

Takazawa, T., Oshima, K. and Saito, S. (2017) Drug-induced anaphylaxis in the emergency room, *Acute Medicine and Surgery*, 4(3): 235–245.

Turner, P., Gowland, M., Sharma, V., Lerodiakonou, D., Harper, N., Garcez, T., Pumphrey, R. and Boyle, R. (2015) Increase in anaphylaxis-related hospitalisations but no increase in fatalities: an analysis of United Kingdom national anaphylaxis data, *Journal of Allergy and Clinical Immunology*, 135(4): 956–963.

World Health Organisation. (2000) *Safety monitoring of medicinal products. Guidelines for setting up and running a pharmacovigilance centre*, London: World Health Organisation.

World Health Organisation. (2002) *The importance of pharmacovigilance: safety monitoring of medicinal products*, Geneva: World Health Organisation.

World Health Organisation. (2010) Growing threat from counterfeit medicines, *Bulletin of the World Health Organisation*, 88(4): 247–248.

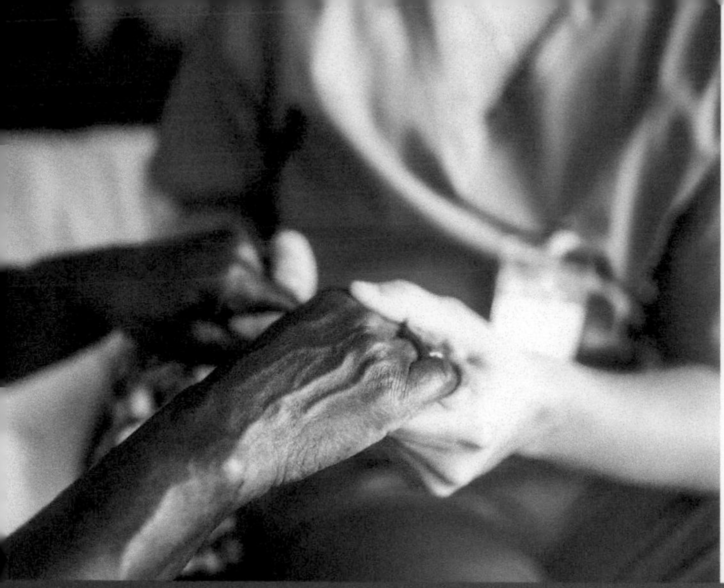

59

Storage, Transportation and Disposal of Medicinal Products

Carol Wills

Northumbria University, UK

Chapter Aim

- This chapter will familiarise the reader with the requirements for safe storage, transportation and disposal of medicinal products in practice.

Learning Outcomes

After reading this chapter, the reader will be able to:

- Demonstrate understanding of the legislation relating to safe storage, transportation and disposal of medicinal products.
- Explain the governance requirements for safe storage, transportation and disposal of medicinal products.
- Recognise and report factors that may impact on safe and effective care provision.

Test Your Knowledge Multiple Choice Questions

1. The security requirements for medicines are directed by:
   A) Their drug classification
   B) The facilities available in the health or social care environment
   C) The size of their containers
2. Toxic, harmful or dangerous medicines are referred to as:
   A) Secure medicines
   B) Hazardous substances
   C) Controlled medicines

The Nursing Associate's Handbook of Clinical Skills, First Edition. Edited by Ian Peate.

Companion website: www.wiley.com/nursingassociate

3. **Medicines need to be stored securely to:**
   A) **Safeguard from unauthorised access and prevent harm**
   B) **Maintain orderly stock control and administration**
   C) **Ensure only senior staff can access**
4. **COSHH refers to the:**
   A) **Central Office for Substances which are Hazardous to Health**
   B) **Community Order for Solutions known to cause Health Hazards**
   C) **Control Of Substances Hazardous to Health regulations**
5. **Vaccines normally need to be stored at temperatures of:**
   A) **−2°C to −8°C (+28°F to +17°F)**
   B) **+2°C to +8°C (+36°F to +46°F)**
   C) **+8°C to +25°C (+46°F to +77°F)**

Introduction

Medicines are an extremely important aspect of modern healthcare with the potential to prevent illness as well as managing and curing conditions and diseases. They also have the potential for considerable harm if misused or of being ineffective if they have not been stored correctly. The supply, storage and disposal of medicines are identified by the Care Quality Commission (CQC) in England (CQC 2019a) as one of the six most common areas for risk. Medicinal products are, therefore, governed by a range of legislation, regulation, policies and individual product requirements to direct their use and ensure their safety and security when stored, transported and disposed of. This chapter will help you to understand the relevant legal, regulatory and governance requirements alongside health and safety legislation related to safe storage, transportation and disposal of medicinal products.

Blue Flag

Relationships are important in any health and social care setting. In September 2016, the CQC successfully prosecuted a care home provider and a registered manager.

A 78-year-old man with vascular dementia relied on the provider and registered manager to make sure he received his medicines safely. They failed to do this; their systems failed to identify that the man's medication was missed for between 30 and 33 days.

Both failed to provide safe care and treatment resulting in avoidable harm. The care home provider and a registered manager had a duty of care to residents; they have entered into a contract with residents; this is a fiscal and professional relationship.

Understanding this will help you to demonstrate proficiency with regard to the standards that have been set by the Nursing and Midwifery Council (NMC) (2018).

The nursing associate is required to apply and understand relevant legal, regulatory and governance requirements, policies and ethical frameworks, including any mandatory reporting duties, in all areas of practice. The principles of health and safety legislation and regulations are paramount; they are required to maintain safe environments and guide storage and disposal of medications.

Legislation

The safe and secure handling of medicines is essential in all health and social care environments to ensure patient and employee safety. Employers are required under the Health and Safety at Work Act etc. 1974 to safeguard their employees and patients from the potential harm involved in handling a range of substances including medicines. All organisations are required to assess the risks to patients and staff and implement a system to manage risks and prevent incidents, which may be hazardous to health (Health and Safety Executive (HSE) 2019).

Medicines must be kept secure and safeguarded from unauthorised access and stored at a level of security appropriate to their proposed use. This means that they must be stored in locked cupboards or storage units that comply with British Standards (BS 6321) or in rooms that are locked when not being accessed. Medicine trolleys must be locked and either fixed to a wall or floor anchor point or in a locked room when not in use (Royal Pharmaceutical Society (RPS) 2018, Appendix A). The medicines for clinical emergencies, such as critical medicines, need to be stored so that they are readily accessible but also secure, tamper-evident and clearly labelled. Patient Safety Wales (2015) highlights the challenges of medicines being accessible but also safe following a practice incident where a patient was choking from accidentally swallowing food thickener, which was left by his bedside for mixing into foods. Healthcare employers and their employees have a responsibility to ensure the safety of patients by reviewing the potential for risk of harm. This includes the storage of patients' own drugs, which must be stored securely and where a personal locker or cabinet is used, the responsibility for the master key is determined by a risk assessment (RPS 2018, Appendix A). This will identify whether the patient is capable of maintaining the security of their medicines and can self-manage their administration or whether the professional staff will need to assume this responsibility on their behalf. Chapter 53 of this text discussed a person's ability to administer their own medicines including storage in more detail. The safe storage of medicines also extends to patients' homes so patients should be advised on good practice.

Violet Flag Safety of medicines in the home

- Patients must be warned to keep all medicines out of the sight and reach of children.
- Medicines should be dispensed in re-closable child-resistant containers where possible.
- Medicines should be stored in a dry atmosphere (preferably not a bathroom).
- Patients should be advised to keep medicines in the containers they were dispensed in.
- Medicines should be stored at the recommended temperature; pharmacy staff will always label medicines to indicate when they will require refrigeration.

The legal classification of the product as well as the product characteristics will define how the product must be handled and stored. The Human Medicines Regulations (2012) consolidates all previous UK laws to define the authorisation, labelling and distribution of prescription only medicines (POMs), general sales list (GSL) and pharmacy (P) products (these classifications are discussed in more depth in Chapter 58). The security requirements for a GSL product, for example glycerol suppositories, are very different from a POM, schedule 2 controlled drug, for example diamorphine hydrochloride, as controlled drugs are considered more dangerous so must be kept in a secure place with restricted access; this means it must be kept in a locked safe, room or locked receptacle, which is accessible only to specific people.

The Misuse of Drugs Act (1971) details drugs which are subject to abuse and misuse and categorises them from Class A to C, according to how harmful they are considered to be. All drugs may be harmful if misused; however, Class A drugs are deemed to be most harmful (e.g. heroin), Class B less harmful (e.g. barbiturates) and Class C least harmful (e.g. tranquilisers). People who illegally manufacture, supply or are in possession of drugs under these categories, for example cannabis or heroin, are subject to prosecution under this Act. Recent changes in legislation, however, in November 2018 (Javid 2018) allowed patients to access Cannabis-Based Products for Medicinal use (CBPMs) under Schedule 2 of the Misuse of Drugs Regulations 2001, where prescribed by or under the direction of doctors on the General Medical Council's Specialist Register (CQC 2019b, p. 3). These patients would, therefore, be legitimately entitled to be in possession of these products. This also highlights that medicines can change their classification status so their storage and security requirements may also change.

Yellow Flag

Social and legal debates may mean that medicines may be reclassified depending on the evidence available, and this will affect their security requirements. Current debates around the reclassification and legalisation of cannabis in the United Kingdom consider the following as important viewpoints:

- Some countries have already legalised the manufacture, supply and possession of cannabis, for example Uruguay in 2013 and Canada in 2018.
- It could have a positive impact on public health as legalisation considers a safer supply through controlled manufacture and monitoring, which may protect vulnerable people.
- There could be financial incentives as it is thought that legalisation could save the treasury money through reduced legal frameworks (e.g. policing) and generate tax income similar to the cigarettes and alcohol tax model.
- CBPMs whilst unlicensed were rescheduled to Schedule 2 and became available for prescription in 2019 by doctors in England, on the General Medical Council Specialist Register. Once licenced products become available, these will be prescribable like other Schedule 2 products
- The Secretary of State for the Home Department (Javid 2019) stated that he has no intention of legalising the recreational use of cannabis in England

Source: Health Poverty Action (2018); Institute for Social and Economic Research (2013); Javid (2019); National Health Service England (2019).

Health professionals are protected from prosecution if they have controlled drugs in their possession in a professional capacity, and the Misuse of Drugs (Safe Custody) Regulations 1973 and subsequent amendments (available at https://www.health-ni.gov.uk/articles/misuse-drugs-legislations) detail who these may be, the conditions in which these activities may be undertaken and the safe custody and storage requirements of the different products. Your organisation will have a medicine policy in place, which outlines who is the Accountable Officer and how all medicines, especially controlled drugs, must be kept secure (National Institute for Health and Care Excellence (NICE) 2016). This includes the responsibilities of staff handling the products as well as the recording of medicines ordered, received and used/disposed of within controlled drug registers. You will need to be familiar with this policy to help you to understand what your role may be in maintaining the security and safe storage of medicinal products in your practice area.

Green Flag

The important legislation, regulation and governance relating to the safe storage, transportation and disposal of medicines include:

- The Human Medicines Regulations (2012)
- Control of Substances Hazardous to Health (COSHH)
- The Medicines and Healthcare Products Regulatory Agency
- RPS Professional guidance for the Safe and Secure Handling of Medicines (2018)
- NMC (2018) Standards of Proficiency for Nursing Associates
- Your employer/organisation's medicine policy

The Care Quality Commission (2019c) reports that theft, diversion and misuse of controlled drugs within the lower schedules, as well as the theft of prescription pads and staff identity badges alongside poor record keeping of controlled drug registers, causes real concerns for safe custody. The potential for the trading, diversion and misuse of controlled drugs in places of detention is also reported by Her Majesty's Inspectorate of Prisons for England and Wales (HMI Prisons) to remain high (CQC 2019a).

The CQC (2019b, p. 4) recommends that '*All healthcare professionals need to remember their responsibility to speak up on areas of concern that might negatively affect patient safety, including prescribing, administering, dispensing, supplying and disposing of controlled drugs*'. This means you should understand the processes for raising any concerns within your organisation so that you will be confident in speaking up.

Regulatory Governance

The RPS professional guidance 'Safe and Secure Handling of Medicines' (2018) extends to all healthcare settings to guide working practices, policies and procedures. The president of the RPS states that, with approximately £20 billion spent in 2017–2018, it was fundamental that the systems were in place to improve care, and that we can account for a medicine from the time of ordering to the time of use (Burns 2018). The RPS (2018) guidance refers to all medicines including cytotoxics, medical gases, vaccines and blood products licensed as medicines, for example immunoglobulins, among many others. It centres around four governance principles, which underpin the safety and security of medicines:

- The first principle sets out the accountability of the management/leadership team within the organisation, risk assessment processes and ensures policies and procedures are in place to ensure the safety and security of medicines. You should, therefore, become familiar with the policies and procedures that are in place within your organisation so that you can demonstrate your achievement of nursing associate Platform 1.2.
- The second outlines roles, responsibilities and the training needed to be knowledgeable and competent as well as the premises and equipment required are fit for purpose. This advises that all individuals who handle medicines must be competent, legally entitled, appropriately trained and authorised to do the job. You should not undertake any medicine processes or procedures without training and having demonstrated competence in handling medicines and associated equipment.
- Principle three details the quality assurance systems and processes, which include audit and risk assessment as well as supporting a leadership culture, which resolves and learns from incidents. You should understand the processes required to report an incident and feel confident that this will be regarded as a learning opportunity for the organisation.
- The final principle requires that learning and improvement is embedded throughout the service with systems and processes in place to support the identification, investigation and reporting of incidents, which are then fed into the regional and/or national reporting schemes. A review of practice is integrated within this process and good practice is encouraged to be shared with other organisations. Figure 59.1 demonstrates the relationship between the 4 principles and the safety of the patient.

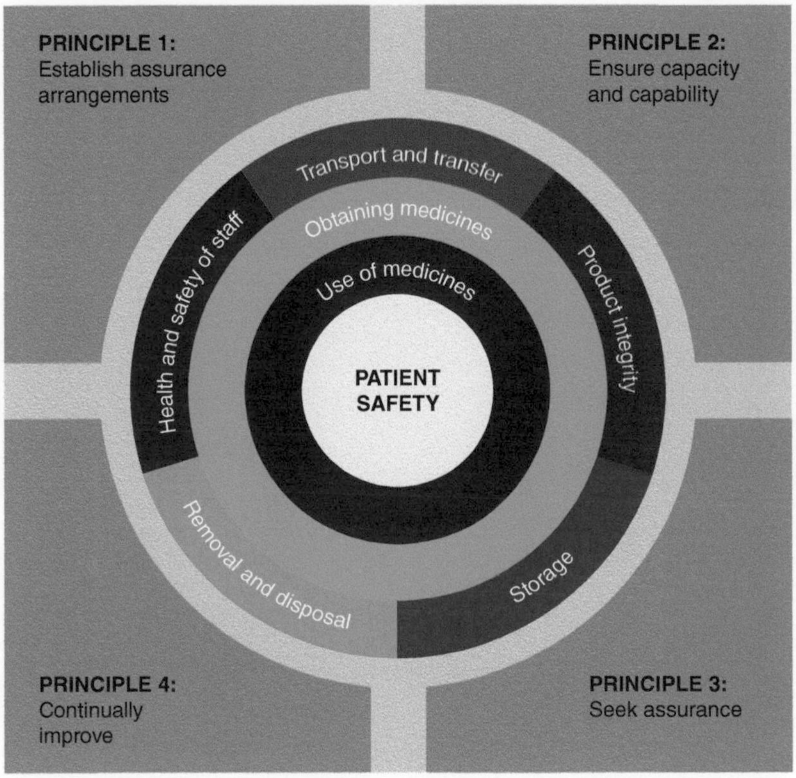

Figure 59.1 4 Governance Principles. *Source:* Creamer & Humpreys (2008).

Each medicine must be stored according to its specific instructions as some may require protecting from light conditions and sealed in airtight containers, their details of which can be found in the electronic Medicines Compendium (https://www.medicines.org.uk/emc). All medicine storage systems should facilitate the separation of similar coloured and packaging designs to avoid mistakes in product choice and administration (RPS 2018). Health and Social Care Northern Ireland (2015) suggests that confirmation bias, where you see what you expect, can lead to mistakes so you must not rely on your recognition of the packaging to confirm the product name.

Red Flag

The risks that are posed by poor medicines management can result in serious or fatal illness, particularly to people who may be vulnerable, for example, older people, those with reduced mental capacity, reduced mobility, a sensory impairment and individuals who depend on others to help take their medicines.

Medicines labelled as flammable must not be stored near a naked flame, direct heat or any equipment that may emit sparks. This includes alcohol gels, which are highly flammable; so, the RPS (2018) advises that community staff should store these within their bags, pockets and/or in the boot of the car and not left in the car in direct sunlight. Simple advice such as ensuring keeping the bottle closed to avoid spillage, replacing caps after use, keeping away from electrical equipment and not storing in the refrigerator aim to reduce the risks of combustion. All flammable products and medical gases must be stored in fire safety approved cupboards, and Control of Substances Hazardous to Health regulations (COSHH) data sheets must be available for all flammable liquids kept on the premises and kept in a central point available to all staff to refer to (RPS 2018, Appendix A).

Supporting Evidence

The Health and Safety Executive website contains a wealth of information governing health and safety at work. This includes the legislation, which governs hazardous medicines and the reporting of dangerous or hazardous incidents.

https://www.medicines.org.uk/emc/ is a free electronic medicines compendium of all products licenced for use in the United Kingdom. Here you can find information about medicines and whether they have specific storage requirements.

The Government web page with full details of medicines regulations can be found at https://www.health-ni.gov.uk/articles/legislation-covering-medicines.

Touch Point

- Medicines must be stored appropriately to maintain their security.
- You must have appropriate training and demonstrate competence in procedures for safe handling of medicines.
- Hazardous substances must be stored and disposed of according to COSSH regulations.

Medicines Requiring Ambient Temperatures

Some products need to be stored at specific temperatures to maintain their integrity, potency and efficacy. This could be room temperatures of no greater than 25°C or a cooler temperature may be required. For example, vaccines and unopened insulin usually need to be stored at temperatures of between +2°C and +8°C (+36° to +46°F) as storage at suboptimal temperatures can cause them to deteriorate. These must be stored in lockable refrigerators, which are monitored at least daily to measure room and refrigerator temperatures and recorded on a room and refrigerator monitoring form. The room and refrigerator maximum and minimum thermometer(s) must be reset on a daily basis although most modern medical refrigerators have integrated temperature monitoring systems, which automatically log and control the temperature, but these must also be checked regularly to ensure they are accurate.

If the temperature range is exceeded, it is the responsibility of the individual to report the incident and immediately seek advice from the pharmacy team. The World Health Organization (WHO) (2006) advises that vaccines degrade over time but this is accelerated by exposure to extremes of heat, cold, sunlight or fluorescent light, and once potency has been lost, it cannot be restored. This not only affects the quality and effectiveness of the vaccine, but there are also concerns about the immune response and the protection afforded if these vaccines are administered. Liquid vaccines have a small heat-sensitive label on the vial/tube called a vaccine vial monitor or VVM, which changes colour when the vaccine has been exposed to heat or has aged. This should normally appear as a dark circle with a white square in the centre. If the square has changed to the same colour or darker than the circle, then it must not be used (WHO 2016). Stock must also be regularly checked and rotated so that those with the shortest expiry dates are used first to minimise wastage from products passing their use by date. The financial costs of wasting these medicines are ill afforded to the NHS; Public Health England (PHE) reported the costs of wasted vaccines in England in 2018 totalled £6.3 million (PHE 2019).

Strict adherence to the storage and transportation of these products must be maintained through the 'cold chain'. This means they must, therefore, be kept at the specific temperature conditions throughout the process from its manufacture to the point of the patient receiving the vaccine. The Green Book (PHE 2014) advises that if they are to be transported offsite, for example to a school, then they must be kept in their original packaging and stored in a validated cool box (with a minimum and maximum temperature thermometer) with the opening kept to a minimum. Only the amounts necessary should be removed from the refrigerator and unused vaccines should be returned to the refrigerator and used at the earliest opportunity, if the cold chain has been adequately maintained. Where this has been compromised, a risk assessment must be undertaken to determine whether the integrity of the product has been affected. The Green Book (PHE 2014) advises that this is the responsibility of the user. Your workplace medicine or vaccine policy will advise on the reporting steps within your organisation.

Touch Point

- Some products require storage at specific temperatures to maintain their efficacy.
- Remember to check the VVM label prior to administration.
- Check your organisation's policy for guidance or reporting of incidents where the integrity of the medicine is in doubt.

Safe Disposal

The safe disposal of medicines will include the disposal of hazardous and non-hazardous medicines and those which are not pharmaceutically active, for example glucose solutions. Pharmacies are obliged to accept expired or unwanted medicines from patients for safe disposal (Department of Health and Social Care 2013). This includes inhalers, which contain gases that can be harmful to the environment so should not be put in waste bins. The pharmacy may then sort them into solids (including ampoules and vials), liquids and aerosols, if required, and the local NHS England team will plan for a waste contractor to collect them from pharmacies at regular intervals.

When disposing of 'sharps', which are required to administer medicines, for example syringes or intra-muscular needles, the Health and Safety (Sharps Instruments in Healthcare) 2013 regulations (Secretary of State 2013) state that needles should not be recapped or re-sheathed where this could pose a risk of accidental skin puncture to the employee as this has an associated risk of transferring any blood-borne virus or biological agent to the employee. 'Safer sharps' should be used where possible as these are designed to incorporate a mechanism or safety feature to prevent injuries. The NHS received over 1800 claims for needlestick injuries between 2012 and 2017 costing the NHS over £4 million for injury claims so far (NHS Resolution 2018). The majority of the successful claims were from ancillary staff who sustained an injury after the primary healthcare worker had not disposed of the needles correctly. Many of these were caused through overfull sharps containers and inadequate disposal of clinical waste. Where an incident needs to be reported, check your local policy for the correct policy and procedure and how you can complete an incident report. Your employer has a duty to report serious or dangerous occurrences, for example where an employee has been accidently exposed to a biological agent, to the Health and Safety Executive under the Reporting of Injuries, Disease and Dangerous Occurrences Regulations (RIDDOR) (2013).

Equipment used for vaccination, including used vials, ampoules or syringes, should be disposed of by placing it in a proper, puncture-resistant 'sharps' box according to local authority regulations and guidance in the technical memorandum 07-01 (Department of Health 2006). The 'sharps' container should be sealed and replaced once it is two-thirds full, or at the level indicated on the box by the manufacturer. The container should not be accessible to any unauthorised individual and disposed in accordance with local contractual procedures.

Additional segregation of some medicines and medical devices is also required under the Hazardous Waste Regulations. Hazardous substances are so called as they are defined as toxic, harmful and dangerous, posing great risk to human health (HSE 2019). Cytotoxic drugs, which are used in treating cancer and rheumatoid arthritis so forth, are governed by the Health and Safety Executive (HSE) (2019) as they present significant risks for those who handle them. They can be absorbed through the skin, aerosols or drug particles may be inhaled or they may be inadvertently ingested or injected through a needlestick injury following drug preparation or administration, transportation or waste disposal (HSE 2019). Handling patient waste and cleaning up spills are also other risks during medicine disposal. The HSE provides guidance on how these substances should be safely handled and disposed of in all health and social care environments. This guidance should be written into your organisation's policies for all staff to follow and the necessary equipment should be available to ensure this is undertaken safely.

Take Note

- Unwanted medicines should be returned to a pharmacy.
- Sharps containers should be sealed and replaced when two-thirds full.
- 'Safer sharps' should be used whenever possible.

Conclusion

The safe storage, transportation and disposal of medicines are governed by a range of legal, governance and professional requirements. This chapter has explored the important laws and supervisions, which are central in ensuring that medicines are stored so that they remain secure to prevent harm or inappropriate access, but that they also maintain their efficacy. It has also highlighted where you need to have accessed your local organisation's medicines and vaccines policies so that you understand the local requirements for safe storage, transportation and disposal of products and medical equipment. You will have learned how to report any serious incidents which may cause harm or where medicine policies have not been adhered to. You should now be able to demonstrate your achievements of the learning outcomes for this chapter and the Standards of Proficiency for Nursing Associates' Platforms (1.2 and 5.1) and Procedure 10.10 'Undertake safe storage, transportation and disposal of medicinal products' (NMC 2018).

Test your learning by completing the following multiple-choice questions.

References

Burns, C. (2018) *Revised guidance on handling of medicines brings multi-disciplinary focus, The Pharmaceutical Journal, [online]*. doi: 10.1211/PJ.2018.20205868.

Care Quality Commission (CQC). *(2019a) Medicines in adult health and social care; Learning from risk and sharing good practice for better outcomes.* [online] Available: https://www.cqc.org.uk/news/stories/medicines-health-adult-social-care-learning-risks-sharing-good-practice-better-outcomes. Accessed September 2020.

Care Quality Commission (CQC). (2019b) *The safer management of controlled drugs: annual update 2018.* [online] Available: https://www.cqc.org.uk/publications/major-report/safer-management-controlled-drugs. Accessed September 2020.

Care Quality Commission (CQC). (2019c) *The safer management of controlled drugs: annual update 2018; 2018 activity report for controlled drugs national group and cross-border group.* [online] Available: https://www.cqc.org.uk/sites/default/files/20190708_controlleddrugs2018_report.pdf. Accessed September 2020.

Creamer, E., Humphreys, H. (2008) The contribution of beds to healthcare associated infection: the importance of adequate decontamination. *Journal of Hospital Infection*, 69(1): 8–23. doi: 10.1016/j.jhin.2008.01.014. Epub 2008 Mar 19.

Department of Health and Social Care. (2013) *Health technical memorandum 07-01 safe management of healthcare waste.* [online] Available: https://www.gov.uk/government/publications/guidance-on-the-safe-management-of-healthcare-waste. Accessed September 2020.

Health and Social Care Northern Ireland. (2015*) Medication safety today, Issue 53 Medicines Governance Team.* [online] Available: http://www.medicinesgovernance.hscni.net/wpfb-file/medication-safety-today-53-pdf/. Accessed September 2020.

Health Poverty Action. (2018) *UK Cannabis Reform*. Available: https://www.healthpovertyaction.org/change-is-happening/campaign-issues/a-21st-century-approach-to-drugs/uk-cannabis-reform/. Accessed September 2020.

Institute for Social and Economic Research. (2013) *A Cost benefit analysis of the legalisation of cannabis*. Institute for Social and Economic Research, University of Essex.

Javid, S. (2019) *(The Secretary of State for the Home Department) Rescheduling of cannabis-based products for medicinal use: written statement HCWS994.* [online] Available: https://www.parliament.uk/. Accessed September 2020.

National Health Service England (2019) *Cannabis-based products for medicinal use*. Available: https://www.england.nhs.uk/medicines-2/support-for-prescribers/cannabis-based-products-for-medicinal-use/. Accessed September 2020.

NMC. (2018) *Standards for proficiency for nursing associates*, London: Nursing and Midwifery Council. [online] Available: www.nmc.org.uk/globalassets/sitedocuments/standards-of-proficiency/nursing-associates/nursing-associates-proficiency-standards.pdf. Accessed September 2020.

NICE. (2016) *Controlled drugs; safe use and management, National Guidance 46, National Institute for Health and Care Excellence.* [online] Available: https://www.nice.org.uk/guidance/ng46/chapter/Recommendations. Accessed September 2020.

NHS Resolution. (2018) *Preventing needlestick injuries*. [online] Available: https://resolution.nhs.uk/wp-content/uploads/2017/05/NHS-Resolution-Preventing-needlestick-injuries-leaflet-final.pdf. Accessed September 2020.

Patient Safety Wales. (2015) *Patient safety notice 008; Risk of death from asphyxiation by accidental ingestion of fluid/food thickener.* [online] Available: www.patientsafety.wales.nhs.uk. Accessed September 2020.

Public Health England. (2013) *Immunisation against infectious disease; The Green Book, Chapter 3, v2-1,p17. Storage, distribution and disposal of vaccines.* [online] Available: www.gov.uk/government/publications/storage-distribution-and-disposal-of-vaccines-the-green-book-chapter-3. Accessed September 2020.

Public Health England. (2019) *Vaccine incident guidance; responding to errors in vaccine storage, handling and administration.* [online] Available: https://www.gov.uk/government/publications/vaccine-incident-guidance-responding-to-vaccine-errors. Accessed September 2020.

Royal Pharmaceutical Society. (2018) *Professional guidance on the safe and secure handling of medicines.* [online] Available: https://www.rpharms.com/recognition/setting-professional-standards/safe-and-secure-handling-of-medicines/professional-guidance-on-the-safe-and-secure-handling-of-medicines. Accessed September 2020.

Secretary of State. (1971) *Misuse of drugs (safe custody) regulations 1971.* [online] Available: https://www.health-ni.gov.uk/articles/misuse-drugs-legislations. Accessed September 2020.

Secretary of State for Health. (2013) *The controlled drugs (supervisions of management and use) regulations*, UK Statutory Instrument no. 373. [online] Available: http://www.legislation.gov.uk/uksi/2013/373. Accessed September 2020.

The Secretary of State and the Minister for Health, Social Services and Public Safety. (2012) *The human medicines regulations*, UK Statutory Instruments 2012 No. 1916. [online] Available: https://www.legislation.gov.uk/uksi/2012/1916/contents/made. Accessed September 2020.

World Health Organization. (2006) *Temperature sensitivity of vaccines, Department of Immunization, vaccines and biologicals.* [online] Available: https://apps.who.int/iris/handle/10665/69387. Accessed September 2020.

World Health Organization. (2016) *What is a VVM and how does it work?* [online] Available: https://www.who.int/immunization/programmes_systems/service_delivery/EN_Information_Bulletin_VVM_assignments.pdf?ua=1. Accessed September 2020.

Answers

Chapter 1 Theories and Models of Communication

Test Yourself Multiple Choice Questions

1. (a); 2. (d); 3. (c); 4. (c); 5. (b).

Chapter 2 Approaches to Effective Communication

Test Yourself Multiple Choice Questions

1. (c); 2. (b); 3. (a); 4. (c); 5. (c).

Chapter 3 Interpersonal Skills and Therapeutic Relationship Skills

Test Yourself Multiple Choice Questions

1. (b); 2. (d); 3. (c); 4. (a); 5. (d).

Chapter 4 Working in a Team

Test Yourself Multiple Choice Questions

1. (b); 2. (a); 3. (c); 4. (a); 5. (b).

Chapter 5 Listening Actively

Test Yourself Multiple Choice Questions

1. (c); 2. (a); 3. (c); 4. (b); 5. (a).

Chapter 6 Information Gathering

Test Yourself Multiple Choice Questions

1. (b); 2. (b); 3. (c); 4. (a); 5. (c).

The Nursing Associate's Handbook of Clinical Skills, First Edition. Edited by Ian Peate.

Companion website: www.wiley.com/nursingassociate

Chapter 7 Escalating Concerns

Test Yourself Multiple Choice Questions

1. (d); 2. (b); 3. (c); 4. (d); 5. (a).

Chapter 8 Written Communication

Test Yourself Multiple Choice Questions

1. (c); 2. (a); 3. (b); 4. (b); 5. (a).

Chapter 9 Addressing Compliments and Complaints

Test Yourself Multiple Choice Questions

1. (c); 2. (b); 3. (a); 4. (d); 5. (b).

Chapter 10 Vital Signs

Test Yourself Multiple Choice Questions

1. (d); 2. (b); 3. (c); 4. (c); 5. (b).

Chapter 11 Venepuncture

Test Yourself Multiple Choice Questions

1. (b); 2. (a); 3. (a); 4. (b); 5. (b).

Chapter 12 ECG Recording

Test Yourself Multiple Choice Questions

1. (d); 2. (b); 3. (d); 4. (b); 5. (a).

Chapter 13 Blood Glucose Assessment

Test Yourself Multiple Choice Questions

1. (c); 2. (c); 3. (a); 4. (d); 5. (d).

Chapter 14 Specimen Collection

Test Yourself Multiple Choice Questions

1. (d); 2. (c); 3. (a); 4. (c); 5. (b).

Chapter 15 Recognising and Escalating Signs of All Forms Abuse

Test Yourself Multiple Choice Questions

1. (c); 2. (b); 3. (b); 4. (a); 5. (b).

Chapter 16 Recognising and Escalating Signs of Self-harm and/or Suicidal Ideation

Test Yourself Multiple Choice Questions

1. (b); 2. (d); 3. (c); 4. (a); 5. (b).

Chapter 17 Basic Mental Health First Aid

Test Yourself Multiple Choice Questions

1. (c); 2. (a); 3. (c); 4. (b); 5. (a).

Chapter 18 Basic First Aid

Test Yourself Multiple Choice Questions

1. (a); 2. (c); 3. (b); 4. (a); 5. (c).

Chapter 19 Pain

Test Yourself Multiple Choice Questions

1. (c); 2. (c); 3. (d); 4. (b); 5. (a).

Chapter 20 Promoting Comfort in Bed

Test Yourself Multiple Choice Questions

1. (e); 2. (a); 3. (b); 4. (a); 5. (c).

Chapter 21 Maintaining Privacy and Dignity

Test Yourself Multiple Choice Questions

1. (a); 2. (a); 3. (d); 4. (b); 5. (d).

Chapter 22 Promoting Sleep

Test Yourself Multiple Choice Questions

1. (a); 2. (b); 3. (c); 4. (d); 5. (c).

Chapter 23 Reassessment of Skin

Test Yourself Multiple Choice Questions

1. (c); 2. (b); 3. (b); 4. (a,b,c,d); 5. (a,b,c,d).

Chapter 24 Supporting a Person's Skin Integrity

Test Yourself Multiple Choice Questions

1. (a); 2. (a,b,c); 3. (b); 4. (a,b); 5. (a,b,c,d).

Chapter 25 Reassessment of Hygiene Status Supporting a Person's Hygiene Needs

Test Yourself Multiple Choice Questions

1. (d); 2. (d); 3. (d); 4. (d); 5. (d).

Chapter 26 Providing Oral and Dental Care

Test Yourself Multiple Choice Questions

1. (a); 2. (c); 3. (b); 4. (a); 5. (b).

Chapter 27 Providing Eye Care

Test Yourself Multiple Choice Questions

1. (a); 2. (d); 3. (c); 4. (b); 5. (d).

Chapter 28 Providing Nail Care

Test Yourself Multiple Choice Questions

1. (c); 2. (b); 3. (c); 4. (a); 5. (c).

Chapter 29 Monitoring of Wounds and Providing Wound Care

Test Yourself Multiple Choice Questions

1. (b); 2. (a); 3. (b); 4. (c); 5. (d).

Chapter 30 Using Nutritional Assessment Tools

Test Yourself Multiple Choice Questions

1. (d); 2. (a); 3. (c); 4. (d); 5. (a).

Chapter 31 Assisting People with Feeding and Drinking

Test Yourself Multiple Choice Questions

1. (b); 2. (a); 3. (d); 4. (d); 5. (d).

Chapter 32 Fluid Balance

Test Yourself Multiple Choice Questions

1. (c); 2. (d); 3. (c); 4. (d); 5. (d).

Chapter 33 Observing and Monitoring Urinary and Bowel Continence

Test Yourself Multiple Choice Questions

1. (a); 2. (d); 3. (a); 4. (d); 5. (d).

Chapter 34 Recognising Bladder and Bowel Patterns

Test Yourself Multiple Choice Questions

1. (a); 2. (d); 3. (c); 4. (c); 5. (a).

Chapter 35 Care and Management of People with Urinary Catheters

Test Yourself Multiple Choice Questions

1. (b); 2. (c); 3. (d); 4. (a); 5. (d).

Chapter 36 Assisting with Toileting, Choosing and Using Appropriate Continence Products

Test Yourself Multiple Choice Questions

1. (c); 2. (c); 3. (a); 4. (b); 5. (a).

Chapter 37 Risk Assessment Tools Associated with Mobility and Falls

Test Yourself Multiple Choice Questions

1. (a); 2. (a); 3. (c); 4. (c); 5. (b).

Chapter 38 Using a Range of Moving and Handling Techniques, Aids and Equipment

Test Yourself Multiple Choice Questions

1. (a); 2. (b); 3. (b); 4. (a); 5. (b).

Chapter 39 Managing the Administration of Oxygen

Test Yourself Multiple Choice Questions

1. (a); 2. (a); 3. (d); 4. (e); 5. (a).

Chapter 40 Measuring Respiratory Status

Test Yourself Multiple Choice Questions

1. (a); 2. (a,b,c); 3. (a); 4. (a); 5. (a,b).

Chapter 41 Using Nasal and Oral Suctioning Techniques

Test Yourself Multiple Choice Questions

1. (a); 2. (a); 3. (e); 4. (a); 5. (a).

Chapter 42 Managing Inhalation, Humidifier and Nebuliser Devices

Test Yourself Multiple Choice Questions

1. (a); 2. (a); 3. (a); 4. (b); 5. (a).

Chapter 43 Recognising and Responding Rapidly to Potential Infection Risk

Test Yourself Multiple Choice Questions

1. (d); 2. (b); 3. (a); 4. (d); 5. (c).

Chapter 44 Using Aseptic Non-Touch Technique

Test Yourself Multiple Choice Questions

1. (b); 2. (b); 3. (c); 4. (b); 5. (b).

Chapter 45 Using Appropriate Personal Protective Equipment

Test Yourself Multiple Choice Questions

1. (b); 2. (a); 3. (d); 4. (d); 5. (c).

Chapter 46 Implementing Isolation Procedures

Test Yourself Multiple Choice Questions

1. (c); 2. (a); 3. (c); 4. (c); 5. (c).

Chapter 47 Using Hand Hygiene Techniques

Test Yourself Multiple Choice Questions

1. (a); 2. (a); 3. (a); 4. (a); 5. (b).

Chapter 48 Decontaminating Equipment and the Environment

Test Yourself Multiple Choice Questions

1. (a); 2. (b); 3. (b); 4. (b); 5. (a).

Chapter 49 Safely Handling Waste, Laundry and Sharps

Test Yourself Multiple Choice Questions

1. (d); 2. (a); 3. (c); 4. (b); 5. (c).

Chapter 50 Recognising and Responding to the Needs of Those at the End of Their Lives

Test Yourself Multiple Choice Questions

1. (b); 2. (d); 3. (d); 4. (a); 5. (c).

Chapter 51 Review of Care for The People and Their Families at the End of Their Lives

Test Yourself Multiple Choice Questions

1. (c); 2. (a); 3. (c); 4. (d); 5. (d).

Chapter 52 Providing Care for the Deceased

Test Yourself Multiple Choice Questions

1. (d); 2. (b); 3. (a); 4. (c); 5. (b).

Chapter 53 Reviewing a Person's Ability to Administer Their Own Medicines

Test Yourself Multiple Choice Questions

1. (a); 2. (b); 3. (c); 4. (c); 5. (b).

Chapter 54 Undertaking Accurate Drug Calculations

Test Yourself Multiple Choice Questions

1. (a); 2. (c); 3. (d); 4. (b); 5. (c).

Chapter 55 Accountability in Ensuring the Safe Administration of Medicines

Test Yourself Multiple Choice Questions

1. (b); 2. (a); 3. (a,c); 4. (b); 5. (b).

Chapter 56 Administering Medicines

Test Yourself Multiple Choice Questions

1. (b); 2. (c); 3. (d); 4. (c); 5. (b).

Chapter 57 Managing the Effectiveness of Symptom Relief Medications

Test Yourself Multiple Choice Questions

1. (c); 2. (b); 3. (b); 4. (d); 5. (c).

Chapter 58 Recognising and Responding to Adverse Effects of Medications

Test Yourself Multiple Choice Questions

1. (c); 2. (a); 3. (a,c); 4. (c,d); 5. (d).

Chapter 59 Storage, Transportation and Disposal of Medicinal Products

Test Yourself Multiple Choice Questions

1. (a); 2. (b); 3. (a); 4. (c); 5. (b).

Index

N.B. – page numbers in *italics* are figures separate from text, page numbers in **bold** are tables.

The Nursing Associate's Handbook of Clinical Skills, First Edition. Edited by Ian Peate.

Companion website: www.wiley.com/nursingassociate